Guidelines for PERINATAL CARE

Eighth Edition

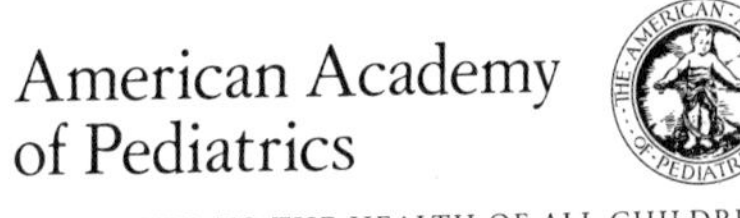

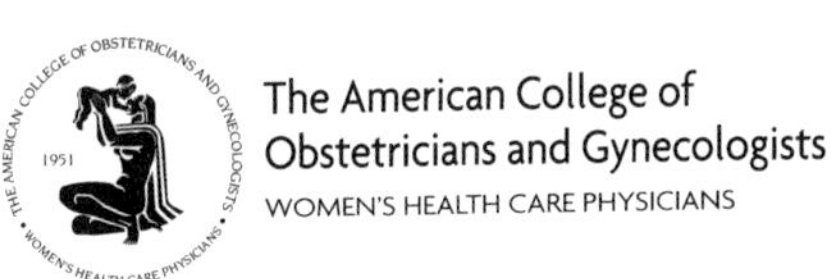

Supported in part by

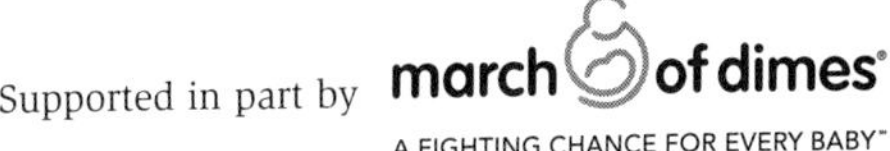

Guidelines for Perinatal Care was developed through the cooperative efforts of the American Academy of Pediatrics (AAP) Committee on Fetus and Newborn and the American College of Obstetricians and Gynecologists (ACOG) Committee on Obstetric Practice. This information is designed as an educational resource to aid clinicians in providing obstetric and gynecologic care, and use of this information is voluntary. This information should not be considered as inclusive of all proper treatments or methods of care or as a statement of the standard of care. It is not intended to substitute for the independent professional judgment of the treating clinician. Variations in practice may be warranted when, in the reasonable judgment of the treating clinician, such course of action is indicated by the condition of the patient, limitations of available resources, or advances in knowledge or technology. The American College of Obstetricians and Gynecologists reviews its publications regularly; however, its publications may not reflect the most recent evidence. Any updates to this document can be found on www.acog.org or by calling the ACOG Resource Center.

While ACOG makes every effort to present accurate and reliable information, this publication is provided "as is" without any warranty of accuracy, reliability, or otherwise, either express or implied. ACOG does not guarantee, warrant, or endorse the products or services of any firm, organization, or person. Neither ACOG nor its officers, directors, members, employees, or agents will be liable for any loss, damage, or claim with respect to any liabilities, including direct, special, indirect, or consequential damages, incurred in connection with this publication or reliance on the information presented.

Library of Congress Cataloging-in-Publication Data

Names: American Academy of Pediatrics, issuing body. | American College of Obstetricians and Gynecologists, issuing body.

Title: Guidelines for perinatal care / American Academy of Pediatrics [and] the American College of Obstetricians and Gynecologists.

Description: Eighth edition. | Elk Grove Village, IL : American Academy of Pediatrics ; Washington, DC : The American College of Obstetricians and Gynecologists, [2017] | Includes bibliographical references and index. | Includes bibliographical references and index.
Identifiers: LCCN 2017020397| ISBN 9781934984697 (ACOG) | ISBN 9781610020879 (AAP)
Subjects: | MESH: Perinatal Care--standards | United States | Practice Guideline
Classification: LCC RG600 | NLM WQ 210 | DDC 618.3/206--dc23
LC record available at https://lccn.loc.gov/2017020397

ISBN: 978-1-61002-087-9 (AAP)
ISBN: 978-1-934984-69-7 (ACOG)

Orders to purchase copies of *Guidelines for Perinatal Care* or inquiries regarding content can be directed to the respective organizations.

American Academy of Pediatrics
141 Northwest Point Boulevard
PO Box 927
Elk Grove Village, IL 60009-0927

The American College of Obstetricians and Gynecologists
409 12th Street, SW
PO Box 96920
Washington, DC 20090-6920

12345/10987

Editorial Committee

Editors

Sarah J. Kilpatrick, MD, PhD, FACOG
Lu-Ann Papile, MD, FAAP

Associate Editors

George A. Macones, MD, FACOG
Kristi L. Watterberg, MD, FAAP

Staff

The American College of Obstetricians and Gynecologists (ACOG)

Christopher M. Zahn, MD, FACOG
Debra Hawks, MPH
Sandra Patterson
Donna Lormand, MPH

American Academy of Pediatrics (AAP)

Jim Couto, MA

The College Committee on Obstetric Practice

Members, 2014–2015

Jeffrey L. Ecker, MD, FACOG (Chair)
James D. Goldberg, MD, FACOG (Vice Chair)
Ann Elizabeth Bryant Borders, MD, FACOG
Yasser Yehia El-Sayed, MD, FACOG
R. Phillips Heine, MD, FACOG
Denise J. Jamieson, MD, MPH, FACOG
Maria Anne Mascola, MD, FACOG
Howard L. Minkoff, MD, FACOG
Alison M. Stuebe, MD, FACOG
James E. Sumners, MD, FACOG
Methodius G. Tuuli, MD, FACOG
Joseph R. Wax, MD, FACOG
Kurt R. Wharton, MD, FACOG
William Grobman, MD, FACOG (Ex Officio)
Tina Clark-Samazan Foster, MD, MPH, MS, FACOG (Ex Officio)

Liaison Representatives

Debra Bingham, DrPh, RN, FAAN
Sean C. Blackwell, MD, FACOG
William M. Callaghan, MD, FACOG
Julia A. Carey-Corrado, MD
Beth Choby, MD, FAAFP
Joshua A. Copel, MD, FACOG
Nathaniel DeNicola, MD, MSc, FACOG
Rhonda Hearns-Stokes, MD, FACOG
Tekoa King, CNM, FACNM
Uma M. Reddy, MD, MPH, FACOG
Kristi L. Watterberg, MD, FAAP
Edward A. Yaghmour, MD
Cathy H. Whittlesey (Ex Officio)

Members, 2015–2016

Jeffrey L. Ecker, MD, FACOG (Chair)
Joseph R. Wax, MD, FACOG (Vice Chair)
Ann Elizabeth Bryant Borders, MD, FACOG
Yasser Yehia El-Sayed, MD, FACOG
R. Phillips Heine, MD, FACOG
Maria Anne Mascola, MD, FACOG
Brigid K. McCue, MD, FACOG
Russell Scott Miller, MD, FACOG
T. Flint Porter, MD, FACOG
Alfred G. Robichaux, MD, FACOG
Alison M. Stuebe, MD, FACOG
James E. Sumners, MD, FACOG
Kurt R. Wharton, MD, FACOG
G. Marc Jackson, MD, FACOG (Ex Officio)
Michael D. Moxley, MD, FACOG (Ex Officio)
Wanda Nicholson, MD, MPH, FACOG (Ex Officio)

Liaison Representatives

Debra Bingham, DrPH, RN, FAAN
William M. Callaghan, MD, FACOG
Beth Choby, MD, FAAFP
Kelly Colden, MD, FACOG
Joshua A. Copel, MD, FACOG
Nathaniel DeNicola, MD, MSc, FACOG
Cynthia Gyamfi-Bannerman, MD, FACOG
Rhonda Hearns-Stokes, MD, FACOG
Tekoa King, CNM, FACNM
Uma M. Reddy, MD, MPH, FACOG
Kristi L. Watterberg, MD, FAAP
Edward A. Yaghmour, MD
Brigid K. McCue, MD, FACOG
Cathy H. Whittlesey (Ex Officio, Ex Bd)

The College Committee on Obstetric Practice *(continued)*

Members, 2016–2017

Joseph R. Wax, MD, FACOG (Chair)
Yasser Yehia El-Sayed, MD, FACOG (Vice Chair)
Meredith Lee Birsner, MD, FACOG
Ann Elizabeth Bryant Borders, MD, FACOG
Alison Gale Cahill, MD, MSCI, FACOG
Angela Brawley Gantt, MD, FACOG
R. Phillips Heine, MD, FACOG
Maria Anne Mascola, MD, FACOG
Brigid K. McCue, MD, FACOG
Russell Scott Miller, MD, FACOG
T. Flint Porter, MD, FACOG
Alfred G. Robichaux, MD, FACOG
Kurt R. Wharton, MD, FACOG
Robert G. Bonebrake, MD, FACOG (Ex Officio)
G. Marc Jackson, MD, FACOG (Ex Officio)
Glenn R. Markenson, MD, FACOG (Ex Officio)
Michael D. Moxley, MD, FACOG (Ex Officio)

Liaison Representatives

William M. Callaghan, MD, FACOG
Beth Choby, MD, FAAFP
Kelly Colden, MD, FACOG
Joshua A. Copel, MD, FACOG
Nathaniel DeNicola, MD, MSc, FACOG
Cynthia Gyamfi-Bannerman, MD, FACOG
Rhonda Hearns-Stokes, MD, FACOG
R. Phillips Heine, MD, FACOG
Tekoa King, CNM, FACNM
Brigid K. McCue, MD, FACOG
Menachem Miodovnik, MD
Elizabeth Rochin, PhD, RN, NE-BC
Kristi L. Watterberg, MD, FAAP
Edward A. Yaghmour, MD
Carl Dunn, MD, FACOG (Ex Officio)

AAP Committee on Fetus and Newborn

Members, 2014–2015

Kristi L. Watterberg, MD, FAAP (Chair)
Susan W. Aucott, MD, FAAP
William E. Benitz, MD, FAAP
James J. Cummings, MD, FAAP
Eric C. Eichenwald, MD, FAAP
Jay P. Goldsmith, MD, FAAP
Brenda B. Poindexter, MD, MS, FAAP
Karen M. Puopolo, MD, PhD, FAAP
Dan L. Stewart, MD, FAAP
Kasper S. Wang, MD

Liaison Representatives

Capt. Wanda D. Barfield, MD, MPH, FAAP
Erin L. Keels APRN, MS, NNP-BC
Maria Anne Mascola, MD, FACOG
Thierry Lacaze-Masmonteil, MD
Tonse N. K. Raju, MD, DCH, FAAP

Members, 2015–2016

Kristi L. Watterberg, MD, FAAP (Chair)
Susan W. Aucott, MD, FAAP
William E. Benitz, MD, FAAP
James J. Cummings, MD, FAAP
Eric C. Eichenwald, MD, FAAP
Jay P. Goldsmith, MD, FAAP
Brenda B. Poindexter, MD, MS, FAAP
Karen M. Puopolo, MD, PhD, FAAP
Dan L. Stewart, MD, FAAP

Liaison Representatives

Capt. Wanda D. Barfield, MD, MPH, FAAP
Erin L. Keels, APRN, MS, NNP-BC
Maria Anne Mascola, MD, FACOG
Thierry Lacaze-Masmonteil, MD
Tonse N. K. Raju, MD, DCH, FAAP

AAP Committee on Fetus and Newborn *(continued)*

Members, 2016–2017

Kristi L. Watterberg, MD, FAAP (Chair)
Susan W. Aucott, MD, FAAP
William E. Benitz, MD, FAAP
James J. Cummings, MD, FAAP
Eric C. Eichenwald, MD, FAAP
Jay P. Goldsmith, MD, FAAP
Brenda B. Poindexter, MD, MS, FAAP
Karen M. Puopolo, MD, PhD, FAAP
Dan L. Stewart, MD, FAAP

Liaison Representatives

RADM Wanda D. Barfield, MD, MPH, FAAP
Erin L. Keels, DNP, APRN, NNP-BC
Thierry Lacaze-Masmonteil, MD
Maria Anne Mascola, MD, FACOG
Tonse N. K. Raju, MD, DCH, FAAP

Consultants

The committee would like to express appreciation to the following consultants:

Susan W. Aucott, MD, FAAP
RADM Wanda D. Barfield, MD, MPH, FAAP
William H. Barth, MD, FACOG
William E. Benitz, MD, FAAP
Debra Bingham, DrPH, RN, FAAN
Ann Elizabeth Bryant Borders, MD, FACOG
William M.Callahan, MD, FACOG
Beth Choby, MD, FAAFP
Kelly Colden, MD, FACOG
James J. Cummings, MD, FAAP
Jeffrey L. Ecker, MD, FACOG
Eric C. Eichenwald, MD, FAAP
Yasser Yehia El-Sayed, MD, FACOG
Tina Clark-Samazan Foster, MD, MPH, MS, FACOG
Jay P. Goldsmith, MD, FAAP
Cynthia Gyamfi-Bannerman, MD, FACOG
R. Phillips Heine, MD, FACOG
Mark L. Hudak, MD, FAAP
G. Marc Jackson, MD, FACOG
Erin L. Keels, DNP, APRN, NNP-BC
Tekoa King, CNM, FACNM
Maria Anne Mascola, MD, FACOG
Brigid K. McCue, MD, FACOG
Russell Scott Miller, MD, FACOG
Brenda B. Poindexter, MD, MS, FAAP
Ronald L. Poland, MD
T. Flint Porter, MD, FACOG
Karen M. Puopolo, MD, PhD, FAAP
Tonse N. K. Raju, MD, DCH, FAAP
Alfred G. Robichaux, MD, FACOG
Dan L. Stewart, MD, FAAP
Alison M. Stuebe, MD, FACOG
James E. Sumners, MD FACOG
Naomi K. Tepper, MD, FACOG
Kasper S. Wang, MD, FAAP
Joseph R. Wax, MD, FACOG
Kurt R. Wharton, MD, FACOG
Edward A. Yaghmour, MD

Contents

Preface

As we have done since the first edition, published in 1983, the eighth edition of *Guidelines for Perinatal Care* provides updated and expanded information from the seventh edition. All updates are taken from existing American Academy of Pediatrics' (AAP) or American College of Obstetricians and Gynecologists' (ACOG) documents as of July 2017. Several chapters have been reorganized and rewritten, and two chapters in the seventh edition ("Preconception and Antepartum Care" and "Intrapartum and Postpartum Care of the Mother") have been split into "Prepregnancy Care," "Antepartum Care," "Intrapartum Care of the Mother," and "Postpartum Care of the Mother" for the current edition to improve the presentation of the expanded content. We continue to focus on reproductive awareness and patient safety as well as quality in obstetrics and neonatology and approach all topics from the vantage point of best care for the mother and newborn.

Guidelines for Perinatal Care represents a cross section of different disciplines within the perinatal community. It is designed for use by all personnel who are involved in the care of pregnant women, their fetuses, and their newborn infants in community programs, hospitals, and medical centers. An intermingling of information in varying degrees of detail is provided to address their collective needs. The result is a unique resource that complements the educational documents listed in Appendix H, which provide more specific information. Readers are encouraged to refer to the appendix for related documents to supplement those listed at the end of each chapter.

The American Academy of Pediatrics and ACOG will continue to update information presented in this guide through policy statements and recommendations that both organizations issue periodically, particularly with regard to rapidly evolving technologies and areas of practice.

Guidelines for Perinatal Care is published as a companion document to the ACOG's *Guidelines for Women's Health Care,* which is in its fourth edition. Although each book is developed with the aid of a separate committee, their contents are coordinated to provide comprehensive reference to all aspects of women's health care with minimal duplication.

The most current scientific information, professional opinions, and clinical practices have been used to create this document, which is intended to offer guidelines, not strict operating rules. Local circumstances must dictate the way in which these guidelines are best interpreted to meet the needs of a particular hospital, community, or system. Emphasis has been placed on identifying those areas to be covered by specific, locally defined protocols rather than on promoting rigid recommendations.

The content of this newest edition of *Guidelines for Perinatal Care* has undergone careful review to ensure accuracy and consistency with the policies of both groups. The guidelines are not meant to be exhaustive, nor do they always agree with those of other organizations; however, they reflect the latest recommendations of AAP and ACOG. The recommendations of AAP and ACOG are based on the best understanding of the data and consensus among authorities in the discipline. The text was written, revised, and reviewed by members of the AAP Committee on Fetus and Newborn and the ACOG Committee on Obstetric Practice. Consultants in a variety of specialized areas also contributed to the content. The pioneering efforts of those who developed the previous editions also must be acknowledged. To each and every one of them, sincere appreciation is extended.

Introduction

Throughout its prior seven editions, *Guidelines for Perinatal Care* has focused on improving the outcomes of pregnancies and reducing maternal and perinatal mortality and morbidity by suggesting sound paradigms for providing perinatal care. Its strong advocacy of regionalized perinatal systems, including effective risk identification, care in a risk-appropriate setting, and maternal or neonatal transport to tertiary care facilities when necessary, has had a demonstrable effect on perinatal outcomes. This eighth edition expands the regionalized care concept further by describing levels of maternal care in detail in Chapter 1. Although a national dialogue about matching levels of hospital care to levels of care required for mothers and neonates has been ongoing since the publication of the March of Dimes Foundation's *Toward Improving the Outcome of Pregnancy* in the 1970s, this concept has only truly been implemented consistently for neonates. In Chapter 1, you can see that the American College of Obstetricians and Gynecologists and the American Academy of Pediatrics now believe it is time to demand such levels for mothers as well. We present the suggested level of maternal care from birth centers to a described level IV institution. This edition also makes evidence-based recommendations on the use of safe and effective diagnostic and therapeutic interventions in maternal–fetal medicine and neonatology.

The full spectrum of high-quality perinatal care is covered by this eighth edition of *Guidelines for Perinatal Care*, from the principles of prepregnancy counseling and the provision of antepartum and intrapartum care in routine and complex settings to guidelines for routine and complex neonatal and postpartum care. The prepregnancy and antepartum care chapters introduce the concept and underscore the importance of interpregnancy care to maternal and fetal health. Chapter 5 from the seventh edition has been split into two chapters one of which includes prepregnancy and interpregnancy care, and the other of which covers antepartum care. We also have added sections on screening for preterm delivery risk to the chapter on antepartum care. Chapter 6 from the previous edition has been split into two chapters: one of which covers intrapartum care, and the other of which covers postpartum care. New guidance concerning the timing of umbilical cord clamping, the need (or not) for bedrest, updates in hypertension, planned home birth, and immersion in the first and second stages of labor is also included. Guidance regarding postpartum contraception recommendations (aligned with the *U.S. Medical Eligibility Criteria for Contraception* published by the Centers for Disease Control and Prevention) and obstetric and medical complications has been expanded to incorporate new information and evidence-based recommendations to guide clinical practice in these specialized areas. The chapter on perinatal infections now includes a section on mosquito-borne illnesses (including Zika) and a section on infections with high-risk infection control issues, emerging infections, and bioterrorism (including a discussion of Ebola).

The chapters on care of healthy and high-risk neonates include updated recommendations on neonatal resuscitation, screening and management of hyperbilirubinemia, and neonatal drug withdrawal. The addition of information on late preterm infants reflects the importance of this group of infants to the rate of prematurity and their increased vulnerability compared with term infants.

Updated recommendations for the conduct of perinatal care in a hospital setting are presented and continue to emphasize family-centered and patient-centered care, wherein patients and families are recognized and respected as true partners in their health care. The roles of hospitalists and laborists also are discussed.

As in previous editions, the concept of quality improvement in all aspects of perinatal care is a focus and we have updated the quality improvement and patient safety chapter and added a discussion of safety bundles. This chapter provides commentary on the need for procedures and policies to ensure effective communication among caregivers and between caregivers and patients, as communication remains a critical component of quality perinatal care. The concepts of team training, simulations and drills, and their roles in improving perinatal care continue to be featured.

Achieving the goal of optimal outcomes for newborns and mothers requires a coordinated system of perinatal care, including a multidisciplinary team of clinicians working in concert with the patient and within a supportive community. This eighth edition of *Guidelines for Perinatal Care* provides a framework of recommendations based on the best available evidence. Wide implementation of these recommendations will bring us closer to our goal.

Guidelines for

PERINATAL CARE

Eighth Edition

Chapter 1

Organization of Perinatal Health Care

The organization of perinatal health care on a regional basis emerged as a model of health care delivery beginning in the 1970s and 1980s. Regional organization of perinatal care was endorsed in a 1976 report by the March of Dimes Foundation, *Toward Improving the Outcome of Pregnancy*, which was prepared by the Committee on Perinatal Health, an ad hoc committee of representatives appointed by participating professional organizations with support from the March of Dimes Foundation. The importance of regional organization was further emphasized in the second edition and third editions of *Toward Improving the Outcome of Pregnancy,* published in 1993 and 2010, respectively. Although a comprehensive, integrated perinatal care delivery system is optimal, this goal has not been attained in many areas of the country, where financial incentives promote competing systems and duplication of services.

Health Care Delivery System

A regionalized system of perinatal care with integrated delivery of services should address the care received by the woman before and during pregnancy, the management of labor and delivery, postpartum care, and neonatal care. A health care system that is responsive to the needs of families, and especially women, requires strategies to:

- ensure access to services
- identify risks early
- provide linkage to the appropriate level of care
- ensure adherence, continuity, and comprehensiveness of care
- promote efficient use of resources

Structural, financial, and cultural barriers to care need to be identified and eliminated. The regionalized organization and integration of perinatal care must evolve within the framework of the general health care delivery system while avoiding unnecessary duplication of services. A successful perinatal health care system has five essential responsibilities: 1) provide access to comprehensive perinatal health care services, 2) embrace a patient-centered and family-centered approach to health care, 3) deliver culturally and linguistically appropriate care, 4) educate the public about reproductive health, and 5) be accountable for all components of the health care delivery system.

Comprehensive Perinatal Health Care Services

The integration of a spectrum of clinical activities, basic care through subspecialty care, within one system or geographic region potentially provides timely access to care at the appropriate level for the entire population. Achieving the primary goal of providing the appropriate level of care is facilitated by early and ongoing risk assessment to prevent, recognize, and treat conditions associated with maternal and neonatal morbidity and mortality. A secondary goal is to improve referral and consultation among institutions that provide different levels of care. When populations that are in need of reproductive health care are widely dispersed, both geographically and economically, a carefully structured, well-organized system of supportive services becomes necessary to ensure access to appropriate care for all pregnant women and newborns. Networks and other forms of vertically integrated systems within a region should be structured to provide all the necessary services, including health care, transportation, public and professional education, research, and outcome evaluations with data organized in a standard format. All components are necessary to minimize perinatal mortality and morbidity while using resources efficiently and effectively.

Patient-Centered and Family-Centered Health Care

The perinatal health care system should be oriented toward providing patient-centered and family-centered health care because the family often is the primary source of support for individuals receiving health services. The Institute for Patient- and Family-Centered Care importantly notes that the term family is defined by the patient, as is the degree to which the family is involved in care. The term "family" as it is used here includes the expectant woman and her support system, which may include any or all of the following individuals: a spouse or partner, relatives, and friends. Health care providers should strive to engage the family as co-providers and decision-making partners, as long as this is in accordance with the pregnant woman's personal situation, beliefs, and desires. Every encounter should build on the expectant woman's strengths, preserve her dignity, and enhance her confidence and competence. Such an approach incorporates family perspectives, offers real choices, and respects the decisions made by the family for themselves and their children. Hospital and program leaders should communicate the concepts of patient-centered and family-centered care consistently and clearly to staff, students, families, and communities through statements of vision, mission, and philosophy and through institutional policies and actions. Providing an environment that is supportive of the family's key role in promoting the health of its members is important in successful health promotion. This includes respecting the choices, values, and cultural backgrounds of expectant women, new mothers, and other family members; communicating honestly and openly; promoting opportunities for mutual support and information sharing; and collaborating in the development and evaluation of services.

Family-centered practices can help expectant families and new families become nurturing caregivers. Efforts should be made throughout the neonatal course to promote continuous contact between newborns and their families. Economic interests and decisions should never take priority over the best interests of the newborn infant, the woman, the family, and the community in keeping the family together. When separation of the family unit is necessitated by the requirement for a higher level of care for the woman or newborn infant, the responsibility for maintaining communication and involvement of the family in decisions relating to care should be shared by the entire health care team. Whenever medically feasible, a woman whose newborn infant has been transferred to another hospital should be discharged or transferred to the same facility. Staff interactions and unit policies at every level should consistently reinforce the importance of family for the health and well-being of their newborn infant. Families' strengths and capabilities should be the foundation on which to build competency and confidence in caregiving abilities. Preserving an individual sense of personal responsibility and identity is important for the optimum outcome of pregnancy and family life.

Culturally and Linguistically Appropriate Care

In addition to being family-centered, perinatal health care systems should be culturally and linguistically appropriate. Communication with patients can be improved and patient care enhanced if health care providers can bridge the divide between the culture of medicine and the beliefs and practices that make up patients' value systems. These may be based on ethnic heritage, nationality of family origin, age, religion, sexual orientation, disability, or socioeconomic status. Reaching out to community cultural leaders can be enormously beneficial in understanding cultural practices.

Large perinatal health disparities exist in racial and ethnic minority groups and in low-income level groups, compared with white and high-income level groups. The publication of *National Standards for Culturally and Linguistically Appropriate Services in Health Care* by the Office of Minority Health of the U.S. Department of Health and Human Services emphasizes the need to address these long-standing disparities through the implementation and evaluation of culturally sensitive and competent health care. These recommendations encourage the coordination of the U.S. Department of Health and Human Services agencies, along with other federal agencies, health care organizations, accreditation bodies, patient communities, and private sector organizations to ensure consistent training for health care providers; increase cultural diversity among health care professionals; and empower minority, vulnerable, and underserved patients to participate as equal partners in the health care process and system.

Education of the Public About Reproductive Health and Life Planning

Insight into the broad social and medical implications of pregnancy and awareness of reproductive risks, health-enhancing behaviors, and family-planning options are essential for improving the outcomes of pregnancy. Education about reproductive health, including reproductive life planning, must be integrated more effectively into the health care system and society at large. A recent report emphasizes that in the United States

- a little more than one half of pregnancies are planned and approximately one half of unintended pregnancies end in abortion.
- unintended pregnancies occur in all segments of society.
- a woman with an unintended pregnancy is less likely to seek early prenatal care and is more likely to expose the fetus to potentially harmful

substances such as alcohol, tobacco, nonmedical use of drugs, and elevated glucose.

- a newborn of an unwanted pregnancy is at higher risk of having a low birth weight and other complications throughout childhood.

Because pregnancy intention and other behavioral health risks—including the use of alcohol, tobacco, and other drugs—occur across all socioeconomic groups, the target group for reproductive education must be all women of childbearing age. Reproductive health screening should be implemented by all health care providers serving women in their reproductive years (see also Chapter 5 and Chapter 6).

Every encounter with the health care system, including those involving adolescents and men, should be viewed as an opportunity to reinforce awareness of reproductive health issues and to encourage reproductive life planning. New messages and marketing techniques regarding responsible reproductive health practices may be helpful in changing attitudes and behaviors in women and men.

In communicating with the patient and the public, it is important to tailor health messages to the appropriate literacy and language level. Low functional literacy may compromise the quality of care received, contribute to medical errors and poor health outcomes, and increase the risk of medical liability litigation. This problem can be minimized by consistent use of simplified language on written documents, such as consent forms and patient instructions, and in face-to-face conversation.

Language and cultural barriers should be examined and addressed. For those who do not speak English, a family member should not be used as an interpreter, but rather efforts should be made to provide assistance, such as offering appropriately trained interpreters and written translations of forms and patient education materials. In some circumstances, federal and state laws and regulations impose responsibilities on health care providers to accommodate individuals with limited English proficiency. Appropriate measures for overcoming communication barriers will depend on the circumstances of the individual practice and patient population. Various options may be available, including hiring bilingual staff for clerical or medical positions, using appropriate community resources, or using translation telephone services.

Accountability

Accountability for actions is a fundamental principle of health care provision applicable to all components of a health care delivery system and is a valuable attribute of professional practice that benefits all patients. This accountability includes, but is not limited to, the care of individual patients by individual health care providers. Within the perinatal health care delivery system, accountability and responsibility must be required equally of all participants, including patients, families, perinatal health care programs and systems, government agencies, insurers, local communities, and health maintenance organizations, all of whose actions and policies influence the delivery of patient care and, thereby, influence outcomes. Accountability includes developing meaningful quality improvement programs, monitoring medical errors, and working to ensure patient safety. Access to high-quality care for all patients is a responsibility that requires a coordinated system with involvement, commitment, and accountability of all parties.

Clinical Components of Regionalized and Integrated Delivery of Perinatal Services

A regionalized system that focuses on integrated delivery of graded levels of hospital-based perinatal care has been shown to be effective and to result in improved outcomes for women and their newborns. Integrated perinatal care programs can be extended to encompass prepregnancy evaluation and early pregnancy risk assessment in both ambulatory and hospital-based settings.

Prepregnancy Care

Prepregnancy care aims to promote the health of women of reproductive age before pregnancy and improve pregnancy outcomes. Integrated perinatal health care programs and systems should place additional emphasis on prepregnancy care through educational programs. All women of childbearing age should have access to prepregnancy care and reproduction life planning. Health care providers in various disciplines (eg, internal medicine, family medicine, and pediatrics) should be made aware of prepregnancy care recommendations and guidelines. Clinical details of prepregnancy care for perinatal health care providers are presented in Chapter 5.

Ambulatory Prenatal Care

The goals for the coordination of ambulatory prenatal care are to provide appropriate care for all women, to ensure good use of available resources, and to improve the outcome of pregnancies. As recommended by the March of Dimes Foundation in the second edition of *Toward Improving the Outcome of Pregnancy*, prenatal care can be delivered more effectively and efficiently by defining the capabilities and expertise (basic, specialty, and subspecialty) of health care providers and ensuring that pregnant women receive risk-appropriate care (Table 1-1). Developments in maternal–fetal

TABLE 1–1. Ambulatory Prenatal Care Provider Capabilities and Expertise

Level of Care	Capabilities	Health Care Provider Types
Basic	Risk-oriented prenatal care record, physical examination and interpretation of findings, routine laboratory assessment, assessment of gestational age and normal progress of pregnancy, ongoing risk identification, mechanisms for consultation and referral, psychosocial support, childbirth education, care coordination (including referral for ancillary services, such as transportation, food, and housing assistance)	Obstetricians, family physicians, certified nurse–midwives, certified midwives, and other advanced practice registered nurses with experience, training, and demonstrated competence
Specialty	Basic care plus fetal diagnostic testing (eg, biophysical tests, amniotic fluid analysis, basic ultrasonography), expertise in management of medical and obstetric complications	Obstetricians
Subspecialty	Basic and specialty care plus advanced fetal diagnostics (eg, targeted ultrasonography, fetal echocardiography); advanced therapy (eg, intrauterine fetal transfusion and treatment of cardiac arrhythmias); medical, surgical, neonatal, and genetic consultation; and management of severe maternal complications	Maternal–fetal medicine specialists and reproductive geneticists with experience, training, and demonstrated competence

Modified with permission from March of Dimes. Toward improving the outcome of pregnancy: the 90s and beyond. White Plains (NY): March of Dimes Birth Defects Foundation; 1993.

risk assessment and diagnosis, as well as the interventions to change behavior, make early and ongoing prenatal care an effective strategy to improve pregnancy outcomes (see also "Triage" in Chapter 7).

Early and ongoing risk assessment should be an integral component of perinatal care. Early identification of high-risk pregnancies allows prevention and treatment of conditions associated with maternal and fetal morbidity and mortality. Risk assessment facilitates development of a plan of care, including referral and consultation as appropriate, among health care providers of basic, specialty, and subspecialty prenatal care on the basis of the patient's circumstances and the capability of the individual health care providers.

The content and timing of prenatal care should be varied according to the needs and risk status of the woman and her fetus. Use of community-based risk assessment tools, such as a standardized prenatal record (see also Appendix A), by all health care providers within a regionalized perinatal care system helps to ensure the integration of care delivery and appropriate implementation of risk assessment and intervention activities. All prenatal health care providers should be able to identify a full range of medical and psychosocial risks and either provide appropriate care or make appropriate referrals (see also Appendix B and Appendix C).

Prenatal care may involve the services of many types of health care providers, including the early involvement of pediatricians and neonatologists as well as other pediatric subspecialists (eg, cardiologists, surgeons, and geneticists). A consultation with a neonatologist and other appropriate specialists to discuss the pediatric implications with the woman and her partner is particularly important when fetal risks or problems have been identified (see also Chapter 7).

In-Hospital Perinatal Care

The conceptual framework of regionalization of perinatal care has focused almost entirely on the newborn. With 39% of hospital births in the United States occurring at hospitals that deliver fewer than 500 newborns each year and an additional 20% occurring at hospitals that deliver between 501 newborns and 1,000 newborns each year, it is likely that the majority of maternal care in the United States is provided at basic care and specialty care hospitals. This likelihood supports recent commentary that noted the need to readdress "perinatal levels of care" to focus specifically on maternal health conditions that warrant designation as high risk, and to define specific clinical and systems criteria to manage such conditions.

Although maternal mortality in high-resource countries improved substantially during the 20th century, maternal mortality rates in the United States have worsened in the past 14 years. Currently, the United States is ranked 60th in the world for maternal mortality. According to a Centers for Disease Control and Prevention study, the leading causes of maternal mortality are associated with chronic conditions that affect women of reproductive age, and common obstetric complications such as hemorrhage. Moreover, maternal mortality in the United States represents a small component of the larger emerging problem of maternal severe morbidities and near-miss mortality that increased by 75% between 1998–1999 and 2008–2009. National increases in obesity, hypertensive disorders, and diabetes among women of reproductive age increase the risk of maternal morbidity and mortality, as does the increasing cesarean delivery rate. Although specific modifications in the clinical management of these conditions have been instituted (eg, the use of thromboembolism prophylaxis and bariatric beds in obstetrics), more can be done to improve the system of care for high-risk women at facility and population levels.

Systematic review of the published literature over the past three decades demonstrates improved neonatal and posthospital discharge survival among very-low-birth-weight and very preterm infants born in hospitals with neonatal intensive care units. Careful documentation of birth-weight-specific neonatal mortality rates by hospital of birth has shown that the chance of survival of preterm, very-low-birth-weight infants is highest when births occur in hospitals with higher-volume neonatal intensive care units. This finding has been reported in the United States and other countries. In addition, multiple reports regarding the outcomes of neonatal surgery support the concentration of resources and patients in a few highly specialized centers for neonatal surgery. Given the weight of the evidence, it must be emphasized that inpatient perinatal health care services should be organized within individual regions or service areas in such a manner that there is a concentration of care for the highest-risk pregnant women and their fetuses and newborns who require the highest level of perinatal care.

Classification System for Levels of Maternal Care

Although there is strong evidence of more favorable neonatal outcomes with regionalized perinatal care, evidence of a beneficial effect on maternal outcome is limited. Maternal mortality is an uncommon event, highlighting the need to focus on severe maternal morbidity to better understand opportunities for improvement in outcomes. Methods for tracking severe morbidity have recently been proposed. Data indicate that obstetric complications are significantly more frequent in hospitals with low delivery volume, and that obstetric care providers with the lowest patient volume have significantly increased rates of obstetric complications compared with high-volume obstetric care providers. Hospital clinical volume likely is a proxy measure for institutional and individual experience that may not be available at hospitals with lower volumes. Also, data indicate that outcomes are better if certain conditions, such as placenta previa or placenta accreta, are managed in a high-volume hospital. It also has been noted that maternal mortality is inversely related to the population density of maternal–fetal medicine subspecialists at the state level, although other factors, such as the presence of obstetrician–gynecologists, nurses, and anesthesiologists who have experience in high-risk maternity care, also may contribute to this trend. Although these findings provide support for an association between availability of resources and favorable maternal outcomes, they do not prove a direct cause-and-effect relationship between levels of care and outcomes. For these reasons, in 2014 the American College of Obstetricians and Gynecologists and the Society for Maternal–Fetal Medicine published an Obstetric Care Consensus document regarding the levels of maternal care. The objectives outlined in the document are to:

1. introduce uniform designations for levels of maternal care, complimentary but distinct from neonatal levels of care that address maternal health needs.
2. develop standardized definitions and nomenclature for facilities providing each level of maternal care, including birth centers.
3. provide consistent standards of service by levels of maternal care for use in quality improvement and health promotion.
4. foster the development and equitable geographic distribution of full service maternal care facilities and systems that promote proactive integration of risk-appropriate perinatal services.

Table 1-2 and Table 1-3 list the expected capabilities of basic, specialty, subspecialty, and regional perinatal health care levels of inpatient perinatal health care services as delineated in Obstetric Care Consensus No. 2,

Levels of Maternal Care, from the American College of Obstetricians and Gynecologists and the Society for Maternal–Fetal Medicine.

TABLE 1-2. Levels of Maternal Care: Definitions, Capabilities, and Types of Health Care Providers *

Birth Center	
Definition	Peripartum care of low-risk women with uncomplicated singleton term pregnancies with a vertex presentation who are expected to have an uncomplicated birth
Capabilities	• Capability and equipment to provide low-risk maternal care and a readiness at all times to initiate emergency procedures to meet unexpected needs of the woman and newborn within the center, and to facilitate transport to an acute care setting when necessary. • An established agreement with a receiving hospital with policies and procedures for timely transport. • Data collection, storage, and retrieval. • Ability to initiate quality improvement programs that include efforts to maximize patient safety. • Medical consultation available at all times.
Types of health care providers	Every birth attended by at least two professionals: • Primary maternal care providers. This includes CNMs, CMs, CPMs, and licensed midwives who are legally recognized to practice within the jurisdiction of the birth center; family physicians; and ob-gyns. • Availability of adequate numbers of qualified professionals with competence in level I care criteria and ability to stabilize and transfer high-risk women and newborns.
Examples of appropriate patients (not requirements)	• Term, singleton, vertex presentation
Level I (Basic Care)	
Definition	Care of uncomplicated pregnancies with the ability to detect, stabilize, and initiate management of unanticipated maternal–fetal or neonatal problems that occur during the antepartum, intrapartum, or postpartum period until patient can be transferred to a facility at which specialty maternal care is available

(continued)

TABLE 1-2. Levels of Maternal Care: Definitions, Capabilities, and Types of Health Care Providers * *(continued)*

Level I (Basic Care) *(continued)*	
Capabilities	Birth center capabilities plus • ability to begin emergency cesarean delivery within a time interval that best incorporates maternal and fetal risks and benefits with the provision of emergency care. • available support services, including access to obstetric ultrasonography, laboratory testing, and blood bank supplies at all times. • protocols and capabilities for massive transfusion, emergency release of blood products, and management of multiple component therapy. • ability to establish formal transfer plans in partnership with a higher-level receiving facility. • ability to initiate education and quality improvement programs to maximize patient safety, and/or collaborate with higher-level facilities to do so.
Types of health care providers	Birth center providers plus • continuous availability of adequate number of RNs with competence in level I care criteria and ability to stabilize and transfer high-risk women and newborns. • nursing leadership has expertise in perinatal nursing care. • obstetric care provider with privileges to perform emergency cesarean available to attend all deliveries. • anesthesia services available to provide labor analgesia and surgical anesthesia.
Examples of appropriate patients (not requirements)	Any patient appropriate for a birth center, plus capable of managing higher-risk conditions such as • term twin gestation • trial of labor after cesarean delivery • uncomplicated cesarean delivery • preeclampsia without severe features at term
Level II (Specialty Care)	
Definition	Level I facility plus care of appropriate high-risk antepartum, intrapartum, or postpartum conditions, both directly admitted and transferred from another facility

(continued)

TABLE 1-2. Levels of Maternal Care: Definitions, Capabilities, and Types of Health Care Providers * *(continued)*

Level II (Specialty Care) *(continued)*	
Capabilities	Level I facility capabilities plus • computed tomography scan and ideally magnetic resonance imaging with interpretation available. • basic ultrasonographic imaging services for maternal and fetal assessment. • special equipment needed to accommodate the care and services needed for obese women.
Types of health care providers	Level I facility health care providers plus • continuous availability of adequate numbers of RNs with competence in level II care criteria and ability to stabilize and transfer high-risk women and newborns who exceed level II care criteria. • nursing leadership and staff have formal training and experience in the provision of perinatal nursing care and should coordinate with respective neonatal care services. • ob-gyn available at all times. • director of obstetric service is a board-certified ob-gyn with special interest and experience in obstetric care. • MFM available for consultation onsite, by telephone, or by telemedicine, as needed. • anesthesia services available at all times to provide labor analgesia and surgical anesthesia. • board-certified anesthesiologist with special training or experience in obstetric anesthesia available for consultation. • medical and surgical consultants available to stabilize obstetric patients who have been admitted to the facility or transferred from other facilities.
Examples of appropriate patients (not requirements)	Any patient appropriate for level I care, plus higher-risk conditions such as • severe preeclampsia • placenta previa with no prior uterine surgery
Level III (Subspecialty Care)	
Definition	Level II facility plus care of more complex maternal medical conditions, obstetric complications, and fetal conditions

(continued)

TABLE 1-2. Levels of Maternal Care: Definitions, Capabilities, and Types of Health Care Providers * *(continued)*

Level III (Subspecialty Care) *(continued)*	
Capabilities	Level II facility capabilities plus • advanced imaging services available at all times. • ability to assist level I and level II centers with quality improvement and safety programs. • provide perinatal system leadership if acting as a regional center in areas where level IV facilities are not available (see level IV). • medical and surgical ICUs accept pregnant women and have critical care providers onsite to actively collaborate with MFMs at all times. • appropriate equipment and personnel available onsite to ventilate and monitor women in labor and delivery until they can be safely transferred to the ICU.
Types of health care providers	Level II health care providers plus • continuous availability of adequate numbers of nursing leaders and RNs with competence in level III care criteria and ability to transfer and stabilize high-risk women and newborns who exceed level III care criteria, and with special training and experience in the management of women with complex maternal illnesses and obstetric complications. • ob-gyn available onsite at all times. • MFM with inpatient privileges available at all times, either onsite, by telephone, or by telemedicine. • director of MFM service is a board-certified MFM. • director of obstetric service is a board-certified ob-gyn with special interest and experience in obstetric care. • anesthesia services available at all times onsite. • board-certified anesthesiologist with special training or experience in obstetric anesthesia in charge of obstetric anesthesia services. • full complement of subspecialists available for inpatient consultations.
Examples of appropriate patients (not requirements)	Any patient appropriate for level II care, plus higher-risk conditions such as • suspected placenta accreta or placenta previa with prior uterine surgery • suspected placenta percreta • adult respiratory syndrome • expectant management of early severe preeclampsia at less than 34 weeks of gestation

(continued)

TABLE 1-2. Levels of Maternal Care: Definitions, Capabilities, and Types of Health Care Providers * *(continued)*

Level IV (Regional Perinatal Health Care Centers)	
Definition	Level III facility plus onsite medical and surgical care of the most complex maternal conditions and critically ill pregnant women and fetuses throughout antepartum, intrapartum, and postpartum care
Capabilities	Level III facility capabilities plus • on-site ICU care for obstetric patients. • on-site medical and surgical care of complex maternal conditions with the availability of critical care unit or ICU beds. • Perinatal system leadership, including facilitation of maternal referral and transport, outreach education for facilities and health care providers in the region, and analysis and evaluation of regional data, including perinatal complications and outcomes and quality improvement.
Types of health care providers	Level III health care providers plus • MFM care team with expertise to assume responsibility for pregnant women and women in the postpartum period who are in critical condition or have complex medical conditions. This includes co-management of ICU-admitted obstetric patients. An MFM team member with full privileges is available at all times for on-site consultation and management. The team is led by a board-certified MFM with expertise in critical care obstetrics. • physician and nursing leaders with expertise in maternal critical care. • continuous availability of adequate numbers of RNs who have experience in the care of women with complex medical illnesses and obstetric complications; this includes competence in level IV care criteria. • director of obstetric service is a board-certified MFM, or board-certified ob-gyn with expertise in critical care obstetrics. • anesthesia services are available at all times onsite. • board-certified anesthesiologist with special training or experience in obstetric anesthesia in charge of obstetric anesthesia services. • adult medical and surgical specialty and subspecialty consultants available onsite at all times to collaborate with MFM care team.

(continued)

TABLE 1-2. Levels of Maternal Care: Definitions, Capabilities, and Types of Health Care Providers * *(continued)*

Level IV (Regional Perinatal Health Care Centers)	
Examples of appropriate patients (not requirements)	Any patient appropriate for level III care, plus higher-risk conditions such as • severe maternal cardiac conditions • severe pulmonary hypertension or liver failure • pregnant women requiring neurosurgery or cardiac surgery • pregnant women in unstable condition and in need of an organ transplant

Abbreviations: CMs, certified midwives; CNMs, certified nurse–midwives; CPMs, certified professional midwives; ICU, intensive care unit; MFMs, maternal–fetal medicine subspecialists; ob-gyns, obstetrician–gynecologists; RNs, registered nurses.

*These guidelines are limited to the maternal needs. Consideration of perinatal needs and the appropriate level of care should occur following existing guidelines. In fact, levels of maternal care and levels of neonatal care may not match within facilities. Additionally, these are guidelines, and local issues will affect systems of implementation for regionalized maternal care, perinatal care, or both.

Levels of maternal care. Obstetric Care Consensus No. 2. American College of Obstetricians and Gynecologists. Obstet Gynecol 2015;125:502–15.

TABLE 1-3. Levels of Maternal Care by Services*

Level of Maternal Care					
Required Service	Birth Centers	Level I	Level II	Level III	Level IV
Nursing	Adequate numbers of qualified professionals with competence in level I care criteria	Continuously available RNs with competence in level I care criteria Nursing leadership has expertise in perinatal nursing care	Continuously available RNs with competence in level II care criteria Nursing leadership has formal training and experience in perinatal nursing care and coordinates with respective neonatal care services	Continuously available nursing leaders and RNs with competence in level III care criteria and have special training and experience in the management of women with complex maternal illnesses and obstetric complications	Continuously available RNs with competence in level IV care criteria Nursing leadership has expertise in maternal intensive and critical care
Minimum primary delivery provider to be available	CNMs, CMs, CPMs, and licensed midwives	Obstetric provider with privileges to perform emergency cesarean delivery	Ob-gyns or MFMs	Ob-gyns or MFMs	Ob-gyns or MFMs
Obstetrics surgeon		Available for emergency cesarean delivery	Ob-gyn available at all times	Ob-gyn onsite at all times	Ob-gyn onsite at all times
MFMs			Available for consultation onsite, by telephone, or by telemedicine, as needed	Available at all times onsite, by telephone, or by telemedicine with inpatient privileges	Available at all times for onsite consultation and management

(continued)

TABLE 1-3. Levels of Maternal Care by Services* *(continued)*

Level of Maternal Care *(continued)*					
Required Service	Birth Centers	Level I	Level II	Level III	Level IV
Director of obstetric services			Board-certified ob-gyn with experience and interest in obstetrics	Board-certified ob-gyn with experience and interest in obstetrics	Board-certified MFM or board-certified ob-gyn with expertise in critical care obstetrics
Anesthesia		Anesthesia services available	Anesthesia services available at all times Board-certified anesthesiologist with special training or experience in obstetrics, available for consultation	Anesthesia services available at all times Board-certified anesthesiologist with special training or experience in obstetrics is in charge of obstetric anesthesia services	Anesthesia services available at all times Board-certified anesthesiologist with special training or experience in obstetrics is in charge of obstetric anesthesia services
Consultants	Established agreement with a receiving hospital for timely transport, including determination of conditions necessitating consultation and referral	Established agreement with a higher-level receiving hospital for timely transport, including determination of conditions necessitating consultation and referral	Medical and surgical consultants available to stabilize	Full complement of subspecialists available for inpatient consultation, including critical care, general surgery, infectious disease, hematology, cardiology, nephrology, neurology, and neonatology	Adult medical and surgical specialty and subspecialty consultants available onsite at all times, including those indicated in level III and advanced neurosurgery, transplant, or cardiac surgery

(continued)

TABLE 1-3. Levels of Maternal Care by Services* *(continued)*

Level of Maternal Care *(continued)*					
Required Service	Birth Centers	Level I	Level II	Level III	Level IV
ICU				Appropriate equipment and personnel available onsite to ventilate and monitor women in labor and delivery until safely transferred to ICU Accepts pregnant women	Collaborates actively with the MFM care team in the management of all pregnant women and women in the post-partum period who are in critical condition or have complex medical conditions Co-manages ICU-admitted obstetric patients with MFM team

Abbreviations: CMs, certified midwives; CNMs, certified nurse–midwives; CPMs, certified professional midwives; ICU, intensive care unit; MFMs, maternal–fetal medicine specialists; ob-gyns, obstetrician–gynecologists; RNs, registered nurses.

Birth Centers

In 1995, the American Association of Birth Centers (www.birthcenters.org/) defined birth centers as "homelike facilities existing within a healthcare system with a program of care designed in the wellness model of pregnancy and birth and providing family-centered care for healthy women before, during, and after normal pregnancy, labor, and birth." This common definition is used in this book and includes birth centers regardless of their location. Birth centers provide peripartum care to low-risk women with uncomplicated singleton term pregnancies with a vertex presentation who are expected to have an uncomplicated birth. Cesarean delivery and operative vaginal delivery are not offered at birth centers. In a freestanding birth center, every birth should be attended by at least two health care providers, one of whom is competent in neonatal resuscitation. The primary maternity care provider who attends each birth is educated and licensed to provide birthing services. Primary maternity care providers include certified nurse–midwives (CNMs), certified midwives, certified professional midwives, and licensed midwives who are legally recognized to practice within the jurisdiction of the birth center; family physicians; and obstetrician–gynecologists. In addition, there should be adequate numbers of qualified professionals available who have completed orientation and demonstrated competence in the care of obstetric patients (women and fetuses) consistent with level I care criteria and are able to stabilize and transfer high-risk women and newborn infants. Medical consultation should be available at all times. These facilities should be ready to initiate emergency procedures (including cardiopulmonary and neonatal resuscitation and stabilization) at all times to meet unexpected needs of the woman and newborn infants within the center, and to facilitate transport to an acute care setting when necessary. To ensure optimal care of all women and their newborn infants, a birth center should have a clear understanding of its capability to provide maternal and neonatal care and the threshold at which it should transfer women to a facility with a higher level of care. A birth center should have an established agreement with a receiving hospital and have policies and procedures in place for timely transport. These transfer plans should include risk identification; determination of conditions necessitating consultation; referral and transfer; and a reliable, accurate, and comprehensive communication system between participating facilities and transport teams. All facilities should have quality improvement programs that include efforts to maximize patient safety. Birth center facility licenses currently are available in more than 80% of states in the United States and state requirements for accreditation for birth centers vary. Three national agencies (Accreditation Association for Ambulatory Health Care [www.aaahc.org/], The Joint Commission [www.jointcommission.org/], and The Commission for the Accreditation of Birth Centers [www.birthcenteraccreditation.org/]) provide accreditation of birth centers. The Commission for the Accreditation of Birth Centers is the only accrediting agency that chooses to use the national American Association of Birth Centers' *Standards for Birth Centers* in its accreditation process.

Level I Facilities

Level I facilities provide care to women who are low risk and are expected to have an uncomplicated birth. Level I facilities have the capability to perform routine intrapartum and postpartum care that is anticipated to be uncomplicated. As in birth centers, maternity care providers, midwives, family physicians, or obstetrician–gynecologists should be available to attend all births. Adequate numbers of registered nurses (RNs) are available who have completed orientation, demonstrated competence in the care of obstetric patients (women and fetuses) consistent with level I care criteria, and are able to stabilize and transfer high-risk women and newborn infants. Nursing leadership should have expertise in perinatal nursing care. An obstetric care provider with privileges to perform an emergency cesarean delivery should be available to attend deliveries. Anesthesia services should be available to provide labor analgesia and surgical anesthesia. Level I facilities have the capability to begin an emergency cesarean delivery within a time interval that best incorporates maternal and fetal risks and benefits with the provision of emergency care. Support services include access to obstetric ultrasonography, laboratory testing, and blood bank supplies at all times. All hospitals with obstetric services should have protocols and capabilities in place for massive transfusion, emergency release of blood products (before full compatibility testing is complete), and for management of multiple component therapy. These facilities and health care providers can appropriately detect, stabilize, and initiate management of unanticipated maternal, fetal, or neonatal problems that occur during the antepartum, intrapartum, or postpartum period until the patient can be transferred to a facility at which specialty maternal care is available. To ensure optimal care of all pregnant women, formal transfer plans should be established in partnership with a higher-level receiving facility. These plans should include risk identification; determination of conditions necessitating consultation; referral and transfer; and a reliable, accurate, and comprehensive communication system between participating hospitals and transport teams. All facilities should have education and quality improvement programs to maximize patient safety, provide such programs through collaboration with facilities with higher levels of care that receive transfers, or both. Examples of women who need at least level I care include women with term twin gestation; women attempting trial of labor after cesarean delivery; women expecting an uncomplicated cesarean delivery; and women with preeclampsia without severe features at term.

Policies should be developed regarding the provision of obstetric anesthesia, including the necessary qualifications of personnel who are to administer anesthesia and their availability for both routine and emergency deliveries.

Cesarean delivery may warrant the assistance of an additional physician or a surgical assistant to provide necessary surgical care, based on the judgment of the primary obstetric surgeon.

In level I maternal care facilities, perinatal care should be coordinated jointly by the chiefs of the obstetric, pediatric, family medicine, nursing, and midwifery services. This administrative approach requires close coordination and unified policy statements. The coordinators of perinatal care are responsible for developing policy, maintaining appropriate guidelines, and collaborating and consulting with the professional staff of hospitals (including anesthesiologists, radiologists, and laboratory personnel) who provide specialty and subspecialty care in the region. In hospitals that do not separate these services, one person may be given the responsibility for coordinating perinatal care.

Level II Facilities

Level II facilities provide care to appropriate high-risk pregnant women, both admitted and transferred to the facility. In addition to the capabilities of a level I (basic care) facility, level II facilities should have the infrastructure for continuous availability of adequate numbers of RNs who have demonstrated competence in the care of obstetric patients (women and fetuses). Orientation and demonstrated competence should be consistent with level II care criteria and include stabilization and transfer of high-risk women and newborn infants who exceed level II care criteria. The nursing leaders and staff at a level II facility should have formal training and experience in the provision of perinatal nursing care and should coordinate with respective neonatal care services. Although midwives and family physicians may practice in level II facilities, an attending obstetrician–gynecologist should be available at all times. A board-certified obstetrician–gynecologist with special interest and experience in obstetric care should be the director of obstetric services. Access to a maternal–fetal medicine subspecialist for consultation should be available onsite, by telephone, or by telemedicine as needed. Anesthesia services should be available at all times to provide labor analgesia and surgical anesthesia. A board-certified anesthesiologist with special training or experience in obstetric anesthesia should be available for consultation. Support services include level I capabilities plus computed tomography scan and, ideally, magnetic resonance imaging with interpretation available; basic ultrasonographic imaging services for maternal and fetal assessment; and special equipment needed to accommodate the care and services needed for obese women. Medical and surgical consultants should be available to stabilize obstetric patients who have been admitted to the facility or transferred from other facilities. Examples of women who need at least level II care include women with severe preeclampsia and women with placenta previa with no prior uterine surgery.

In level II maternal care facilities, the director of obstetric service and the chief of neonatal care services should coordinate the hospital's perinatal care services and, in conjunction with other medical, anesthesia, nursing, midwifery, respiratory therapy, and hospital administration staff, develop policies concerning staffing, procedures, equipment, and supplies. In addition, the coordinators of perinatal care at a hospital that delivers level II maternal care are responsible for collaborating and consulting with the professional staff of hospitals who provide specialty and subspecialty care in the region.

Level III Facilities

Level III facilities (subspecialty care) provide all level I (basic care) and level II (specialty care) services, and have subspecialists available onsite, by telephone, or by telemedicine to assist in providing care for more complex maternal and fetal conditions. Level III facilities will function as the regional perinatal health care centers for some areas of the United States if there are no level IV facilities available. In these areas, the level III facilities will be responsible for the leadership, facilitation of transport and referral, educational outreach, and data collection and analysis outlined in the Regionalization section discussed later in this chapter. Designation of level III should be based on the demonstrated experience and capability of the facility to provide comprehensive management of severe maternal and fetal complications. An obstetrician–gynecologist is available onsite at all times and a maternal–fetal medicine subspecialist is available at all times, either onsite, by telephone, or by telemedicine, and should have inpatient privileges. The director of the maternal–fetal medicine service should be a board-certified maternal–fetal medicine subspecialist. A board-certified obstetrician–gynecologist with special interest and experience in obstetric care should direct obstetric services. Anesthesia services should be available at all times onsite. A board-certified anesthesiologist with special training or experience in obstetric anesthesia should be in charge of obstetric anesthesia services. A full complement of subspecialists, including subspecialists in critical care, general surgery, infectious disease, hematology, cardiology, nephrology, neurology, and neonatology should be available for inpatient consultations. An on-site intensive care unit (ICU) should accept pregnant women and have critical care providers onsite to actively collaborate with maternal–fetal specialists at all times. Equipment and personnel with expertise must be available onsite to ventilate and monitor women in the labor and delivery unit until they can be safely transferred to the ICU. Level III facilities have nursing leaders and adequate numbers of RNs who have completed orientation and demonstrated competence in the care of obstetric patients (women and fetuses) consistent with level III care criteria, including transfer of high-risk women and newborn infants who exceed level III care criteria, and who have special training and experience in the management of women with complex maternal illnesses and obstetric complications. These nursing personnel continuously are available. Level III facilities should be able to provide imaging services, including basic interventional radiology, maternal echocardiography, computed tomography, and magnetic resonance imaging, and nuclear medicine imaging. These imaging services with interpretation should be available at all times. Level III facilities should have the ability to perform detailed obstetric ultrasonography and fetal assessment, including Doppler studies. These facilities also should provide evaluation of new technologies and therapies. Examples of women who need at least level III care include those women with extreme risk of massive hemorrhage at delivery, such as those with suspected placenta accreta or placenta previa with prior uterine surgery; women with suspected placenta percreta; women with adult respiratory distress syndrome; and women with rapidly evolving disease, such as planned expectant management of severe preeclampsia at less than 34 weeks of gestation.

Level IV Facilities

Level IV facilities (regional perinatal health care centers) include the capabilities of level I, level II, and level III facilities with additional capabilities and considerable experience in the care of the most complex and critically ill pregnant women throughout antepartum, intrapartum, and postpartum care. Although level III and level IV may seem to overlap, a level IV facility is distinct from a level III facility in the approach to the care of pregnant women and women in the postpartum period with complex and critical illnesses. In addition to having ICU care onsite for obstetric patients, a level IV facility must have evidence of a maternal–fetal medicine care team that has the expertise to assume responsibility for pregnant women and women in the postpartum period who are in critical condition or have complex medical conditions. The maternal–fetal medicine team collaborates actively in the co-management of all obstetric patients who require critical care and ICU services. This includes co-management of ICU-admitted obstetric patients. A maternal–fetal medicine team member with full privileges is available at all times to come in for on-site consultation and management. The team should be led by a board-certified maternal–fetal medicine subspecialist with expertise in critical care obstetrics. The maternal–fetal medicine team must have expertise in critical care at the physician level, nursing level, and ancillary services level. A key principle of caring for critically ill pregnant and peripartum women is the facility's recognition of the need for seamless communication between maternal–fetal medicine subspecialists and other subspecialists in the planning and facilitation of care for women with the most high-risk complications of pregnancy. There should be institutional support for the routine involvement of a maternal–fetal medicine care team with the critical care units and specialists. There also should be a commitment to having physician and nursing leaders with expertise in maternal intensive and critical care, as well as adequate numbers of available RNs in level IV facilities who have experience in the care of women with complex medical illnesses and obstetric complications; this includes completed orientation, demonstrated competence in the care of obstetric patients (women and fetuses) consistent with level IV care criteria. The director of obstetric services is a board-certified maternal–fetal medicine subspecialist or a board-certified obstetrician–gynecologist with expertise in critical care obstetrics. As in level III facilities, anesthesia services are available onsite at all times. A board-certified anesthesiologist with special training or experience in obstetric anesthesia should be in charge of obstetric anesthesia services. Level IV facilities should include the capability for on-site medical and surgical care of complex maternal conditions (eg, congenital maternal cardiac lesions, vascular injuries, neurosurgical emergencies, and transplants) with the availability of critical (or intensive) care unit beds. There should be adult medical and surgical specialty and subspecialty consultants (a minimum of those listed in level III) available onsite at all times to collaborate with the maternal–fetal medicine care team. The designation of level IV also may pertain only to a particular specialty in that advanced neurosurgery, transplant, and cardiovascular capabilities may not all be available in the same regional facility. Examples of women who would need level IV care (at least at the time of delivery) include pregnant women with severe maternal cardiac conditions, severe pulmonary hypertension, or liver failure; pregnant women in need of neurosurgery or cardiac surgery; or pregnant women in unstable condition and in need of an organ transplant.

In level III and level IV maternal care facilities, the director of obstetric service, the director of neonatal intensive care unit, and the director of maternal–fetal medicine service should co-direct the perinatal medical service. These physicians are responsible for maintaining practice guidelines and, in cooperation with nursing and hospital administration, are responsible for developing the operating budget; evaluating and purchasing equipment; planning, developing, and coordinating in-hospital and outreach educational programs; and participating in the evaluation of perinatal care. If they are in a regional center, they should coordinate the services provided at their hospital with those provided at institutions delivering level I and level II care in the region or system.

Regionalization

Regional centers, which include any level III facility that functions in this capacity and all level IV facilities, should coordinate regional perinatal health care services; provide outreach education to facilities and health care providers in their region; and provide analysis and evaluation of regional data, including perinatal complications and outcomes, as part of collaboration with lower-level care facilities in the region. Community outreach and data analysis and evaluation will require additional resources in personnel and equipment within these facilities. Although specific supporting data are not currently available in maternal health, it is believed that concentrating the care of women with the most complex pregnancies at designated regional perinatal health care centers will allow these centers to maintain the expertise needed to achieve optimal outcomes. Regionalization of maternal health care services requires that there be available and coordinated specialized services, professional continuing education to maintain competency, facilitation of opportunities for transport and back-transport, and collection of data on long-term outcomes to evaluate the effectiveness of delivery of perinatal health care services and the safety and efficacy of new therapies. Because the health statuses of women and fetuses may differ, referral should be organized to meet the needs of both. In some cases with specific care needs, optimal coordination of care will not be delineated by geographic area, but rather by availability of specific expertise (eg, transplant services or fetal surgery).

In general, each hospital should have a clear understanding of the categories of perinatal patients that can be managed appropriately in the local facility and those that should be transferred to a higher-level facility. Preterm labor and impending delivery at less than 32 weeks of gestation usually warrant maternal transfer to a facility with neonatal intensive care. In some states, because of geographic distances or demographics, hospitals may be approved for a level of neonatal care higher than that for the perinatal service as a whole. In such circumstances, transfer to a facility with a higher level of perinatal care may be appropriate (see also Chapter 4).

Levels of Neonatal Care

The American Academy of Pediatrics published a policy statement regarding levels of neonatal care in 2004, with a subsequent revision in 2012. The levels of neonatal care are illustrated in Table 1-4. Note that each higher level includes the capabilities of the previous level. Levels of maternal and neonatal care may not match within facilities. However, a pregnant woman should be cared for at the facility that best meets both her and her newborn infant's needs (see also Chapter 4).

Level I Neonatal Care

Level I neonatal care units offer a basic level of newborn care to infants at low risk. These units have personnel and equipment available to perform neonatal resuscitation at every delivery and to evaluate and provide routine postnatal care for healthy term newborn infants. In addition, level I neonatal units have personnel who can care for physiologically stable infants who are born at 35 weeks of gestation or more, and can stabilize ill newborn infants who are born at less than 35 weeks of gestation until they can be transferred to a facility where the appropriate level of neonatal care is provided.

A facility providing level I neonatal care should have the personnel and equipment to perform neonatal resuscitation. At least one caregiver whose primary responsibility is for the newborn infant should be present at every delivery, and a person who has successfully completed the American Heart Association and American Academy of Pediatrics' Neonatal Resuscitation Program should be immediately available to perform neonatal resuscitation, including endotracheal intubation and administration of medications, if needed. When required, one or two additional persons should be available to assist with neonatal resuscitation (for more information on neonatal resuscitation, see Chapter 10).

TABLE 1-4. Definitions, Capabilities, and Health Care Provider Types: Neonatal Levels of Care

Level of Care	Capabilities	Health Care Provider Types*
Level I well newborn nursery	Provide neonatal resuscitation at every delivery Evaluate and provide postnatal care to stable term newborn infants Stabilize and provide care for infants born at 35–37 weeks of gestation who remain physiologically stable Stabilize newborn infants who are ill and those born before 35 weeks of gestation until transfer to a higher level of care	Pediatricians, family physicians, newborn nurse practitioners, and other nursery advanced practice registered nurses
Level II special care nursery	Level I capabilities plus: Provide care for infants born at 32 weeks of gestation or later and weigh 1,500 g or more who have physiologic immaturity or who are moderately ill with problems that are expected to resolve rapidly and are not anticipated to need subspecialty services on an urgent basis Provide care for infants convalescing after intensive care Provide mechanical ventilation for brief duration (less than 24 hours) or continuous positive airway pressure or both Stabilize infants born before 32 weeks of gestation and weigh less than 1,500 g until transfer to a neonatal intensive care facility	Level I health care providers plus: Pediatric hospitalists, neonatologists, and neonatal nurse practitioners

(continued)

TABLE 1-4. Definitions, Capabilities, and Health Care Provider Types: Neonatal Levels of Care *(continued)*

Level of Care	Capabilities	Health Care Provider Types*
Level III neonatal intensive care unit	Level II capabilities plus: Provide sustained life support Provide comprehensive care for infants born before 32 weeks of gestation and weigh less than 1,500 g and infants born at all gestational ages and birth weights with critical illness Provide prompt and readily available access to a full range of pediatric medical subspecialists, pediatric surgical specialists, pediatric anesthesiologists, and pediatric ophthalmologists Provide a full range of respiratory support that may include conventional ventilation and/or high-frequency ventilation and inhaled nitric oxide Perform advanced imaging, with interpretation on an urgent basis, including computed tomography, magnetic resonance imaging, and echocardiography	Level II health care providers plus: Pediatric medical subspecialists†, pediatric anesthesiologists†, pediatric surgeons, and pediatric ophthalmologists†

(continued)

TABLE 1-4. Definitions, Capabilities, and Health Care Provider Types: Neonatal Levels of Care *(continued)*

Level of Care	Capabilities	Health Care Provider Types*
Level IV regional neonatal intensive care unit	Level III capabilities plus: Located within an institution with the capability to provide surgical repair of complex congenital or acquired conditions Maintain a full range of pediatric medical subspecialists, pediatric surgical subspecialists, and pediatric anesthesiologists at the site Facilitate transport and provide outreach education	Level III health care providers plus: Pediatric surgical subspecialists

*Includes all health care providers with relevant experience, training, and demonstrated competence

†At the site or at a closely related institution by prearranged consultative agreement

Reprinted from Levels of neonatal care. Policy statement. American Academy of Pediatrics. Committee on Fetus and Newborn. Pediatrics 2012;130:587–97.

Level II Neonatal Care

Level II neonatal care should be reserved for infants born at 32 weeks of gestation or more and weighing 1,500 g or more at birth who have physiologic immaturity or who are moderately ill with problems that are expected to resolve rapidly and who would not be anticipated to need subspecialty-level services on an urgent basis. These situations usually occur as a result of relatively uncomplicated preterm labor or preterm rupture of membranes.

Level II nurseries may provide assisted ventilation for a brief duration (less than 24 hours) until the infant's condition either soon improves or the infant can be transferred to a higher-level facility. A facility that provides level II neonatal care must have readily available experienced personnel who are capable of providing either continuous positive airway pressure or mechanical ventilation for a brief period (less than 24 hours) or both (Table 1–4). Level II nurseries must have equipment (eg, portable X-ray equipment, blood gas laboratory) and personnel, such as physicians, specialized nurses, respiratory therapists, radiology technicians, and laboratory technicians (see "Support Health Care Providers" in Chapter 2), continuously available to provide ongoing care and to address emergencies. Referral to a higher level of care should occur for all infants when needed for subspecialty surgical or medical intervention.

A board-certified neonatologist or board-certified pediatrician with experience in the care of newborn infants should be chief of the neonatal care service. Care of newborn infants at high risk should be provided by appropriately qualified personnel including pediatricians, neonatologists, pediatric hospitalists, and neonatal nurse practitioners (see "Advanced Practice Registered Nurses in Perinatal Care" in Chapter 2). When an infant is maintained on a ventilator, these specialized personnel should be available onsite to manage respiratory emergencies.

A general pediatrician or pediatric hospitalist should have sufficient training and expertise to assume responsibility for the care of newborn infants who require Level II care. In collaboration with, or under the supervision of, a physician, care may be provided by qualified advanced practice registered nurses who have completed a formal neonatal educational program and are certified by an accepted national body, such as the National Certification Corporation (see also "Advanced Practice Registered Nurses in Perinatal Care" in Chapter 2).

Level III Neonatal Care

Evidence suggests that infants who are born at less than 32 weeks of gestation or weigh less than 1,500 g at birth or have complex medical or surgical conditions, regardless of gestational age, should be cared for at a level III facility. Designation of level III care should be based on clinical experience, as demonstrated by large patient volume, increasing complexity of care, and availability of pediatric medical subspecialists and pediatric surgical specialists. Subspecialty care services should include expertise in neonatology and, ideally, maternal–fetal medicine if women are referred for the management of potential preterm birth. Level III neonatal intensive care units (NICUs) are defined by having continuously available personnel (neonatologists, neonatal nurses, respiratory therapists) and equipment to provide life support for as long as needed. Facilities should have advanced respiratory support and physiologic monitoring equipment, laboratory and imaging facilities, nutrition and pharmacy support with pediatric expertise, social services, and pastoral care.

Level III facilities should be able to provide ongoing assisted ventilation for periods longer than 24 hours, which may include conventional ventilation, high-frequency ventilation, and inhaled nitric oxide. Level III facility capabilities also should be based on a region's consideration of geographic constraints, population size, and personnel resources. If geographic constraints for land transportation exist, the level III facility should ensure availability of rotor and fixed-wing transport services to quickly and safely transfer infants requiring subspecialty intervention. Potential transfer to higher-level facilities or children's hospitals, as well as return transport of recovering infants to lower-level facilities, should be considered as clinically indicated.

A broad range of pediatric medical subspecialists and pediatric surgical specialists should be readily accessible onsite or by prearranged consultative agreements. Prearranged consultative agreements can be performed using, for example, telemedicine technology, or telephone consultation, or both from a distant location. Pediatric ophthalmology services and an organized program for the monitoring, treatment, and follow-up of retinopathy of prematurity should be readily available in level III facilities. Level III units should have the capability to perform major surgery (including anesthesiologists with pediatric expertise) onsite or at a closely related institution, ideally in geographic proximity. Because the outcomes of less complex surgical procedures in children, such as appendectomy or pyloromyotomy, are better when performed by pediatric surgeons compared with general surgeons, it is recommended that pediatric surgical specialists perform all procedures in newborn infants.

Level III facilities should have the capability to perform advanced imaging with interpretation on an urgent basis, including computed tomography, magnetic resonance imaging, and echocardiography. Level III facilities should collect data to assess outcomes within their facility and to compare with other levels.

The director of the neonatal intensive care unit (NICU) should be a full-time, board-certified neonatologist. A neonatologist should be continuously available for consultation 24 hours per day. Personnel qualified to manage the care of infants with complex or critical illnesses, including emergencies, should be in-house.

Level IV Neonatal Care

Level IV units include the capabilities of level III units with additional capabilities and considerable experience in the care of the most complex and critically ill newborn infants and should have pediatric medical and pediatric surgical specialty consultants continuously available 24 hours per day. Level IV facilities also would include the capability for surgical repair of complex conditions. Further evidence is needed to assess the risk of morbidity and mortality by level of care for newborn infants with complex congenital cardiac malformations. A recent study was not able to note a difference in postoperative morbidity or mortality associated with dedicated pediatric cardiac intensive care units versus NICUs and pediatric intensive care units, but the study did not separately assess the newborn and postneonatal periods. Although specific supporting data are not currently available, it is thought that concentrating the care of such infants at designated level IV centers will allow these centers to develop the expertise needed to achieve optimal outcomes.

Not all level IV hospitals need to act as regional centers; however, regional organization of perinatal health care services requires that there be coordination in the development of specialized services, professional continuing education to maintain competency, facilitation of opportunities for transport and return transport, and collection of data on long-term outcomes to evaluate both the effectiveness of delivery of perinatal health care services and the safety and efficacy of new therapies. These functions usually are best achieved when responsibility is concentrated in a single regional center with both perinatal and neonatal subspecialty services.

Maternal and Newborn Postdischarge Care

Perinatal health care at all levels should include ambulatory care of the woman and the newborn infant after hospital discharge. Increasing economic pressure for early discharge and decreased length of hospital stay after delivery has increased the importance of organization and coordination of continuing care as well as the need for evaluation and monitoring of outcomes. In most cases, healthy term infants discharged before 72 hours of age should be evaluated by a qualified health care provider within 1–2 days of discharge. Late preterm infants need additional care and monitoring (see also Chapter 10). Postdischarge care for an infant who has survived a complicated perinatal course should include care by a health care provider with expertise and experience in caring for such infants. Infants who have been discharged from the NICU also should be enrolled in an organized follow-up program that tracks and records medical and neurodevelopmental outcomes to allow later analysis. Such a follow-up program is an essential component of level III and level IV neonatal services. Service components for follow-up care for women are discussed in Chapter 8 and for newborn infants in Chapter 10 and Chapter 11.

When prolonged infant hospitalization far from the woman's home is anticipated, it is recommended that a local maternity health care provider be identified to provide the standard postpartum care and support that she would have received in her home environment, even if delivery did not take place at a local hospital.

Planned Home Birth

In the United States, approximately 35,000 births (0.9%) of births per year occur in the home. Approximately one fourth of these births are unplanned or unattended. Among women who originally intend to give birth in a hospital or those who make no provisions for professional care during childbirth, unplanned home births are associated with high rates of perinatal and neonatal mortality. The relative risk versus benefit of a planned home birth, however, remains the subject of debate. Women inquiring about planned home birth should be informed of its risks and benefits based on recent evidence (Table 1-5 and Table 1-6). Specifically, they should be informed that although planned home birth is associated with fewer maternal interventions than planned hospital birth, it is also associated with a more than twofold increased risk of perinatal death (1–2 in 1,000) and a threefold risk of neonatal seizures or serious neurologic dysfunction (0.4–0.6 in 1,000). These observations may reflect fewer obstetric risk factors among women planning home birth compared with those planning hospital birth. Although the American College of Obstetricians and Gynecologists believes that hospitals and accredited birth centers are the safest settings for birth, each woman has the right to make a medically informed decision about delivery.

Women should be informed that several factors are critical to reducing perinatal mortality rates and achieving favorable home birth outcomes. These factors include the appropriate selection of candidates for home birth; the availability of a certified nurse–midwife, certified midwife, or midwife whose education and licensure meet International Confederation of Midwives' Global Standards for Midwifery Education, or physicians practicing obstetrics within an integrated and regulated health system; ready access to consultation; and access to safe and timely transport to nearby hospitals. Fetal malpresentation, multiple gestation, or prior cesarean delivery should be considered absolute contraindications to planned home birth.

TABLE 1-5. Maternal Outcomes Associated with U.S. Planned Out of Hospital Births Versus Hospital Births*

Outcome	Planned Out of Hospital Birth (events per 1,000 births)	Planned Hospital Birth (events per 1,000 births)	Adjusted Odds Ratio	95% CI
Labor induction	48	304	0.11	0.09–0.12
Labor augmentation	75	263	0.21	0.19–0.24
Operative vaginal delivery	10	35	0.24	0.17–0.34
Cesarean delivery	53	247	0.18	0.16–0.22
Blood transfusion/ hemorrhage	6	4	1.91	1.25–2.93
Severe perineal lacerations	9	13	0.69	0.49–0.98

*Data from Snowden JM, Tilden EL, Snyder J, Quigley B, Caughey AB, Cheng YW. Planned out-of-hospital birth and birth outcomes. N Engl J Med 2015;373:2642–53.

TABLE 1-6. Adverse Perinatal Outcomes Associated with U.S. Planned Home Births Versus Hospital Births

Outcome	Planned Home Birth (events per 1,000 births)	Planned Birth (events per 1,000 births)	Odds Ratio	95% CI
5-minute Apgar Score	24.2*	11.7*	2.42*	2.13–2.74*
	23†§	18†	1.31†	1.04–1.66†
<7	3.7*	2.43*	1.87*	1.36–2.58*
<4	6†§	4†	1.56†	0.98–2.47*
0	1.63‡	0.16‡	10.55‡	8.62–12.93‡
Neonatal seizures (or serious neurologic dysfunction‡)	0.58*	0.22*	3.08*	1.44–6.58*
	0.86‡	0.22‡	3.80‡	2.80–5.16‡
	1.3†§	0.4†	3.60†	1.36–9.50†

(continued)

TABLE 1-6. Adverse Perinatal Outcomes Associated with U.S. Planned Home Births Versus Hospital Births *(continued)*

Outcome	Planned Home Birth (events per 1,000 births)	Planned Birth (events per 1,000 births)	Odds Ratio	95% CI
Perinatal mortality (fetal death and neonatal mortality)	3.9[†§]	1.8[†]	2.43[†]	1.37–4.30[†]

Abbreviation: CI, confidence interval

Data from *Cheng YW, Snowden JM, King TL, Caughey AB. Selected perinatal outcomes associated with planned home births in the United States. Am J Obstet Gynecol 2013;209:325.e1–8.

Data from †Grunebaum A, McCullough LB, Sapra KJ, Brent RL, Levene MI, Arabin B, et al. Apgar score of 0 at 5 minutes and neonatal seizures or serious neurologic dysfunction in relation to birth setting. Am J Obstet Gynecol 2013;209:323.e1–6.

Data from ‡Snowden JM, Tilden EL, Snyder J, Quigley B, Caughey AB, Cheng YW. Planned out-of-hospital birth and birth outcomes. N Engl J Med 2015;373:2642–53.

§Includes planned birth center and home births

Workforce: The Distribution and Supply of Perinatal Care Providers

The distribution and supply of physicians who provide perinatal health care services have been changing. Although the number of physicians has increased substantially over the past 20 years, the percentage of all physicians who provide obstetric care has decreased. In addition, obstetricians who provide care for high-risk patients, maternal–fetal medicine specialists, and neonatologists are unevenly distributed among geographic areas and types of facilities. Good data are lacking on the number of obstetricians who provide care for high-risk patients and the number of neonatologists needed to serve a given population.

In perinatal health care delivery, a team-based model of care that strives to meet patient needs and preferences by actively engaging patients as full participants in their care while encouraging all health care providers to function to the full extent of their education, certification, and experience is essential to improve the outcome of pregnancy. Optimally implemented, the team-based approach provides integrated care over the course of a specific experience, as well as across a patient's lifespan within a regionalized care system. The care team for a given patient is composed of health care providers with the training and skills needed to provide high-quality, coordinated care specific to the patient's clinical needs and circumstances. A team may span multiple practices and locations, especially through the use of telemedicine. Certified nurse–midwives, certified midwives, laborists, obstetric and gynecologic hospitalists, family practitioners, physician assistants, advanced practice registered nurses, respiratory therapists, perinatal social workers, lactation consultants, and other professionals also are important health care providers of perinatal services.

Strategies aimed at increasing recruitment of perinatal health care providers are needed, particularly in rural and urban medically underserved areas. More than 2,000 federal Health Professional Shortage Areas have been designated; most of the people in need of services in these areas are women of childbearing age and young children. Lack of sufficient funding to support perinatal health care services contributes to the number of underserved women.

Examples of regional programs that have been successfully used to increase access to care include liability cost relief, locum tenens programs, satellite practice models, financial incentives to establish or maintain a practice, innovative approaches to continuing education, and programs to provide technical support. The Health Resources and Services Administration, National Health Service Corps, and state scholarship and loan repayment programs for the education of health care professionals, which include a special requirement for service in underserved areas, provide another important incentive. Such programs should be strengthened, adequately funded, and encouraged to give priority to perinatal health care providers.

The obstetrician–gynecologist hospitalist model is one method hospitals can employ to improve the quality and safety of their obstetric–gynecologic services and reduce the incidence of adverse events. Standardization of medical care has been shown to lead to improved outcomes, and ob-gyn hospitalists can serve as a driving force behind the implementation of these protocols in labor units. Effective patient handoffs, updates on progress, and clear follow-up instructions between ob-gyn hospitals and patients, nurses, and other health care providers, are vital to maintaining patient safety (see Chapter 3). Hospitals and other health care organizations should ensure that candidates for positions as obstetrician–gynecologist hospitalists are drawn from those with documented training and experience appropriate for the management of the acute and potentially emergent clinical circumstances that may be encountered in obstetric care.

Bibliography

Alper J. Health literacy and consumer-facing technology: workshop summary. Roundtable on Health Literacy, Board on Population Health and Public Health Practice, Institute of Medicine, The National Academies of Sciences, Engineering, Medicine. Washington, DC: The National Academies Press; 2015.

American College of Obstetricians and Gynecologists. Collaboration in practice: implementing team-based care. Washington, DC: American College of Obstetricians and Gynecologists; 2016. Available at: http://www.acog.org/Resources-And-Publications/Task-Force-and-Work-Group-Reports/Collaboration-in-Practice-Implementing-Team-Based-Care. Retrieved September 30, 2016.

Blackmon LR, Barfield WD, Stark AR. Hospital neonatal services in the United States: Variation in definitions, criteria, and regulatory status, 2008. J Perinatol 2009;29:788–94.

Burstein DS, Jacobs JP, Li JS, Sheng S, O'Brien SM, Rossi AF, et al. Care models and associated outcomes in congenital heart surgery. Pediatrics 2011;127:e1482–9.

Cultural sensitivity and awareness in the delivery of health care. Committee Opinion No. 493. American College of Obstetricians and Gynecologists. Obstet Gynecol 2011;117:1258–61.

Cummings J. Antenatal counseling regarding resuscitation and intensive care before 25 weeks of gestation. Committee on Fetus and Newborn. Pediatrics 2015;136: 588–95.

Effective patient–physician communication. Committee Opinion No. 587. American College of Obstetricians and Gynecologists. Obstet Gynecol 2014;123:389–93.

Engle WA, Tomashek KM, Wallman C. "Late-preterm" infants: a population at risk. Committee on Fetus and Newborn, American Academy of Pediatrics [published erratum appears in Pediatrics 2008;121:451]. Pediatrics 2007;120:1390–401.

Family-centered care and the pediatrician's role. Committee on Hospital Care. American Academy of Pediatrics. Pediatrics 2003;112:691–7.

Finer LB, Zolna MR. Declines in unintended pregnancy in the United States, 2008–2011. N Engl J Med 2016;374:843–52.

Health literacy to promote quality of care. Committee Opinion No. 676. American College of Obstetricians and Gynecologists. Obstet Gynecol 2016;128:e183–6.

Howell EM, Richardson D, Ginsburg P, Foot B. Deregionalization of neonatal intensive care in urban areas. Am J Public Health 2002;92:119–24.

Institute for Patient- and Family-Centered Care. Bethesda (MD): IPFCC; 2016. Available at: http://www.ipfcc.org/. Retrieved September 21, 2016.

Johnson K, Posner SF, Biermann J, Cordero JF, Atrash HK, Parker CS, et al. Recommendations to improve preconception health and health care—United States. A report of the CDC/ATSDR Preconception Care Work Group and the Select Panel on Preconception Care. CDC/ATSDR Preconception Care Work Group; Select Panel on Preconception Care. MMWR Recomm Rep 2006;55:1–23.

Lasswell SM, Barfield WD, Rochat RW, Blackmon L. Perinatal regionalization for very low-birth-weight and very preterm infants: a meta-analysis. JAMA 2010;304:992–1000.

Levels of maternal care. Obstetric Care Consensus No. 2. American College of Obstetricians and Gynecologists. Obstet Gynecol 2015;125:502–15.

Levels of neonatal care. American Academy of Pediatrics Committee on Fetus and Newborn. Pediatrics 2012;130:587–97.

MacDorman MF, Matthews TJ, Declercq E. Trends in out-of-hospital births in the United States, 1990–2012. NCHS Data Brief 2014;(144):1–8.

March of Dimes. Toward improving the outcome of pregnancy III: enhancing perinatal health through quality, safety and performance initiatives. Committee on Perinatal Health. White Plains (NY): National Foundation—March of Dimes; 2010.

March of Dimes. Toward improving the outcome of pregnancy: the 90s and beyond. Committee on Perinatal Health. White Plains (NY): National Foundation—March of Dimes; 1993.

March of Dimes. Toward improving the outcome of pregnancy: recommendations for the regional development of maternal and perinatal health services. Committee on Perinatal Health. White Plains (NY): National Foundation—March of Dimes; 1976.

Optimizing postpartum care. Committee Opinion No. 666. American College of Obstetricians and Gynecologists. Obstet Gynecol 2016;127:e187–92.

Planned home birth. Committee Opinion No. 697. American College of Obstetricians and Gynecologists. Obstet Gynecol 2017;129:e117–22.

Roter DL. Physician/patient communication: transmission of information and patient effects. Md State Med J 1983;32:260–5.

The importance of preconception care in the continuum of women's health care. ACOG Committee Opinion No. 313. American College of Obstetricians and Gynecologists. Obstet Gynecol 2005;106:665–6.

The obstetric and gynecologic hospitalist. Committee Opinion No. 657. American College of Obstetricians and Gynecologists. Obstet Gynecol 2016;127:e81–5.

United States. Office of Minority Health. National standards for culturally and linguistically appropriate services in health care: final report. Washington, DC: U.S. Dept. of Health and Human Services; 2001. Available at: http://minorityhealth.hhs.gov/assets/pdf/checked/finalreport.pdf. Retrieved September 21, 2016.

Vaginal birth after previous cesarean delivery. Practice Bulletin No. 115. American College of Obstetricians and Gynecologists. Obstet Gynecol 2010;116:450–63.

Wax JR, Pinette MG, Cartin A. Home versus hospital birth—process and outcome. Obstet Gynecol Surv 2010;65:132–40.

Weinstein L. The laborist: a new focus of practice for the obstetrician. Am J Obstet Gynecol 2003;188:310–2.

Chapter 2

Inpatient Perinatal Care Services

Inpatient perinatal care services are dependent upon the education, training, and experience of hospital personnel (ie, medical care providers and support staff) as well as the functional capabilities of the physical facilities required for providing care. To achieve optimal outcomes, regionalized systems are recommended to ensure that each woman is cared for in a facility appropriate for her health needs, and that each infant is delivered and cared for in a facility appropriate for his or her health care needs.

Personnel

Factors critical to planning and evaluating the quality and level of personnel required to meet patients' needs in perinatal settings include the mission, philosophy, geographic location, and design of the facility; the patient population; the scope of practice; the qualifications of staff; and obligations for education or research. Perinatal care program personnel include medical care providers (ie, physicians, nurses, certified nurse–midwives, certified midwives, nurse practitioners, and physician assistants), lactation support (ie, professional International Board-Certified Lactation Consultants, certified counselors and educators, peer support), and support staff. Medical and nursing directors for obstetric, family medicine, and pediatric services should jointly coordinate perinatal care programs.

Perinatal Medical Care Providers

Perinatal medical care providers include obstetricians, pediatricians, family physicians, laborists, obstetric–gynecologic and pediatric hospitalists, certified nurse–midwives, certified midwives, nurse practitioners, and physician assistants.

Obstetricians, Pediatricians, Family Physicians, Advanced Practice Providers, Certified Nurse–Midwives, and Certified Midwives

Credentialing and granting privileges to members of its medical and advanced practice provider staff are among the most important responsibilities of any health care facility. Credentialing is a multifaceted process that involves verification of identification (such as National Provider Identification), licensure, education, training, specialty board certification, medical liability coverage, and experience. Other criteria for effective credentialing include review of official source data, such as the National Practitioner Data Bank, data from state licensing boards, data from other facilities where the individual has privileges, and references from peers. Hospitals must query the National Practitioner Data Bank at the time of application, every 2 years for renewal of clinical privileges, and when considering expansion of existing privileges.

A more difficult, yet critical, aspect of the credentialing process is the actual determination of which requested privileges should be granted. The granting of privileges is based on training, experience, and demonstrated current clinical competence. For obstetric care providers, care may be stratified into different levels of complexity. New equipment or technology may improve health care outcomes, provided that practitioners and other hospital staff use the tools as specified for the conditions for which they are designed. Institutions should consider granting privileges for new skills only when the appropriate training has been completed and documented and the competency level has been achieved with adequate supervision (see also Appendix D).

For pediatric providers, the credentials required and the privileges extended will depend on the level of care that is provided. Verification of training, experience, credentialing, and current clinical competence is similar to that for obstetric providers.

Laborists and Hospitalists

The term "laborist" most commonly refers to a physician who is employed by a hospital or physician group and whose primary role is to care for laboring patients and to manage obstetric emergencies. The term "hospitalist" refers to physicians whose primary professional focus is the general medical care of hospitalized patients.

In contrast to internal medicine hospitalists who have essentially replaced their practice-based colleagues in the hospital, obstetrician–gynecologists (laborists) and pediatric hospitalists may replace, but also can assist and complement, their colleagues. Responsibilities of the obstetrician–gynecologist hospitalist may be broad or narrow in focus, ranging from providing only triage and care for unassigned patients, to admitting and providing the full spectrum of labor and delivery and postpartum care for some or all obstetric patients. Depending on the hospital, obstetrician–gynecologist hospitalists may directly supervise and teach residents and students, provide surgical and consultative support to certified nurse–midwives, certified midwives, and family physicians, or manage unassigned patients in the emergency department or medical floors, including gynecologic emergencies and surgeries. Other responsibilities may include assisting in cesarean or multiples' deliveries, providing coverage for precipitous births, managing obstetric emergencies such as postpartum hemorrhage, and providing coverage for obstetrician–gynecologists during scheduled clinic hours. The obstetrician–gynecologist hospitalists also may provide assistance for scheduled operative cases and could support fatigued obstetrician–gynecologists. The obstetrician–gynecologist hospitalists may also work with nursing leadership to ensure effective resource use and to monitor quality metrics, such as elective delivery before 39 weeks of gestation. It is estimated that in 2014, there were more than 1,700 obstetrician–gynecologist hospitalists working at more than 243 hospitals in the United States, which represents approximately 10% of hospitals that offer obstetric services, though penetration of the model may vary by region. Similarly, the responsibilities of the pediatric hospitalist can vary widely, depending on the needs of the program and the capabilities and credentialing of the individual.

Certified Nurse–Midwives and Certified Midwives

Certified nurse–midwives are registered nurses who have graduated from a midwifery education program accredited by the Accreditation Commission for Midwifery Education and have passed a national certification examination administered by the American Midwifery Certification Board, Inc. Certified midwives do not start with a nursing degree, but receive the relevant nursing education as part of a midwifery program accredited by the Accreditation Commission for Midwifery Education. They then undergo the same certification process as certified nurse–midwives. Certified nurse–midwives and certified midwives manage the care of low-risk women in the antepartum, intrapartum, and postpartum periods; manage healthy newborns; and provide primary gynecologic services in accordance with state laws or regulations. In collaboration with obstetricians or family physicians, certified nurse–midwives and certified midwives also may be involved in the care of women with medical or obstetric complications. Certified nurse–midwives and certified midwives work in a variety of settings, including private practice, community health facilities, clinics, hospitals, and accredited birth centers. In some hospital settings, a certified nurse–midwife or certified midwife may also function as a laborist in conjunction with an obstetrician–gynecologist or family physician (see also Appendix E).

Capabilities of Perinatal Medical Care Providers

Advanced Practice Registered Nurses in Perinatal Care. Trends in maternal and neonatal care have resulted in the increased use of advanced practice registered nurses. Nationally recognized standards mandate that an advanced practice registered nurse (nurse practitioner, clinical nurse specialist, certified nurse–midwife, and nurse anesthetist) complete an educational program of study and supervised practice beyond the level of basic nursing. As of January 1, 2000, this preparation must include the attainment of a master's or doctoral degree, usually in the nursing specialty. Nurses who entered the profession before the year 2000 without a graduate degree, but who are certified in their field, should be allowed to maintain their practice and are encouraged to complete their formal graduate education. Nationally recognized certification examinations are required for each category of advanced practice nursing within one of six population foci: Adult–Gerontology, Family, Pediatrics, Psychiatric–Mental Health, Neonatal, or Women's Health. The Advanced Practice Registered Nurses Consensus Model acknowledges that strict adherence to these age-based categories may create barriers and limit access to care. There may be situations when a patient's care falls outside of the traditional population focus for an advanced practice registered nurse, but the patient may be best served through continued care by that practitioner. As licensed health care providers, advanced practice registered nurses are subject to the scope of practice rules and regulations established by and pursuant to the nurse practice act in their state of practice. Commonly, advanced practice registered nurses within perinatal care are the certified nurse–midwife (described earlier in this chapter), the neonatal clinical nurse specialist, the women's health clinical nurse specialist (which now includes those specializing in perinatal nursing care), and the neonatal and women's health nurse practitioners.

Clinical Nurse Specialist. Neonatal and women's health clinical nurse specialists are registered nurses with master's or doctoral degrees who, through study and supervised practice at the graduate level, have become experts in the theory and practice of neonatal or women's health, with a focus on perinatal nursing. Responsibilities of the clinical nurse specialist include fostering continuous quality improvement in nursing care, developing and educating staff to provide evidence-based care, mentoring and team building, leadership of multidisciplinary teams, case management of high-risk perinatal patients, and research. The clinical nurse specialist models expert nursing practice, participates in administrative functions within the hospital setting, serves as a consultant external to the unit, and applies and promotes evidence-based nursing practice.

Nurse Practitioner. Nurse practitioners are advanced practice registered nurses who have achieved licensure and credentialing beyond their role as registered nurses. Nurse practitioners diagnose and manage acute and chronic conditions, emphasizing health promotion and disease prevention. Nurse practitioners' services include, but are not limited to the following: ordering, conducting, supervising, and interpreting diagnostic and laboratory tests; prescribing or furnishing pharmacologic agents and nonpharmacologic therapies; and teaching and counseling. Within this framework, women's health nurse practitioners and neonatal nurse practitioners are prepared through academic and clinical study to practice as advanced practice registered nurses specific to women's health population or the neonatal population.

Scope of Practice. The spectrum of duties performed by an advanced practice registered nurse is determined by state nursing practice statutes and will vary according to the institution. Inpatient care privileges are granted by individual institutions. Each institution should develop a procedure for the initial granting and subsequent maintenance of privileges for advanced practice registered nurses, ensuring that the proper professional credentials are in place. Each institution must ensure that the advanced practice registered nurse has the formal education and national certification to function within the requested scope of practice. That procedure is best developed by the collaborative efforts of the nursing administration and the medical staff governing body.

Women's Health Nurse Practitioner. The women's health nurse practitioner is a primary care nurse practitioner who has completed a formal women's health educational program and has national certification as a women's health nurse practitioner. This practitioner focuses on providing care for conditions unique to women from menarche through the remainder of their lives and on reproductive health care for men. The role of the women's health nurse practitioner is to provide evidence-based assessment, diagnosis, treatment, and management in wellness promotion, care of women's common primary care nongynecologic problems, well-woman gynecologic care, prepregnancy care for women and men, male sexual and reproductive health care, and normal prenatal and postpartum care. Examples of women's health nurse practitioner services specific to the perinatal continuum include providing prepregnancy and interpregnancy care, contraceptive services, prenatal and postpartum care for women with low-risk pregnancies, recognition and early intervention for maternal mental health and behavioral health conditions, antepartum and intrapartum triage and evaluation, and collaboration in providing care to women with high-risk pregnancies. The women's health nurse practitioner is an integral part of the obstetric care team and practices autonomously and in collaboration with other health care professionals to manage women's health needs across the perinatal continuum. For a more comprehensive description of the women's health nurse practitioner role, please see: *the WHNP: Guidelines for Practice and Education* (7th Ed); available at: www.npwh.org/pages/clinicalguidelines. Women's health nurse practitioners manage the care of women in collaboration with a physician, usually an obstetrician–gynecologist or a maternal–fetal medicine specialist. The women's health nurse practitioner training includes didactic and clinical education and includes a demonstrated competency in pharmacology.

Neonatal Nurse Practitioner. The neonatal nurse practitioner manages a caseload of neonatal patients in collaboration with a physician, usually a pediatrician or neonatologist. Neonatal nurse practitioners caring for neonates in the neonatal intensive care unit (NICU) must demonstrate completion of a formal neonatal educational program, which includes a minimum of 200 neonatal-specific didactic hours and at least 600 supervised clinical hours in the care of the at-risk and critically ill newborn in the delivery room and level II, level III, or level IV NICU, and must have national certification as a neonatal nurse practitioner.

The following guidelines are recommended for neonatal nurse practitioners:

- Clinical care by the neonatal nurse practitioner for infants receiving level II, level III, and level IV care is provided in collaboration with, or under the supervision of, a physician, usually a neonatologist. Clinical care by neonatal nurse practitioners for infants receiving level I neonatal care is provided in collaboration with, or under the supervision of, a physician with special interest and experience in neonatal medicine; usually this is a pediatrician.

- Clinical care by the neonatal nurse practitioner is provided in collaboration with all members of the health care team.
- Whether the neonatal nurse practitioner practices in collaboration with or under supervision of a physician should be determined in accordance with the board of nursing regulations in the state in which the neonatal nurse practitioner is practicing and by the hospital guidelines where they are practicing.
- The neonatal nurse practitioner must maintain certification by a nationally recognized organization.

Physician Assistants. Trends in neonatal care have resulted in an increased use of physician assistants in addition to advanced practice registered nurses. Physician assistants are health care professionals licensed to practice medicine with physician supervision. Within the physician–physician assistant relationship, physician assistants exercise autonomy in medical decision making and provide a broad range of diagnostic and therapeutic services. A physician assistant's responsibilities also may include education, research, and administrative services.

Physician assistants are educated and trained in programs accredited by the Accreditation Review Commission on Education for the Physician Assistant. The length of physician assistant programs averages approximately 26 months, and students must complete more than 2,000 hours of supervised clinical practice before graduation. Graduation from an accredited physician assistant program and passage of the national certifying examination are required for state licensure. A number of postgraduate physician assistant programs also have been established to provide practicing physician assistants with advanced education or master's level education in medical specialties.

The responsibilities of a physician assistant depend on the practice setting, education, and experience of the physician assistant, on state laws and regulations, and on specific hospital guidelines. Regardless of background training, the following guidelines are recommended:

- Physician supervision should be provided by a neonatologist in subspecialty NICUs. In level I and level II neonatal units, a board-certified pediatrician with special interest and experience in neonatal medicine may provide supervision.
- The physician assistant is responsible for maintaining clinical expertise and knowledge of current therapy by participating in continuing medical education and scholarly activities.
- The physician assistant must maintain national certification, which includes 100 hours of continuing medical education every 2 years and a recertification examination given by the National Commission on Certification of Physician Assistants every 6 years.

Perinatal Nursing

Nursing responsibilities in individual hospitals vary according to the level of care provided by the facility, practice procedures, number of professional registered nurses and ancillary staff, and professional nursing activities in continuing education and research. Intrapartum care requires the same labor intensiveness and expertise as any other intensive care unit and, accordingly, perinatal units should have the same adequately trained personnel and fiscal support. Trends in medical management and technologic advances influence and may increase the nursing workload. Each hospital should determine the scope of nursing practice for each nursing unit and specialty department. The scope of practice should be based on national nursing guidelines for the specialty area of practice and should be in accordance with state laws and regulations and the recommended staffing patterns for the particular type of health care provider. The health care provider-to-patient ratio should take into account the role expected at the individual unit, acuity of patients, procedures performed, and participation in deliveries or neonatal transport. A multidisciplinary committee, including representatives from hospital, medical, and nursing administrations, should follow published professional guidelines, consult state nurse practice acts and any accompanying regulations, identify the types and numbers of procedures performed in each unit, and delineate the direct and indirect nursing care activities.

Nurse–Patient Ratios

Delivery of safe and effective perinatal nursing care requires appropriately qualified registered nurses in adequate numbers to meet the needs of each patient. The number of staff and level of skill required are influenced by the scope of nursing practice and the degree of nursing responsibilities within an institution. Patient and health care system factors, such as the acuity of the patient population, nursing skill mix, availability and number of support staff, and physical layout of the unit, will also affect the number of nursing staff needed. Patient variables that can affect acceptable nurse–patient ratios include birth weight, gestational age, and diagnoses of patients; patient turnover; acuity of patients' conditions; patient or family education needs; bereavement care; mixture of the staff; environment; types of delivery; and use of anesthesia. In addition, all newborns, including well newborns, require the care of a registered nurse, and this should be considered when making nursing staff decisions. The Association of Women's Health, Obstetric and Neonatal Nurses has developed guidelines for nurse–patient ratios for various antepartum, intrapartum, and postpartum scenarios (Table 2-1).

TABLE 2-1. Summary of Guidelines for Professional Registered Nursing Staffing for Perinatal Units*†

Nurse-to-Woman or Nurse-to-Baby Ratio	Care Provided
Antepartum	
1 to 2–3	Women during nonstress testing
1 to 1	Woman presenting for initial obstetric triage
1 to 2–3	Women in obstetric triage after initial assessment and in stable condition
1 to 3	Woman with antepartum complications in stable condition
1 to 1	Woman with antepartum complications who is unstable
1 to 1	Continuous bedside attendance for woman receiving IV magnesium sulfate for the first hour of administration for preterm labor prophylaxis and no more than one additional couplet or woman for a nurse caring for a woman receiving IV magnesium sulfate in a maintenance dose
1 to 2	Woman receiving pharmacologic agents for cervical ripening

(continued)

TABLE 2-1. Summary of Guidelines for Professional Registered Nursing Staffing for Perinatal Units*† *(continued)*

Nurse-to-Woman or Nurse-to-Baby Ratio	Care Provided
Intrapartum	
1 to 1	Woman with medical (such as diabetes, pulmonary or cardiac disease, or morbid obesity) or obstetric (such as preeclampsia, multiple gestation, fetal demise, indeterminate or abnormal fetal heart rate pattern, women having a trial of labor attempting vaginal birth after cesarean birth) complications during labor
1 to 1	Woman receiving oxytocin during labor
1 to 1	Woman laboring with minimal to no pain relief or medical interventions
1 to 1	Woman whose fetus is being monitored via intermittent auscultation
1 to 1	Continuous bedside nursing attendance to woman receiving IV magnesium sulfate for the first hour of administration; one nurse to one woman ratio during labor and until at least 2 hours postpartum and no more than one additional couplet or woman in the patient assignment for a nurse caring for a woman receiving IV magnesium sulfate during postpartum
1 to 1	Continuous bedside nursing attendance during initiation of regional anesthesia until condition is stable (at least for the first 30 minutes after initial dose)
1 to 1	Continuous bedside nursing attendance to a woman during the active pushing phase of second-stage labor
1 to 2	Women in labor without complications
2 to 1	Birth; one nurse responsible for the mother and one nurse whose sole responsibility is the baby
Postpartum and Newborn Care	
1 to 1	Continuous bedside nursing attendance to a woman in the immediate postoperative recovery period (for at least 2 hours)
1 to 3	Mother–baby couplets after the first 2-hour recovery period (with consideration for assignments with mixed acuity rather than all recent postcesarean cases)

(continued)

TABLE 2-1. Summary of Guidelines for Professional Registered Nursing Staffing for Perinatal Units*† *(continued)*

Nurse-to-Woman or Nurse-to-Baby Ratio	Care Provided
Postpartum and Newborn Care **(continued)**	
1 to 2	Women on the immediate postoperative day who are recovering from cesarean birth as part of the nurse-to-patient ratio of one nurse to three mother–baby couplets
1 to 5–6	Women postpartum without complications (no more than two to three women on the immediate postpartum day who are recovering from cesarean birth as part of the nurse-to-patient ratio of one nurse to five to six women without complications)
1 to 3	Women postpartum with complications who are stable
1 to 5–6	Healthy newborns in the nursery requiring only routine care whose mothers cannot or do not desire to keep their baby in the postpartum room
1	At least one nurse physically present at all times in each occupied basic care nursery when babies are physically present in the nursery
1 to 1	Newborn undergoing circumcision or other surgical procedures during the immediate preoperative, intraoperative, and immediate postoperative periods
1 to 3–4	Newborns requiring continuing care
1 to 2–3	Newborns requiring intermediate care
1 to 1–2	Newborns requiring intensive care
1 to 1	Newborns requiring multisystem support
1 to 1 or greater	Unstable newborn requiring complex critical care
1	At least one nurse available at all times with skills to care for newborns who may develop complications or need resuscitation

(continued)

TABLE 2-1. Summary of Guidelines for Professional Registered Nursing Staffing for Perinatal Units*† *(continued)*

Nurse-to-Woman or Nurse-to-Baby Ratio	Care Provided
Minimum Staffing	
2	A minimum of two nurses as minimum staffing even when there are no perinatal patients, in order to be able to safely care for a woman who presents with an obstetric emergency that may require cesarean birth (one nurse circulator; one baby nurse, one or both of whom should have obstetric triage, labor and fetal assessment skills). A scrub nurse or surgical technician should be available in-house or on call such that an emergent birth can be accomplished within 30 minutes of the decision to proceed. Another labor nurse should be called in to be available to care for any other pregnant woman who may present for care while the first two nurses are caring for the woman undergoing cesarean birth and during postanesthesia recovery.

Abbreviation: IV, intravenous.

*See the full text for assumptions and conditions that may affect the stated ratios in each instance.

†It should be recognized that these staffing ratios represent minimal staffing, require further consideration based on acuity and needs of service, and assume that there will be ancillary personnel to support the nurse.

Reprinted with permission from Association of Women's Health, Obstetric and Neonatal Nurses. Guidelines for professional registered nurse staffing for perinatal units. Washington, DC: AWHONN; 2010.

Levels of Perinatal Nursing Care

Basic Perinatal Care and Level I Neonatal Care. Perinatal nursing care in a facility at this level of care should be under the direction of a registered nurse. The registered nurse's responsibilities include directing perinatal nursing services, guiding the development and implementation of perinatal policies and procedures, collaborating with medical staff, and consulting with hospitals that provide higher levels of care in the region or system.

For perinatal care, it is recommended that there be two registered nurses continuously available, in order to care for a woman who presents with an obstetric emergency. Their responsibilities include the organization and supervision of antepartum, intrapartum, and neonatal nursing services. The presence of two or more registered nurses with demonstrated knowledge and clinical competence in the nursing care of women, fetuses, and newborn infants during labor, delivery, and the postpartum and neonatal periods is suggested. The nursing staff should be formally trained and competent in neonatal resuscitation (Neonatal Resuscitation Program®). Ancillary personnel, supervised by a registered nurse, may provide support to the patient and attend to her personal comfort. Nursing leadership should have expertise in perinatal nursing care.

Intrapartum care should take place under the direct supervision of a registered nurse. Responsibilities of the registered nurse include triage (the initial assessment and prioritization for evaluation by the qualified medical provider), admission of patients in labor; continuing assessment and evaluation of patients in labor, including supporting the patient, checking the status of the fetus, recording vital signs, monitoring the fetal heart rate, performing obstetric examinations, and observing uterine contractions; determining the presence or absence of complications; supervising the performance of nurses with less training and experience and of ancillary personnel; and staffing at the time of birth. A licensed practical nurse or nurse assistant, supervised by a registered nurse, may provide support to the patient and attend to her personal comfort.

Postpartum care of the woman should be supervised by a registered nurse in collaboration with the obstetrician–gynecologist, family physician, or certified nurse–midwife/certified midwife. The nurse's responsibilities include initial and ongoing assessment, early initiation and ongoing support for breastfeeding, newborn care education, support for the attachment process, preparation for healthy parenting, preparation for discharge, and follow-up of the woman and her newborn infant based on her and her family's needs. This registered nurse should have training and experience in the recognition of normal and abnormal physical and emotional signs or symptoms exhibited by a woman or newborn infant. Again, a licensed practical nurse or nurse assistant, supervised by a registered nurse, may provide support to the woman and attend to her personal comfort in the postpartum period.

Routine newborn care delivered by the registered nurse is provided in collaboration with a pediatrician or family physician. The nurse monitors the infant's adaptation to extrauterine life, keeping the mother and infant together unless separation is medically necessary.

Specialty Perinatal Care and Level II Neonatal Care. Hospitals at this level of care should have a director of perinatal and neonatal nursing services who has overall responsibility for inpatient activities in the respective obstetric and neonatal areas. This registered nurse should have formal training and experience in perinatal nursing care and should coordinate with respective neonatal care services.

In addition to fulfilling basic perinatal care nursing responsibilities, nursing staff in the labor, delivery, and recovery unit should be able to identify and respond to the obstetric and medical complications of pregnancy, labor, and delivery. A registered nurse with adequate training and experience in routine obstetric care and high-risk obstetric care should be assigned to the labor, delivery, and recovery unit at all times. In the postpartum period, a registered nurse should be responsible for providing support for women and families with newborn infants who require intensive care and for facilitating visitation and communication with the NICU.

Licensed practical nurses and unlicensed personnel who have appropriate training in perinatal care and are supervised by a registered nurse may provide assistance with the delivery of care, provide support to the patient, assist with lactation support, and attend to the woman's personal comfort.

All nurses caring for ill newborn infants must possess demonstrated knowledge in the observation and treatment of newborn infants, including cardiorespiratory monitoring. Furthermore, the registered nursing staff of a level II neonatal unit in a hospital that provides specialty perinatal care takes on a greater responsibility for monitoring the preterm newborn infant or the newborn infant who is having difficulty in adapting to extrauterine life. The neonatal nurse provides the newborn infant with frequent observation and monitoring and should demonstrate competency in monitoring and maintaining the stability of cardiopulmonary, neurologic, metabolic, and thermal functions, either independently or in conjunction with the physician; assist with specialized procedures, such as lumbar puncture, endotracheal intubation, and umbilical vessel catheterization; and perform emergency resuscitation. The nurse should be trained and able to initiate, modify, or stop treatment when appropriate, according to established protocols or orders, even when a physician or advanced practice nurse is not present. In units where newborn infants receive mechanical ventilation, staff with demonstrated competency to intubate the trachea, manage assisted ventilation, and decompress a pneumothorax should be available continually. The nursing staff should be formally trained and competent in neonatal resuscitation (Neonatal Resuscitation Program®). The unit's medical director, in conjunction with other personnel, should define and supervise the delegated medical functions, processes, and procedures performed by various categories of personnel.

Subspecialty and Regional Perinatal Care and Level III and Level IV Neonatal Care. The director of perinatal and neonatal nursing services at a facility providing this level of care should have overall responsibility for inpatient activities in the maternity–neonatal care units. This registered nurse should have experience and training in obstetric nursing, neonatal nursing, or both, as well as in the care of women with complex maternal illnesses and obstetric complications. Preferably, this individual should have at least a master's degree. For regional perinatal health care centers, maternal nursing leadership should have expertise in maternal intensive and critical care.

For antepartum care, a registered nurse should be responsible for the direction and supervision of nursing care. All nurses working with antepartum patients at high risk should have documented continuing education in maternal–fetal nursing. An advanced practice registered nurse with advanced clinical training should be on staff to coordinate education.

For intrapartum care, a registered nurse should be in attendance within the labor and delivery unit at all times. This registered nurse should be skilled in the recognition and nursing management of complications of labor and delivery.

For postpartum care, a registered nurse should be in attendance at all times. This registered nurse should be skilled in the recognition and nursing management of complications in women.

Registered nurses in NICUs should have specialty certification or advanced training and experience in the nursing management of newborn infants at high risk and their families. These nurses should have competence in caring for unstable newborn infants with multiorgan system problems and in specialized care technology. Neonatal nurses in level III and level IV NICUs provide direct care to preterm or term infants who require complex care, including intensive life support, inhaled nitric oxide therapy, high-frequency ventilation, extracorporeal membrane oxygenation, and other advanced specialty care, as well as care for chronically technology-dependent infants, and should have appropriate training and competency.

An advanced practice registered nurse should be available to the staff for consultation, education, and support on nursing care issues. Additional nurses with special training are needed to fulfill regional center responsibilities, such as outreach and transport (see also "Transport Procedure" and "Outreach Education" in Chapter 4).

The obstetric and neonatal areas may be staffed by a mix of professional and technical personnel. Assessment and monitoring activities should remain the responsibility of a registered nurse or an advanced practice registered nurse, even when personnel with a mixture of skills are used. The responsibilities of a physician assistant depend on the practice setting, education, and experience of the physician assistant, and on state laws and regulations.

Support Health Care Providers

All Facilities

Personnel who are capable of determining blood type, crossmatching blood, and performing antibody testing should be available on a 24-hour basis. Facilities should have protocols and capabilities for massive transfusion, emergency release of blood products, and management of multiple component therapy. The hospital's infection control personnel are responsible for surveillance of infections in women and newborn infants as well as for the development of an appropriate environmental control program (see also Chapter 13). A radiologic technician should be available 24 hours per day to perform portable X-rays.

All maternity facilities should implement evidence-based practices that support initiation of breastfeeding (see Box 2-1). Clinicians providing maternal or infant care should be competent in supporting breastfeeding and providing basic breastfeeding education. The World Health Organization Baby Friendly Hospital Initiative recommends maternity staff receive at least 20 hours of training in breastfeeding support and management. International board-certified lactation consultants have completed specific training in the clinical management of complex problems with lactation, including didactic education and supervised clinical care. International board-certified lactation consultants undergo a certification exam every 10 years. Effective inpatient lactation care requires adequate staffing, which varies with patient acuity. In addition to working with maternity patients and NICU infants, inpatient lactation consultants can provide consultation to sustain breastfeeding for children or mothers who are hospitalized on pediatric or adult medical/surgical units.

Box 2-1. Ten Hospital Practices to Encourage and Support Breastfeeding*

1. Have a written breastfeeding policy that is routinely communicated to all health care staff.
2. Train all health care staff in the skills necessary to implement this policy.
3. Inform all pregnant women about the benefits and management of breastfeeding.
4. Help women initiate breastfeeding within 1 hour of birth.
5. Show women how to breastfeed and how to maintain lactation, even if they are separated from their newborns.
6. Give newborns no food or drink other than breast milk, unless medically indicated.
7. Practice rooming in — allow mothers and newborns to remain together 24 hours a day.
8. Encourage breastfeeding on demand.
9. Give no pacifiers or artificial nipples to breastfeeding infants[†].
10. Foster the establishment of breastfeeding support groups and refer mothers to them on discharge from the hospital or birth center and foster the establishment of these services when they are not available.

*The 1994 report of the Healthy Mothers, Healthy Babies National Coalition Expert Work Group recommended that the UNICEF-WHO Baby Friendly Hospital Initiative be adapted for use in the United States as the United States Breastfeeding Health Initiative, using the adapted 10 steps above.

[†]The American Academy of Pediatrics endorsed the UNICEF-WHO Ten Steps to Successful Breastfeeding but does not support a categorical ban on pacifiers because of their role in reducing the risk of sudden infant death syndrome and their analgesic benefit during painful procedures when breastfeeding cannot provide the analgesia.

Data from Baby-Friendly USA. Guidelines and Evaluation Criteria for Facilities Seeking Baby-Friendly Designation. Albany (NY): Baby Friendly USA; 2016. Available at: https://www.babyfriendlyusa.org/get-started/the-guidelines-evaluation-criteria. Retrieved December 7, 2016.

The need for other support personnel depends on the intensity and level of sophistication of the other support services provided. An organized plan of action that includes personnel and equipment should be established for identification and immediate resuscitation of newborn infants in need of intervention (see also Chapter 10 for information on neonatal resuscitation).

High-Level Care Facilities

The following support personnel should be available to the perinatal care service of hospitals providing specialty and subspecialty perinatal care and level III and level IV neonatal care:

- At least one full-time, master's degree-level, medical social worker for every 30 beds who has experience with the socioeconomic and psychosocial problems of both women and fetuses at high risk, ill newborn infants, and their families. Additional medical social workers are required when there is a high volume of medical or psychosocial needs.
- At least one occupational or physical therapist with neonatal expertise
- At least one individual skilled in evaluation and management of neonatal feeding and swallowing disorders (eg, speech–language pathologist)
- At least one registered dietitian or nutritionist who has special training in perinatal nutrition and can plan diets that meet the special needs of both women and newborn infants at high risk as well as expertise in the storage and preparation of human milk for medically fragile infants. One dietitian/nutritionist should be available to serve only the NICU
- Qualified personnel for support services, such as diagnostic laboratory studies, radiologic studies, and ultrasound examinations (available 24 hours per day)
- Respiratory therapists who can supervise the assisted ventilation of newborn infants
- Pharmacy personnel with pediatric expertise who can work to continually review their systems and processes of medication administration to ensure that patient care policies are maintained
- Personnel skilled in pastoral care, available as needed

The hospital's engineering department should include air-conditioning, electrical, and mechanical engineers and biomedical technicians who are responsible for the safety and reliability of the equipment in all perinatal care areas.

Education

In-Service and Continuing Education

The medical and nursing staff of any hospital providing perinatal care at any level should maintain knowledge about and competency in current maternal and neonatal care through joint in-service sessions, which ideally should include simulation drills and debriefs. These sessions should cover the diagnosis and management of perinatal emergencies, as well as the management of routine problems and family-centered care. The staff of each unit should have regular multidisciplinary conferences at which patient care problems are presented and discussed. Ongoing review of policies and procedures, as well as regular emergency drills and simulations, can assist in maintaining readiness for unanticipated emergency events.

The staff of regional centers should be capable of assisting with the in-service programs of other hospitals in their region on a regular basis. Such assistance may include periodic visits to those hospitals as well as periodic review of the quality of patient care provided by those hospitals. Regional center staff should be accessible for consultation at all times. The medical and nursing staff of hospitals that provide care beyond basic and level I should participate in formal courses or conferences. Regularly scheduled conferences may include the following subjects:

- Review of the major perinatal conditions, their medical treatment, and nursing care
- Review of electronic fetal monitoring, including maternal–fetal outcomes, toward a goal of standardizing nomenclature and patient care
- Review of perinatal statistics, the pathology related to all deaths, and significant surgical specimens
- Review of current imaging studies
- Review of perinatal and neonatal complications (severe maternal and neonatal morbidity and mortality) and outcomes (see Chapter 3).
- Structured team debriefs after adverse events
- Review of patient satisfaction data, complaints, and compliments

Perinatal Outreach Education

Design and coordination of a program for perinatal outreach education should be provided by neonatal and obstetric physicians and advanced practice registered nurses. Responsibilities may include assessing educational needs; planning curricula; teaching, implementing, and evaluating the program; collecting and using perinatal data; providing patient follow-up information to referring community personnel; writing reports; and maintaining informative working relationships with community personnel and outreach team members. Ideally, the perinatal outreach team would include a maternal–fetal medicine specialist, a certified nurse–midwife or certified midwife, an obstetric nurse, a neonatologist, and a neonatal nurse. Other professionals (eg, a social worker, respiratory therapist, occupational and physical therapist, lactation consultant, or nutritionist) also may be assigned to the team. Each member is responsible for teaching, consulting with community professionals as needed, and maintaining communication with the program coordinator and other team members.

Each subspecialty care center in a regionalized or integrated system may organize an education program that is tailored to meet the needs of the perinatal health professionals and institutions within the network. The various educational strategies that have been found to be effective include seminars, audiovisual and media programs, self-instruction booklets, and clinical practice rotations. Establishment of a routine time and place for perinatal outreach education meetings can promote standardization and continuity of communication among community professionals and regional center personnel. As mandated by the subspecialty boards and the Accreditation Council for Graduate Medical Education, a facility providing subspecialty care that has a fellowship training program must have an active research program.

Quality Improvement

Support for outcomes measurement, including data collection and membership in a multi-institutional collaborative quality improvement database, should be incorporated in the NICU and maternity care budget. Support also should be available for at least one ongoing, active quality improvement initiative (see also Chapter 3).

Physical Facilities

The physical facilities for perinatal care should be conducive to meeting the unique physiologic and psychosocial needs of newborn infants and their families (see also "Patient-Centered and Family-Centered Health Care" in Chapter 1). Special facilities should be available when clinical conditions require continuous physiologic, biochemical, and clinical observation of patients throughout the perinatal period. Labor, delivery, and newborn care facilities should be located in proximity to each other. When these facilities are distant from each other, provisions should be made for appropriate transitional areas.

The following recommendations are intended as general guidelines and should be interpreted with consideration given to local needs. Individual limitations of physical facilities for perinatal care may impede strict adherence to these recommendations. Furthermore, every facility will not have each of the functional units described. Provisions for individual units should be consistent with a regionalized perinatal care system and state and local public health regulations.

Obstetric Functional Units

The patient's personal needs, as well as those of her newborn infant and family, should be considered when obstetric service units are planned. The service should be located in an area that is physically designed to prohibit unrelated traffic through the service unit. The obstetric facility should incorporate the following components of maternity and newborn care:

- Antepartum care for patient stabilization or hospitalization before labor
- Fetal diagnostic testing
- Observation and evaluation for patients who are not yet in active labor or who must be observed to determine whether labor has actually begun; hospital obstetric services should develop a casual, comfortable area ("early labor lounge") for patients in prodromal labor
- Labor
- Birth
- Infant resuscitation and stabilization
- Postpartum maternal and newborn care

Where rooms are suitably sized, located, and equipped, some or all of the components of maternity care listed previously can be combined in one or more rooms. Combining functions into labor, delivery, and recovery rooms can maximize economy and flexibility of staff and space (*Guidelines for Design and Construction of Health Care Facilities* has more detailed information on facility design).

The following facilities should be available to the antepartum unit and the postpartum unit and may be shared, if appropriate:

- Unit director and head nurse's office
- Nurses' station
- Medical records area with a flat writing surface and computers with access to electronic medical records
- Conference room
- Patient education area
- Staff lounge, locker rooms, and on call sleeping rooms
- Examination and treatment room(s)
- Secure area for storage of medications
- Instrument cleanup area
- Soiled workroom and holding room
- Area and equipment for bedpan cleansing
- Kitchen and pantry
- Clean workroom or clean supply room
- Equipment and supply storage area
- Sibling and family visiting area

The need for care of extremely obese patients is growing for all medical and surgical units in the United States, including maternity units. These patients require more space for antenatal, intrapartum, and postpartum care; staff; and equipment able to support heavier weights. (For more information, see "Obesity" in Chapter 9.)

The labor and delivery area should be used for nonobstetric patients only during periods of low occupancy. The obstetric department, in conjunction with the hospital administration, should establish written policies consistent with state and local regulations indicating which nonobstetric patients may be admitted to the labor and delivery suite. Under all circumstances, however, labor and delivery patients must take precedence over nonobstetric patients in this area. Clean gynecologic operations may be performed in the delivery rooms if patients are adequately screened to eliminate infectious cases and if enough personnel are present to prevent any compromise in the quality of obstetric care.

Combined Units

Each labor, delivery, and recovery room is a single-patient room containing a toilet and shower with optional bathtub. A sink should be located in each room for scrubbing and handwashing. A window with an outside view is desirable in the labor, delivery, and recovery room. Each room should contain a birthing bed that is comfortable during labor and can be readily converted to a delivery bed and transported to the cesarean delivery room when necessary. A bassinet for the newborn infant should be readily available. A designated area within the room, containing a radiant warmer, distinct from the laboring woman's area, should be provided for neonatal stabilization and resuscitation (see also "Neonatal Functional Units" later in this chapter). Separate oxygen, air, and suction facilities for the woman and her newborn infant should be provided in two separate locations. Gas outlets and wall-mounted equipment should be easily accessible but may be covered with a panel. Either a ceiling mount or a portable delivery light may be used, depending on the preference of the obstetric staff.

Proper care of the woman in labor requires sufficient space for a sphygmomanometer, stethoscope, fetal monitor, infusion pump, regional anesthesia administration, and resuscitation equipment at the head of the bed. Proper care of the newborn infant requires access to the newborn infant from three sides and capability for quick transport to the nursery or NICU. The family area should be farthest from the entry to the room, and there should be a comfortable area for the support person, including a recumbent sleeping surface.

Equipment needed for labor, delivery, newborn resuscitation, and newborn care should be stored in the room or in a nearby central storage or supply area immediately available to the labor, delivery, and recovery room. For ease of movement, space below the foot of the bed should be adequate to accommodate staff and equipment brought into the room. Standard major equipment held in this area for delivery should include a fetal monitor, delivery case cart, linen hamper, and portable examination lights. A unit equipped for neonatal stabilization and resuscitation (described in "Neonatal Functional Units" later in this chapter) should be available during delivery.

The workable size of a labor, delivery, and recovery room measures 340 net ft^2 (31.57 m^2), including an infant stabilization and resuscitation area of 40 ft^2 (3.7 m^2) of floor space that is distinct from the mother's area. This room should be able to accommodate six to eight people comfortably during the childbirth process.

Labor. Each labor, delivery, and recovery room should have—or have immediate access to—the following equipment and supplies necessary for women in labor:

- Sterilization equipment (if there is no central sterilization equipment)
- X-ray view box or a computer and monitor to review digital images
- Stretchers with side rails
- Equipment for pelvic examinations
- Emergency drugs
- Suction apparatus, either operated from a wall outlet or portable equipment
- Immediate access to a cardiopulmonary resuscitation cart (maternal and neonatal)
- Protective gear for personnel exposed to body fluids
- Warming cabinets for solutions and blankets
- A labor or birthing bed that allows variations in position and a footstool
- A storage area for the patient's clothing and personal belongings
- Sufficient work space for information management systems
- One or more comfortable chairs
- Adjustable lighting that is pleasant for the patient and adequate for examinations
- An adjustable mirror
- An emergency signal and intercommunication system
- Adequate ventilation and temperature control
- Equipment to measure and monitor blood pressure
- Mechanical infusion equipment

- Fetal monitoring equipment
- Oxygen and air outlets
- Adequate electrical outlets
- Access to at least one shower for use by patients in labor
- A writing surface for medical records, computer hookup for medical record purposes, or both
- Storage facilities for supplies and equipment

There should be adequate space for the patient to ambulate in labor, as well as for support persons, personnel, and equipment such as telemetry. Design or renovation should include planning for bedside and workstation information management systems and for computer management of medical information.

It is recommended that birth occur on land, not in water. However, facilities that plan to offer immersion during labor and delivery need to establish rigorous protocols for candidate selection, maintenance and cleaning of tubs and immersion pools, infection control procedures including standard precautions and personal protective equipment for health care personnel, monitoring of mothers and fetuses at appropriate intervals while immersed, and moving women from tubs if urgent maternal or fetal concerns or complications develop (see also Chapter 7).

Patients with significant medical or obstetric complications should be cared for in a labor, delivery, and recovery room that is specially equipped with cardiopulmonary resuscitation equipment and other monitoring equipment necessary for observation and special care. Rooms used for intensive care of patients at high risk in hospitals with no designated high-risk units are best located in the labor and delivery area and should meet the physical standards of other intensive care rooms in the hospital, with a minimum of 200 net ft^2 (18.58 m^2) of floor space and at least three oxygen and three suction outlets. When patients with significant medical or obstetric complications receive care in the labor and delivery area, the capabilities of the unit should be identical to those of an intensive care unit.

Delivery. Delivery can be performed in a properly sized and equipped labor, delivery, and recovery room. A comfortable waiting area for families should be adjacent to the labor, delivery, and recovery room, and restrooms should be nearby.

Traditional delivery rooms and cesarean delivery rooms are similar in design to operating rooms. Vaginal deliveries can be performed in a labor, delivery, and recovery room or cesarean delivery room; cesarean delivery rooms are designed especially for that purpose and therefore are larger. A cesarean delivery room should measure 440 net ft^2 (40.85 m^2). Each room should be well lit and environmentally controlled to prevent chilling of the woman and the newborn infant. The consensus committee on NICU design standards recommends that ambient temperature be kept between 72°F and 78°F (22–26°C) during the delivery, resuscitation, and stabilization of a newborn infant, especially for low-birth-weight preterm infants. Cesarean deliveries should be performed in the obstetric unit or designated operating unit, and postpartum sterilization capabilities should be available in that area when appropriate. At least one support person should be present at the time of delivery as long as the mother is awake.

Each cesarean delivery room should have the following equipment and supplies:

- Operating room table
- Birthing bed that allows variations in position for delivery
- Instrument table and solution basin stand
- Instruments and equipment for vaginal delivery and repair of lacerations
- Solutions and equipment for the intravenous administration of fluids
- Equipment for administration of all types of anesthesia, including equipment for emergency resuscitation of the patient
- Individual oxygen, air, and suction outlets for the mother and newborn infant
- An emergency call system
- Adequate lighting
- Mirrors for patients to observe the birth
- Wall clock with a second hand or digital clock
- Equipment for fetal heart rate monitoring
- Designated area for neonatal resuscitation and stabilization (as defined in "Neonatal Functional Units" later in this chapter)
- Scrub sinks strategically placed to allow observation of the patient

Carts containing drugs and equipment necessary for emergency treatment of the mother and the newborn infant should be kept in the delivery room area. Equipment necessary for cardiopulmonary resuscitation also should be easily accessible.

A workroom should be available for washing instruments. Instruments should be prepared and sterilized in a separate room; alternatively, these services may be performed in a separate area or by a central supply facility. There also should be a room for the storage and preparation of anesthetic equipment; a room or unit for medication storage, preparation, and distribution; a clean workroom and supply room; and an environmental services room for housekeeping supplies and equipment. Scales for weighing the newborn infant and measuring blood loss should be readily available.

Cesarean delivery rooms should additionally have available the following support areas: a control and nurse station, a soiled workroom, and a fluid waste disposal room or area.

Postpartum and Newborn Care. The postpartum unit should permit the comfortable accommodation of patients when the patient census is at its peak and allow the use of beds for alternate functions when the patient census is low. The patient and her newborn infant should be admitted to the room together to facilitate bonding, feeding on demand, and education on infant care. Ideally, rooms are occupied by a single family and equipped for newborn care. Each room in the postpartum unit should have a handwashing sink, a mobile bassinet unit, and supplies necessary for the care of the newborn infant. If possible, each room should have a toilet and shower. When this is not possible and it is necessary for patients to use common facilities, patients should be able to reach them without leaving the postpartum suite. Siblings may visit in the patient's room or in a designated space in the antepartum area or postpartum area.

Larger services may have a specific recovery room for postpartum patients and a separate area for patients at high risk. The equipment needed is similar to that needed in any surgical recovery room and includes equipment for monitoring vital signs, suctioning, administering oxygen, and infusing fluids intravenously, with cardiopulmonary resuscitation equipment immediately available. Equipment for pelvic examinations also should be available. Recovery rooms should be configured so that the newborn infant and mother can stay together, unless medically contraindicated.

Bed Need Analysis

Historically, the calculation of the number of patient rooms needed for all phases of the birth process was based on a simple ratio including the number of births, the average length of stay, and the accepted occupancy level. To best estimate patient room needs, each delivery service should thoroughly analyze functions, philosophies, and projections that will determine the types and quantities of rooms needed. An analysis of the present patterns of care should be reviewed, and consideration should be given to the following types of information:

- Projected birth rates and regional population changes
- Projected cesarean delivery rates
- Occupancy projections that address "peaks and valleys" in the census
- Present (and projected) number of women in the unit during peak periods, as well as the length and frequency of the peak periods
- Numbers and types of high-risk births
- Anticipated length of stay for women during labor, delivery, and recovery
- Anticipated changes in technology

One planning method is to carefully analyze the activities that will occur in each type of room. For example, labor, delivery, and recovery rooms should not be used routinely to accommodate care such as outpatient testing when another room would provide a more appropriate setting. Rooms that allow adequate privacy are recommended for the entire birth process, from labor through discharge.

Planning the number of labor, delivery, and recovery rooms requires that consideration be given to these additional questions:

- Will patients scheduled for cesarean delivery use labor, delivery, and recovery rooms or other rooms for their preoperative, recovery, and postpartum stays?
- Are the labor, delivery, and recovery rooms to be used for other purposes, such as triage or short-term observation for false labor or antepartum admission? If so, the length of stay and volume of all these activities must be considered in the calculation of bed need.

Once the data have been accumulated, the following normative formula can be used to calculate the number of rooms needed by type of room (note that "patient episodes," including all activities [eg, admissions, observations and transitional care] is used, rather than only the number of births):

$$\frac{\text{Number of patient episodes}}{\text{365 days} \times \text{occupancy for the room type}} \times \text{Mean overall length of stay}$$

This formula will provide only a crude estimate of bed needs. For more precise estimates, computerized simulation models are available commercially. However, many of these software packages are expensive and require a significant investment of time for adequate training and use. This software may be purchased by a hospital planning department to develop models for each service as needed. Alternatively, some consulting firms that specialize in maternal–child services can provide an on-site assessment of obstetric capacity and perform a bed need analysis using proprietary simulation software.

Neonatal Functional Units

All neonatal services in a birthing hospital should have facilities available to perform the following functions:

- Resuscitation and stabilization
- Admission and observation
- Normal newborn care (in the mother's room, or in a neonatal observation unit, when the mother is not able to care for her infant)
- Isolation
- Visitation
- Supporting service areas

Level II, level III, and level IV NICUs require facilities for intermediate and intensive care. These may be separate or contiguous. Local circumstances should be considered in the design and management of these care areas.

Resuscitation and Stabilization Area

The resuscitation area should contain the following items:

- Infant warmer or overhead source of radiant heat
- Noncompressible resuscitation and examination mattress that allows access on three sides

- Wall clock with second hand or digital clock
- Flat working surface for medical records
- Table or flat surface for trays and equipment
- Dry, warmed linens
- Stethoscope with neonatal head
- Compressed air and oxygen source
- Oxygen blender with flow meter and tubing
- Pulse oximeter and oximeter probe
- An electrocardiogram monitor may be helpful in accurately determining heart rate
- Resuscitation equipment, including bulb syringe, mechanical suction, tubing, and suction catheters; feeding tubes and large syringes; laryngoscope with blades and extra bulbs and batteries; endotracheal tubes and tape; meconium aspirator; ventilation device (self-inflating bag, flow-inflating bag, or T-piece resuscitator that is capable of delivering 90–100% oxygen and continuous positive airway pressure; a self-inflating bag should be available as a back-up for the latter two devices); laryngeal mask airway; oropharyngeal airways; masks for term newborn infants and preterm infants; carbon dioxide detector; and umbilical vessel catheterization supplies
- Syringes, medications (epinephrine, dextrose solution), fluid for volume expansion, and normal saline for flushes
- Equipment for examination, immediate care, and identification of the newborn infant
- Protective gear to prevent exposure to body fluids
- Special equipment for surgical care (eg, bowel bag for gastroschisis, donut for neural tube defect) or special circumstances (plastic wrap or bag for very preterm infants and transport incubator to maintain temperature during the move to the NICU)
- Task lighting that is capable of providing no less than 2,000 lux at the plane of the infant bed, framed so that no more than 2% of the light output extends beyond the lumination field. Task lighting should be adjustable so that lighting at less than maximal levels can be provided whenever possible.

The resuscitation area usually is within the labor, delivery, and recovery room, although it may be in a contiguous, separate room. If resuscitation takes place in the labor, delivery, and recovery room, the area should be large enough to allow for proper resuscitation of the newborn infant without interference with the care of the mother. Items contaminated with maternal blood, urine, and stool should be kept physically distant from the neonatal resuscitation area. The thermal environment for infant resuscitation should be maintained by use of an infant warmer or overhead source of radiant heat. When delivery of a preterm infant is anticipated, the temperature of the room should be increased (for more information on neonatal resuscitation, see Chapter 10).

Within a labor, delivery, and recovery room, a resuscitation area should be allotted a minimum of 40 net ft^2 (3.7 m^2) of floor space. This space may be used for multiple purposes, including resuscitation, stabilization, observation, examination, or other infant needs. A total of one oxygen, one air, one vacuum, and six simultaneously accessible electrical outlets should be provided. In an operative delivery room, a minimum of 80 net ft^2 (7.5 m^2) of floor space should be provided, with a total of three oxygen, three air, three vacuum, and 12 simultaneously accessible electrical outlets. A separate resuscitation room should have approximately 150 net ft^2 (13.94 m^2) of floor space. These areas should have adequate suction, oxygen, compressed air, and electrical outlets to accommodate simultaneous resuscitation of twins. A separate resuscitation room also should have an electrical outlet that can accommodate a portable X-ray machine. Electrical outlets should conform to regulations for areas in which anesthetic agents are administered.

Admission and Observation (Transitional and Stabilization Care) Area

Healthy newborn infants should be monitored without being separated from their mothers during the first 4–8 hours after birth. If physical separation is medically necessary, admission and observation should occur in an area near or adjacent to the delivery area and cesarean delivery room, if possible. No special or separate isolation facilities are required for infants born at home or in transit to the hospital.

An estimated 40 net ft^2 (3.7 m^2) of floor space is needed for each newborn infant in the admission and observation area. The capacity required depends on the size of the delivery service and the duration of close observation. The number of observation stations required depends on the birth rate and the length of stay in the observation area. There should be a minimum of two observation stations. The admission and observation area should be well lit and should contain a wall clock and emergency resuscitation equipment similar to that in the designated resuscitation area. Outlets also should be similar to those in the resuscitation area.

The health care provider's assessment of the infant's condition determines the subsequent level of care. When the admission and observation area is in a labor, delivery, and recovery room, the newborn infant remains in the room with the mother for skin-to-skin care to facilitate maternal–infant bonding and initiation of breastfeeding. Healthy newborn infants are never separated from their healthy mothers, and they are kept with their mothers in the labor, delivery, and recovery room at all times. In facilities where the mother must be transferred from the delivery room to a postpartum room, her newborn infant also is admitted to the postpartum room. Some newborn infants require transfer to an intermediate or intensive care area.

Neonatal Care Units

Within each perinatal care facility there may be several types of units for newborn care. These units are defined by the content and complexity of care required by a specific group of infants. As in the resuscitation and stabilization area and the admission and observation area, equipment for emergency resuscitation is required in all neonatal care areas. Recommendations regarding the intensity of care are made in the following paragraphs.

Newborn Observation Unit. Care for healthy term newborn infants should be provided in the mother's room unless there are extenuating circumstances. Late preterm infants also should remain with their mothers when physiologically stable in order to ensure prompt feeding in response to infant cues. These newborn infants are not ill but may require frequent feeding and more hours of nursing care than healthy term newborn infants, and units should use evidence-based guidelines to address the monitoring and care of this population. A separate newborn observation unit should be available for infants who require closer observation or whose mothers cannot care for them. Level I units in hospitals without higher-level units also need to have equipment and personnel to stabilize newborn infants who are ill or are born at less than 35 weeks of gestation until they can be transferred to a higher-level facility.

Because relatively few staff members are needed to provide care in the neonatal observation unit and bulky equipment is not needed, 24 net ft^2 (2.23 m^2) of floor space for each infant should be adequate. Bassinets should be at least 3 ft (approximately 1 m) apart in all directions, measured from the edge of one bassinet to the edge of the neighboring bassinet. In this setting, one neonatal registered nurse is recommended for every 6–8 newborn infants requiring routine care, and a registered nurse should be available in each newborn-occupied area at all times (see also "Nurse–Patient Ratios" earlier in this chapter). During decreased patient occupancy, central neonatal observation units use nursing staff inefficiently. Direct care of those newborn infants remaining in the unit may be provided by licensed practical nurses and unlicensed nursing personnel under the registered nurse's direct supervision.

The neonatal observation unit should be well lit, have a large wall clock and a sink for handwashing, and be equipped for emergency resuscitation. One pair of wall-mounted electrical outlets is recommended for every two neonatal stations. One oxygen outlet, one compressed-air outlet, and one suction outlet are recommended for every four neonatal stations. Cabinets and counters should be available within the newborn care area for storage of routinely used supplies, such as diapers, formula, and linens. If circumcisions are performed in the unit, an appropriate table with adequate lighting is required. Electrical outlets to power portable X-ray machines are highly recommended.

Special Care Unit. Sick newborn infants who do not require intensive care but who require a higher level of surveillance should be cared for in a special care unit. A special care unit also may be used for convalescing newborn infants who have returned to specialty facilities from an intensive care unit in an outside facility or have been transferred from a higher level of care within the institution. The special care area may be separate from, adjacent to, or combined with a level III or level IV NICU in hospitals where these exist. Back transport is encouraged where appropriate in terms of care for the sick infant in order to facilitate bonding and the maintenance of the maternal–infant dyad.

The neonatal special care area optimally is close to the delivery area, cesarean delivery room, and the intensive care area (if there is one) and away from general hospital traffic. It should have radiant heaters or incubators for maintaining body temperature, as well as infusion pumps, cardiopulmonary monitors, oximeters, and equipment to provide phototherapy.

In facilities with level II and level III units, infants who need assisted ventilation should be cared for in the level III unit. In facilities where the level II NICU is the highest level of neonatal care, equipment should be available to provide continuous positive airway pressure and, in some units, equipment may be available to provide short-term assisted ventilation. In that case, newborns requiring complex care or assisted ventilation for greater than 24 hours should be transferred to a facility with a level III or level IV NICU.

Single-family rooms should have a minimum of 165 ft^2 (15.3 m^2) of clear floor area for single infants, and at least 240 net ft^2 (22.4 m^2) of floor space for twins. Provisions for family members should include a reclining chair suitable for skin-to-skin care, a recumbent sleep surface for at least one parent, a desk or writing surface for a laptop computer, at least four electrical outlets for use and charging of electronic devices, and at least 6 ft^3 (0.2m^3) of storage space.

In multipatient rooms, each infant space requires at least 120 ft^2 (11.2 m^2) of floor space, and there should be at least 8 ft (2.4 m) between each incubator, warmer, bassinet, or crib. At each infant space, there should be a chair that allows the parent to be seated, reclining or fully recumbent, with privacy curtains or other separations to allow extended, intimate parental contact with the infant. Aisles should be at least 4 ft (1.2 m) wide to accommodate passage of personnel and equipment. Space needed for other purposes (eg, desks, counters, cabinets, corridors, and treatment rooms) should be added to the space needed for patients. In multipatient rooms, each room should accommodate some multiple of three to four newborn stations because one registered neonatal nurse is required for every three to four infants who require intermediate care.

Each infant bed should have a minimum of 20 simultaneously accessible electrical outlets, three oxygen outlets, three compressed-air outlets, and three suction outlets. In addition, the area should have a special outlet to power the neonatal unit's portable X-ray machine. All electrical outlets for each patient station should be connected to regular and auxiliary power. An oxygen tank for emergency use should be stored but readily available for each infant receiving wall-supplied oxygen. All equipment and supplies for resuscitation should be immediately available within the intermediate care unit. These items may be conveniently placed on an emergency cart.

Large, open rooms allow greater flexibility in the use of equipment, enhanced communication between staff and families, and more efficient assignment of personnel, but offer less privacy for family involvement. Single family rooms may enhance breastfeeding, facilitate family visitation, and potentially improve neurodevelopmental outcomes, if the family is able to be present on a regular basis and the proper supports, including nursing care workflows, are in place. However, there is not sufficient evidence to recommend single-family units as a standard at this time.

Additional Provisions for Neonatal Intensive Care Units. Constant nursing and continuous cardiopulmonary and other support for severely ill infants should be provided in the intensive care unit. Because emergency care is provided in this area, laboratory and radiologic services should be readily available 24 hours per day. The results of blood gas analyses should be available shortly after sample collection. In many centers, a laboratory adjacent to the intensive care unit provides this service.

The neonatal intensive care area should ideally be located near the delivery area and cesarean delivery room(s) and should be easily accessible from the hospital's ambulance entrance. It should be located away from routine hospital traffic. Intensive care may be provided in individual patient rooms, in a single area, or in two or more separate rooms.

The number of nursing, medical, and surgical personnel required in the neonatal intensive care area is greater than that required in less acute perinatal care areas. The nurse-to-patient ratio should be 1:2 or 1:1, depending on acuity. In some cases, such as during extracorporeal life support, additional nursing personnel are required. The amount and complexity of equipment required also are considerably greater. In addition, the educational responsibilities of a neonatal intensive care facility require that the design include space for instructional activities and, for those facilities also serving as regional centers, office space for files on the region's perinatal experience.

Equipment and supplies in the intensive care area should include all those needed in the resuscitation and intermediate care areas. Immediate availability of emergency oxygen is essential. In addition, equipment for long-term ventilatory support should be provided. Ventilators should be equipped with nebulizers or humidifiers with heaters. Equipment for manual-assisted ventilation, including appropriately sized face masks and T-piece resuscitators, flow-inflating or self-inflating bags should be available at each bed space. Continuous, online monitoring of oxygen concentrations, body temperature, heart rate, respiration, oxygen saturation, and blood pressure measurements should be available for each patient. If wireless transmission is not available, provisions can be made at each bedside to allow data transmission from cardiorespiratory monitors to a remote location. Supplies should be kept close to the patient bed space so that nurses are not away from the infant unnecessarily and may use their time and skills efficiently. A central modular supply system can enhance efficiency.

In some cases, surgical procedures (eg, ligation of a patent ductus arteriosus) are performed in an area in or adjacent to the NICU. Specific policies should address preparatory cleaning, physical preparation of the unit, presence of other newborn infants and staff, venting of volatile anesthetics, and quality assessment. Ideally, procedures, equipment, facilities, and supplies for this area should be comparable to those required for similar procedures in the surgical department of the hospital.

Supporting Service Areas

Milk and Formula Preparation Areas. Unless performed elsewhere in the hospital (eg, in a milk bank), a specialized area or room to prepare feedings should be provided in the NICU, away from the bedside, to accommodate mixing of additives to human milk or formula. This area should be equipped with a hands-free handwashing station, counter workspace, and storage areas for supplies, formula, and refrigerated and frozen human milk. Bar coding of maternal milk may reduce errors in providing expressed milk to infants.

Utility Rooms. Both clean and soiled utility rooms are needed in neonatal care areas. Separate storage areas should be available for foodstuffs, medications, and clean supplies. Clean utility rooms should not have direct lighting because some of the formulas, medications, and supplies may be light sensitive. The maintenance of soiled utility rooms should conform to the guidelines and state regulations of the Facility Guidelines Institute.

Storage Areas. A three-zone storage system is desirable. The first storage area should be the central supply department of the hospital. The second storage area should be adjacent to the patient care areas or within the patient care areas. In this area, routinely used supplies and clean utilities, such as diapers, formula, linen, cover gowns, medical records, and information booklets, may be stored. Generally, space is required in this area only for the amount of each item used between deliveries from the hospital's central supply department (eg, daily or three times weekly). The third area is needed for the storage of items frequently used at the infant's bedside. There should be a bedside cabinet storage area for each bed–patient unit in the mother–baby unit or neonatal observation unit, intermediate care area, and intensive care area. The neonatal observation unit requires secondary storage of items such as linen and formula. In the resuscitation and stabilization area, the admission and observation area, the intermediate care area, and the intensive care areas, there should be space for secondary storage of syringes, needles, intravenous infusion sets, and sterile trays needed in procedures, such as umbilical vessel catheterization, lumbar puncture, and thoracostomy.

Large equipment items (eg, bassinets, incubators, warmers, radiant heaters, phototherapy units, breast pumps, and infusion pumps) should be stored in a clean, enclosed storage area in close proximity to, but not within, the immediate patient care area. Easily accessible electrical outlets are desirable in this area for recharging equipment.

Treatment Rooms. Many facilities have developed areas for resuscitation and stabilization, admission and observation, intermediate care, and intensive care in which each patient station constitutes a treatment area. This largely has eliminated the need for a separate treatment room for procedures, such as lumbar punctures, intravenous infusions, venipuncture, and minor surgical procedures. A separate treatment area may be necessary, however, if infants in the newborn nursery or postpartum mother–baby unit are to undergo certain procedures (eg, circumcision). The facilities, outlets, equipment, and supplies in the treatment area should be similar to those of the resuscitation area. The amount of space required depends on the procedures performed.

Scrub Areas

At the entrance to each neonatal care area, there should be a scrub area that can accommodate all personnel and families entering the area. It should have a sink that is large enough to prevent splashing, with faucets operated by hands-free controls. A backsplash should be provided to prevent standing or retained water. Waterless antiseptics often are available at these sinks. Sinks for handwashing should not be built into counters used for other purposes. Soap and towel dispensers and appropriate trash receptacles should be available. The scrub areas also should contain racks, hooks, or lockers for storing clothing and personal items, as well as cabinets for clean gowns, a receptacle for used gowns, and a large wall clock with a sweep second hand, or digital clock, to time handwashing.

Scrub sinks should have hands-free faucets and should be large enough to control splashing and to prevent retained water. These hands-free sinks should be provided at a minimum ratio of one for at least every eight patient stations in the newborn nursery. In the intermediate care or intensive care areas, every bed should be within 20 ft (6.10 m) of a hands-free washing station. In addition, one scrub sink is needed in the resuscitation and stabilization area, and one is needed for every three to four patient stations in the admission and observation area. Alcohol-based hand hygiene solutions should be available at all entry points and at each bed space.

Nursing Areas

Space should be provided at the bedside not only for patient care but also for instructional and medical record activities. For electronic documentation, computer terminals should be readily accessible, and policies should be in place to ensure cleaning of keyboards. If manual documentation is performed, a flat writing surface (eg, a clipboard or loose-leaf notebook) is needed.

A nurses' area or desk for tasks, such as compiling more detailed records, completing requisitions, and handling specimens is useful. Primary care providers also may perform medical record and clerical activities in this area. However, in level III or level IV and many level II care units, documentation needs to take place at or near the bedside. Maintaining medical records should be considered an unclean procedure, and personnel who have been working on medical records should perform hand hygiene before they have further contact with an infant.

The unit director or nurse manager should have an office close to the newborn care areas. Nurses' dressing rooms preferably should be adjacent to a lounge and should contain lockers, storage for clean and soiled scrub attire (in hospitals that provide and launder staff scrubs), a dressing area, toilets, and showers.

Family Areas

Space should be available for families of infants hospitalized in the NICU, preferably including a family lounge, rest room facilities, space for a play area with educational materials and toys for children, and a nourishment area. Family education resources should be available.

Consultation room. A private room with comfortable seating should be available for family meetings with the infant's care team.

Lactation support. Private space for lactation consultation and milk expression should be available that includes a hand-washing sink, a hospital-grade breast pump, and comfortable seating. Certified lactation consultants should be available to assist mothers of NICU infants with establishing and maintaining lactation.

Education Areas

A conference room suitable for educational purposes is highly desirable, particularly for facilities with level II, level III, and level IV units. It may be in or adjacent to the maternal–newborn areas.

Clerical Areas

The control point for patient care activities is the clerical area. It should be located near the entrance to the neonatal care areas so that personnel can supervise traffic and limit unnecessary entry into these areas. It should have telephones and communication devices that connect to the various neonatal care areas and the delivery suite. In addition, patients' medical records, computer terminals, and hospital forms may be located in the clerical area.

General Considerations

Safety and Environmental Control

Because of the complexities of environmental control and monitoring, a hospital environmental engineer must ensure that all electrical, lighting, air composition, and temperature systems function properly and safely. A regular maintenance program should be specified to ensure that systems continue to function as designed after initial occupancy.

The environmental temperature in newborn care areas should be independently adjustable, and control should be sufficient to prevent hot and cold spots, particularly when heat-generating equipment (eg, a radiant warmer) is in use. The air temperature should be kept at 22–26°C (72–78°F). Humidity should be kept between 30% and 60% and should be controlled through the hospital heating and air-conditioning system. Condensation on wall and window surfaces should be avoided.

A minimum of six air changes per hour is recommended, and a minimum of two changes should be outside air. The ventilation pattern should inhibit particulate matter from moving freely in the space, and intake and exhaust vents should be placed so as to minimize drafts on or near the patient beds. Ventilation air delivered to the NICU should be filtered at 90% efficiency, or as specified in the most current edition of the Facilities Guidelines Institute's *Guidelines for Design and Construction of Health Care Facilities*. Filters should be located outside the infant care area so that they can be changed easily and safely. Fresh-air intake should be located at least 25 ft (7.6 m) from exhaust outlets of ventilating systems, combustion equipment stacks, medical or surgical vacuum systems, plumbing vents, or areas that may collect vehicular exhausts or other noxious fumes.

Radiation exposure to infants, families, and staff is another safety concern (see also "Radiation Risk" in Chapter 11). Radiation exposure to personnel is negligible at a distance of more than 1 ft (0.30 m) lateral to the primary vertical roentgen beam. Care should be taken to ensure that only the patient and the area of interest being examined is in the primary beam, and staff needed to assist in patient positioning should wear appropriate shielding. It is unnecessary for families or personnel to leave the area during the roentgen exposure.

Illumination

Ambient lighting levels in all infant care areas should be adjustable. Both natural and artificial light sources should have controls that allow immediate darkening of any bed position sufficient for transillumination or ultrasonography when necessary. Artificial light sources should have a color rendering index of no less than 80, and a full-spectrum color index of no less than 55. Artificial light sources should have a visible spectral distribution similar to that of daylight but should avoid unnecessary ultraviolet or infrared radiation by the use of appropriate lamps, lenses, or filters. Newly constructed or renovated NICUs should be able to provide ambient lighting at levels recommended by the Illuminating Engineering Society. Separate procedure lighting should be available at each patient care station. Procedure lighting should minimize shadows and glare, and it should be controlled with a rheostat so that it can be provided at less than maximal levels whenever possible. Light should be highly framed so that newborns at adjacent bed stations will not experience any increase in illumination.

Illumination of support areas within the NICU, including medical records areas, medication preparation areas, reception desks, and handwashing areas, should conform to the specifications of the Illuminating Engineering

Society. Illumination should be adequate in the areas of the NICU where staff perform important or critical tasks. In locations where these functions overlap with patient care areas (eg, proximity of the nurse documentation area to patient beds), the design should permit separate light sources with independent controls so that the very different needs of sleeping newborns and working nurses can be accommodated to the greatest possible extent.

Windows

Windows may provide an important psychological benefit to staff and families in the NICU and for women with a prolonged hospital admission. Properly designed natural light is the most desirable illumination for nearly all nursing tasks, including updating medical records and evaluating newborn skin tone. However, placing infants too close to external windows can cause serious problems with temperature control and glare, so providing windows in the NICU requires careful planning and design.

At least one source of natural light should be visible from each patient care area. External windows in patient care rooms should be glazed with insulating glass to minimize heat gain and loss. They should be situated at least 2 ft (0.60 m) away from any part of a patient bed to minimize radiant heat loss from the infant. All external windows should be equipped with shading devices that are easily controlled to allow flexibility at various times of day. These shading devices should be contained within the window or easily cleanable. Windows in neonatal care areas should have opaque shades that make it possible to darken the area to reduce inappropriate radiant heat gain or loss, or for procedures that require reduced light, such as transillumination or ultrasonography examination.

Wall Surfaces

Wall surfaces should be easily cleanable, provide protection at point of contact with moveable equipment, and be free of substances known to be teratogenic, mutagenic, carcinogenic, or otherwise harmful to human health.

Oxygen and Compressed-Air Outlets

Newborn care areas should have oxygen and compressed air piped from a central source at a pressure of 50–60 psi, with an alarm system that warns of any critical reduction in line pressure. Reduction valves and mixers should produce adjustable concentrations of 21–100% oxygen at atmospheric pressure for head hoods and 50–60 psi for mechanical ventilators.

Acoustic Characteristics

Infant rooms (including airborne infection isolation rooms), staff work areas, family areas, staff lounge, sleeping areas, and spaces opening into them should be designed to produce minimal background noise and to contain and absorb much of the transient noise that arises within them. The ventilation system, monitors, incubators, suction pumps, mechanical ventilators, and staff produce considerable noise, and the noise level should be monitored intermittently. Mechanical systems and equipment in infant rooms and adult sleep rooms should conform to Noise Criteria 25. The construction and redesign of neonatal care areas and adult sleep areas should include acoustic absorption units or other means to ensure that the combination of continuous background sound and transient sound in any bed space or patient care area does not exceed an hourly 'equivalent continuous sound level' (L_{eq}) of 45 dB and an hourly L_{10} of 50 dB (ie, no more than 10% of the time at greater than 50 dB), both A-weighted slow response.

Transient sounds or L_{max}, should not exceed 65 dB, A-weighted slow response. Staff members should take particular care to avoid noise pollution in enclosed patient spaces (eg, incubators). Care should be taken to avoid spaces shaped so as to focus or amplify sound levels, thus creating "hot spots" that exceed the maximum recommended noise levels. In staff work areas, staff lounge areas, and family areas, the combination of continuous background and operational sound should not exceed an hourly L_{eq} of 50 dB and an hourly L_{10} of 55 dB, both A-weighted slow response. The transient sounds should not exceed 70 dB, A-weighted slow response in these areas.

Electrical Outlets and Electrical Equipment

All electrical outlets should be attached to a common ground. All electrical equipment should be checked for current leakage and grounding adequacy when first introduced into the neonatal care area, after any repair, and periodically while in service. Current leakage allowances, preventive maintenance standards, and equipment quality should meet the standards developed by the Joint Commission. There should be both emergency and normal power for all electrical outlets per National Fire Protection Association recommendations. Personnel should be thoroughly and repeatedly instructed on the potential electrical hazards within the neonatal care areas.

General Disaster Preparedness and Evacuation Plan

An overall disaster preparedness plan is essential for all areas of the hospital and all personnel. A plan addressing natural and terrorist disasters should be in place for each perinatal care area. This should include an evacuation plan; a relocation plan; triage principles; immediate measures for utilities and water supply; emergency supply of medical gases, essential medications, and equipment; and the role of each staff member in the plan. A floor plan that indicates designated evacuation routes should be posted in a conspicuous place in each unit. The policy and floor plan should be reviewed with the staff at least annually.

Disasters disproportionally affect vulnerable, technology-dependent people, including preterm and critically ill newborn infants. It is important for health care providers to be aware of and prepared for the potential consequences of disasters for the NICU. Neonatal intensive care personnel can provide specialized expertise for their hospital, community, and regional emergency preparedness plans and can help develop institutional surge capacity for mass critical care, including equipment, medications, personnel, and facility resources.

Specific Considerations for Overflow and Disaster Planning

- Appoint an obstetrician to direct disaster planning for maternity services
  - Pediatrician involvement (or co-director) recommended
  - Maternity and pediatric nursing also recommended
- Consider regional patterns of obstetric care provision and disaster scenarios
- Consider obstetric and neonatal needs with high obstetric patient surge
- Establish policies for visitation and lactation that balance infection control concerns with patient/familial desires for involvement in the birthing process
- Foster functional working relationships with local and regional critical care clinicians
- Have a working algorithm for ethical resource allocation when demand outstrips supply that considers obstetric and pediatric specifics

- Develop a surge capacity plan with the realization that control of patient volume is challenging during pregnancy
- Consider the option of temporary alterations to usual standards of obstetric care and mechanisms to optimize obstetric services with less resource usage. Examples include, but are not limited to:
  - Early discharge after delivery
  - Enhanced telephone triage with attention to documentation requirements
  - Rapid credentialing of health care providers to enable delivery of obstetric care when there are work force limitations

Bibliography

American Academy of Pediatrics, American Heart Association. Textbook of neonatal resuscitation. 7th ed. Elk Grove Village (IL): AAP; Dallas (TX): AHA; 2016.

American College of Obstetricians and Gynecologists, American College of Nurse-Midwives. Joint statement of practice relations between obstetricians-gynecologists and certified nurse-midwives/certified midwives. College Statement of Policy. Washington, DC: American College of Obstetricians and Gynecologists; 2011. Available at: https://www.acog.org/-/media/Statements-of-Policy/Public/sop1102.pdf?dmc = 1&ts = 20160923T1632030516. Retrieved September 23, 2016.

Association of Women's Health, Obstetric and Neonatal Nurses. Guidelines for professional registered nurse staffing for perinatal units. Washington, DC: AWHONN; 2010.

Association of Women's Health, Obstetric and Neonatal Nurses, National Association of Clinical Nurse Specialists. Women's health clinic nurse specialist competencies. Washington, DC; Philadelphia (PA): AWHONN; NACNS; 2014. Available at: http://www.nacns.org/professional-resources/practice-and-cns-role/cns-competencies. Retrieved September 23, 2016.

Association of Women's Health, Obstetric and Neonatal Nurses, National Association of Nurse Practitioners in Women's Health. Women's health nurse practitioner: guidelines for practice and education. Washington, DC: AWHONN; NPWH; 2014.

Barfield WD, Krug SE, Committee on Fetus and Newborn, Disaster Preparedness Advisory Council. Disaster Preparedness in Neonatal Intensive Care Units. Pediatrics 2017:139:e1–11.

Beauman SS, Ikuta LM, editors. Policies, procedures, and competencies for neonatal nursing care. Chicago (IL): National Association of Neonatal Nurses; 2011.

Dilaura DL, Houser KW, Mistrick RG, Steffy GR, editors. The lighting handbook: Reference and application. 10th ed. New York (NY): Illuminating Engineering Society; 2011.

Facility Guidelines Institute. Guidelines for design and construction of health care facilities. Chicago (IL): American Society for Healthcare Engineering of the American Hospital Association; 2014.

Guiding principles for pediatric hospital medicine programs. Section on Hospital Medicine. Pediatrics 2013;132:782–6.

Hospital disaster preparedness for obstetricians and facilities providing maternity care. Committee Opinion No. 555. American College of Obstetricians and Gynecologists. Obstet Gynecol 2013;121:696–9.

Illuminating Engineering Society of North America. Lighting for hospitals and health care facilities. ANSI/IESNA RP-29-06. New York (NY): IESNA; 2006.

Lathrop JK, Bielen RP, editors. Health care facilities code: NFPA 99. 2015th ed. Quincy (MA): National Fire Prevention Association; 2015.

Levels of neonatal care. American Academy of Pediatrics Committee on Fetus and Newborn. Pediatrics 2012;130:587–97.

Levels of maternal care. Obstetric Care Consensus No. 2. American College of Obstetricians and Gynecologists. Obstet Gynecol 2015;125:502–15.

National Association of Neonatal Nurses. Advanced practice registered nurse: role, preparation, and scope of practice. Position Statement #3059. Chicago (IL): NANN; 2014. Available at: http://nann.org/uploads/Membership/NANNP_Pubs/APRN_Role_Preparation_position_statement_FINAL.pdf. Retrieved September 28, 2016.

National Association of Neonatal Nurses. Education standards and curriculum guidelines for neonatal nurse practitioner programs. Chicago (IL): NANN; 2014. Available at: http://nann.org/uploads/About/PositionPDFS/1.4.8_Education%20Standards%20and%20Curriculum%20Guidelines%20for%20Neonatal%20Nurse%20Practitioner%20Programs.pdf. Retrieved September 28, 2016.

National Association of Neonatal Nurses. RN staffing in the neonatal intensive care unit. Position Statement #3061. Chicago (IL): NANN; 2014. Available at: http://nann.org/uploads/About/PositionPDFS/1.4.6_RN%20Staffing%20in%20the%20NICU.pdf. Retrieved September 28, 2016.

National Association of Neonatal Nurses. Standard for maintaining the competence of neonatal nurse practitioners. Position Statement #3062. Chicago (IL): NANN; 2015. Available at: http://nann.org/uploads/About/PositionPDFS/1.4.4_Standard%20for%20Maintaining%20the%20Competence%20of%20NNPs.pdf. Retrieved September 28, 2016.

Nurse Practitioners in Women's Health: Clinical Guidelines. Washington, DC: NPWH; 2015. Available at: https://www.npwh.org/pages/clinicalguidelines. Retrieved December 7, 2016.

Optimizing postpartum care. Committee Opinion No. 666. American College of Obstetricians and Gynecologists. Obstet Gynecol 2016;127:e187–92.

Optimizing support for breastfeeding as part of obstetric practice. Committee Opinion No. 658. American College of Obstetricians and Gynecologists. Obstet Gynecol 2016;127:e86–92.

Ortenstrand A. The role of single-patient neonatal intensive care unit rooms for preterm infants. Acta Paediatr 2014;103:462–3.

Phillips RM, Goldstein M, Hougland K, Nandyal R, Pizzica A, Santa-Donato A, et al. Multidisciplinary guidelines for the care of late preterm infants. National Perinatal Association. J Perinatol 2013;33(suppl):S5–22.

Rea M, Deng L, Wolsey R. Light Sources and Color. NLPIP Lighting Answers 2004;8(1):1–38. Available at: http://www.lrc.rpi.edu/programs/NLPIP/index.asp. Retrieved September 28, 2016.

Reynolds EW, Bricker JT. Nonphysician clinicians in the neonatal intensive care unit: meeting the needs of our smallest patients. Pediatrics 2007;119:361–9.

Robbins ST, Meyers R, editors. Infant feedings: guidelines for preparation of formula and breastmilk in health care facilities. Pediatric Nutrition Practice Group. 2nd ed. Chicago (IL): American Dietetic Association; 2011.

Shahheidari M, Homer C. Impact of the design of neonatal intensive care units on neonates, staff, and families: a systematic literature review. J Perinat Neonatal Nurs 2012;26:260–6; quiz 267–8.

Steele C, Bixby C. Centralized breastmilk handling and bar code scanning improve safety and reduce breastmilk administration errors. Breastfeed Med 2014;9:426–9.

United States Lactation Consultant Association. International Board Certified Lactation Consultant staffing recommendations for the inpatient setting. Washington, DC: USLCA; 2010. Available at: http://uslca.org/wp-content/uploads/2013/02/IBCLC_Staffing_Recommendations_July_2010.pdf. Retrieved September 28, 2016.

Wallman C. Advanced practice in neonatal nursing. Committee on Fetus and Newborn. Pediatrics 2009;123:1606–7.

Weinstein L. The laborist: a new focus of practice for the obstetrician. Am J Obstet Gynecol 2003;188:310–2.

White RD, Smith JA, Shepley MM. Recommended standards for newborn ICU design, eighth edition. Committee to Establish Recommended Standards for Newborn ICU Design. J Perinatol 2013;33(suppl):S2–16.

Women's Health Nurse Practitioner: Guidelines for Practice and Education - 7th Edition. Association of Women's Health, Obstetric, and Neonatal Nurses. 2014.

Chapter 3

Quality Improvement and Patient Safety

The Health and Medicine Division of the National Academies of Sciences, Engineering, and Medicine (previously known as the Institute of Medicine) and other organizations have stressed the urgency of "transforming hospitals into places where each patient receives the best quality care, every single time." In studies of progress in quality improvement (QI) and patient safety, a recurring theme emerges: hospitals need to change systems to increase reliability. The success of obstetric and neonatal services depends on an awareness of the high-risk nature of the organization's activities, a commitment to resilience after failure, sensitivity to issues facing health care providers immediately involved with care and, finally, development of a culture of safety and continuous quality improvement. The key features of a culture of safety, according to the Agency for Healthcare Research and Quality (AHRQ), include:

- acknowledgment of the high-risk nature of an organization's activities and the determination to achieve consistently safe operations;
- a blame-free environment where individuals are able to report errors or near misses without fear of reprimand or punishment; and
- encouragement of collaboration and commitment of resources to address safety concerns.

In its 2001 report, *Crossing the Quality Chasm*, the Institute of Medicine (now the Health and Medicine Division of the National Academies of Science, Engineering, and Medicine) set forth a list of performance characteristics that, if addressed and improved, would lead to better health and function for the people of the United States (see "Bibliography"). In 2016, the American College of Obstetricians and Gynecologists (ACOG) released a report further elaborating that building collaboration through a team-based model of care was essential in order to manage large amounts of information and multiple handoffs, promote seamless communication and transitions among health care providers (within a team or among teams), and support wellness and care for patients with complex health conditions. However, the following six specific qualities of good care still are not met routinely and should be the focus of designing a QI program:

1. Safe—avoiding injuries to patients from the care that is intended to help
2. Effective—providing services based on scientific knowledge to all who could benefit and refraining from providing services to those not likely to benefit (avoiding underuse and overuse)
3. Patient centered—providing care that is respectful of and responsive to individual patient preferences, needs, and values, and ensuring that patient values guide all the clinical decisions
4. Timely—reducing waiting times and sometimes harmful delays for those who receive and those who provide care
5. Efficient—avoiding waste, in particular, waste of equipment, supplies, ideas, and energy
6. Equitable—providing care that does not vary in quality because of personal characteristics, such as gender, ethnicity, geographic location, and socioeconomic status

Quality Improvement

Quality improvement is an approach to quality management that builds upon traditional quality assurance methods by emphasizing the organization and its systems. It focuses on processes rather than individuals, recognizes internal and external factors, and promotes the need for objective data to analyze and improve care processes. The QI process assists the health care team at all levels of care and includes ongoing monitoring and evaluation of clinical patient care. The QI process must focus on the total care delivered to the patient by an institution, thus involving outpatient care leading up to hospital admission and the patient's discharge and transition of care to outpatient facilities; care from physicians, midwives, nurses, and support staff; administration; and all components of care that contribute to a patient's hospital experience. However, it does not eliminate individual responsibility and accountability for care. The Just Culture framework recognizes that safety is an organizational value, but that adverse events and human errors are potential outputs. System design and behavioral choices, however, are the inputs.

The Just Culture model identifies three types of behavioral choices that every person makes and needs to manage:

1. Human error, which are inadvertent actions (slips, lapses, or mistakes), and which require that the employee be consoled.
2. At-risk behavior, a choice where the risk is believed to be insignificant or justified, which can be managed by coaching.
3. Reckless behavior, which is conscious disregard of substantial and unjustifiable risk, and which must be managed by punishment.

If individual health care provider issues are identified, they may need to be referred to the institution's peer review process. The Just Culture framework provides helpful guidance on understanding and improving individual accountability when needed; available at: www.chpso.org/sites/main/files/file-attachments/marx_primer.pdf.

Quality improvement starts from the premise that although much medical care is good; it always can be better. The goal is to reduce inappropriate variations in care and improve performance. Quality improvement accepts that good care depends upon more than just the judgment of the individual. Important components of a well-designed QI program include leadership, peer review, root cause analysis, methods to reduce variation, quality measures and indicators, and data collection and analysis.

Leadership

A QI program requires effective, responsive clinical and administrative leadership. The chair of the department is ultimately responsible for QI activities. However, with the increasing complexity of care, the growing awareness of obstetric and neonatal care units as high-reliability organizations, and the increased reporting requirements of local, state, and national organizations, the responsibilities related to patient safety and quality in perinatal health care are substantial. Larger departments may benefit from designation of a patient safety officer and quality improvement manager who report directly to the department chair/chief of service. When physicians accept these leadership positions, their primary purpose is to establish an environment in which quality care and a culture of patient safety can thrive.

Peer Review

Peer review is a quality assessment process in which a retrospective analysis of cases is undertaken using outcomes data to assess adherence to guidelines or other standards of care. Cases typically referred to peer review or QI review are those that meet a specific clinical indicator such as those listed in Box 3-1. Although initial screening may be performed by nonphysicians, peer

BOX 3-1. Sample Clinical Indicators of Quality and Safety in Perinatal Care

Maternal Indicators

1. Maternal mortality
2. Elective delivery at less than 39 weeks of gestation
3. Unplanned maternal postpartum readmission within 14 days
4. Maternal cardiopulmonary arrest, resuscitated
5. In-hospital initiation of antibiotics 24 hours or more following term vaginal delivery
6. Unplanned removal, injury, or repair of organ during operative procedure
7. Excessive maternal blood loss
   a. Required transfusion of four or more units of blood
   b. Postpartum anemia hematocrit less than 22%, hemoglobin less than 7 g (decline of antepartum hematocrit of 11% or hemoglobin decline of 3.5 g)
8. Maternal length of stay in excess of 1 day greater than the local standard after vaginal or cesarean delivery
9. Eclampsia
10. Delivery unattended by the responsible physician*
11. Unplanned postpartum return to the delivery room or operating room for management or admission of a pregnant or postpartum woman to an intensive care unit
12. Cesarean delivery for uncertain fetal status
13. Cesarean delivery for failure to progress

Neonatal Indicators

1. Deaths of infants weighing 500 g or more subcategorized by intrahospital neonatal deaths, total stillborn fetuses, and intrapartum stillborn fetuses
2. Delivery of an infant at less than 32 weeks of gestation in an institution without a neonatal intensive care unit
3. Transfer of a newborn to a neonatal intensive care unit

*To be defined by each institution

Modified from American College of Obstetricians and Gynecologists. Quality and safety in women's health care. 2nd ed. Washington, DC: American College of Obstetricians and Gynecologists; 2010.

review is performed by physicians with similar background and training. Peer review may result in recommendations for individual practice changes or systems and process changes. The American College of Obstetricians and Gynecologists supports a multidisciplinary approach to departmental peer review. Consideration might be given to having the vice chair of the department serve as the QI committee chair, with other possible members to include:

- Representative obstetric care providers and obstetric nurses with varying levels of clinical experience within the department
- Representative anesthesia providers
- Representative subspecialists, when available
- House staff member, when appropriate

This expanded committee is likely to add a fuller perspective to the QI evaluation process. In addition, The Joint Commission includes cases of severe maternal morbidity as a sentinel event meriting review, and facilities and systems should adopt existing criteria or develop their own criteria to review such cases of severe maternal morbidity.

Facilities should have a screening process in place to detect cases of severe maternal morbidity for review. The American College of Obstetricians and Gynecologists and the Society for Maternal–Fetal Medicine recommend using two criteria to screen for women with severe morbidity: 1) transfusion of four or more units of blood, and 2) admission of a pregnant or postpartum woman to an intensive care unit. Institutions may choose to incorporate additional screening criteria. Facilities should review all cases that meet these two screening criteria for severe maternal morbidity and all cases of maternal mortality to determine if they represent cases of the facilities' definitions of severe maternal morbidity. Those cases should be reviewed in greater depth to determine if opportunities for improvement or opportunities that could be addressed within system exist or other changes designed to promote improved future performance could be implemented. Not all cases that meet criteria for review will have true morbidity; even among those that do, some morbidities reflect the underlying health of a mother or pregnancy complication and are thus not avoidable. Therefore, simply meeting one of the screening criteria recommended does not constitute a sentinel event, and the prevalence of such events should not be used as a quality metric, but should be trended.

Small hospitals may face difficulty conducting peer review because of competitive interests or interpersonal issues that have a real or perceived effect on the efficacy of the review. Therefore, it may be helpful to develop a relationship with another hospital or outside independent reviewer or consultant to conduct peer review. The American College of Obstetricians and Gynecologists' Voluntary Review of Quality of Care Program provides peer consultations to departments of obstetrics and gynecology, assesses the quality of care provided, and suggests possible alternative actions for improvement. This is accomplished by a site visit, using various quality assessment techniques, including an evaluation based on ACOG guidelines. It is important to remember that responsibility for peer review and QI rests with the hospital medical staff and, ultimately, the governing board. It is imperative to remember that the focus of peer review should not be punitive, but instead be directed toward system and process improvements that lead to better patient outcomes.

Root Cause Analysis

It is our duty as health care providers to learn from each adverse outcome with the goal of preventing similar events from occurring. In addition, it is our responsibility to ourselves and our patients to design systems to help individuals avoid errors and minimize the effect errors have on our patients, recognizing that human errors are inevitable and unavoidable.

A properly performed root cause analysis is a powerful tool through which teams can investigate an adverse event and try to prevent its recurrence. The Joint Commission requires that organizations perform a root cause analysis for every sentinel event, but root cause analysis also may be used to investigate near misses in which a patient was at risk of, but did not actually sustain, harm. During a root cause analysis, each component of patient care is evaluated, and its potential contribution to the adverse event is assessed. The root cause analysis process is designed to answer four basic questions:

1. What happened in this case?
2. What usually happens?
3. Why did this event occur?
4. What, if anything, can be done to prevent it from happening again?

If contributors to an adverse event are identified, corrective action plans can then be designed. The steps in performing a root cause analysis include the following:

- Establishment of a no-blame culture, in which the common goal of improving patient safety is explicit

- Identification of an event that requires further investigation
- Formation of a multidisciplinary team (include participation by both leadership of the organization and those most closely involved in the relevant processes and systems)
- Identification of all causes potentially associated with the undesirable outcome
- Development of targeted and measurable recommendations to prevent similar events in the future
- Effective communication to others in the organization about lessons learned from the root cause analysis and a plan for implementation of the recommendations

The unexpected birth of a compromised newborn infant is one example of a situation in which obstetric and pediatric teams, including resident physicians, may learn to improve patient outcomes. In addition, every unexpected maternal death should have a root cause analysis or full review.

Reducing Variation

Experts suggest that substantial quality improvements can be achieved by eliminating unnecessary variation in treatment plans and patient outcomes. Although care always must be customized to specific patient needs, unnecessary variation can hamper patient safety efforts, decrease reliability, and increase costs. One approach to reducing variation is the development and implementation of clinical guidelines and bundles. Per the AHRQ, sound clinical practice guidelines are developed from evidence-based research. The Institute for Healthcare Improvement defines a *bundle* as "a structured way of improving the processes of care and patient outcomes: a small, straightforward set of evidence-based practices—generally three to five—that, when performed collectively and reliably, have been proven to improve patient outcomes."

There are currently two national initiatives working in conjunction to develop maternal safety bundles. The Council on Patient Safety in Women's Health Care is a multidisciplinary partnership spearheaded by ACOG that strives to continually improve patient safety in women's health care and drive culture change. The American College of Obstetricians and Gynecologists' Alliance for Innovation on Maternal Health (AIM) is a national maternal safety and quality improvement initiative designed to implement the safety bundles developed by the Council on Patient Safety and to reduce severe maternal morbidity and maternal mortality. The Council's series of patient safety bundles can be found at www.safehealthcareforeverywoman.org.

Guidelines and bundles provide the physician or health care provider with clear guidance that is problem specific. The QI committee can develop best practice guidelines that address particular issues, review them with the entire staff, and amend them to meet the staff's needs. Once a guideline has been finalized, staff may deviate from the guideline as long as the medical record documents the reason for alternative management. Guidelines must be reviewed and updated on a regular basis; ideally, guidelines would be refined on a continuing basis by ongoing observation and assessment of reasons for deviations. Best practices guidelines have been shown to improve clinical care processes by identifying steps in diagnosis as well as treatments.

Quality Measures and Indicators

Quality improvement programs must focus on measurable dimensions of care when selecting indicators to track for identifying processes in need of improvement. The AHRQ maintains an updated list of possible quality measures, including those in obstetrics and neonatology. Their National Quality Measures Clearinghouse is available at www.qualitymeasures.ahrq.gov/. Sample clinical indicators proposed by ACOG are shown in Box 3-1. Pragmatic considerations in developing and deploying valid measures of quality and safety in obstetrics are addressed in ACOG's resource, *Quality and Safety in Women's Health Care*, second edition.

Data Collection and Analysis

The QI process requires accurate collection and analysis of both process and outcome data. Care has been improved by focusing on specific outcomes, such as maternal and neonatal morbidity and mortality. Significant progress has been made in methodologies for collection of data and vital statistics (eg, prenatal records, linked birth and death certificate data, linked birth and hospital discharge data). All states should follow the most current National Center for Health Statistics requirements for issuing standard certificates and reports for birth, death, and fetal death (www.cdc.gov/nchs/nvss/vital_certificate_revisions.htm). The 2003 revision included new recommendations for reporting antenatal treatment (eg, corticosteroids) and postnatal care (eg, neonatal intensive care unit [NICU) admission (Appendix F). The concept of key indicators has been used to assess access to early and continuous perinatal care and to predict or measure poor pregnancy outcome (eg, rates of unintended pregnancy, use of prenatal care services, and fetal, neonatal, and maternal mortality). Many states now use the Centers for Disease Control and Prevention's Pregnancy Risk Assessment Monitoring System or similar surveys to measure population-based health indicators before, during, and after pregnancy (available at www.cdc.gov/prams/). An example of a highly successful data collection system is the California Maternal Data Center (accessed at www.cmqcc.org).

New and improved tools in evaluative clinical sciences should be used to monitor performance and provide the basis for improvement in clinical care and outcomes. Perinatal health care providers and facilities must play an active role by participating in regional data collection, developing standardized data collection tools, supporting analysis, benchmarking, and using the resulting information for individual, institutional, and professional QI. As outlined in the ACOG and Society for Maternal–Fetal Medicine *Levels of Maternal Care*, Level IV/Regional Perinatal Health Care Centers are responsible for analyzing regional data, including perinatal complications and outcomes and quality improvement. Thorough and systematic collection of data on long-term outcomes is essential to evaluate changes in perinatal care delivery systems and new technologies and therapies. Regional care collaboratives can facilitate data collection and sharing and provide an opportunity for learning new approaches. Examples of such collaboratives include the California Maternal Quality Care Collaborative (www.cmqcc.org/) and Perinatal Quality Care Collaborative, (www.cpqcc.org), the Northern New England Perinatal Quality Improvement Network (www.nnepqin.org), the Ohio Perinatal Quality Collaborative (www.opqc.net/), and the CDC Perinatal Quality Collaboratives (www.cdc.gov/reproductivehealth/maternalinfanthealth/pqc.htm). In addition, the development of regional relationships between hospitals that provide different levels of care may also be beneficial for data collection, confidential review, and analysis of cases for quality improvement. This also will increase the likelihood that infants are born in a hospital equipped with an appropriate level of maternal and neonatal care.

In addition to the efforts of individual hospitals and perinatal care systems, the National Fetal and Infant Mortality Review (NFIMR) program provides an opportunity for QI efforts to review fetal, infant, and maternal deaths. The NFIMR process is a broad type of analysis that is valuable at the community level. The program brings together key members of the community, including prenatal and pediatric providers, public health professionals, social service agency representatives, grief professionals, consumer advocates, consumers, and others. They review de-identified information from individual cases of fetal and infant death to identify factors associated with those deaths, determine if they represent service system problems that require change, develop recommendations for change, and assist in the implementation of change. Currently, NFIMR is being implemented in over 37 states and the Pacific Basin. The NFIMR program was initiated as a collaborative effort between ACOG and the federal Maternal and Child Health Bureau, Health Resources and Services Administration. (For more information about the NFIMR process or to learn if there is a NFIMR program in your community, go to www.nfimr.org.)

Although maternal deaths attributable to pregnancy remain relatively rare, the rate of pregnancy-related maternal mortality continues to be on the rise in the United States. Therefore, it is important that each death be identified and carefully reviewed at the local and state level. The lessons learned from reviews of these deaths need to be shared with those who have the opportunity to influence policies and practices related to the systems of care in place for women in the prepregnancy, antepartum, and postpartum periods.

Patient Safety

According to the AHRQ, patient safety refers to freedom from accidental or preventable injuries produced by medical care. Thus, practices of interventions that improve patient safety are those that reduce the occurrences of preventable adverse events. Patient safety emphasizes a systems analysis of medical errors and minimizes individual blame and retribution while still maintaining individual accountability. Patient safety is an explicit principle that must be embraced as a core value in patient care. It is an ongoing effort that requires health care professionals to continually strive to learn from problems, identify system deficiencies, redesign processes, and implement change in processes and systems of practice. Patient-centered and family-centered care, open communication, and teamwork provide the foundation for optimal patient care and safety. Although health care aims to be highly reliable it is equally important to consider resilience; ie, the ability to detect, respond to, and mitigate the effects of errors. Patient safety focuses on systems of care, not individuals. Confidential analysis and reporting of errors and near misses will reveal areas that require remediation to improve patient safety. State and federal laws may direct the level of confidentiality and the manner of reporting.

National Patient Safety Goals

The Joint Commission recognizes the importance of patient safety. In 2003, The Joint Commission created the first set of National Patient Safety Goals (see "Bibliography" in this chapter). These goals, derived from Sentinel Event Alerts and other sources, are designed to be explicit, evidence based, and measurable, and are updated each year based on comment and evidence (www.jointcommission.org/standards_information/npsgs.aspx).

Patient Safety Principles

The American College of Obstetricians and Gynecologists and the American Academy of Pediatrics also have a long-standing commitment to quality and patient safety. To improve patient care and reduce medical errors, they encourage all health care providers to promote the following four principles:

1. Commit to a culture of patient safety
2. Implement safe medication practices
3. Reduce the likelihood of surgical errors
4. Improve communication

Commit to a Culture of Patient Safety

A culture of patient safety should be the framework for every effort to reduce medical errors. Development of such culture starts at the top of administration with strong leadership that provides the necessary human and financial resources to achieve patient safety. Additionally, a culture of safety recognizes the importance of team function in optimizing individual performance. A culture of patient safety fosters open communication and welcomes input from every team member at every level. Care must be taken to ensure that hierarchical systems do not hamper free communication. Competing demands, interruptions, and distractions are inherent in clinical practice, but all attempts should be made to minimize these. It requires specific effort to ensure that issues are understood and that meaningful information is transferred. Certain clinical communications should be verified, such as reading back medication orders. Inaccurate information and missing clinical data can result in serious medical errors and patient injury. Any significant communications should be documented appropriately (see section on "Handoff Communication" later in this chapter).

Specific training on patient safety principles and practices is critical. This could include a program such as TeamSTEPPS (Team Strategies and Tools to Enhance Performance and Patient Safety) available free from AHRQ (www.ahrq.gov/teamstepps/index.html) or regular drills and simulations. The participation of all team members is fundamental to the creation of a safe unit. This applies to inpatient and outpatient settings; for the ambulatory environment, the ACOG Safety Certification in Outpatient Practice Excellence (SCOPE) for Women's Health Program outlines many important safety principles (www.scopeforwomenshealth.org/).

Implement Safe Medication Practices

Medication errors are one of the most common types of preventable adverse events. Automated systems for prescribing and dispensing medication can greatly reduce these errors, but there are many low technology solutions that can be implemented rapidly with minimal cost, such as the following:

- If an electronic ordering system is used within an electronic medical record, formats that clarify appropriate dosages/intervals and facilitate weight-based dosing should be included. Such systems can also warn prescribers of medication conflicts and potentially inappropriate use of medications in pregnancy.
- If no electronic medical record is available, improve the legibility of written orders.
- Do not use unapproved abbreviations, as recommended by The Joint Commission (see "Bibliography").
- Always use a leading 0 for doses less than 1 unit (eg, 0.1 not .1) and never use a trailing 0 after a decimal point (eg, 1 mg not 1.0 mg): "always lead, never follow."
- Require that all verbal orders be written by the individual receiving the order and then read back to the prescriber. An effort should be made to eliminate most verbal orders.

Reduce the Likelihood of Surgical Errors

The American College of Obstetricians and Gynecologists and the American Academy of Pediatrics, along with other specialty societies and other organizations, have endorsed The Joint Commission's Universal Protocol to Prevent Wrong Site, Wrong Procedure, and Wrong Patient Surgery. The Joint Commission now requires this protocol as part of a preoperative time out, which involves all members of the operating room team, including the patient (see "Bibliography"). In obstetrics, the time out process does not need to be limited to patient identification and planned procedure, but also may provide an opportunity to ensure the completion of other patient safety or clinical recommendations, such as administration of antibiotics before cesarean delivery, communication of important fetal or neonatal information with the neonatal care provider, or the possible need for and availability of blood products. At the completion of vaginal delivery, the time out could include a correct sponge and needle account, as with any surgical procedure. A time out also is required for all invasive procedures performed in the NICU.

Improve Communication

Effective communication among team members (including the patient) is a core concept of high-functioning teams and safe and reliable patient care. Team communication serves the dual purpose of providing an opportunity to relay important information about the task-related responsibilities of the team and providing evidence about the nature of the team's interprofessional performance. It creates a culture that enables a continuous learning environment within the practice and translates to better and more efficient care. Physicians should be aware that complete and accurate communication of relevant clinical information is critical to reduce preventable medical errors. Improving communication skills merits the same attention as improving clinical skills. According to information gathered by The Joint Commission regarding sentinel events, the most common cause of preventable adverse outcomes is communication error. Optimal communication to improve patient safety has many dimensions including the following:

- Communication with the patient and the family
- Communication among all those caring for the patient
- Availability of information necessary for coordination of care

Physician–Patient Communication. Patients should receive complete, timely information about their care and changes in their care. Team members should assume the best motives of others. They should recognize that their initial assumptions may reflect their own world views and should first seek to understand others' views and then to be understood. Active listening is also an important aspect of successful interprofessional collaboration and connotes respect when communicating with patients, families, and colleagues.

The U.S. Preventive Services Task Force defines *shared decision making* as a process in which both the patient and physician share information, participate in the decision-making process, and agree on a course of action (see "Bibliography" in this chapter). The American College of Obstetricians and Gynecologists recommends that care always should be patient centered; ie, it is focused on the health needs of the patient; respects the patient's values, preferences, and goals; is based on an enduring personal relationship; and sees the patient as a partner in managing his or her health and making health care decisions. Patient-centered care should be as valued as clinical outcomes. This can be accomplished by establishing shared, clearly articulated goals for the process and outcomes of care, driven by the values and preferences of the patient. These goals should be mutually decided and agreed upon by the patient, the family (according to patient preference), and the health care team.

Open communication facilitates the gathering of complete information, a more accurate diagnosis, and patient adherence. This type of communication, based on negotiation and consensus building, is referred to as the partnership model. Communication tools that can be of assistance include AIDET® and RESPECT (Box 3-2 and Box 3-3), as well as the five steps for patient-centered interviewing (Table 3-1).

Another factor potentially limiting communication is health literacy, which may be related or unrelated to level of education or social status. In order to have a meaningful discussion with an individual about her health care, the patient's level of understanding and knowledge must be considered.

BOX 3-2. AIDET® Five Fundamentals of Patient Communication

Acknowledge	Being attentive and greeting the patient in a positive manner
Introduce	Giving your name, your role, and your skill set
Duration	Giving a reasonable time expectation
Explanation	Making sure the patient is knowledgeable and informed
Thank you	Showing appreciation to the patient for her cooperation

Studer Group is the author and owner of this work. AIDET® is a trademark of Studer Group. Reprinted with permission.

BOX 3-3. The RESPECT Model

Rapport

- Connect on a social level.
- See the patient's point of view.
- Consciously attempt to suspend judgment.
- Recognize and avoid making assumptions.

Empathy

- Remember that the patient has come to you for help.
- Seek out and understand the patient's rationale for her behaviors or illness.
- Verbally acknowledge and legitimize the patient's feelings.

Support

- Ask about and try to understand barriers to care and compliance.
- Help the patient overcome barriers.
- Involve family members if appropriate.
- Reassure the patient you are and will be available to help.

Partnership

- Be flexible with regard to issues of control.
- Negotiate roles when necessary.
- Stress that you will be working together to address medical problems.

Explanations

- Check often for understanding.
- Use verbal clarification techniques.

Cultural Competence

- Respect the patient and her culture and beliefs.
- Understand that the patient's view of you may be defined by ethnic or cultural stereotypes.
- Be aware of your own biases and preconceptions.
- Know your limitations in addressing medical issues across cultures.
- Understand your personal style and recognize when it may not be working with a given patient.

Trust

- Self-disclosure may be an issue for some patients who are not accustomed to Western medical approaches.
- Take the necessary time and consciously work to establish trust.

Reprinted from Toward Culturally Competent Care: A Toolbox for Teaching Communication Strategies by permission of the Center for Health Professions, University of California, San Francisco, 2002.

TABLE 3-1. Five Step Patient-Centered Interviewing

Step 1. Set the stage for the interview (30–60 s)	1. Welcome the patient 2. Use the patient's name 3. Introduce yourself and identify specific role 4. Ensure patient readiness and privacy 5. Remove barriers to communication (sit down) 6. Ensure comfort and put the patient at ease
Step 2. Elicit chief concern and set an agenda (1–2 min)	7. Indicate time available 8. Forecast what you would like to have happen in the interview 9. Obtain a list of all issues the patient wants to discuss 10. Summarize and finalize the agenda
Step 3. Begin the interview with nonfocusing skills that help the patient to express herself (30–60 s)	11. Start with open-ended request/question 12. Use nonfocusing open-ended skills (attentive listening) 13. Obtain additional data from nonverbal sources
Step 4. Use focusing skills to learn three things: Symptom Story, Personal Context, and Emotional Context (3–10 min)	14. Elicit symptom story 15. Elicit personal context 16. Elicit emotional context 17. Respond to feelings/emotions 18. Expand the story
Step 5. Transition to middle of the interview (clinician-centered phase) (30–60 s)	19. Brief summary 20. Check accuracy 21. Indicate that both content and style of inquiry will change if the patient is ready

Reprinted with permission from Fortin AH 6th, Dwamena FC, Frankel RM, Smith RC. Smith's patient-centered interviewing: an evidence-based method. 3rd ed. New York (NY): McGraw Hill; 2012.

The following guidance can improve communication, increase the level of understanding, and improve health literacy:

- Tailor speaking and listening skills to individual patients.
  - Ask open-ended questions using the words "what" or "how" to start the sentence. (For example: "What questions do you have for me?" rather than "Do you have any questions?")
  - Use medically trained interpreters when necessary.
  - Check for comprehension by asking patients to restate the health information given in their own words. (For example: "Tell me how you are going to take this medication.") This is particularly useful during the informed consent process.
  - Encourage staff and colleagues to use plain language that is culturally sensitive and to obtain training in improving communication with patients.
- Tailor health information to the intended user.
  - When developing health information, make sure it reflects the target group's age, social and cultural diversity, language, and literacy skills.
  - When developing information and services, include the target group in the development (pretest) and implementation (posttest) phases of the process to ensure the program is effective.
  - When preparing health information, consider cultural factors and the influence of culture on health, including race, ethnicity, language, nationality, religion, age, gender, sexual orientation, income level, and occupation.
- Develop written materials.
  - Keep the messages simple.
  - Limit the number of messages (general guideline is four main messages).
  - Focus on action. Give specific recommendations based on behavior rather than the medical principle. (For example, "Take a warm water bath two times a day" instead of "Sitz baths may help healing.")
  - Use the active voice instead of the passive voice. (For example, "These pills can make you sick to your stomach" instead of "Nausea may be caused by this medication.")
  - Use familiar language and avoid jargon. (For example, "You may have itching" instead of "You may experience pruritus.")

- — Use visual aids such as drawings or models for key points. Make sure the visual messages are culturally relevant.
- — Use at least a 12-point type size to make the messages easy to read.
- — Leave plenty of white space around margins and between sections.

A very important part of physician–patient communication is when and how to disclose medical errors. The Joint Commission requires that accredited hospitals inform patients of adverse events. According to The Joint Commission Standard RI.01.02.01, "the licensed independent practitioner responsible for managing the patient's care, treatment, and services, or his or her designee, informs the patient about unanticipated outcomes of care, treatment and services." When an error contributed to an injury, the patient and the family or representative should receive a truthful and compassionate explanation about the error and the remedies available to the patient. They should be informed that the factors involved in the injury will be investigated so that steps can be taken to reduce the likelihood of similar injury to other patients. Improving the disclosure process through policies, programmatic training, and available resources will enhance patient satisfaction, strengthen the physician–patient relationship, potentially decrease litigation, and most importantly promote higher quality health care.

Handoff Communication. Good provider-to-provider patient handoffs require accurate communication, and can prevent discontinuity of care, eliminate preventable errors, and provide a safe patient environment. A structured handoff (such as the "I-PASS" framework, available at: www.ahrq.gov/teamstepps/instructor/essentials/pocketguide.html) can ensure that information is not inadvertently omitted and can give the oncoming provider the chance to ask questions and clarify information. In the ambulatory setting, outgoing providers must ensure that someone is designated to review results and answer incoming questions. Regular, scheduled team meetings also can facilitate effective communication by ensuring timely, consistent, and reliable group communication. These meetings should address patient care (ie, appropriate monitoring of care, the patient's condition, and collaborative problem solving) and, distinct from patient care, team functioning (ie, discussion of team member contributions, peer feedback on communication patterns, and performance). Regular, scheduled team meetings also can facilitate effective communication by ensuring timely, consistent, and reliable group communication.

Physician Fatigue and Patient Safety

Individuals who are tired are more likely to make mistakes. Reducing fatigue may improve patient care and safety as well as improve a health care provider's performance satisfaction and increase communication. Although there are no current guidelines placing any limits on the volume of deliveries and procedures performed by a single physician or the length of time physicians may be on call and still perform procedures, it is imperative that all team members recognize any limitations caused by fatigue.

The National Sleep Foundation recommends 8 hours of sleep per night for an adult. Sleep deprivation can result from insufficient sleep, fragmented sleep, or both. Recovery from a period of insufficient sleep generally requires at least two or three full nights of adequate uninterrupted sleep.

Individual practitioners and group practices should examine their sleeping habits and work schedules to ensure an optimal balance between fatigue and continuity of patient care. Although there may be an economic effect of such considerations, patient safety should take precedence.

Physician/Practitioner Impairment

Impairment presents a sensitive problem in all settings in which physicians and licensed independent practitioners practice. Practitioners are considered impaired if they are unable to practice medicine with reasonable skill and safety because of physical or mental illness (including alcohol or other chemical drug dependencies) or mood disorders. Any condition that may affect decision-making capabilities, medical judgment, and competence—including diseases of an organic nature—may contribute to impairment.

Early recognition of chemical dependency or other impairment can be difficult. Denial is common. The following are some of the manifestations of impairment:

- Failure to monitor patients appropriately
- Poor quality of medical care
- Incomplete or poor-quality medical records
- Frequent absences
- Increased isolation from colleagues and other staff members
- Self-prescribing of drugs

Intervention as soon as impairment is suspected, or before professional performance is impaired, is encouraged. Providers should know whom to contact to address an emergency related to an impaired colleague. The chief medical officer and on-call administrator are often the designated authorities. Impaired physician or diversion programs, usually operated through the state medical licensing board, are an excellent source of information regarding the evaluation and treatment of impaired health care providers and any applicable legal requirements.

The American Medical Association has recommended that institutions develop a policy on reporting and investigating suspected impairment. In addition, The Joint Commission has specific requirements regarding the institution's method for identifying and managing matters of individual health for licensed independent practitioners, including physicians.

Drills and Simulations

The principle that standardization of care can improve patient outcomes applies to emergencies as well as to routine care. Thus, each service should consider a guideline for management of common and uncommon emergencies. Guidelines can be reinforced by prominent display as posters, pocket cards, other cognitive aids, and simulation.

Simulation should include the following components: standardized procedures, effective communication among team members, and nonhierarchical teamwork with discussion of near or actual errors in a nonjudgmental setting. Drills and simulations may use a sophisticated simulated environment, but also can use the everyday workspace for a mock event. The environment should ensure the availability of the following:

- Availability of appropriate emergency supplies in a resuscitation cart (crash cart) or kit
- Development of a rapid response team
- Development of protocols that include clinical triggers
- Use of standardized communication tools for huddles and briefs (eg, Situation, Background, Assessment, Recommendation [SBAR])
- Implementation of emergency drills and simulations

Using drills to train the care team to respond to emergencies has several theoretical advantages. Adult learning theory supports the importance of experiential learning. Emergencies occur in a specific physical setting and may involve a group of nurses, physicians, and other health care providers attempting to respond. By conducting a drill in a realistic simulator or in the actual patient care setting, issues related to the physical environment become obvious.

Emergency drills also allow participants to practice principles of effective communication in a crisis. Many aspects of the medical environment work against effective communication, including the often hierarchical hospital structure, the nature of the training, the work setting, and the different educational backgrounds and levels of understanding of the health care team members. Many physicians are accustomed to directing nurses and others. Although this is sometimes necessary in an emergency, effective teamwork also requires talking with each other. It requires that there be a team leader coordinating the response, but it also should empower all members of the team to share information. By practicing together, barriers hindering communication and teamwork can be overcome.

Simulation training also may be beneficial with respect to identifying common clinical errors made during emergencies and correcting those deficiencies. Although this is promising, there are limited data to suggest that improved proficiency with simulation models correlates with increased proficiency during actual emergencies.

Quality Improvement and Patient Safety in Neonatal Intensive Care

All of the topics discussed in the preceding text are of critical importance in the NICU, where the complexity and severity of illnesses highlight the consequences of errors and gaps in communication. A well-functioning, coordinated team is essential to address emergent or urgent situations, such as the delivery of a compromised infant or a sudden deterioration in the intensive care unit, and to promote QI and a culture of safety to improve outcomes. Development and updating of clinical guidelines, careful and comprehensive handoffs, and regular drills and simulations for emergencies are essential for good patient care. The communication principles outlined earlier in this chapter apply particularly to discussions with families of sick infants.

The number of medications received by infants in the NICU, together with the extremely wide variation in dosing weights, significantly increases the possibility of medication errors. In one large prospective database, extremely low-birth-weight infants were exposed, on average, to 17 different medications during their hospital stay. Thus, the practices outlined earlier in this chapter to decrease medication errors are of utmost importance in the NICU. Electronic medical records can be particularly useful, with the use of standardized order sets and dosing weight checks. The presence of a pharmacist in the NICU can help reduce medication errors. All medication orders should be checked by a pharmacist before administration except in emergency circumstances. Use of bar codes and bedside medication verification also decreases the risk of medication errors. Changes as simple as more frequent simulations and including a pharmacist on daily rounds can have a demonstrable positive effect on patient care outcomes.

The introduction of guidelines and bundles to reduce variation in practice and improve outcomes has been shown effective in numerous situations, such as improving nutrition, reducing health care-associated infections, and improving delivery room care ("the Golden Hour"). Participation in a multi-institutional collaborative (such as the Vermont–Oxford Network, https://public.vtoxford.org/) or the California Perinatal Quality Care Collaborative (www.cpqcc.org) allows individual institutions to compare their morbidities and outcomes to other similar institutions. The CDC also maintains a list of all Perinatal Quality Collaboratives (available at www.cdc.gov/reproductivehealth/maternalinfanthealth/pqc.htm). Areas of increased morbidity can then be evaluated for a QI program, identifying and implementing best practices and using rigorous improvement methodology. Every NICU should strive to reduce variation in processes and outcomes. Although some variation may be explained by baseline risk, often differences between NICUs persist even after adjustment for case mix. Transparency with process and outcome data and use of evidence-based decision making remain essential to ensure that every patient at every encounter receives appropriate care that is supported by the literature.

Care in the NICU today remains a complex system with many opportunities for medical errors to occur. The neonatologist and the clinical care team should facilitate development of an environment that encourages investigation of actual and averted (near-miss) events and learning from errors. Significant variations in care and outcomes, and gaps in the capability of physicians to engage in and lead QI, still exist. These deficiencies could be remedied by increasing the availability of improvement curricula, training opportunities, and skilled faculty.

Bibliography

American College of Obstetricians and Gynecologists. Collaboration in practice: implementing team-based care. Washington, DC: American College of Obstetricians and Gynecologists; 2016. Available at: http://www.acog.org/Resources-And-Publications/Task-Force-and-Work-Group-Reports/Collaboration-in-Practice-Implementing-Team-Based-Care. Retrieved September 30, 2016.

American College of Obstetricians and Gynecologists. Guidelines for women's health care: a resource manual. 4th ed. Washington, DC: American College of Obstetricians and Gynecologists; 2014.

American College of Obstetricians and Gynecologists. Quality and safety in women's health care. 2nd ed. Washington, DC: American College of Obstetricians and Gynecologists; 2010.

Barfield WD; Committee On Fetus and Newborn. Standard Terminology for Fetal, Infant, and Perinatal Deaths. Pediatrics 2016 May;137(5).

Centers for Disease Control and Prevention. Infant Mortality. Atlanta (GA): CDC 2016. Available at: https://www.cdc.gov/reproductivehealth/maternalinfanthealth/infantmortality.htm. Retrieved April 3, 2017.

Communication strategies for patient handoffs. Committee Opinion No. 517. American College of Obstetricians and Gynecologists. Obstet Gynecol 2012;119:408–11.

Disclosure and discussion of adverse events. Committee Opinion No. 681. American College of Obstetricians and Gynecologists. Obstet Gynecol 2016;128:e257–61.

Effective patient–physician communication. Committee Opinion No. 587. American College of Obstetricians and Gynecologists. Obstet Gynecol 2014;123:389–93.

Fatigue and patient safety. Committee Opinion No. 519. American College of Obstetricians and Gynecologists. Obstet Gynecol 2012;119:683-5.

Fortin AH 6th, Dwamena FC, Frankel RM, Smith RC. Smith's patient-centered interviewing: an evidence-based method. 3rd ed. New York (NY): McGraw Hill; 2012.

Health literacy. Committee Opinion No. 585. American College of Obstetricians and Gynecologists. Obstet Gynecol 2014;123:380–3.

Institute of Medicine (U.S.). Crossing the quality chasm: a new health system for the 21st century. Washington, D.C.: National Academy Press; 2001.

Levels of maternal care. Obstetric Care Consensus No. 2. American College of Obstetricians and Gynecologists. Obstet Gynecol 2015;125:502–15.

March of Dimes. Toward improving the outcome of pregnancy III: enhancing perinatal health through quality, safety and performance initiatives. Committee on Perinatal Health. White Plains (NY): National Foundation--March of Dimes; 2010. Available at: http://www.marchofdimes.org/materials/toward-improving-the-outcome-of-pregnancy-iii.pdf. Retrieved September 30, 2016.

Markenson D, Reynolds S. The pediatrician and disaster preparedness. American Academy of Pediatrics Committee on Pediatric Emergency Medicine Task Force on Terrorism. Pediatrics 2006;117:e340–62.

Martin JA, Kirmeyer S, Osterman M, Shepherd RA. Born a bit too early: recent trends in late preterm births. NCHS Data Brief 2009;(24):1–8.

Martin JA, Osterman MJ, Sutton PD. Are preterm births on the decline in the United States? Recent data from the National Vital Statistics System. NCHS Data Brief 2010;(39):1–8.

National Sleep Foundation. Arlington (VA): National Sleep Foundation; 2016. Available at: http://www.sleepfoundation.org. Retrieved October 3, 2016.

National Transportation Safety Board. Factors that affect fatigue in heavy truck accidents. Safety Study NTSB/SS-95/01. Washington, DC: NTSB; 1995. Available at: http://www.ntsb.gov/safety/safety-studies/Documents/SS9502.pdf. Retrieved October 3, 2016.

Partnering with patients to improve safety. Committee Opinion No. 490. American College of Obstetricians and Gynecologists. Obstet Gynecol 2011;117:1247–9.

Patient safety in obstetrics and gynecology. ACOG Committee Opinion No. 447. American College of Obstetricians and Gynecologists. Obstet Gynecol 2009;114:1424–7.

Patient safety in the surgical environment. Committee Opinion No. 464. American College of Obstetricians and Gynecologists. Obstet Gynecol 2010;116:786–90.

Preparing for clinical emergencies in obstetrics and gynecology. Committee Opinion No. 590. American College of Obstetricians and Gynecologists. Obstet Gynecol 2014;123:722–5.

Sheridan SL, Harris RP, Woolf SH. Shared decision making about screening and chemoprevention. a suggested approach from the U.S. Preventive Services Task Force. Shared Decision-Making Workgroup of the U.S. Preventive Services Task Force. Am J Prev Med 2004;26:56–66.

Severe maternal morbidity: screening and review. Obstetric Care Consensus No. 5. American College of Obstetricians and Gynecologists. Obstet Gynecol 2016;128:e54-60.

Studer Q. AIDET five fundamentals of patient communication [DVD]. Gulf Breeze (FL): Fire Starter Publishing; 2005.

The Joint Commission. Comprehensive accreditation manual for hospitals: CAMH. Oakbrook Terrace (IL): The Commission; 2016.

The Joint Commission. Facts about the official "do not use" list. Oakbrook Terrace (IL): The Joint Commission; 2016. Available at: https://www.jointcommission.org/facts_about_do_not_use_list. Retrieved September 30, 2016.

The Joint Commission. Introduction to the universal protocol for preventing wrong site, wrong procedure, and wrong person surgery. In: Comprehensive accreditation manual for hospitals: CAMH. Oakbrook Terrace (IL): The Commission; 2016. p. NPSG-18-NPSG-24.

The Joint Commission. 2016 National patient safety goals. Oakbrook Terrace (IL): The Joint Commission; 2016. Available at: https://www.jointcommission.org/standards_information/npsgs.aspx. Retrieved September 30, 2016.

The Women's and Children's Health Policy Center. Evaluation of Fetal and Infant Mortality Review (FIMR) Programs nationwide. Baltimore (MD): Johns Hopkins University; Available at: http://www.jhsph.edu/research/centers-and-institutes/womens-and-childrens-health-policy-center/projects/fimr.html. Retrieved September 30, 2016.

Resources

American Medical Association. Clinical practice improvement and patient safety. Chicago (IL): AMA; 2011.

California Maternal Quality Care Collaborative. Stanford (CA): CMQCC; 2016. Available at: https://www.cmqcc.org. Retrieved December 9, 2016.

Centers for Disease Control and Prevention. Pregnancy Risk Assessment Monitoring System (PRAMS). Atlanta (GA): CDC; 2016. Available at: http://www.cdc.gov/prams. Retrieved October 4, 2016.

Managing Obstetrical Risk Efficiently: MOREob. Society of Obstetricians and Gynaecologists of Canada; Healthcare Insurance Reciprocal of Canada. London, Ontario: Salus Global Corporation; 2016. Available at: http://moreob.com/. Retrieved October 4, 2016.

National Fetal–Infant Mortality Review Program. Washington, DC: NFIMR; 2016. Available at: http://www.nfimr.org/home. Retrieved December 16, 2016.

National Quality Measures Clearinghouse. Rockville (MD): Agency for Healthcare Research and Quality; 2011. Available at: http://www.qualitymeasures.ahrq.gov/. Retrieved December 9, 2016.

The Joint Commission. Reviewing maternal morbidity. Quick Safety. Oakbrook Terrace (IL): The Joint Commission; 2014. Available at: http://www.jointcommission.org/assets/1/23/Quick_Safety_Issue_Six_Sep_2014_FINAL.pdf. Retrieved April 4, 2017.

Chapter 4

Maternal and Neonatal Interhospital Transfer

The primary goal of regionalized perinatal care is for women and newborn infants at high risk to receive care in facilities that are prepared to provide the required level of specialized care. It is essential that each facility has a clear understanding of its capability to handle increasingly complex levels of maternal and neonatal care and has a well-defined threshold for transferring women and newborn infants to facilities that offer a higher level of care. A pregnant woman should be cared for at the facility that best meets her needs and those of her infant. Delivery in a center providing high level maternal and neonatal care offers availability of obstetric and pediatric subspecialists for early diagnosis and treatment of life-threatening conditions. Antepartum transport avoids separation of mother and infant in the immediate postpartum period, allows mothers to communicate directly with neonatal intensive care unit health care providers, and supports the goal of family-centered health care. Because all hospitals cannot provide all levels of perinatal and neonatal care, interhospital transport of pregnant women and newborn infants is an essential component of a regionalized perinatal health care system. Receiving hospitals should openly accept transfers; the appropriate care level for patients should be driven by their medical need for that care and not limited by financial constraint.

Both facilities and professionals providing health care to pregnant women need to understand their obligations under federal and state law. The Emergency Medical Treatment and Labor Act (EMTALA) defines the responsibilities of transferring and receiving facilities and practitioners. Federal law requires all Medicare-participating hospitals to provide an appropriate medical screening examination for any individual seeking medical treatment at an emergency department to determine whether the patient has an emergency medical condition (Appendix G). Some states have similar statutory requirements. These laws also place strict requirements on the transfer of these patients. However, there have been misinterpretations of these laws that have been barriers to optimal health care. For example, the medical condition of a woman having contractions is not considered an emergency if there is adequate time for her safe transfer before delivery or if the transfer will not pose a threat to the health or safety of the woman or the fetus.

Types of Transport

There are three types of perinatal patient transport: 1) maternal transport, 2) neonatal transport, and 3) return transport. Maternal and neonatal transport programs are typically considered separately because they each have particular characteristics and requirements and are generally overseen by their respective specialists.

Maternal Transport

Maternal transport refers to the transport of a pregnant woman during the antepartum period, intrapartum period, or the postpartum period for a higher level of care of the woman, her newborn infant, or both. Occasionally, the same system is used to transport a postpartum woman and her newborn infant so that the mother can be with her newborn infant or receive a higher level of care for severe postpartum complications. Depending on the severity of the maternal illness, a team from the receiving hospital may go to the referring hospital to pick up the patient, or the patient may be sent by one-way ambulance from the referring hospital to the receiving hospital.

All attempts need to be made to ensure that women and infants at high risk receive care in a facility that provides the required level of specialized obstetric and newborn care. Women who develop high-risk medical conditions need to receive obstetric care in a hospital with a high level of maternal care, regardless of the gestational age of the fetus. Likewise, women whose fetus is determined to be high risk need to receive care in a facility that has appropriate resources to care for the newborn infant. Delivery hospitals that do not have a level III or level IV maternal or neonatal care need to develop affiliation(s) with facilities that provide higher levels of care. It is essential that formal transfer agreements be in place that clearly outline the responsibilities of each facility. The American Academy of Pediatrics has developed general guidance based on neonatal gestational age and potential complications to help determine the most optimal level of newborn care for a given gestational age and estimated fetal weight (see Table 1-4 in Chapter 1). More recently the American College of Obstetricians and Gynecologist in collaboration with the Society for Maternal–Fetal Medicine has developed a similar document to help determine the most optimal level of maternal care (see Table 1-2 in Chapter 1).

Neonatal Transport

The interhospital transfer of a newborn infant who requires specialized or intensive care generally proceeds according to one of the following approaches:

- A team is sent from one hospital, often a regional center, to the referring hospital to evaluate and stabilize the infant at the referring hospital and then transfer the infant to the team's hospital.
- A team is sent from the referring hospital with an infant who is being transferred to another hospital for specialized or intensive care.
- A team is sent from one hospital to the referring hospital to evaluate and stabilize the infant and then transfer the infant to a third hospital. Such a transfer may be necessary because of bed constraints or the need for specialized care available only at the third hospital. (For more information, see "Levels of Neonatal Care" in Chapter 1 and the American Academy of Pediatrics' resource *Guidelines for Air and Ground Transport of Neonatal and Pediatric Patients*.)

Return Transport

After receiving intensive or specialized care at a referral center, a woman or her infant may be returned to the original referring hospital or to a local hospital for continuing care after the problems that required the transfer have been resolved. This needs to be done in consultation with the referring physician.

Transport Program Components and Responsibilities

Components

To ensure optimal care of patients at high risk, the following components need to be part of a regional referral program:

- Formal transfer plans for mothers and newborn infants with receiving hospitals that are established by facilities that provide lower levels of care
- A method of risk identification and assessment of problems that are expected to benefit from consultation and transport
- Assessment of the perinatal capabilities and determination of conditions necessitating consultation, referral, transfer, and return transfer of each participating hospital
- Resource management to maximize efficiency, effectiveness, and safety
- Adequate financial and personnel support
- A reliable, accurate, and comprehensive communication system between participating hospitals and transport teams available 24 hours per day
- Determination of responsibility for each of these functions

An interhospital transport program must provide 24-hour service. It needs to include a receiving or program center responsible for ensuring that patients at high risk receive the appropriate level of care, a dispatching unit to coordinate the transport of patients between facilities, an appropriately equipped transport vehicle, and a specialized transport team. The program also needs to have a system for providing a continuum of care by various health care providers, including the personnel and equipment required for the level of care needed, as well as outreach education and program evaluation.

Responsibilities

Each of the functional components of an interhospital transport program has specific responsibilities. If the transport is done by the referring hospital, the referring physician and hospital retain responsibility until the transport team arrives with the patient at the receiving hospital. If the transport team is sent by the receiving hospital, the receiving physician or designee assumes responsibility for patient care from the time the patient leaves the referring hospital. It needs to be emphasized that during the preparation for transport by the transport team, the referring physician and hospital retain responsibility for the patient unless there have been other prior agreements. Transport services must work with their referring hospital to delineate clearly the primary medical responsibility for the patient when the patient is still within the referring hospital but is being cared for by the transport team. Regardless of the site of origin of the transport team, qualified staff needs to accompany the patient to the receiving hospital.

Medical–Legal Aspects

Many legal details of perinatal transport are not well defined and are subject to interpretation. In addition, many transport teams provide service in more than one state and, therefore, must comply with the laws of the state in which they are practicing and cannot be guided solely by their home state or area. Legal consult needs to be sought when developing a service to ensure compatibility with existing laws, and periodic review is encouraged to maintain compliance with laws and regulations. It is clear that all involved parties (eg, the referring hospital and personnel, the receiving hospital and personnel, and the transportation carriers or corporations) assume a number of responsibilities for which they are accountable:

- Each transport system must comply with the standards and regulations set forth by local, state, and federal agencies.
- Informed consent for transfer, transport, and admission to and care at the receiving hospital needs to be obtained before the transport team moves the patient. All federal and state laws regulating patient transfer need to be followed. The completed consent form needs to be signed by the patient or parent or guardian and witnessed; a copy needs to be placed in the patient's medical record. If the neonatal patient will require an emergency procedure before the parents' arrival at the receiving facility, the informed consent for this procedure needs to be obtained before departure from the referring facility if this action will not adversely delay the transport.
- Consent for any neonatal surgical procedures needs to be obtained by the surgical staff by telephone if parents are not at the receiving facility.

- Formal protocols need to be developed by hospitals that provide lower levels of care to outline procedures for transport and to clarify responsibilities for care of the patient being transported.
- Hospital medical staff policies need to delineate the level of capability of their maternal and newborn units, which conditions need prompt consultation, and which patients need to be considered for transfer.
- Relevant personal identification is to be provided for the patient to wear during transport.
- Patient care guidelines, standing orders, and verbal communication with the designated supervising transport physician are to be used to initiate and maintain patient care interventions during transport.

The professional qualifications and actions of the transport team are the responsibility of the institution that employs the team. Insurance must be adequate to protect patients and transport team members.

Director

The director of the transport program (neonatal or maternal) needs to be a board-certified/board-eligible subspecialist in neonatology or a board-certified (or active candidate for board certification) specialist in maternal–fetal medicine, respectively. In select cases, the director can be a pediatrician or obstetrician–gynecologist with special expertise in these respective subspecialty areas. As noted previously, typically the programs are organized and directed separately. The program director's responsibilities include the following:

- Training and supervising staff
- Ensuring appropriate review of all transport records
- Developing and implementing protocols for patient care
- Developing and maintaining standardized patient records and a database to track the program
- Establishing a program for performance quality
- Identifying trends and effecting improvements in the transport system by regularly reviewing the following elements:
  - operational aspects of the program, such as response times, effectiveness of communications, and equipment issues
  - evaluation forms completed by the referring and receiving hospitals soon after each transport

- Developing protocols for programs that use multiple modes of transport (ground, helicopter, and airplane)
- Determining which mode of transport to be used and any conditions, such as weather, that would preclude the use of a particular form of transport
- Developing alternative plans for care of the patient if a transport cannot be accomplished
- Ensuring that proper safety standards are followed during transport
- Requiring the transportation services to follow established guidelines regarding maintenance and safety

The director may delegate specific responsibilities to other persons or groups but retains the responsibility of ensuring that these functions are addressed appropriately.

Referring Hospital

Referring physicians need to be familiar with the transport system, including how to gain access to its services and appropriately use its services. The referring physician is responsible for evaluating the patient's condition and initiating stabilization procedures before the transport team arrives. Within the referring hospital, the transport team continues resuscitation and care in collaboration with the referring physician and staff. Transfer generally is performed when the patient is clinically stable, although there are circumstances when ongoing stabilization is necessary during the transfer to the accepting hospital.

A maternal or neonatal transport form needs to accompany each patient. The form contains general information about the patient, including the reason for referral, the transport mode, and any additional information that may enhance understanding of the patient's needs. Also provided is relevant patient medical information that maximizes the opportunity for appropriate and timely care and minimizes duplication of tests and diagnostic procedures at the receiving hospital.

The newborn infant must have appropriate identification bands in place, and the following items need to be sent with the infant:

- Properly labeled, red-topped tubes of clotted maternal and umbilical cord blood with label identification consistent with the newborn identification bands

- Copies of all relevant maternal antepartum, intrapartum, and postpartum records
- All recent or new diagnostic or clinical information for the infant, including imaging studies

The referring team and the transport team need to delineate who is responsible for the care of the pregnant woman or newborn infant. Parental consent needs to be obtained for transfer to and treatment of the newborn infant at the receiving hospital. The referring physician needs to personally transfer care to the transport team or needs to designate another physician to transfer care. A status report regarding the patient's care needs to be provided by the referring hospital's nursing staff to the appropriate transport team member.

Receiving Center

The receiving center is responsible for the overall coordination of the regional program. It needs to make sure that interhospital transport is organized in a way that ensures that patients will receive the appropriate level of care. The receiving hospital for maternal transports typically decides whether the woman's condition warrants a team going to pick her up or if she can be safely transported by one-way ambulance. Programs that use one-way ambulances must have procedures in place that identify the ambulance company, level of ambulance, and how to initiate the transport.

Contingency plans need to be in place to avoid a shortage of beds for patients needing tertiary or quaternary care. The plans need to include provisions for accepting or transferring patients among the cooperating centers or to an alternate receiving center, when special circumstances warrant (eg, patient census or need for specialized services).

The receiving center is responsible for providing referring physicians with the following services:

- Access by telephone on a 24-hour basis to communicate with receiving obstetric and neonatal units
- Follow-up on the patient by telephone, letter, or fax, provided all federal, state, and local requirements are met
- A complete summary, including diagnosis, an outline of the hospital course, and recommendations for ongoing care for each patient at discharge
- Ongoing communication and follow-up

Dispatching Units

Dispatching units are responsible for the following activities:

- Providing rapid coordination of vehicles and staff
- Serving as a communication link between the transport team and the referring and receiving hospitals
- Communicating the transport team's estimated time of arrival at the referring hospital so that any planned therapeutic or diagnostic interventions can be completed in time
- Communicating the patient's estimated time of arrival at the receiving center so that all resources can be mobilized and ready
- Coordinating any connections that need to be made between air transport and ground ambulances

Personnel

The transport teams need to have the expertise necessary to provide supportive care for a wide variety of emergency conditions that can arise with pregnant women and newborn infants at high risk. Team members may include physicians, neonatal nurse practitioners, registered nurses, respiratory therapists, and emergency medical technicians. The composition of the transport team needs to be consistent with the expected level of medical need of the patient being transported. Transport personnel also need to be thoroughly familiar with the transport equipment to ensure that any malfunction en route can be handled.

Equipment

Safe and successful patient transfer depends on the equipment available to the transport team. The kinds and amounts of equipment, medications, and supplies needed by the transport team depend on the type of transport (maternal or neonatal), the distance of the transfer, the type of transport vehicle used, and the resources available at the referring medical facility. The transport equipment and supplies need to be based on the needs of the most seriously ill patients and need to include essential medications and special supplies needed during stabilization and transfer.

The transport team generally needs the following items to perform its functions:

- Equipment for monitoring physiologic functions (heart rate, blood pressure levels [invasive or noninvasive], temperature [skin or axillary], respiratory rate, and noninvasive pulse oximetry)
- Resuscitation and support equipment (intravenous pumps, suction apparatus, mechanical ventilators) and isolettes for neonatal transport
- Portable medical gas tanks attached to a flowmeter, with a blender that can be easily integrated with vehicle or building sources of pressurized gas during transport, if patients dependent on ventilators are transported
- Electrical equipment that is capable of operating on alternating current, extended direct current, or both, and is compatible with the sources in the transport vehicle or medical facility. Additional specialized equipment and supplies may be needed for individual clinical situations.

The performance characteristics of transport equipment need to be tested for the most extreme environmental conditions that may be encountered. Equipment performance may not perform optimally if there is a harsh electromagnetic environment, altitude changes, vibration, forces of acceleration, or extremes of temperature and humidity. Hospital-based equipment may cause electromagnetic interference with aircraft navigation or communication systems. Altered performance of medical or aircraft systems could affect the safety of the transport team and the patient.

All equipment needs to be tested to ensure accuracy and safety in flight. The Federal Aviation Administration and the U.S. Food and Drug Administration have no known comprehensive testing guidelines. The Federal Aviation Administration has guidance regarding equipment for operators of emergency medical services or helicopters. The U.S. Department of Defense has discovered flaws in hospital-based medical equipment that could affect safety when used in air transport. The Department of Defense has comprehensive testing guidelines for electronic and electric component parts and electromagnetic interference characteristics of subsystems and equipment. ASTM International (formerly known as the American Society for Testing and Materials) has developed standards for fixed and rotary wing aircraft operating as air ambulances.

The following organizations also can offer assistance in choosing medical equipment suitable for use in aircraft:

Association of Air Medical Services
909 N. Washington Street, Suite 410
Alexandria, VA 22314
Tel: (703) 836-8732, Fax: (703) 836-8920
www.aams.org

Emergency Care Research Institute
5200 Butler Pike
Plymouth Meeting, PA 19462-1298
Tel: (610) 825-6000, Fax: (610) 825-1275
www.ecri.org

Federal Aviation Administration
800 Independence Avenue, SW
Washington, DC 20591
Tel: (866) 835-5322
www.faa.gov

National Aeronautics and Space Administration
300 E. Street SW, Suite 5R30
Washington, DC 20546-0001
Tel: (202) 358-0001, Fax: (202) 358-4338
www.nasa.gov

Several factors need to be considered in selecting vehicles for an interhospital transport system. Ground transportation is most appropriate for short-range transport. The use of airplanes allows for coverage of a large referral area but is more expensive, requires skilled operators and specially trained crews, and may actually prolong the time required for response and transport over relatively short distances because of the time needed to prepare for flight and the time required for transport to and from the airport. Helicopters can shorten response and transport times over intermediate distances or in highly congested areas but are very expensive to maintain and operate.

The decision to use an aircraft in a patient-transport system requires special commitments from the director and members of the transport team. The pilot's decision needs to be based solely on flight safety. Therefore, the pilot needs to be included in appropriate decision making and needs to have the authority to change, modify, or cancel the mission for safety reasons.

Transport Procedure

Interhospital transport needs to be considered if the necessary resources or personnel for optimal patient outcomes are not available at the facility currently providing care. The resources available at the referring and the receiving hospitals need to be considered. The risks and benefits of transport, as well as the risks and benefits associated with not transporting the patient, need to be assessed. Transport may be undertaken if the health care provider determines that the well-being of the woman, the fetus, or the infant will not be adversely affected or that the benefits of transfer outweigh the foreseeable risks. The staff of the referring hospital needs to consult with the receiving hospital as soon as the need for the transport of a woman or her newborn infant is considered.

Transportation of patients to an alternate receiving center solely because of third-party payer issues (eg, conflicts between managed care plans and referring and receiving hospital affiliations) need to be strongly discouraged and may be illegal in certain situations. All transfers need to be based on medical need. If the patient to be transported is pregnant, pretreatment evaluation needs to include the following:

- Maternal vital signs
- Fetal assessment by electronic fetal monitoring or Doppler, depending on gestational age
- Maternal cervical examination, if the woman is having contractions

It may be necessary to stabilize the mother before transport. Initiation of blood pressure medication, intravenous fluids, or tocolytics may be started at the referring hospital. The level of care to be provided in the referring hospital is dependent on the time required for transport, method of transport, and maternal medical condition. The level of care needs to be determined locally between the referring and receiving hospitals' medical personnel.

If the patient to be transferred is a newborn infant, the family needs to be given an opportunity to see and touch the infant before the transfer. A transport team member needs to meet with the family to explain what the team will be doing en route to the receiving hospital. The patient, personnel, and all equipment need to be safely secured inside the transport vehicle.

Patient Care and Interactions

The following important components of patient care need to be implemented during transport:

- The patient needs to be observed continuously.
- Vital signs need to be monitored and recorded.
- Intravenous fluids and medications need to be given, monitored, and recorded as required.

The following components of care are specific for a maternal patient or a newborn infant:

Maternal patients

- Uterine activity of maternal patients and fetal heart rates need to be monitored before and after transport; continuous uterine activity or fetal heart rate monitoring during transport need to be individualized.

Newborn infants

- The infant needs to be kept in a neutral thermal environment and needs to receive appropriate respiratory support and additional monitoring, such as assessment of oxygen saturation and blood glucose, as clinically indicated.
- If ventilator support is required, ventilator parameters and inspired oxygen percentages need to be monitored.
- The team needs to be prepared to perform lifesaving invasive procedures, such as placement of a chest tube and intubation.

On arrival at the receiving hospital, the following activities are recommended:

- The receiving staff needs to be prepared to address any unresolved problems or emergencies that involved the transported patient.
- The transport team needs to report the patient's history and clinical status to the receiving staff.
- The receiving staff needs to inform the patient's family, as well as the referring physician and staff at the referring hospital, of the condition of the patient on arrival to the receiving hospital and periodically thereafter.

- On completion of the patient transfer, the transport team or other designated personnel needs to immediately restock and re-equip the transport vehicle in anticipation of another call.

Transfer for Critical Care

The care of any pregnant women who requires intensive care unit services needs to be managed in a facility with obstetric adult and neonatal intensive care unit capabilities (see Table 1-4 in Chapter 1). Guidelines for perinatal transfer have been published and follow the federal Emergency Medical Treatment and Labor Act guidelines. General recommendations include antenatal rather than neonatal transfer. In the event that maternal transport is unsafe or impossible, alternative arrangements for neonatal transfer may be necessary. In the event of imminent delivery, transfer needs to be held until after delivery of the placenta.

The minimal monitoring required for a critically ill patient during transport includes continuous pulse oximetry, electrocardiography, and regular assessment of vital signs. All critically ill patients must have secure venous access before transfer. Patients who are mechanically ventilated must have endotracheal tube position confirmed and secured before transfer. In the obstetric patient, left uterine displacement and supplemental oxygen need to be applied routinely during transport. The utility of continuous fetal heart rate monitoring or tocodynamic monitoring is unproven; therefore, its use needs to be individualized.

Return Transport

Infants whose conditions have stabilized and who no longer require specialized services need to be considered for return transport. Transporting the infant back to the referring hospital is important for the following reasons:

- It allows the family to return to their home, often permitting more frequent interactions between the family and the infant.
- It involves the health care providers who ultimately will be responsible for the continuing care of the infant earlier in the care process.
- It preserves specialized services for patients who require them and allows for a better distribution of resources.
- It enhances the integrity of the regionalized care system and emphasizes the partnership between the hospitals in the system.

Economic barriers, including those imposed by managed care organizations, that restrict or raise barriers to this movement of newborn infants are detriments to optimal patient care. Every effort needs to be made to eliminate these artificial constraints.

Transfer is best accomplished after detailed communication between physicians and nursing services at both hospitals that outlines the infant's care requirements and the anticipated course of the patient to ensure that the hospital receiving the return transport can provide the needed services. These services must not only be available but they must be provided in a consistent fashion and be of the same quality as those that the infant is receiving in the regional center. Further, if special equipment or treatment is required at the hospital receiving the infant, arrangements need to be made before the infant is transferred. Lastly, there also must be an understanding that if problems arise that cannot be managed in an appropriate manner at the receiving hospital, the infant will be returned to the regional center, or the regional center will participate in developing an alternative care plan.

It is important that parents consent to the return transfer of the infant and understand the benefits to them and their infant. Their comfort with this process will be enhanced if they realize that the regional center and the referring hospital are working together in a regionalized system of care, that there is frequent communication between the staff of the two hospitals, that there will be continuing support after the return transport, and that the infant will be returned to the regional center if necessary. It also may be helpful if parents visit the facility to which the infant will be transported before transfer.

A comprehensive plan for follow-up of the infant after return transfer and after discharge from the hospital needs to be developed. This plan needs to outline the required services and identify the party bearing the responsibility for follow-up.

To ensure optimal care during a return transfer, the following guidelines are recommended:

- The parents' informed consent for return transfer needs to be obtained.
- Return transfer needs to be accomplished through an adequately equipped vehicle with trained personnel so that the level of care received by the infant remains the same during transport.
- Staffing at both hospitals needs to be adequate to ensure a safe transition of care.

- The family needs to be notified of the transfer so that they may be present at the accepting facility when the transfer occurs.
- Appropriate records, including a summary of the hospital course, diagnosis, treatments, recommendations for ongoing care, and follow-up, need to accompany the infant.
- The transport team needs to call the referring hospital and the infant's parents to inform them of the completion of the transport and to report the newborn's condition.
- The center that provided the higher level of care needs to provide easily accessible consultation on current or new problems to professional staff at the return transfer facility.

Outreach Education

Critical to the appropriate use of a regional referral program is a program to educate the public and users about its capabilities. The receiving center and receiving hospitals need to participate in efforts to educate the public about the kinds of services available and their accessibility.

Outreach education needs to reinforce cooperation between all individuals involved in the interhospital care of perinatal patients. Receiving hospitals need to provide all referring hospitals with information about their response times and clinical capabilities and need to ensure that health care providers know about the specialized resources that are available through the perinatal care network. Primary physicians need to be informed as changes occur in indications for consultation and referral of perinatal patients at high risk and for the stabilization of their conditions. Each receiving hospital also needs to provide the outcomes of all transported patients, continuing education, and information to referring physicians about current treatment modalities for high-risk situations. Effective outreach programs will improve the care capabilities of referring hospitals and may allow for some patients to be retained or, if transferred, to be returned earlier in their course of care.

Program Evaluation

Ideally, the director of a regional transport program needs to coordinate program evaluation based on patient outcome data and logistic information. Program monitoring needs to include the following information:

- Unexpected maternal or neonatal morbidity or mortality during transport

- Deliveries during transport or immediately after arriving at the receiving hospital
- Morbidity or mortality of patients at the receiving hospital
- Frequency of failure to transfer patients generally considered to require a higher level of care
- Availability of all the services that may be needed by the perinatal patient
- Accessibility of services, capability to connect the patient quickly and appropriately with the services needed, and programs to promote patient and community awareness of available and appropriate regional referral programs

These data need to be tracked as part of the ongoing quality improvement programs of the transport team and the receiving hospital (see also Chapter 3).

Bibliography

American College of Obstetricians and Gynecologists. Guidelines for women's health care: a resource manual. 4th ed. Washington, DC: American College of Obstetricians and Gynecologists; 2014.

ASTM International. Standard specification for rotary wing basic life support, advanced life support, and specialized medical support air ambulances. Designation: F2318-15. West Conshocken (PA): ASTM; 2015.

Department of Defense. Electronic and electrical component parts: test method standard. DLA Land and Maritime MIL-STD-202H. Columbus (OH): DOD; 2015. Available at: http://quicksearch.dla.mil/Transient/DA9286207EDE41238D2FEECEAB36690B.pdf. Retrieved October 18, 2016.

Department of Defense. Electronic and electrical component parts: test method standard. DLA Land and Maritime MIL-STD-202H. Revision H. Columbus (OH): DOD; 2015. Available at: http://quicksearch.dla.mil/qs/DocDetails.aspx?ident_number=35612. Retrieved June 29, 2017.

Federal Aviation Administration. Helicopter air ambulance operations. Advisory Circular No. 135-14B. Washington, DC: FAA; 2015. Available at: http://www.faa.gov/documentLibrary/media/Advisory_Circular/AC_135-14B.pdf. Retrieved October 18, 2016.

Hospital-based triage of obstetric patients. Committee Opinion No. 667. American College of Obstetricians and Gynecologists. Obstet Gynecol 2016;128:e16–9.

Insoft RM, Schwartz HP, Romito J, editors. Guidelines for air and ground transport of neonatal and pediatric patients. American Academy of Pediatrics. Section on

Transport Medicine. 4th ed. Elk Grove Village (IL): American Academy of Pediatrics; 2015.

March of Dimes. Toward improving the outcome of pregnancy: the 90s and beyond. Committee on Perinatal Health. White Plains (NY): National Foundation—March of Dimes; 1993.

March of Dimes. Toward improving the outcome of pregnancy III: enhancing perinatal health through quality, safety and performance initiatives. Committee on Perinatal Health. White Plains (NY): National Foundation—March of Dimes; 2010. Available at: http://www.marchofdimes.org/materials/toward-improving-the-outcome-of-pregnancy-iii.pdf. Retrieved September 30, 2016.

Section on Transport Medicine. American Academy of Pediatrics. Elk Grove Village (IL): American Academy of Pediatrics; 2016. Available at: https://www.aap.org/en-us/about-the-aap/Committees-Councils-Sections/section-transport-medicine/Pages/default.aspx. Retrieved October 18, 2016.

Stroud MH, Trautman MS, Meyer K, Moss MM, Schwartz HP, Bigham MT, et al. Pediatric and neonatal interfacility transport: results from a national consensus conference. Pediatrics 2013;132:359–66.

Warren J, Fromm RE Jr, Orr RA, Rotello LC, Horst HM. Guidelines for the inter- and intrahospital transport of critically ill patients. American College of Critical Care Medicine. Crit.Care Med 2004;32:256–62. Available at: http://www.learnicu.org/Docs/Guidelines/Inter-IntrahospitalTransport.pdf. Retrieved October 18, 2016.

Resources

ECRI Institute. Plymouth Meeting (PA): ECRI; 2016. Available at: https://www.ecri.org/Pages/default.aspx. Retrieved December 16, 2016.

Federal Aviation Administration. Washington, DC: FAA; 2016. Available at: https://www.faa.gov/. Retrieved December 16, 2016.

Levels of maternal care. Obstetric Care Consensus No. 2. American College of Obstetricians and Gynecologists. Obstet Gynecol 2015;125:502–15.

National Aeronautics and Space Administration. Washington, DC: NASA; 2016. Available at: https://www.nasa.gov/. Retrieved December 16, 2016.

The Association of Air Medical Services. Alexandria (VA): AAMS; 2015. Available at: http://aams.org/. Retrieved December 16, 2016.

Chapter 5

Prepregnancy Care

Optimizing a woman's health, health behavior, and knowledge before she plans to and becomes pregnant is known as prepregnancy care. It is a component of a larger health care goal—optimizing the health of every woman. Because reproductive capacity spans almost four decades for most women, optimizing women's health before and between pregnancies is an ongoing process that requires access to and the full participation of all segments of the health care system. Although a specific visit for prepregnancy counseling would be the ideal, few women actually do so. Therefore, all health encounters during a woman's reproductive years should include discussion of a woman's preference for contraception and counseling about health lifestyle changes a woman can make to improve her health status before pregnancy. Women still should be encouraged to seek a specific prepregnancy visit if they are planning a pregnancy.

Obstetrician–gynecologists and other obstetric care providers should engage each patient in supportive, respectful conversation about her pregnancy intentions and provide prepregnancy or contraceptive counseling based on the woman's desires and preferences. Questions, such as the One Key Question® "Would you like to become pregnant in the next year?" (Box 5-1), can initiate several evidence-based prepregnancy care interventions and lifestyle modifications to optimize health status if the answer is "yes," including those listed as follows:

- An evaluation of her overall health and opportunities to improve her health
- Education about the important effect that social, environmental, occupational, behavioral, and genetic factors have on pregnancy
- Identification of factors associated with a high risk of an adverse pregnancy outcome, with interventions recommended to improve a women's risk profile before pregnancy

BOX 5-1. Questions to Assess Women's Pregnancy Intentions

One Key Question®

- Would you like to become pregnant in the next year?

The Centers for Disease Control and Prevention's Quality Family Planning Recommendations

- Do you have any children now?
- Do you want to have (more) children?
- How many (more) children would you like to have and when?

Reproductive life planning to reduce unintended pregnancy. Committee Opinion No. 654. American College of Obstetricians and Gynecologists. Obstet Gynecol 2016;127:e66–9.

Prepregnancy Counseling and Interventions

During episodic or focused health care visits of women who could become pregnant, in addition to performing a physical exam and obtaining her obstetric and gynecologic histories, there are core topics in prepregnancy care that should be addressed. The following topics may serve as the basis for such counseling (Table 5-1):

- Family planning and pregnancy spacing
- Immunization status
- Risk factors for sexually transmitted infections (STIs)
- Substance use, including alcohol, tobacco, and recreational and illicit drugs
- Exposure to violence and intimate partner violence
- Medical, surgical, and psychiatric histories
- Current medications (prescription and nonprescription)
- Family history
- Genetic history (maternal and paternal)
- Nutrition, body weight, and exercise
- Teratogens; environmental and occupational exposures (available at www.acog.org/toxicchemicals)
- Assessment of socioeconomic, educational, and cultural context

TABLE 5-1. Health Screening for Women of Reproductive Age

Selective Reproductive Health Screening	Done	Referred
Reproductive awareness		
Pregnancy prevention counseling		
Prepregnancy and nutrition counseling		
Medical diseases (counsel regarding effects on future pregnancies)		
Diabetes mellitus		
Hypertension		
Epilepsy		
Other chronic illness		
Infectious diseases (counsel, test, or refer)		
Sexually transmitted diseases, including human immunodeficiency virus (HIV)		
Hepatitis A		
Hepatitis B (immunize if at high risk)		
Rubella (test; if nonimmune, immunize)		
Varicella		
Teratogens and genetics (counsel regarding effects on future pregnancies)		
Hemoglobinopathy		
Medication and vitamin use (eg, isotretinoin and vitamin A [retinoic acid])		
Self or prior child with congenital defect		
Family history of genetic disease		
Environmental exposure at home or in workplace (see www.acog.org/toxicchemicals)		
Uterine anomaly/diethylstilbestrol (DES)		
Behavior (counsel regarding effects on future pregnancies)		
Alcohol use		
Tobacco use (ie, smoking, chewed, electronic nicotine delivery system [ENDS], vaped)		
Use of illicit substances (eg, prescription opioid use, cocaine)		
Social support		
Safety (eg, domestic violence)		
Personal resources (eg, transportation or housing)		

Modified with permission from March of Dimes Birth Defects Foundation, Committee on Perinatal Health. Toward improving the outcome of pregnancy: the 90s and beyond. White Plains (NY): March of Dimes Birth Defects Foundation; 1993.

In addition, women should be counseled regarding the benefits of enhancing their personal health status and practicing safe sex to avoid STIs, including human immunodeficiency virus (HIV).

Reproductive Life Plan

A reproductive life plan is a set of personal goals regarding whether, when, and how to have children based on individual priorities, resources, and values. Such a plan addresses the individual's or couple's desire for a child or children (or desire not to have children); the optimal number, spacing, and timing of children; and age-related changes in fertility. Because many women's plans change over time, creating a reproductive life plan requires an ongoing assessment of the desirability of a future pregnancy, determination of steps that need to be taken to prevent or to plan for and optimize a pregnancy, and evaluation of current health status and other issues relevant to the health of a pregnancy. Health care providers should counsel that the optimal interval between delivery and subsequent pregnancy is 18 months to 5 years; the greatest risk of low-birth-weight and preterm birth occurs when the interpregnancy interval is less than 6 months. The patient's reproductive life plan provides context for discussing contraceptive options.

If pregnancy is not desired, clinicians can discuss pregnancy prevention, if appropriate or relevant, including education and counseling on all available contraceptive options, and help each woman arrive at an appropriate choice based on her health status, personal values, and preferences. Counseling should include guidance on the correct use of the chosen contraceptive method and the need for consistent use. Physicians and other health care providers have the duty to refer patients in a timely manner to other health care providers if they do not feel that they can in conscience provide the standard of reproductive services that their patients request. In an emergency in which referral is not possible or might negatively affect a patient's physical or mental health, health care providers have an obligation to provide medically indicated and requested care regardless of the health care provider's personal moral objections.

Prepregnancy Immunization

Prepregnancy care offers the opportunity to review immunization status. Ideally, vaccinations should be administered before pregnancy, although there is no evidence of adverse fetal effects from vaccinating pregnant women with an inactivated virus or bacterial vaccines or toxoids. Live vaccines pose a theoretical risk for the fetus, and women who receive a live-virus vaccination should be advised to avoid pregnancy for at least 1 month after vaccination.

The Advisory Committee on Immunization Practices of the Centers for Disease Control and Prevention (CDC) recommends vaccination with the inactivated influenza vaccine for all women who will be pregnant through the influenza season (typically October through May in the United States). No study to date has shown an adverse consequence of the inactivated influenza vaccine in pregnant women or their offspring. Vaccination early in the season and regardless of gestational age is optimal, but unvaccinated pregnant women should be immunized at any time during the influenza season as long as the vaccine is available. Women who have not been immunized with the tetanus toxoid, reduced diphtheria toxoid, and acellular pertussis (Tdap) vaccine, women whose vaccine status is unknown, and those who are due for a Tdap booster should be offered immunization with Tdap.

In addition, vaccination(s) should be offered to women found to be not immune to measles, mumps, rubella, varicella, hepatitis A, hepatitis B, meningococcus, and pneumococcus. The human papillomavirus vaccination should be offered to appropriate nonpregnant women. The target age for human papillomavirus vaccine is 11–12 years, but for those not vaccinated at the target age, catch-up vaccination is recommended up through 26 years.

Sexually Transmitted Infections

Chlamydia trachomatis and *Neisseria gonorrhoeae* have been strongly associated with ectopic pregnancy, infertility, and chronic pelvic pain. Annual screening for chlamydial infection in all sexually active women younger than 25 years is recommended, as is screening of older women with risk factors (eg, those who have a new sex partner or multiple sex partners). Targeted screening for gonorrhea is recommended for women younger than 25 years who are at increased risk of infection (eg, women with previous gonorrhea, other STIs, new or multiple sex partners, and inconsistent condom use; those who engage in commercial sex work and drug use; women in certain demographic groups; and those who live in communities with a high prevalence of disease). Dual method use, the use of both condoms and more effective methods as protection against STIs and unwanted pregnancy, is the ideal contraceptive practice for adolescents. Women who have a positive test result for gonorrhea, chlamydial infection, or both should be treated in accordance with current CDC guidelines (see also "Chlamydial Infection" and

"Gonorrhea" in Chapter 12). With regard to HIV testing, it is recommended that females aged 13–64 be tested at least once in their lifetime and annually thereafter based on factors related to risk of HIV. Testing in the prepregnancy period allows the woman to make informed decisions regarding treatment and timing of pregnancy.

Substance Use and Substance Use Disorders

Cessation of tobacco use (ie, smoking, chewed, electronic nicotine delivery system [ENDS], vaped) is recommended before pregnancy. Women who smoke cigarettes or use any other form of tobacco product should be identified and encouraged and supported in an effort to quit before becoming pregnant. There is a strong association between tobacco use during pregnancy and sudden infant death syndrome. Women who wish to quit tobacco use benefit from a brief counseling session, such as the 5As intervention (Box 5-2). Training in the use of the 5As tobacco cessation tool and knowledge of health care support systems, including the National Cancer Institute's Smoking Quitline (1-877-44U-QUIT or 1-877-448-7848), and pharmacotherapy add to the techniques health care providers can use to support tobacco cessation.

Other important behavioral issues to address include alcohol use and the use of prescription and nonprescription recreational drugs. All women should be asked about the quantity and frequency of their alcohol use and should be counseled that there is no known absolutely safe quantity, frequency, type, or timing of alcohol consumption during pregnancy. Referral relationships with appropriate resources should be established and used as needed. Women counseled concerning their alcohol or drug use should

BOX 5-2. Five Major Steps to Intervention (The "5As")

1. Ask about tobacco use.
2. Advise to quit through clear, personalized messages.
3. Assess willingness to quit.
4. Assist to quit.
5. Arrange follow up and support.

Modified from Treating tobacco use and dependence: December 2012 update. Clinical Guidelines and Recommendations. Rockville (MD): Agency for Healthcare Research and Quality. Available at: http://www.ahrq.gov/professionals/clinicians-providers/guidelines-recommendations/tobacco/5steps.html. Retrieved July 15, 2016.

be monitored by appropriate health care providers to assess adherence to recommendations. Before as well as during pregnancy, all women routinely should be asked about their use of all drugs, including prescription opioids and other medications used for nonmedical reasons. This routine screening should be performed annually and should rely on validated screening tools, such as questionnaires including 4Ps (Box 5-3), CRAFFT (Box 5-4), and the NIDA Quick Screen. These tools have been well studied and demonstrate high sensitivity for detecting substance use and misuse. They can be used in direct interview format by physicians as well as nonphysicians, and can be streamlined into clinical practice by using computer-based approaches.

Chronic Medical Conditions

Certain chronic medical conditions, such as diabetes, thyroid disease, and maternal phenylketonuria, should be controlled before pregnancy. It has been shown that achieving prepregnancy and early pregnancy blood sugar control can decrease the risk of spontaneous abortion and birth defects. By achieving a hemoglobin A_{1C} level at or below 6.0 mg per dL before pregnancy, women with diabetes can reduce the risk of birth defects in their offspring to a level comparable to that of nondiabetic women. Women with hyperthyroidism (most often Graves disease) or hypothyroidism should be appropriately treated so that they are euthyroid before attempting

BOX 5-3. Clinical Screening Tools for Prenatal Substance Use and Abuse

4 Ps

Parents: Did any of your parents have a problem with alcohol or other drug use?

Partner: Does your partner have a problem with alcohol or drug use?

Past: In the past, have you had difficulties in your life because of alcohol or other drugs, including prescription medications?

Present: In the past month have you drunk any alcohol or used other drugs?

Scoring: Any "yes" should trigger further questions.

Modified from Ewing H. A practical guide to intervention in health and social services, with pregnant and postpartum addicts and alcoholics: theoretical framework, brief screening tool, key interview questions, and strategies for referral to recovery resources. Martinez (CA): The Born Free Project, Contra Costa County Department of Health Services; 1990.

BOX 5-4. CRAFFT—Substance Abuse Screen for Adolescents and Young Adults

C: Have you ever ridden in a CAR driven by someone (including yourself) who was high or had been using alcohol or drugs?

R: Do you ever use alcohol or drugs to RELAX, feel better about yourself, or fit in?

A: Do you ever use alcohol or drugs while you are by yourself, or ALONE?

F: Do you ever FORGET things you did while using alcohol or drugs?

F: Do your FAMILY or FRIENDS ever tell you that you should cut down on your drinking or drug use?

T: Have you ever gotten in TROUBLE while you were using alcohol or drugs?

Scoring: Two or more YES answers suggest a serious problem and need for further assessment.

Reproduced with permission from the Center for Adolescent Substance Abuse Research, Children's Hospital Boston. The CRAFFT screening interview. Boston (MA): CeASAR; 2009. Available at: http://www.ceasar.org/CRAFFT/pdf/CRAFFT_English.pdf. Retrieved September 27, 2016. For more information, contact ceasar@childrens.harvard.edu.

pregnancy. Inadequately treated hyperthyroidism or hypothyroidism is associated with adverse pregnancy outcomes, including miscarriage and preterm delivery. Women in whom phenylketonuria was diagnosed and treated during infancy and childhood are at risk of having children who are cognitively impaired if they do not adhere to a low-phenylalanine diet before pregnancy and during pregnancy. Other conditions that should be addressed include epilepsy, asthma, hemoglobinopathies, inherited thrombophilias, obesity, a history of bariatric surgery, and hypertension (for more information, see "Medical Complications Before Pregnancy" in Chapter 9).

Medication Use

All medications (prescription and over-the-counter), supplements, and herbal therapies should be noted. In general, using the lowest effective dose of only necessary medications is recommended. The use of known or potentially teratogenic medications, including warfarin, valproic acid, carbamazepine, isotretinoin, and angiotensin-converting enzyme inhibitors, should be addressed. Physician and patient information about known teratogenic medications, can be found on the Organization of Teratology

Information Specialists' website, available at www.otispregnancy.org, or on the Reproductive Toxicology Center website, Reprotox available at www.reprotox.org.

The effectiveness of folate supplementation in the prevention of drug-associated neural tube defects (NTDs) has not been documented; however, folate supplementation of 4 mg per day should be offered before pregnancy to women taking anticonvulsant medications and for the first trimester.

For women with a psychiatric illness, advising a pregnant or breastfeeding woman to discontinue medication exchanges the fetal or neonatal risks of medication exposure for the risks of untreated maternal illness. Maternal psychiatric illness, if inadequately treated or untreated, may result in poor adherence to prenatal care, inadequate nutrition, exposure to additional medication or herbal remedies, increased alcohol and tobacco use, deficits in mother–infant bonding, and disruptions within the family environment. Further, discontinuing antidepressant medication in women with depression further increases their already heightened risk of peripartum depression. Optimally, shared decision making among obstetric and mental health clinicians and the patient should occur before pregnancy. Whenever possible, multidisciplinary management involving the obstetrician, mental health clinician, primary health care provider, and pediatrician is recommended to facilitate care.

Prepregnancy Genetic Screening

Carrier screening and counseling ideally should be performed before pregnancy. Ethnic-specific, panethnic, and expanded carrier screening are acceptable strategies for prepregnancy and prenatal carrier screening. Each obstetrician–gynecologist or other obstetric care provider or practice should establish a standard approach that is consistently offered to and discussed with each patient. After counseling, a patient may decline any or all carrier screening. If a patient requests a screening strategy other than the one used by the obstetrician–gynecologist or other obstetric care provider, the requested test should be made available to her after counseling on its limitations, benefits, and alternatives. If a woman is found to be a carrier for a specific condition, her reproductive partner should be offered screening to provide accurate genetic counseling for the couple with regard to the risk of having an affected child. Additional genetic counseling should be provided to discuss the specific condition, residual risk, and options for prenatal testing. If a carrier couple (ie, carriers for the same condition) is identified before pregnancy, genetic counseling is encouraged so that reproductive options (eg, donor gametes, preimplantation genetic diagnosis, prenatal diagnosis) can be discussed. All patients who are considering pregnancy or are already pregnant, regardless of screening strategy and ethnicity, should be offered carrier screening for cystic fibrosis and spinal muscular atrophy, as well as a complete blood count and screening for thalassemias and hemoglobinopathies. Fragile X permutation carrier screening is recommended for women with a family history of fragile X-related disorders or intellectual disability suggestive of fragile X syndrome, or women with a personal history of ovarian insufficiency. Additional screening also may be indicated based on family history or specific ethnicity. Screening for Tay–Sachs disease should be offered when considering pregnancy or during pregnancy if either member of a couple is of Ashkenazi Jewish, French–Canadian, or Cajun descent. Those with a family history consistent with Tay–Sachs disease also should be offered screening (see also "Antepartum Genetic Screening and Diagnosis" in Chapter 6).

Pretest counseling should be provided by trained personnel. The information about genetic screening should be provided in a clear, objective, and nondirective manner. Printed educational materials or access to electronic resources may be provided at the prenatal or prepregnancy visit for the woman and her partner. If an obstetrician–gynecologist or other obstetric care provider does not have the necessary knowledge or expertise in genetics to counsel a patient appropriately, referral to a genetic counselor, medical or gynecologic oncologist, maternal–fetal medicine specialist, or other genetics specialist should be considered, as appropriate, for the condition examined. This may include determining risks, evaluating a family history of such abnormalities, interpreting laboratory test results, or providing counseling.

Several methods have been established to obtain family medical histories, each with its own advantages and disadvantages. A common tool used in general practice is the family history questionnaire or checklist. Any positive responses on the questionnaire should be followed up by the health care provider to obtain more detail, including the relationship of the affected family member(s) to the patient, exact diagnosis, age of onset, and severity of disease. Another family history assessment tool, commonly used by genetics professionals, is the pedigree. A pedigree ideally shows at least three generations using standardized symbols and clearly marks individuals affected with a specific diagnosis to allow for easy identification. The pedigree may visibly assist in determining the size of the family and the mode of inheritance of a specific condition, and may facilitate identification of members at increased risk of developing the condition or who may be carriers of a certain disease. The screening tool selected should be tailored to the practice setting and patient population, taking into consideration patient education level and cultural competence. Whether the pedigree or questionnaire is used, it is important to review and update the family history periodically for new diagnoses within the family and throughout pregnancy as appropriate.

Prepregnancy Nutritional Counseling

Consumption of a balanced diet with the appropriate distribution of the basic food pyramid groups is especially important during pregnancy. Diet can be affected by food preferences, cultural beliefs, and eating patterns. A woman who has special dietary restrictions will require special dietary measures as well as vitamin and mineral supplements. Women who frequently diet to lose weight, fast, skip meals, or have eating disorders or unusual eating habits should be identified and counseled. Additional risk factors for nutritional problems include adolescence, tobacco and substance use, history of pica during a previous pregnancy, high parity, and mental illness. Finally, the patient's access to food and the ability to purchase food should be ascertained.

Optimal control of obesity begins before pregnancy. Weight loss before pregnancy, achieved by surgical or nonsurgical methods, has been shown to be the most effective intervention to improve medical comorbidities. Obese women who have even small weight reductions before pregnancy may have improved pregnancy outcomes. Motivational interviewing techniques involve an individualized, patient-centered approach toward exploring and resolving ambivalence. The goal of motivational interviewing is to help patients move through the stages of dealing with unhealthy behavior. Motivational interviewing has been used successfully within the clinical setting to promote weight loss, dietary modification, and exercise. Although achieving a normal body mass index (BMI) is the ideal, a weight loss of 5–7% over time can significantly improve metabolic health. The U.S. Preventive Services Task Force recommends that all adults aged 18 years and older with a BMI of 30 or greater be offered or referred to intensive multicomponent behavior interventions. Obese women should be advised regarding their increased risk of adverse perinatal outcomes, including spontaneous abortion, stillbirth, preterm delivery, diabetes, cesarean delivery, hypertensive disease, and thromboembolic disease. Nutrition consultation and encouragement to undertake a weight-reduction program should be offered to overweight and obese women. An exercise program that leads to an eventual goal of moderate-intensity exercise for at least 20–30 minutes per day on most or all days of the week should be developed with the patient and adjusted as medically indicated.

Dietary supplements, including folic acid, are particularly important during the prepregnancy period. Folic acid supplementation is recommended for all reproductive-aged women and is especially important during prepregnancy and pregnancy, because the amount of folic acid in fortified grain products in the United States may be less than the amount recommended to prevent NTDs. In light of this, the U.S. Preventive Services Task Force recommends that all women who are planning or able to become pregnant take a daily supplement containing 400–800 micrograms of folic acid. Similarly, the Centers for Disease Prevention and Control (CDC) and the U.S. Public Health Service recommend the daily intake of 400 micrograms of folic acid, and the CDC urges women to start this daily intake at least 1 month before getting pregnant in order to reduce the risk of NTDs by 50–70%. Women planning a pregnancy who have previously had a fetus or baby with an NTD should be advised to follow the 1991 U.S. Public Health Service guideline, which recommends the daily consumption of 4,000 micrograms (4 mg) of folic acid beginning 1 month before trying to become pregnant and continuing through the first 3 months of pregnancy. This dosage should be prescribed by the health care provider.

Assisted Reproductive Therapy

Over the past decades, the use of assisted reproductive technology (ART) has increased dramatically worldwide and has made pregnancy possible for many infertile couples. The American Society for Reproductive Medicine defines ART as treatments and procedures involving the handling of human oocytes and sperm, or embryos, with the intent of establishing a pregnancy.

Perinatal risks that may be associated with ART and ovulation induction include multifetal gestations, prematurity, low birth weight, small for gestational age, perinatal mortality, cesarean delivery, placenta previa, abruptio placentae, preeclampsia, and birth defects. Although these risks are much higher in multifetal gestations, even singletons achieved with ART and ovulation induction may be at higher risk of these outcomes than singletons achieved spontaneously—although it remains unclear to what extent these associations might be related to the underlying cause(s) of infertility.

With both ART and ovulation induction, higher-order multifetal pregnancy may occur. Multifetal pregnancy and its associated outcomes are the greatest risk of ART and ovulation induction and, consequently, every effort should be made to achieve a singleton gestation. These efforts include following professional society guidelines for number of embryos to be transferred, such as those from the American Society of Reproductive Medicine, and continuing to encourage and expand use of single embryo transfer. Patients and couples should be counseled about the risks of multifetal gestation with these techniques.

Before initiating ART or ovulation induction procedures, clinicians should complete a thorough medical evaluation to ensure that patients are in good health and counsel these women about the risks associated with treatment. Any maternal health problems or inherited conditions should be addressed. Couples at risk of passing genetic conditions on to their offspring, including those due to infertility-associated conditions, should be counseled appropriately.

When a higher-order (triplet or more) multifetal pregnancy is encountered, the option of multifetal reduction should be discussed. In the case of a continuing higher-order multifetal pregnancy, ongoing obstetric care should be with providers and at facilities capable of managing anticipated risks and outcomes.

Bibliography

Adolescent pregnancy, contraception, and sexual activity. Committee Opinion No. 699. American College of Obstetricians and Gynecologists. Obstet Gynecol 2017; 129:e142–9.

American College of Obstetricians and Gynecologists. Access to reproductive health care for women with disabilities. In: Special issues in women's health. Washington, DC: ACOG; 2005. p. 39–59.

At-risk drinking and alcohol dependence: obstetric and gynecologic implications. Committee Opinion No. 496. American College of Obstetricians and Gynecologists. Obstet Gynecol 2011;118:383–8.

Atrash HK, Johnson K, Adams M, Cordero JF, Howse J. Preconception care for improving perinatal outcomes: the time to act. Matern Child Health J 2006;10:S3–11.

Carrier screening for genetic conditions. Committee Opinion No. 691. American College of Obstetricians and Gynecologists. Obstet Gynecol 2017;129:e41–55.

Counseling and interventions to prevent tobacco use and tobacco-caused disease in adults and pregnant women: U.S. Preventive Services Task Force reaffirmation recommendation statement. U.S. Preventive Services Task Force. Ann Intern Med 2009;150:551–5.

Cunniff C, Hudgins L. Prenatal genetic screening and diagnosis for pediatricians. Curr Opin Pediatr 2010;22:809–13.

Exposure to toxic environmental agents. Committee Opinion No. 575. American College of Obstetricians and Gynecologists. Obstet Gynecol 2013;122:931–5.

Family history as a risk assessment tool. Committee Opinion No. 478. American College of Obstetricians and Gynecologists. Obstet Gynecol 2011;117:747–50.

Fiore MC, Jaen CR, Baker TB, Bailey WC, Benowitz NL, Curry SJ, et al. Treating tobacco use and dependence: 2008 update. Clinical Practice Guideline. Rockville (MD): U.S. Department of Health and Human Services; 2008. Available at: https://www.ahrq.gov/sites/default/files/wysiwyg/professionals/clinicians-providers/guidelines-recommendations/tobacco/clinicians/update/treating_tobacco_use08.pdf. Retrieved June 12, 2017.

Genetics and molecular diagnostic testing. Technology Assessment No. 11. American College of Obstetricians and Gynecologists. Obstet Gynecol 2014;123:394–413.

Hook EB. Rates of chromosome abnormalities at different maternal ages. Obstet Gynecol 1981;58:282–5.

Informed consent. ACOG Committee Opinion No. 439. American College of Obstetricians and Gynecologists. Obstet Gynecol 2009;114:401–8.

Intimate partner violence. Committee Opinion No. 518. American College of Obstetricians and Gynecologists. Obstet Gynecol 2012;119:412–7.

March of Dimes. Toward improving the outcome of pregnancy III: enhancing perinatal health through quality, safety and performance initiatives. Committee on Perinatal Health. White Plains (NY): National Foundation—March of Dimes; 2010.

Methamphetamine abuse in women of reproductive age. Committee Opinion No. 479. American College of Obstetricians and Gynecologists. Obstet Gynecol 2011;117:751–5.

Morris JK, Wald NJ, Mutton DE, Alberman E. Comparison of models of maternal age-specific risk for Down Syndrome live births. Prenat Diagn 2003;23:252–8.

National Institute for Health and Care Excellence. Diabetes in pregnancy: management from preconception to the postnatal period. NICE Guideline NG3. London: NICE; 2015. Available at: https://www.nice.org.uk/guidance/ng3?unlid=634501629201610123565 5. Retrieved October 26, 2016.

Nonmedical use of prescription drugs. Committee Opinion No. 538. American College of Obstetricians and Gynecologists. Obstet Gynecol 2012;120:977–82.

Obesity in pregnancy. Practice Bulletin No. 156. American College of Obstetricians and Gynecologists. Obstet Gynecol 2015;126:e112–26.

Opioid abuse, dependence, and addiction in pregnancy. Committee Opinion No. 524. American College of Obstetricians and Gynecologists. Obstet Gynecol 2012;119:1070–6.

Otten JJ, Hellwig JP, Meyers LD, editors. DRI, Dietary Reference Intakes: the essential guide to nutrient requirements. Institute of Medicine. Washington, D.C.: National Academies Press; 2006.

Perinatal risks associated with assisted reproductive technology. Committee Opinion No. 671. American College of Obstetricians and Gynecologists. Obstet Gynecol 2016;128:e61–8.

Physical activity and exercise during pregnancy and the postpartum period. Committee Opinion No. 650. American College of Obstetricians and Gynecologists. Obstet Gynecol 2015;126:e135–42.

Prenatal and perinatal human immunodeficiency virus testing: expanded recommendations. Committee Opinion No. 635. American College of Obstetricians and Gynecologists. Obstet Gynecol 2015;125:1544–7.

Prenatal diagnostic testing for genetic disorders. Practice Bulletin No. 162. American College of Obstetricians and Gynecologists. Obstet Gynecol 2016;127:e108–22.

Reproductive life planning to reduce unintended pregnancy. Committee Opinion No. 654. American College of Obstetricians and Gynecologists. Obstet Gynecol 2016;127:e66–9.

Ross AC, Taylor CL, Yaktine AL, Del Valle HB, editors. Dietary Reference Intakes for Calcium and Vitamin D. Committee to Review Dietary Reference Intakes for Vitamin D and Calcium, Food and Nutrition Board, Institute of Medicine. Washington, D.C.: National Academies Press; 2011.

Routine human immunodeficiency virus screening. Committee Opinion No. 596. American College of Obstetricians and Gynecologists. Obstet Gynecol 2014;123: 1137–9.

Screening for fetal aneuploidy. Practice Bulletin No. 163. American College of Obstetricians and Gynecologists. Obstet Gynecol 2016;127:e123–37.

Siu AL. Behavioral and pharmacotherapy interventions for tobacco smoking cessation in adults, including pregnant women. U.S. Preventive Services Task Force Recommendation Statement. U.S. Preventive Services Task Force. Ann Intern Med 2015;163:622–34.

Smokefree.Gov. Bethesda (MD): NIH; 2016. Available at: https://smokefree.gov/talk-to-an-expert. Retrieved December 16, 2016.

The importance of preconception care in the continuum of women's health care. ACOG Committee Opinion No. 313. American College of Obstetricians and Gynecologists. Obstet Gynecol 2005;106:665–6.

The limits of conscientious refusal in reproductive medicine. ACOG Committee Opinion No. 385. American College of Obstetricians and Gynecologists. Obstet Gynecol 2007;110:1203–8.

Toriello HV, Meck JM. Statement on guidance for genetic counseling in advanced paternal age. Professional Practice and Guidelines Committee. Genet Med 2008;10:457–60.

U.S. Dept. of Health and Human Services. The health consequences of smoking: 50 years of progress. A report of the Surgeon General. Atlanta (GA): U.S. Department of Health and Human Services, Centers for Disease Control and Prevention, National Center for Chronic Disease Prevention and Health Promotion, Office on Smoking and Health; 2014. Available at: http://www.surgeongeneral.gov/library/reports/50-years-of-progress/full-report.pdf. Retrieved October 26, 2016.

Use of psychiatric medications during pregnancy and lactation. ACOG Practice Bulletin No. 92. American College of Obstetricians and Gynecologists. Obstet Gynecol 2008;111:1001–20.

Williams JF, Smith VC. Fetal alcohol spectrum disorders. Committee on Substance Abuse. Pediatrics 2015;136:e1395–406.

Resources

American College of Obstetricians and Gynecologists. Genetics. Washington, DC: American College of Obstetricians and Gynecologists; 2017. Available at: http://www.acog.org/About-ACOG/ACOG-Departments/Genetics. Retrieved March 6, 2017.

American College of Obstetricians and Gynecologists. Immunization for women. Washington, DC: American College of Obstetricians and Gynecologists; 2016. Available at: http://immunizationforwomen.org. Retrieved October 26, 2016.

American Psychiatric Association (APA). Arlington (VA): APA; 2016. Available at: https://www.psychiatry.org. Retrieved October 26, 2016.

Centers for Disease Control and Prevention. Preconception health and health care. Atlanta (GA): CDC; 2016. Available at: https://www.cdc.gov/preconception/index.html. Retrieved October 26, 2016.

Centers for Disease Control and Prevention. Preconception health and health care. Atlanta (GA): CDC; 2017. Available at: https://www.cdc.gov/preconception/index.html. Retrieved March 6, 2017.

Centers for Disease Control and Prevention. Reproductive life plan tool for health professionals: Atlanta (GA): CDC; 2014. Available at: https://www.cdc.gov/preconception/rlptool.html. Retrieved March 6, 2017.

Centers for Disease Control and Prevention. Vaccines and immunizations. Atlanta (GA): CDC; 2016. Available at: http://www.cdc.gov/vaccines. Retrieved October 26, 2016.

Fetal alcohol spectrum disorders. Chicago, IL: American Academy of Pediatrics; 2015. Available at: http://pediatrics.aappublications.org/content/early/2015/10/13/peds.2015-3113.abstract?sid=22f04c16-1473-4774-b2a3-cb6b53934fd4.

Institute for Patient- and Family-Centered Care. Bethesda (MD): IPFCC; 2016. Available at: http://www.ipfcc.org. Retrieved September 21, 2016.

National Center for Complementary and Integrative Health. National Institutes of Health. Bethesda (MD): NIH; 2016. Available at: https://nccih.nih.gov. Retrieved October 26, 2016.

National Heart, Lung, and Blood Institute. Aim for a healthy weight. Calculate your body mass index. BMI calculator. Bethesda (MD): NHLBI; 2016. Available at: http://www.nhlbi.nih.gov/health/educational/lose_wt/BMI/bmicalc.htm. Retrieved October 26, 2016.

March of Dimes. Planning your pregnancy. White Plains (NY): March of Dimes; 2017. Available at: http://www.marchofdimes.org/pregnancy/planning-your-pregnancy.aspx. Retrieved March 6, 2017.

March of Dimes. Toward improving the outcome of pregnancy: the 90s and beyond. Committee on Perinatal Health. White Plains (NY): National Foundation—March of Dimes; 1993.

McKusick-Nathans Institute of Genetic Medicine. Online Mendelian inheritance in man (OMIM). Baltimore (MD): Johns Hopkins University School of Medicine; 2016. Available at: http://www.omim.org. Retrieved October 26, 2016.

Organization of Teratology Information Services. MotherToBaby: medications and more during pregnancy and breastfeeding. Brentwood (TN): OTIS; 2010; 2016. Available at: http://mothertobaby.org. Retrieved October 26, 2016.

Organization of Teratology Information Specialists. MotherToBaby fact sheets. Brentwood (TN): OTIS; 2016. Available at: http://mothertobaby.org/fact-sheets-parent. Retrieved October 26, 2016.

Siu AL. Behavioral and pharmacotherapy interventions for tobacco smoking cessation in adults, including pregnant women. U.S. Preventive Services Task Force Recommendation Statement. U.S. Preventive Services Task Force. Ann Intern Med 2015;163:622–34.

Toxic Environmental Agents. Washington, DC: American College of Obstetricians and Gynecologists; 2016. Available at: http://www.acog.org/toxicchemicals. Retrieved December 16, 2016.

U.S. Department of Agriculture, United States Department of Health and Human Services. 2015–2020 dietary guidelines for Americans. 8th ed. Washington, D.C.: U.S. Dept. of Agriculture; U.S. Dept. of Health and Human Services; 2015. Available at: https://health.gov/dietaryguidelines/2015/resources/2015-2020_Dietary_Guidelines.pdf. Retrieved October 26, 2016.

Chapter 6

Antepartum Care

A comprehensive antepartum care program involves a coordinated approach to medical care, continuous risk assessment, and psychosocial support that optimally begins before pregnancy and extends throughout the postpartum and interpregnancy period. Health care professionals should integrate the concept of family-centered care into antepartum care (see also "Patient-Centered and Family-Centered Health Care" in Chapter 1). Care includes an assessment of the expectant mother's attitude toward her pregnancy (as well as the family's attitudes, if this is so desired by the expectant mother), the support systems available, and the need for parenting education. To the extent it is desired by the expectant mother, she and her family should be encouraged to work with her caregivers in order to make well-informed decisions about pregnancy, labor, delivery, the postpartum period, and the interpregnancy period. The health care team should assess the level of support for each woman and refer her appropriately to agencies if she does not have a spouse, partner, or other individuals with whom to share this experience and to provide support.

Women who receive early and regular prenatal care are more likely to have healthy infants. Prenatal care includes a process of ongoing risk identification and assessment in order to develop appropriate care plans. This plan of care should take into consideration the medical, nutritional, psychosocial, cultural, and educational needs of the patient, and it should be periodically reevaluated and revised in accordance with the progress of the pregnancy. Obstetrician–gynecologists and other obstetric care providers of antepartum care should be able to either primarily provide or easily refer to others to provide a wide array of services. These services include the following:

- Readily available and regularly scheduled obstetric care, beginning in early pregnancy and continuing through the postpartum period
- Access to unscheduled visits or emergency visits on a 24-hour basis. Timing of access varies depending on the nature of the problem

- Timely transmittal of prenatal records to the site of the woman's planned delivery so that her records are readily accessible at the time of delivery. The use of electronic medical records should facilitate this.
- Medical interpretation services (exclusive of family members) for women with limited English language ability
- Referral network of reliable, competent, culturally sensitive, accessible social service, mental health, and specialist medical care providers.

Prenatal Care Visits

The first visit for prenatal care typically occurs in the first trimester. The frequency of follow-up visits is determined by the individual needs of the woman and an assessment of her risks.

Frequency

The frequency of obstetric visits should be individualized. Women with poor pregnancy outcomes in earlier pregnancies, known medical problems, vaginal bleeding before initiation of routine prenatal care, and those who achieved a pregnancy through infertility treatments and are known to be carrying multiple gestations should be seen as early as possible.

Typically, a woman with an uncomplicated first pregnancy is examined every 4 weeks for the first 28 weeks of gestation, every 2 weeks until 36 weeks of gestation, and weekly thereafter. Women with medical or obstetric problems, as well as women at the extremes of reproductive age, will likely require closer surveillance; the appropriate intervals between scheduled visits are determined by the nature and severity of the problems (see also Appendix B and Appendix C). Likewise, parous women with prior normal pregnancy outcomes and without medical and obstetric problems during the current pregnancy may be able to be seen less frequently as long as additional visits on an as-needed basis are available.

The frequency and regularity of scheduled prenatal visits should be sufficient to enable health care providers to accomplish the following activities:

- Assess the well-being of the woman and her fetus
- Provide ongoing, timely, and relevant prenatal education
- Complete recommended health screening studies and review results
- Detect medical and psychosocial issues and institute indicated interventions
- Reassure the woman

First Visit

Unless there was a recent prepregnancy visit, risk assessment and patient education are initiated at the first prenatal visit, at which time the obstetrician–gynecologist begins to compile obstetric information. Appendix A contains a format for documenting information and the database recommended by the American College of Obstetricians and Gynecologists (ACOG). Whatever format is used, the record should display the data in a longitudinal manner clearly and concisely to prompt the obstetrician–gynecologist to complete the appropriate evaluations and screening steps, and to communicate the results in a clear fashion to the users of the chart.

During the first prenatal visit, the following general information should be discussed with each woman:

- Scope of care that is provided
- Laboratory studies and their indications
- Expected course of the pregnancy
- Signs and symptoms to be reported to the health care team and how to report them
- Role of the members of the health care team
- Anticipated schedule of visits
- Physician or midwife schedule and labor and delivery coverage
- Cost to the patient of prenatal care and delivery; patients should be encouraged to discuss this with their insurer and specific plan
- Practices to promote health maintenance (eg, use of safety restraints, including lap and shoulder belts)
- Risk counseling, including substance use and substance use disorders
- Psychosocial topics in pregnancy and the postpartum period
- Review of family history and genetic testing options

Patient education early in pregnancy also includes specialized counseling on topics, such as nutrition, exercise, nausea and vomiting, vitamin and mineral toxicity, teratogens, dental care, working, and air travel (see also "First-Trimester Patient Education" later in this chapter).

For women who have had past pregnancies, a history of prior pregnancies should be reviewed including outcomes and complications. This will allow health care providers to anticipate recurrent complications and consider appropriate surveillance and screening, or treatment, or both, to minimize the risk of recurrent complications. Examples of such conditions that may be highlighted by review of past obstetric history include:

- Prior preterm delivery: treatment with intramuscular progesterone beginning in the second trimester is recommended for women with a history of prior spontaneous preterm birth or preterm premature rupture of membranes (also known as prelabor rupture of membranes).
- Previous preeclampsia: treatment with low-dose (81 mg) aspirin may reduce risk of recurrence and is recommended in women who are considered to be at high risk of preeclampsia. This includes women with a history of early-onset preeclampsia, especially if accompanied by an adverse outcome; multifetal gestation; chronic hypertension; diabetes (type 1 or type 2); renal disease; or autoimmune disease (such as systematic lupus erythematosus, antiphospholipid syndrome).
- Prior gestational diabetes: screening for glucose intolerance is suggested early in pregnancy for women with a history of prior gestational diabetes.
- Prior midtrimester loss or cervical insufficiency: a history of a midtrimester loss may indicate a need to consider cervical cerclage (see Box 6-1).

BOX 6-1. Indications for Cervical Cerclage in Women With Singleton Pregnancies

History

- History of one or more second-trimester pregnancy losses related to painless cervical dilation and in the absence of labor or abruptio placentae
- Prior cerclage due to painless cervical dilation in the second trimester

Physical Examination

- Painless cervical dilation in the second trimester

Ultrasonographic Finding With a History of Prior Preterm Birth

Current singleton pregnancy, prior spontaneous preterm birth at less than 34 weeks of gestation, and short cervical length (less than 25 mm) before 24 weeks of gestation.

As carrier screening becomes more prevalent, it will be important to determine if patients have been screened previously for specific disorders to avoid repeat screens and unnecessary costs. Although screening technology inevitably will advance over time, carrier screening for a specific genetic condition, in general, should be performed only once in a person's lifetime. The decision to rescreen a patient should be undertaken only with the guidance of a genetics professional who can best assess the incremental benefit of repeat testing for additional mutations.

Routine Visits

During each regularly scheduled visit, the obstetrician–gynecologist or other obstetric care provider should evaluate the woman's blood pressure, weight, uterine size for progressive growth and consistency with the estimated due date (EDD), and presence of fetal heart activity at appropriate gestational ages. After the woman reports quickening and at each subsequent visit, she should be asked about fetal movement. She should be queried about contractions, leakage of fluid, or vaginal bleeding. The time-honored inclusion of routine urine dipstick assessment for all pregnant women can be modified according to site-specific protocols. A baseline screen for urine protein content to assess renal status is recommended. However, in the absence of risk factors for urinary tract infections, renal disease, and preeclampsia and in the absence of symptoms of urinary tract infection, hypertension, or unusual edema, there has not been shown to be a benefit in routine urine dip-stick testing.

Later in pregnancy, important topics to discuss during routine visits include childbirth education classes, choosing a newborn care provider, anticipating labor, preterm labor, options for intrapartum care, umbilical cord banking, breastfeeding, choice of a postpartum contraception method, and preparation for hospital discharge (see also "Second-Trimester and Third-Trimester Patient Education" later in this chapter). Immediate postpartum long-acting reversible contraception (LARC) should be offered as an effective option for postpartum contraception for most women, and women should be counseled about the convenience and effectiveness of immediate postpartum LARC, as well as the benefits of reducing unintended pregnancy and lengthening interpregnancy intervals. They also should be counseled about the increased risk of expulsion, including unrecognized expulsion, with immediate postpartum intrauterine device insertion compared with interval intrauterine device insertion, contraindications, and alternatives to allow for informed decision making.

Group Prenatal Care

Group, or shared, medical visits have been used in a variety of medical settings and have been associated with improved health outcomes. Currently, there are several models of group prenatal care that show promise.

In group prenatal care, health care providers deliver prenatal health services and information to groups of women during regularly scheduled shared visits. The group visits are begun after the first prenatal assessment and physical examination, and groups usually are composed of women with similar estimated delivery dates. The typical group visit includes 8–12 women and usually lasts 1–2 hours. The visit typically begins with physical assessments, (including fundal height measurements), assessment of fetal heart tones, maternal–fetal well-being questions, and appropriate testing. Individual issues may be raised at this time. The physical assessment is followed by an informational group discussion facilitated by an obstetrician–gynecologist, a certified nurse–midwife, or a family medicine practitioner. Health care providers are assisted by a variety of other health care professionals, who may serve as a co-facilitator or a guest for a specific topic. Visits are billed as traditional prenatal visits.

The group model is a promising innovation in prenatal care delivery and has been shown in some studies to improve preparation for childbirth, reduce the incidence of preterm delivery, and increase rates of breastfeeding initiation. Additional research and evaluation of patient outcomes to confirm benefit are needed. Practitioners need to approach group prenatal care with deliberate planning and research. Resources are available in the literature as well as on the internet.

Routine Antepartum Care

Determining Gestational Age

An accurately assigned estimated due date (EDD) is among the most important results of evaluation and history taking early in prenatal care. This information is vital for timing of appropriate obstetric care, scheduling and interpretation of certain antepartum tests, determining the appropriateness of fetal growth, and designing interventions to prevent preterm births, post-term births, and related morbidities. A consistent and exacting approach to accurate dating is also a research and public health imperative because of the influence of dating on investigational protocols and vital statistics. There is great utility in using a single, uniform standard within and between institutions that have access to high-quality ultrasonography (as most, if not all, U.S. obstetric facilities do). Accordingly, in creating recommendations and the associated summary table (Table 6-1) single-point cutoffs were chosen based on expert review.

The American College of Obstetricians and Gynecologists, the American Institute of Ultrasound in Medicine, and the Society for Maternal–Fetal Medicine make the following recommendations regarding the method for estimating gestational age and due date:

- Ultrasound measurement of the embryo or fetus in the first trimester (up to and including 13 6/7 weeks of gestation) is the most accurate method to establish or confirm gestational age.
- If pregnancy resulted from assisted reproductive technology, the assisted reproductive technology-derived gestational age should be used to assign the EDD. For instance, the EDD for a pregnancy resulting from in vitro fertilization should be established using the age of the embryo and the date of transfer.
- As soon as data from the last menstrual period (LMP), the first accurate ultrasound examination, or both, are obtained, the gestational age and the EDD should be determined, discussed with the patient, and documented clearly in the medical record. Subsequent changes to the EDD should be reserved for rare circumstances, discussed with the patient, and documented clearly in the medical record.

When determined from the methods outlined in this document for estimating the due date, gestational age at delivery represents the best obstetric estimate for the purpose of clinical care and should be recorded on the birth certificate. For the purposes of research and surveillance, the best obstetric estimate, rather than estimates based on the LMP alone, should be used as the measure for gestational age.

Pregnancies *without* an ultrasound assessment confirming or revising the EDD before 22 0/7 weeks of gestational age should be considered suboptimally dated. In a woman with a suboptimally dated pregnancy:

- The timing of delivery should be based on the best clinical estimate of gestational age.
- There is no role for elective delivery.
- Amniocentesis for fetal lung maturity is not recommended as a routine component of decision making when considering the delivery.

- During the antenatal care, it is reasonable to consider an interval ultrasonographic assessment of fetal weight and gestational age 3–4 weeks after the initial ultrasonographic study. Although this follow-up examination is intended to support the working gestational age, interval fetal growth assessment potentially may detect cases of fetal growth restriction.
- Given a concern that a full-term or late-term suboptimally dated pregnancy could actually be weeks further along than it is believed to be, initiation of antepartum fetal surveillance at 39 weeks of gestation may be considered.

TABLE 6-1. Guidelines for Redating Based on Ultrasonography

Gestational Age Range*	Method of Measurement	Discrepancy Between Ultrasound Dating and LMP Dating That Supports Redating
≤13 6/7 wk	CRL	
• ≤ 8 6/7 wk		More than 5 d
• 9 0/7 wk to 13 6/7 wk		More than 7 d
14 0/7 wk to 15 6/7 wk	BPD, HC, AC, FL	More than 7 d
16 0/7 wk to 21 6/7 wk	BPD, HC, AC, FL	More than 10 d
22 0/7 wk to 27 6/7 wk	BPD, HC, AC, FL	More than 14 d
28 0/7 wk and beyond†	BPD, HC, AC, FL	More than 21 d

Abbreviations: AC, abdominal circumference; BPD, biparietal diameter; CRL, crown–rump length; FL, femur length; HC, head circumference; LMP, last menstrual period.

*Based on last menstrual period.

†Because of the risk of redating a small fetus that may be growth restricted, management decisions based on third-trimester ultrasonography alone are especially problematic and need to be guided by careful consideration of the entire clinical picture and close surveillance.

Fetal Ultrasound Imaging

Ultrasonography is the most commonly used fetal imaging tool and is an accurate method of determining gestational age, fetal number, viability, and placental location. Ultrasonography should be performed by technologists or physicians who have undergone specific training and only when there is a valid medical indication for the examination. Physicians who perform, evaluate, and interpret diagnostic obstetric ultrasound examinations need to be licensed medical practitioners with an understanding of the indications for such imaging studies, the expected content of a complete obstetric ultrasound examination, and a familiarity with the limitations of ultrasound imaging. A physician is responsible for the interpretation of all studies; ultrasonographers may not interpret the studies nor bill for them.

At various gestational ages, ultrasound examination is an accurate method of determining gestational age, fetal number, viability, and placental location, and it is recommended for all pregnant patients. The timing and type of ultrasonography performed should be such that the clinical question being asked is answered. In order to select the best time for a particular woman to receive her scan, health care providers must balance the types and accuracy of information to be gained at different gestational ages with the financial reality of limitations to the number of scans many insurance carriers will pay for. In the absence of other specific indications, the optimal time for a single ultrasound examination is at 18–22 weeks of gestation. In the obese patient, expectations regarding visualization of fetal anatomy should be tempered.

Each type of ultrasound examination should be performed only when indicated and should be appropriately documented. A first-trimester ultrasound examination is performed before 14 0/7 weeks of gestation. Scanning in the first trimester can be performed transabdominally or transvaginally. Some indications for performing first-trimester ultrasound examinations are listed in Box 6-2. Second-trimester and third-trimester ultrasound examinations include the following three types:

1. Standard—Evaluation of fetal presentation, amniotic fluid volume, cardiac activity, placental position, fetal biometry, and fetal number, plus an anatomic survey.
2. Limited—A limited examination is performed when a specific question, such as fetal presentation or amniotic volume assessment, requires investigation.

3. Specialized—A detailed or targeted anatomic examination is performed when an anomaly is suspected on the basis of history, laboratory abnormalities, or the results of the limited examination or standard examination.

Women with an abnormal fetal ultrasound examination result should be referred for evaluation and management to a health care provider who can accurately and thoroughly assess the fetus, communicate the findings to the patient and health care provider, and coordinate further management if needed. The care of a multidisciplinary team may be helpful. Some conditions may require the involvement of a maternal–fetal medicine subspecialist, geneticist, pediatrician, neonatologist, anesthesiologist, or other medical specialist in the evaluation, counseling, and care of the woman. Relationships with appropriate maternal–fetal care specialists should be developed.

Fetal Magnetic Resonance Imaging

If additional imaging modalities are required, magnetic resonance imaging (MRI) may be chosen. Unlike computed tomography, MRI does not involve

BOX 6-2. Indications for First-Trimester Ultrasonography

- To confirm the presence of an intrauterine pregnancy
- To evaluate a suspected ectopic pregnancy
- To evaluate vaginal bleeding
- To evaluate pelvic pain
- To estimate gestational age
- To diagnosis or evaluate multiple gestations
- To confirm cardiac activity
- As adjunct to chorionic villus sampling, embryo transfer, or localization and removal of an intrauterine device
- To assess for certain fetal anomalies, such as anencephaly, in patients at high risk
- To evaluate maternal pelvic or adnexal masses or uterine abnormalities
- To screen for fetal aneuploidy
- To evaluate suspected hydatidiform mole

Data from American College of Radiology. ACR-ACOG-AIUM-SRU practice parameter for the performance of obstetrical ultrasound. ACR Resolution 17. Reston (VA): ACR; 2013. Available at: http://www.acr.org/~/media/f7bc35bd59264e7cbe648f6d1bb8b8e2.pdf. Retrieved October 28, 2016.

radiation exposure. The most common use of MRI is to further delineate a fetal anomaly or to further evaluate abnormal placentation in selected cases.

Routine Laboratory Testing in Pregnancy

Certain laboratory tests are performed routinely in pregnant women in order to identify conditions that may affect the outcome of the pregnancy for the mother or fetus. The results of these tests should be reviewed in a timely manner, communicated to the woman, and documented in the medical record. Abnormal test results prompt some action on the part of the health care provider.

The Centers for Disease Control and Prevention (CDC) recommends screening all pregnant women for human immunodeficiency virus (HIV), hepatitis B, syphilis, and chlamydial infection during the first prenatal visit. In addition, the CDC recommends that, when indicated, pregnant women should be screened for *Neisseria gonorrhoeae* at the first prenatal visit. Women at a high risk of tuberculosis also should be screened early in pregnancy. Other laboratory tests that are routinely performed early in pregnancy are listed in Table 6-2 and Appendix A. Table 6-2 also suggests actions to

TABLE 6-2. Routine Laboratory Tests Early in Pregnancy

Laboratory Test	Potential Actions for Abnormal Results
Blood type	There is no abnormal result here. Blood type is documented for information only, should urgent blood transfusion be necessary at a later time and in order to communicate to the pediatric care provider the risk of ABO blood incompatibility in the neonatal period.
D (Rh) type	Patients who are Rh negative are at risk of developing isoimmunization to D antigen. Further steps depend on results of the antibody screening. Weak rhesus-positive (formerly Du-positive) patients are not at risk of isoimmunization.
Antibody screen	Any positive antibody test result requires obtaining a titer and further action by the health care provider.
Complete blood count (Hematocrit/hemoglobin for iron deficiency, or treated with supplemental iron, or both MCV and platelets)	Women with microcytic anemia should be evaluated further and retested in 3–4 weeks. Women who are of African descent, Asian, or Mediterranean should have a hemoglobin electrophoresis test performed to rule out thalassemia or sickle cell disease. Further testing may be warranted pending the results of these interventions and tests.

(continued)

TABLE 6-2. Routine Laboratory Tests Early in Pregnancy *(continued)*

Laboratory Test	Potential Actions for Abnormal Results
VDRL/RPR (nontreponemal tests)	Evaluate to confirm active syphilis status with treatment as needed. False-negative serologic test results may occur in early primary infection, and infection after the first prenatal visit is possible. False-positive nontreponemal test results can be associated with various medical conditions unrelated to syphilis; therefore, persons with a reactive VDRL or RPR test result should receive a treponemal test to confirm the diagnosis of syphilis.
Urine culture (if performed)	Treat asymptomatic bacteriuria and then do a test of cure*. If results are positive for GBS bacteriuria, document this on the patient's chart and do not perform third-trimester GBS screening but administer prophylactic antibiotics in labor instead.
Urine screening	Obtain baseline screening for urine protein content (dipstick) to assess renal status.
HBsAg	If positive, counsel patient regarding her health risks; document clearly in the chart so that the infant's physicians know to treat the infant with hepatitis B vaccination and hepatitis B immune globulin.
HIV counseling/testing	Affirm your state's laws. If the patient is HIV positive, counsel and refer her to an infectious disease clinic or maternal–fetal medicine specialist for further management. Discuss safe-sex practices.
Chlamydia	Women found to have chlamydial infection during the first trimester should be retested within approximately 3–6 months, preferably in the third trimester.
Gonorrhea (when indicated)	Pregnant women found to have gonococcal infection during the first trimester should be retested within approximately 3–6 months, preferably in the third trimester. Uninfected pregnant women who remain at high risk for gonococcal infection also should be retested during the third trimester.
Mantoux tuberculin skin test or interferon-gamma release assay (when indicated)	Women with a positive or intermediate test result should be evaluated with a chest X-ray and review of their pertinent history to determine the need for additional evaluation.

Abbreviations: GBS, group B streptococci; HBsAg, hepatitis B surface antigen; HIV, human immunodeficiency virus; MCV, mean corpuscular volume; RPR, rapid plasma reagin; VDRL, venereal disease research laboratory.

*In this case, test of cure refers to retesting the patient's urine after completion of antibiotic therapy to determine if the bacteria have been eliminated. Although this practice is recommended in the literature, more data are needed to determine the effectiveness of this strategy.

be considered if results are abnormal. Recommended intervals for additional tests that are indicated after the first prenatal visit are detailed in ACOG's Antepartum Record (see also Appendix A). A more detailed explanation of the CDC recommendations is provided as follows:

- *Human immunodeficiency virus*—Testing for HIV infection, with patient notification, should be part of the routine battery of prenatal blood tests unless a woman declines the test (ie, opt-out approach), as permitted by local and state regulations. Refusal of testing should be documented. In some states, it is necessary to obtain the woman's written authorization before disclosing her HIV status to health care providers who are not members of her health care team (see also "Human Immunodeficiency Virus" in Chapter 12). Women at high risk of HIV infection (eg, women who use nonmedical drugs, have sexually transmitted infections during pregnancy, have multiple sex partners during pregnancy, live in areas with high HIV prevalence, or have HIV-infected partners) should be retested during the third trimester, ideally before 36 weeks of gestation. Testing of women with unknown HIV status using rapid HIV testing in labor and delivery is recommended, and repeat testing in women from high-HIV-prevalent areas should be considered. State laws vary and should be followed.
- *Hepatitis B*—All pregnant women should be routinely tested for hepatitis B surface antigen during the first trimester, even if they have been previously vaccinated or tested. Women who were not screened prenatally, those who engage in behavior that put them at high risk of infection (eg, having had more than one sex partner in the previous 6 months, evaluation or treatment for an STI, recent or current injection-drug use, and a hepatitis B surface antigen-positive sex partner), and those with clinical hepatitis should be retested at the time of admission to the hospital for delivery. Pregnant women at risk of hepatitis B infection also should be vaccinated (see also "Hepatitis B Virus" in Chapter 12).
- *Syphilis*—A serologic test for syphilis should be performed on all pregnant women at the first prenatal visit. Women who are at high risk of syphilis, live in areas of high syphilis morbidity, or are previously untested need to be screened again early in the third trimester (at approximately 28 weeks of gestation) and at delivery, as well as after exposure to an infected partner. Some states require all women to be

screened at delivery. Any woman who gives birth to a stillborn fetus should be tested for syphilis (see also "Syphilis" in Chapter 12).

- *Chlamydial infection*—The CDC recommends that all pregnant women be routinely screened for *Chlamydia trachomatis* during the first prenatal visit. Women 25 years or younger and those at increased risk of chlamydia (eg, women who have a new sex partner or more than one sex partner) should be retested during the third trimester to prevent maternal postnatal complications and chlamydial infection in the infant. Women found to have chlamydial infection during the first trimester should be retested within approximately 3–6 months, preferably in the third trimester (see also "Chlamydial Infection" in Chapter 12).
- *Gonorrhea*—All pregnant women at risk of gonorrhea or living in an area in which the prevalence of *N gonorrhoeae* is high should be screened for *N gonorrhoeae* at the first prenatal visit. Women 25 years or younger are at highest risk of gonorrhea infection as are those living in a high morbidity area. Other risk factors for gonorrhea include a previous infection of gonorrhea, other STIs, new or multiple sex partners, inconsistent condom use, commercial sex work, and drug use. Pregnant women found to have gonococcal infection during the first trimester should be retested within approximately 3–6 months, preferably in the third trimester. Uninfected pregnant women who remain at high risk of gonorrhea also should be retested during the third trimester (see also "Gonorrhea" in Chapter 12).
- *Tuberculosis*—Women at high risk of tuberculosis (TB) should be screened early in pregnancy with a TB skin test. A TB blood test (also called interferon-gamma release assays) is also available and preferred for people who have received the TB vaccine bacillus Calmette–Guérin (BCG) or for people who have a difficult time returning for a second appointment to look for a reaction to the skin test. Screening women at low risk is not indicated. High risk factors include the following:
  - Known HIV infection
  - Close contact with individuals known or suspected to have TB
  - Medical risk factors known to increase the risk of disease if infected (such as diabetes, lupus, cancer, alcoholism, and drug addiction)
  - Birth in or emigration from high-prevalent countries
  - Being medically underserved

  - — Homelessness
  - — Living or working in long-term care facilities, such as correctional institutions, mental health institutions, and nursing homes

  The Mantoux tuberculin skin test should be used and read by a health care professional within 48–72 hours, although it can be accurately read up to 7 days after application. In the United States, induration (not erythema) measuring greater than 10 mm in diameter is a positive test result except in patients who have HIV, have received an organ transplant, are immunosuppressed, or have had recent close contact with others with infectious TB; in these individuals, induration greater than 5 mm is a positive test result. A positive TB blood test means that the person has been infected with TB bacteria. Although the patient does not have to return to have the test read, additional tests are needed to determine if the person has latent TB or TB disease. A positive or intermediate test result should be evaluated by obtaining three induced sputum cultures or with a chest X-ray.

- *Antibody testing*—Antibody tests should be obtained at the time of the first prenatal visit; a woman who is unsensitized and D-negative should receive anti-D immune globulin at the time of any of the following:
  - — Ectopic gestation
  - — Abortion (either threatened, spontaneous, or induced)
  - — Procedures associated with possible fetal-to-maternal bleeding, such as chorionic villus sampling (CVS) or amniocentesis
  - — Conditions associated with fetal–maternal hemorrhage (eg, abdominal trauma or abruptio placentae)
  - — Unexplained vaginal bleeding during pregnancy
  - — Delivery of a newborn who is D-positive. Antibody testing should be repeated in unsensitized, D-negative women at 28–29 weeks of gestation. These women also should receive anti-D immune globulin at a dose of 300 micrograms prophylactically at that time

- *Diabetes mellitus screening*—All pregnant women should be screened for gestational diabetes mellitus (GDM) with a laboratory-based screening test(s) using blood glucose levels. Glucose screening is performed at 24–28 weeks of gestation and can be done in the fasting state or fed state. A 50-g oral glucose challenge test is given followed in 1 hour by a plasma test for glucose level. Different screening thresholds (ranging from 130 mg/dL to 140 mg/dL) are used, and women meeting or exceeding this threshold undergo a 100-g, 3-hour diagnostic oral glucose tolerance test (see also "Gestational Diabetes Mellitus Diagnosis and Management" in Chapter 9).

- *Group B streptococcal disease*—In its 2010 updated guidelines for the prevention of perinatal group B streptococcal disease (GBS), the CDC continues to recommend screening of all women at 35–37 weeks of gestation (see the complete recommendations at www.cdc.gov/groupbstrep/guidelines/guidelines.html). This includes women who are planning cesarean deliveries because onset of labor or rupture of membranes may occur before the recommended administration of prophylactic antibiotics. A single swab specimen (not by speculum examination) is obtained from the lower vagina (introitus) and rectum (through the anal sphincter) and placed in selective broth media. Women who have group B streptococcal bacteriuria during the current pregnancy or who have previously given birth to a newborn infant with early-onset GBS need not be cultured, but rather need to receive intrapartum prophylactic antibiotics. Because GBS carriage is intermittent, women who had GBS colonization during a previous pregnancy require culture evaluation for GBS with each pregnancy. These women do not need intrapartum prophylactic antibiotics unless there is an indication for GBS prophylaxis during the current pregnancy (see also "Bacterial Infections" in Chapter 12). Among those with a history of anaphylaxis to penicillin, sensitivities of any cultured GBS to erythromycin and clindamycin should be obtained to inform selection of alternated treatment regiments.

Antepartum Immunizations

A routine assessment of each pregnant woman's immunization status is recommended, with appropriate immunization if indicated. There is no evidence of risk from vaccinating pregnant women with an inactivated virus or bacterial vaccines or toxoids, and these should be administered, if indicated. Although perinatal harms related to live vaccines have not been demonstrated, they pose a theoretic risk to the fetus and generally should be avoided during pregnancy. The benefits of vaccines outweigh any unproven potential concerns about traces of thimerosal preservative. When deciding whether or not to immunize a pregnant woman with a vaccine not routinely recommended in pregnancy, the risk of exposure to disease as well as the benefits of vaccination for reducing the deleterious effects on the woman and the fetus should be balanced against unknown risks of vaccine exposure. All vaccines administered should be fully documented in the women's permanent medical record. Information on the safety of vaccines given during pregnancy is frequently updated and may be verified from the CDC website at www.cdc.gov/vaccines/index.html. Additional information on immunization during pregnancy can be found on the ACOG's Immunization for Women website, available at www.immunizationforwomen.org/.

The influenza vaccine is recommended to all women who will be pregnant during the influenza season, regardless of their stage of pregnancy. Pregnant women with medical conditions that increase their risk of complications from influenza such as asthma, diabetes, or immunodeficiency should be offered the vaccine before the influenza season. Administration of the injectable, inactivated influenza vaccine is considered safe at any stage of pregnancy. Because of theoretic risk, the live attenuated intranasal influenza vaccine should not be used in pregnant women.

Tetanus toxoid, reduced diphtheria toxoid, and acellular pertussis (Tdap) vaccination is recommended in pregnancy even if a woman has been previously vaccinated. To optimize transplacental transfer of protective antibodies, vaccination at 27–36 weeks of gestation is recommended. Vaccination is also recommended for other family members and planned direct caregivers for the newborn.

Other vaccines that are recommended in pregnancy include hepatitis A, hepatitis B, and pneumococcal (recommended for pregnant patients with prior splenectomy or functional asplenia). According to the CDC, pregnancy does not preclude vaccination with the meningococcal polysaccharide vaccine, if indicated. In studies of meningococcal vaccination with the meningococcal polysaccharide vaccine during pregnancy, adverse effects have not been documented in pregnant women or their newborn infants. However, no data are available on the safety of meningococcal conjugate vaccines during pregnancy.

Although the use of the bivalent or quadrivalent human papilloma virus (HPV) vaccine during pregnancy is not recommended, no teratogenic effects have been reported in animal models. The manufacturer's pregnancy registry should be contacted if pregnancy is detected during the vaccination schedule, and completion of the series should be delayed until pregnancy is completed. Lactating women can receive the quadrivalent HPV vaccine because inactivated vaccines, such as the HPV vaccine, do not affect the safety of breastfeeding for mothers or infants. The CDC recommendations on vaccination precautions during breastfeeding are available at www.cdc.gov/breastfeeding/recommendations/vaccinations.htm#modalIdString_CDCTable_0.

Because of the theoretic risks of live-virus vaccines, both the varicella and the measles–mumps–rubella vaccine are contraindicated during pregnancy. Pregnant women should be assessed for evidence of varicella and rubella immunity: such assessment may include antibody titer or, in the case of varicella, reporting a history of varicella illness or previous immunization. The CDC recommends that women who do not have evidence of immunity receive the first dose of varicella vaccine and the measles–mumps–rubella vaccine during the postpartum period before discharge from the health care facility. (For more information on immunization during pregnancy, see Chapter 12.)

Antepartum Genetic Screening and Diagnosis

There are ever-increasing ways to screen pregnant women for fetal birth defects or genetic abnormalities and to provide diagnostic testing for those who desire it. Obstetrician–gynecologists and other obstetric care providers must be knowledgeable about the choices available to patients in general and either provide that screening themselves or have established referral sources for doing so. It is the responsibility of the obstetrician–gynecologist or other obstetric care provider to educate the woman and make her aware of available options.

Genetic Screening

Carrier screening and counseling ideally should be performed before pregnancy. If this does not occur before pregnancy, a discussion of the risks, benefits, and alternatives for prenatal screening and diagnostic testing should occur with all pregnant women. Counseling should be provided by trained personnel (see also "Prepregnancy Genetic Screening" in Chapter 5).

Family history plays a critical role in assessing risk of inherited medical conditions and single-gene disorders. It is important to review and update the family history periodically for new diagnoses within the family and throughout pregnancy as appropriate.

- *Single-gene (mendelian inheritance) disorders*—Disorders inherited as a result of autosomal dominant, autosomal recessive, or X-linked mutations of single genes are typically referred to as mendelian inheritance disorders. Health care providers should be aware that the list of the genes or genetic regions responsible for many single-gene disorders continues to grow and an updated list can be found using internet databases, such as Online Mendelian Inheritance in Man (www.omim.org/) or GeneTests (www.genetests.org/). One way to screen for these disorders is to obtain a family history including the patient's ethnic background. The same information should be gained about the father of the baby. Certain disorders are more common in different ethnic groups, although it is essential to note that there are no disorders found uniquely in a certain ethnic or racial group and that many families may be of mixed ethnicity and not have an obvious predominant heritage. Recognizing that many women and couples will be of mixed or uncertain ethnic background, paradigms and testing panels that offer broad carrier screening have been introduced.

Pretest and posttest counseling is important whether targeted or expanded carrier screening is used to review the risks, benefits, and limitations of genetic testing. Especially in women who have been pregnant before, it is prudent to determine if she has been screened previously. If so, screening results should be documented and the tests generally should not be repeated. Because of the rapid evolution of genetic testing, additional mutations may be included in newer screening panels. The decision to rescreen a patient should be undertaken only with the guidance of a genetics professional who can best assess the incremental benefit of repeat testing for additional mutations. After counseling, a patient may decline any or all carrier screening.

If carrier testing is to be done, it is reasonable to offer this to the woman first and then test the father only if the mother is positive. Concurrent screening of the patient and her partner is suggested if there are time constraints for decisions about prenatal diagnostic evaluation. If testing is being considered on the basis of an affected relative, it is best to offer testing to the family member of the affected individual first. In such cases it is also important, if possible, to obtain information about the affected individual to determine, for example, if a specific identifiable genetic mutation to target with testing has been identified. Carrier screening does not identify all potential mutations associated with a genetic disorder, therefore knowledge of familial mutations is important in interpreting carrier screening results and counseling of residual risk.

Some health care providers may offer all patients broader panels, called "expanded carrier screening," that provide carrier screening for a multitude of disorders. Expanded carrier screening is a disease screening that evaluates an individual's carrier state for multiple conditions at once and regardless of ethnicity. Expanded carrier screening panels offered by laboratories typically include options to screen from 5–10 conditions to as many as several hundred conditions. Ethnic-specific, panethnic, and expanded carrier screening are acceptable strategies for prepregnancy and prenatal carrier screening (see also "Prepregnancy Genetic Screening" in Chapter 5).

- *Chromosomal abnormalities*—There are many strategies available to screen for chromosomal abnormalities. These incorporate maternal age and a variety of first-trimester and second-trimester ultrasonography and biochemical markers that include nuchal translucency measurement and pregnancy-associated plasma protein A, human chorionic gonadotropin, maternal serum alpha-fetoprotein (MSAFP), estriol, and inhibin levels. More recently, screening tests based on detecting cell-free DNA (cfDNA) in maternal blood, including cfDNA from the pregnancy, have been used. The choice of screening test depends on many factors, including gestational age at first prenatal visit, number of fetuses, previous obstetric history, family history, availability of nuchal translucency measurement, test sensitivity and limitations, risk of invasive diagnostic procedures, desire for early test results, and reproductive options. The goal is to offer screening tests with high detection rates and low false-positive rates that also provide women with the diagnostic options they might want to consider. Cell-free DNA will screen only for the common trisomies and, if requested, sex chromosome composition. However, the scope of conditions detectable and the performance of cfDNA tests continues to evolve; therefore, health care providers who offer this screening need to be familiar with the performance of the particular test used.
- *Aneuploidy*—Down syndrome (trisomy 21) and other autosomal trisomies are primarily the result of meiotic nondisjunction, which increases with maternal age. Fetuses with aneuploidy may have major anatomic malformations that often are discovered during an ultrasound examination performed for another indication. Abnormalities involving a major organ or structure, with a few notable exceptions, or the finding of two or more minor structural abnormalities in the same fetus indicate increased risk of fetal aneuploidy.

Aneuploidy screening or diagnostic testing should be discussed and offered to all women early in pregnancy, ideally at the first prenatal visit (Table 6-3). Women should be counseled regarding the differences between screening and invasive diagnostic testing. Regardless of which screening tests a woman is offered, information about the detection and false-positive rates, advantages, disadvantages, and limitations, as well as the risks and benefits of diagnostic procedures, should be available so that she can make informed decisions. Some women may benefit from an in-depth discussion with an obstetrician–gynecologist or other obstetric care provider with genetics expertise, especially if there is a family history of a chromosome abnormality, genetic disorder, or congenital malformation.

Ideally, women seen early in pregnancy can be offered first-trimester aneuploidy screening or integrated or sequential aneuploidy screening that combines first-trimester and second-trimester testing. Each has its own detection and false-positive rates. The options for women who are first seen during the second trimester include quadruple (or "quad") screening, cfDNA screening, and ultrasound examination (Table 6-3).

Women who have had first-trimester screening for aneuploidy should not undergo independent second-trimester serum screening in the same pregnancy. Instead, women who want a higher detection rate for common aneuploidies can undergo integrated or sequential screening or can consider cfDNA screening alone.

Integrated screening uses both first-trimester and second-trimester markers to adjust a woman's age-related risk of having a child with Down syndrome. The results are reported only after both first-trimester and second-trimester screening tests are completed. Integrated screening best meets the goal of screening by providing a high sensitivity with a low false-positive rate. The low false-positive rate results in fewer invasive tests and, thus, fewer procedure-related losses of normal fetuses.

Sequential screening has a high detection rate as with integrated screening but identifies very high-risk patients early in gestation. In the stepwise sequential screening, women determined to be at high risk of Down syndrome risk above a predetermined cutoff after the first-trimester screening are offered genetic counseling and the option of invasive diagnostic testing or cfDNA, and women below the cutoff are offered second-trimester screening. The sequential approach takes advantage of the higher detection rate achieved by incorporating the first-trimester and second-trimester results with only a marginal increase in the false-positive rate.

TABLE 6-3. Characteristics, Advantages, and Disadvantages of Common Screening Tests for Aneuploidy

Screening Test	Approximate Gestational Age Range for Screening (Weeks)	Detection Rate for Down Syndrome (%)	Screen Positive Rate* (%)	Advantages	Disadvantages	Method
First trimester[†]	10–13 6/7[‡]	82–87	5	1. Early screening 2. Single test 3. Analyte assessment of other adverse outcome	Lower DR than combined tests NT required	NT+PAPP-A and hCG
Triple screen[†]	15–22	69	5	1. Single test 2. No specialized US required 3. Also screens for open fetal defects 4. Analyte assessment for other adverse outcomes	Lower DR than with first-trimester or quad screening Lowest accuracy of the single lab tests	hCG, AFP, uE3
Quad screen[†]	15–22	81	5	1. Single test 2. No specialized US required 3. Also screens for open fetal defects 4. Analyte assessment for other adverse outcomes	Lower DR than combined tests	hCG, AFP, uE3, DIA
Integrated[†]	10–13 6/7[‡], then 15–22	96	5	Highest DR of combined tests Also screens for open fetal defects	Two samples needed before results are known	NT+PAPP-A, then quad screen
Sequential[§]: Stepwise	10–13 6/7[‡], then 15–22	95	5	First-trimester results provided; Comparable performance to integrated, but FTS results provided; also screens for open fetal defects; analyte assessment for other adverse outcomes.	Two samples needed	NT+hCG+PAPP-A, then quad screen
Contingent screening[§]		88–94	5	First-trimester test result: Positive: diagnostic test offered Negative: no further testing Intermediate: second-trimester test offered Final: risk assessment incorporates first- and second-trimester results	Possibly two samples needed	NT+hCG+PAPP-A, then quad screen

Serum Integrated[†]	10–13 6/7[‡], then 15–22	88	5	1. DR compares favorably with other tests. 2. No need for NT	Two samples needed; no first-trimester results	PAPP-A+quad screen
Cell-free DNA[‖]	10 to term	99 (in patients who receive a result)	0.5	1. Highest DR for Down syndrome 2. Can be performed at any gestational age after 10 weeks 3. Low false-positive rate in high-risk women (or women at high risk of Down syndrome)	1. NPV and PPV not clearly reported 2. Higher false-positive rate in women at low risk of Down syndrome 3. Limited information about three trisomies and fetal sex 4. Results do not always represent a fetal DNA result	Three roughly equivalent molecular methods
Nuchal translucency[†]	10–13 6/7[‡]	64–70	5	Allows individual fetus assessment in multifetal gestations Provides additional screening for fetal anomalies and possibly for twin–twin transfusion syndrome	1. Poor screen in isolation 2. Ultrasound certification necessary	US only

Abbreviations: AFP, alpha fetoprotein; DIA, dimeric inhibin-A; DR, detection rate; FTS, first-trimester screening; hCG, human chorionic gonadotropin; NPV, negative predictive value; NT, nuchal translucency; PAPP-A, pregnancy-associated plasma protein A; PPV, positive predictive value; uE3, unconjugated estriol; US, ultrasonography.

*A screen positive test result includes all positive test results: the true positives and false positives.

[†]First-trimester combined screening: 87%, 85%, and 82% for measurements performed at 11 weeks, 12 weeks, and 13 weeks, respectively; Malone FD, Ball RH, Nyberg DA, Comstock CH, Saade GR, Berkowitz RL, et al. First-trimester septated cystic hygroma: prevalence, natural history, and pediatric outcome. FASTER Trial Research Consortium. Obstet Gynecol 2005;106:288–94.

[‡]Because of variations in growth and fertilization timing, some fetuses at the lower and upper gestational age limits may fall outside the required crown–rump length range. Also, different laboratories use slightly different gestational age windows for their testing protocol.

[§]Cuckle H, Benn P, Wright D. Down syndrome screening in the first and/or second trimester: model predicted performance using meta-analysis parameters. Semin Perinatol 2005;29:252–7.

[‖]Bianchi DW, Platt LD, Goldberg JD, Abuhamad AZ, Sehnert AJ, Rava RP. Genome-wide fetal aneuploidy detection by maternal plasma DNA sequencing. MatErnal BLood IS Source to Accurately diagnose fetal aneuploidy (MELISSA) Study Group [published erratum appears in Obstet Gynecol 2012;120:957]. Obstet Gynecol 2012;119:890–901 *and* Palomaki GE, Kloza EM, Lambert-Messerlian GM, Haddow JE, Neveux LM, Ehrich M, et al. DNA sequencing of maternal plasma to detect Down syndrome: an international clinical validation study. Genet Med 2011;13:913–20.

Parallel or simultaneous testing with multiple screening methodologies for aneuploidy is not cost-effective and should not be performed. Laboratories that report aneuploidy screening test results may provide the health care provider with numerical information regarding the woman's revised risk of aneuploidy using maternal age, serum analyte levels, and nuchal translucency measurement as well as other factors, such as maternal weight, diabetes status, and ethnicity. Communicating a numerical risk assessment after screening enables women and their partners to balance the consequences of having a child with the particular disorder against the risk of an invasive diagnostic test. It is often useful to contrast this risk with the general population risk and their age-related risk before screening. Other screening tests, including those using cell-free fetal DNA, may be reported simply as positive or negative, but it is important to emphasize that these too are screening tests. Given the potential for inaccurate results and to understand the type of trisomy for recurrence-risk counseling, a diagnostic test should be recommended for a patient who has a positive cfDNA test result. Women whose results are not reported, indeterminate, or uninterpretable (a "no call" test result) from cfDNA screening should receive further genetic counseling and be offered comprehensive ultrasound evaluation and diagnostic testing because of an increased risk of aneuploidy. A calculator has been developed that allows estimation of the positive predictive value of cfDNA screening based on estimates of population prevalence (available at www.perinatalquality.org/vendors/nsgc/nipt).

Women found to have an increased risk of aneuploidy with first-trimester screening should be offered genetic counseling and diagnostic testing by CVS or a second-trimester genetic amniocentesis. Patients who decline CVS or amniocentesis can be offered cfDNA. Neural tube defect screening should be offered in the second trimester to women who elected to have only first-trimester screening for aneuploidy, including screening with cfDNA, or who have had a normal result from CVS; this is best performed between 16–18 weeks of gestation with serum alpha-fetoprotein screening, targeted second-trimester ultrasonography, or both. Women who have an enlarged fetal nuchal translucency measurement in the first trimester, despite a negative test result on an aneuploidy screening, normal fetal chromosomes, or both, should be offered a targeted ultrasound examination and fetal echocardiogram because such fetuses are at a significant risk of nonchromosomal anomalies, including congenital heart defects and some genetic syndromes.

Women with abnormal first-trimester or second-trimester serum markers or an increased nuchal translucency measurement also may be at increased risk of an adverse pregnancy outcome, such as spontaneous fetal loss before 24 weeks of gestation, fetal demise, preeclampsia, low birth weight, or preterm birth. At the present time, there are no data indicating whether or not fetal surveillance in the third trimester will be helpful in the care of these women.

- *Neural tube defects*—Second-trimester MSAFP testing, targeted ultrasound, or both, may be used to screen for neural tube defects and other open fetal defects. Under ideal circumstances, second-trimester ultrasonography will detect approximately 100% of anencephaly and 95% of spina bifida anomalies. When using MSAFP, a standard screening cutoff (2.5 multiples of the median) will detect approximately 80% of cases of open spina bifida and greater than 95% of cases of anencephaly. Women with increased MSAFP levels should be evaluated by ultrasonography to detect identifiable causes of false-positive test results (eg, fetal death, multiple gestation, underestimation of gestational age) and for targeted study of fetal anatomy for neural tube defects and other defects associated with increased MSAFP values (eg, omphalocele or gastroschisis). Amniocentesis may be recommended to confirm the presence of open defects or to obtain a fetal karyotype. Amniocentesis may be offered even when ultrasound examination results do not reveal an identifiable defect or cause for the increased MSAFP level, particularly if the ultrasound examination was suboptimal because of maternal obesity or abdominal scarring.

Diagnostic Testing

For women who choose to have a diagnostic test for aneuploidy, either in addition to or in place of a screening test, there are two primary options: 1) chorionic villus sampling and 2) amniocentesis.

- *Chorionic villus sampling*—Chorionic villus sampling is a technique for removing a small sample (5–40 mg) of placental tissue (chorionic villi) for performing chromosomal, metabolic, or DNA studies. It generally is performed between 10 weeks and 13 weeks of gestation, either by a transabdominal or a transcervical approach. Chorionic villi, however, cannot be used for the prenatal diagnosis of neural tube defects. Therefore, women who have undergone cytogenetic testing by CVS should be offered MSAFP, detailed ultrasound examinations, or both for the detection of neural tube defects. Most prospective studies have shown that the procedure-related risk of pregnancy loss after CVS is not significantly different from that associated with amniocentesis. The pregnancy loss rate from CVS has been reported to be 0.22% (1 in 455).

- *Amniocentesis*—Amniocentesis is the technique most commonly used for obtaining fetal cells for genetic studies. This well-established, safe, and reliable procedure usually is offered between 15 weeks and 20 weeks of gestation. The fluid obtained through amniocentesis can be used for chemical, metabolic, and microbiologic testing and the cells in the fluid can be isolated for cytogenetics and other DNA testing.

  Multicenter studies have confirmed the safety of genetic amniocentesis as well as its cytogenetic diagnostic accuracy (greater than 99%). The rate of procedure-related pregnancy loss that is attributable to a prenatal diagnostic procedure currently is estimated to be approximately 0.1–0.3% in procedures performed by experienced health care providers and complications (transient vaginal spotting or amniotic fluid leakage) occur in approximately 1–2% of all cases. Spontaneous cessation of amniotic fluid leakage occurs in the majority of cases and is not associated with pregnancy loss.

  Amniocentesis at less than 14 weeks of gestation (also called "early amniocentesis") should not be performed because it results in significantly higher rates of pregnancy loss and complications than later amniocentesis. Chorionic villus sampling is the preferred diagnostic test before 14 weeks of gestation.

In certain situations, when diagnostic testing is undertaken, chromosomal microarray testing is recommended. Microarray allows for the detection of smaller deletions and duplications than those detectable with standard karyotype. Indications for microarray analysis include women with a fetus that has one or more major structural abnormalities identified on ultrasonographic examination, and those with a fetal death or stillbirth and who desire additional genetic testing to detect causative abnormalities. However, microarray testing may be considered whenever diagnostic testing is performed because it may identify additional clinically significant abnormalities in approximately 6% of fetuses with ultrasonographic abnormalities and a normal conventional karyotype result. Further, it may identify abnormalities in 1.7% of fetuses with an abnormal screening test result and a normal karyotype result. Different microarray platforms (sometimes referred to as "chips") will look for different panels of deletions, including, in some cases, the entire aspect of the genome including duplications or deletions of unknown significance. Finding such variations of unknown significance can render counseling regarding clinical significance challenging. Additionally, microarray is currently significantly more expensive that a traditional karyotype and may not be covered by some insurers. Counseling regarding decisions to undertake or in the interpretation of microarray analysis may be facilitated by referral to maternal–fetal medicine physicians, geneticists, or genetic counselors with expertise in this area. Chromosomal microarray can be performed on either CVS or amniocentesis specimens.

Invasive Diagnostic Testing in Women Who Are Rh D Negative

Because both amniocentesis and CVS can result in fetal-to-maternal transfusion, the administration of anti-D immune globulin is indicated for women who are Rh-D negative, unsensitized, and undergo either of these procedures. Chorionic villus sampling should not be performed in women who are red cell antibody sensitized whether to Rh or other antigens because it may worsen the antibody response.

Psychosocial Risk Screening and Counseling

Psychosocial issues are nonbiomedical factors that affect mental and physical well-being. Screening for psychosocial risk factors may help predict a woman's attentiveness to personal health matters, her use of prenatal services, and the health status of her offspring. Such screening should be done for all pregnant women and should be performed regardless of social status, educational level, race, and ethnicity. Past obstetric events and infant outcomes, medical considerations in a current pregnancy, beliefs about and experience with breastfeeding, and family circumstances (among other factors) influence the experience of labor, delivery, and early neonatal and postpartum adjustment. Additionally, some women experience social, economic, and personal difficulties in pregnancy. Given the sensitive nature of psychosocial assessment, every effort should be made to screen women in private. Even then, women may not be comfortable discussing problems with health care providers until a trusting relationship has been formed. Other clinical staff may be trained to provide this screening, with results communicated to the health care provider.

Addressing the broad range of psychosocial issues with which pregnant women are confronted is an essential step toward improving women's health and birth outcomes. An effective system of referrals is helpful in augmenting the screening and brief intervention that can be carried out in an office or clinic setting. Although some psychosocial issues are present before pregnancy, others arise during the course of pregnancy or may not be disclosed early on. To increase the likelihood of successful interventions, psychosocial screening should be performed on a regular basis and documented in the women's prenatal record. Positive screening before delivery may highlight an increased risk of postpartum depression and identify women who may benefit from closer monitoring or intervention after delivery. Screening should include assessment of a woman's desire for pregnancy, tobacco use, substance use, depression, safety, intimate partner violence, stress, barriers to care, unstable housing, communication barriers, and nutrition.

When screening is completed, every effort should be made to identify areas of concern, validate major issues with the woman, provide information, and, if indicated, make suggestions for possible changes. Screening positive for a condition often necessitates referral to community resources for further evaluation or intervention. Health care providers need to be aware of individuals and community agencies to which women can be referred for additional counseling and assistance when necessary.

Desire for Pregnancy

If the woman indicates that the pregnancy is unwanted, she should be fully informed in a balanced manner about all options, including raising the child, placing the child for adoption, and abortion. The information conveyed should be appropriate to the gestational age. The health care provider should make every effort to avoid introducing personal bias. Some women may feel more comfortable having a discussion of this type with someone who is not involved with their ongoing medical care. The health care provider should evaluate the woman's available psychosocial support and refer her to appropriate counseling or other supportive services. Health care providers often may best fulfill their obligations to women through referral to other practitioners who have the appropriate skills and expertise to address these difficult issues.

Substance Use and Substance Use Disorders

Screening for substance use should be a part of comprehensive obstetric care and should be done at the first prenatal visit in partnership with the pregnant woman. Screening based only on factors such as poor adherence to prenatal care or prior adverse pregnancy outcome can lead to missed cases, and may add to stereotyping and stigma. Therefore, it is essential that screening be universal. Routine screening for substance use disorder should be applied equally to all people, regardless of age, sex, race, ethnicity, or socioeconomic status. Routine screening should rely on validated screening tools. (see Chapter 5). Both before pregnancy and in early pregnancy, all women should be routinely asked about their use of alcohol and drugs, including prescription opioids and other medications used for nonmedical reasons. To begin the conversation, the patient should be informed that these questions are asked of all pregnant women to ensure they receive the care they require. Maintaining a caring and nonjudgmental approach, as well as screening when the patient is alone, are important and will yield the most inclusive disclosure. Obstetric care providers should protect patient autonomy, confidentiality, and the integrity of the patient–physician relationship to the extent allowable by laws regarding disclosure of substance use disorder (available at www.guttmacher.org/state-policy/explore/substance-abuse-during-pregnancy). Physicians should be aware that reporting mandates vary widely and be familiar with the legal requirements within their state or community. This includes awareness that laws in some states consider in utero drug exposure to be a form of child abuse or neglect under civil child-welfare statutes and require that positive drug test results in pregnant women or their newborn infants be reported to the state's child protection agency. States vary in their requirements for the evidence of drug exposure to the fetus or newborn infants in order to report a case to the child welfare system. Legally mandated testing and reporting put the therapeutic relationship between the health care provider and the woman at risk, potentially placing the health care provider in an adversarial relationship with the woman.

Routine laboratory testing of biologic samples is not required. Urine drug testing has been used to detect or confirm suspected substance use, but should be performed only with the patient's consent and in compliance with state laws. Pregnant women must be informed of the potential ramifications of a positive test result, including any mandatory reporting requirements. Routine urine drug screening is controversial for several reasons. A positive drug test result is not, in itself, diagnostic of opioid use disorder or its severity. Urine drug testing assesses only for current or recent substance use; therefore, a negative test does not rule out sporadic substance use. Also, urine toxicology testing may not detect many substances, including synthetic opioids, some benzodiazepines, and designer drugs. False-positive results can occur with immune-assay testing and legal consequences can be devastating to the patient and her family. Health care providers should be aware of their laboratory's test characteristics and request that confirmatory testing with mass spectrometry and liquid or gas chromatography be performed as appropriate. Some centers have implemented universal urine toxicology screening, with one study finding improved rates of detection of maternal substance use compared with standard methods. However, this study did not use validated verbal screening tools, which limits the usefulness of these results. For these reasons, validated verbal screening tools (see Chapter 5 for examples of screening tools) are the preferred method for initial screening. History taking and verbal screening tools provide the opportunity for the prenatal provider to offer a brief intervention to educate patients and use principles of motivational interviewing to bring about a desire to change high-risk behavior, when appropriate. If toxicologic testing is indicated, the information should be used to assist the pregnant woman or new mother to receive the treatment she needs and not as a vehicle for punishment. More severe substance use disorders warrant a referral to specialized treatment.

If a woman acknowledges the use of tobacco, alcohol, cocaine, opioids, amphetamines, or other mood-altering drugs or if chemical dependence is suspected, she should be counseled about the perinatal implications of their use during pregnancy and offered referral to an appropriate treatment program. Health care providers should, when possible, advocate for evidence-based and consensual interventions related to substance use disorder. Efforts should be designed to help treat women and, in so doing, optimize pregnancy and neonatal outcomes. Obstetric providers should be knowledgeable about local resources for substance use treatment. Enlisting the help of social service agencies to facilitate patient referral and communicating with substance use treatment providers optimize patient care. Separation of parents from their children solely based on substance use disorder, either suspected or confirmed, should be discouraged.

Tobacco. Inquiry into tobacco use, including smoked, chewed, electronic nicotine delivery system (ENDS), and vaped, and smoke exposure should be a routine part of the prenatal visit. Women should be strongly discouraged from tobacco use, including smoking. Multiple studies have demonstrated a clear association between maternal smoking and perinatal morbidity and mortality. This includes intrauterine growth restriction (IUGR), placenta previa, abruptio placentae, preterm premature rupture of membranes (also known as prelabor rupture of membranes), low birth weight, perinatal mortality, ectopic pregnancy, and sudden infant death syndrome. Children born to mothers who smoke during pregnancy are at increased risk of asthma, infantile colic, and childhood obesity. Secondhand prenatal exposure to tobacco smoke also increases the risk of having an infant with low birth weight by as much as 20%.

The U.S. Preventive Services Task Force has concluded that the use of nicotine replacement products, including electronic nicotine delivery systems, or other pharmaceuticals for smoking cessation aids during pregnancy and lactation have not been sufficiently evaluated to determine their efficacy or safety. Therefore, the use of nicotine replacement therapy should be undertaken with close supervision and after careful consideration and discussion of the known risks of continued smoking and the possible risks of nicotine replacement therapy. If nicotine replacement is used, it should be with the clear resolve of the woman to quit tobacco use. A protocol that systematically identifies pregnant women who use tobacco and offers treatment or referral has proved to increase tobacco cessation rates. A short counseling session with pregnancy-specific educational materials and a referral to the smokers' quit line is an effective smoking cessation strategy. The 5As is an intervention that can be used in the office or clinic under the guidance of trained practitioners (See Box 5-2 in Chapter 5).

Alcohol. Alcohol is a teratogen. Women should be advised to abstain from alcohol consumption during pregnancy. There is no known absolutely safe quantity, frequency, type, or timing of alcohol consumption during pregnancy. Health care providers should advise women that low-level consumption of alcohol in early pregnancy is not an indication for pregnancy termination. However, women who have already consumed alcohol during a current pregnancy should be advised to stop in order to minimize further risk.

Women should be informed that prenatal alcohol consumption is a preventable cause of birth defects, including intellectual disability. Fetal alcohol syndrome is characterized by three conditions: 1) growth restriction, 2) facial abnormalities, and 3) central nervous system dysfunction. Even moderate alcohol consumption during pregnancy may alter psychomotor development, contribute to cognitive defects, and produce emotional and behavioral problems in children.

Mood-Altering Drugs. It is not unusual for women of childbearing age to use potentially addictive and mood-altering drugs. Use of cocaine, marijuana, diazepam, opioids (including morphine, heroin, codeine, meperidine, methadone, and oxycodone), other prescription drugs, and approximately 150 other substances can lead to chemical dependency. Depending on geographic location, it is estimated that 1–40% of pregnant women have used one of these substances during pregnancy and approximately 1 in 10 newborn infants are exposed to one or more mood-altering drugs during pregnancy; the number varies only slightly for publicly versus privately insured women.

The onset and intensity of effect will vary based on how the drug was taken and the formulation; however, all have the potential for causing respiratory depression, overdose, and death. The risk of respiratory depression, overdose, and death is greater for full opioid agonists (such as fentanyl) than for partial agonists (such as buprenorphine). Injection of opioids also carries the risk of cellulitis and abscess formation at the injection site, sepsis, endocarditis, osteomyelitis, hepatitis B, hepatitis C, and HIV infection. Sharing of snorting implements has also been identified as a risk factor for hepatitis C and other virus transmission in a group of pregnant women with hepatitis C.

Opioid use disorder is a chronic treatable disease that can be managed successfully by combining medications with behavioral therapy and recovery support. Elements of prenatal care for women with opioid use or use disorder will depend on each patient's particular situation and comorbid conditions. Several issues to consider include the following:

- Testing for STIs and other infectious agents such as HIV, hepatitis B and C, chlamydia, gonorrhea, syphilis, and tuberculosis should be considered. Repeat testing in the third trimester may be indicated if the woman is considered at increased risk. Hepatitis B vaccination is recommended for pregnant women who are negative for the hepatitis B surface antigen (HBsAg) but at high risk of hepatitis B infection.
- Screening for depression and other behavioral health conditions should be conducted.
- In addition to an ultrasound examination for fetal assessment in mid second trimester, consideration should be given to first trimester ultrasonography for best determination of the estimated due date and an interval ultrasonographic assessment of fetal weight later in pregnancy if there is concern for fetal growth abnormalities.

- Consultations with anesthesia, addiction medicine specialists, pain management specialists, pediatrics, maternal–fetal medicine, behavioral health, nutrition, and social services should be conducted as needed.
- Because breastfeeding should be encouraged in mothers who are stable on their opioid agonists, who are not using illicit drugs, and who have no other contraindications, obstetrician–gynecologists and other obstetric care providers should provide anticipatory breastfeeding guidance during the antepartum period.
- Close communication between the obstetric care provider and pediatric team before delivery is necessary for optimal management of the newborn infant. Neonatal consultation, if available, can be considered prenatally to discuss postdelivery care of the infant.
- Use of other substances, particularly tobacco use, is common in women with opioid use disorder; screening for and discussion about this and other substances are important, and cessation services should be offered.

For women, including pregnant women, with an opioid use disorder, opioid agonist pharmacotherapy (also referred to as medication-assisted treatment) is the standard of care. This includes methadone and buprenorphine (as a monoproduct or in a combined formulation with naloxone). Opioid agonist pharmacotherapy is preferable to medically supervised withdrawal because withdrawal is associated with high relapse rates and poorer outcomes. If a woman refuses treatment with an opioid agonist, or treatment is unavailable, medically supervised withdrawal can be considered under the care of a physician experienced in perinatal addiction treatment and with informed consent; however, it often requires prolonged inpatient care and intensive outpatient behavioral health follow-up in order to be successful. In some areas, access to opioid agonist pharmacotherapy is limited, and efforts should be made to improve availability of local resources.

Naltrexone is a nonselective opioid receptor antagonist that in therapeutic doses blocks the euphoric effects of opioids, and it has been used to help nonpregnant patients with opioid use disorder in their effort to maintain abstinence. To date, information regarding its use in pregnancy is limited to small case series and case reports, with normal birth outcomes reported. However, significant concerns exist regarding unknown fetal effects, as well as risk of relapse and treatment dropout with subsequent return to opioid use and risk of overdose. The decision whether or not to continue naltrexone treatment for a woman already using naltrexone before pregnancy should involve a careful discussion with the patient, comparing the limited safety data versus the potential risk of relapse with treatment discontinuation.

Naloxone is a short-acting opioid antagonist that can rapidly reverse the effects of opioids and can be life-saving in the setting of opioid overdose. Although induced withdrawal may possibly contribute to fetal stress, naloxone should be used in pregnant women in the case of maternal overdose in order to save the woman's life.

Infants born to women with a history of chronic opioid use whether from prescription medications (used as prescribed or nonmedically), heroin, or opioid replacement (methadone, buprenorphine, naloxone) are at risk of neonatal abstinence syndrome, an expected and treatable condition that does not appear to pose permanent risks to the infant if treated. Ideally these women will be identified and counseled in advance of delivery. The possibility of an infant developing neonatal abstinence syndrome should be discussed with patients and may include consultation with the health care provider who will be monitoring and caring for the infant after birth. Obstetrician–gynecologists and other obstetric care providers caring for pregnant women receiving medical or using nonmedical opioids should arrange for delivery at a facility prepared to monitor, evaluate for, and treat neonatal abstinence syndrome. In instances when travel to such a facility would present an undue burden on the pregnant woman, it is appropriate to deliver locally, monitor and evaluate the newborn infant for neonatal abstinence syndrome, and transfer the newborn infant for additional treatment if needed. Women should be counseled about the need to suspend breastfeeding in the event of a relapse and should be counseled on the safe preparation and feeding of infant formula. Families should be encouraged to visit and care for their infants, and mothers should be supported in their effort to breastfeed their infants, if appropriate. Several perinatal collaborative quality initiatives have developed valuable resources for health care providers and patients to optimize the diagnosis and treatment of neonatal abstinence syndrome and promote collaboration between obstetric and neonatal care providers. Close communication between the obstetrician and pediatrician is necessary for optimal management of the newborn infant. (See also "Neonatal Drug Withdrawal" in Chapter 11.)

Clinical Depression

Clinical depression is common in reproductive-aged women. A recent retrospective cohort analysis in a large U.S. managed care organization found that one in seven women was treated for depression between the year before pregnancy and the year after pregnancy. According to the World Health Organization, depression is the leading cause of disability in women, which accounts for $30–50 billion in lost productivity and direct medical costs in the United States each year.

Screening for, diagnosing, and treating depression and anxiety have the potential to benefit a woman and her family and are recommended for all pregnancies. Infants of women who are depressed display delayed psychologic, cognitive, neurologic, and motor development. Furthermore, children's mental and behavioral disorders improve when maternal depression is in remission. Women with current depression or anxiety or a history of perinatal mood disorders warrant particularly close monitoring and evaluation. Pregnancy and the postpartum period represent an ideal time during which consistent contact with the health care delivery system will allow women at risk to be identified and treated. There are multiple depression screening tools available for use. These tools usually can be completed in less than 10 minutes. Examples of highly sensitive screening tools include the Edinburgh Postnatal Depression Scale, Postpartum Depression Screening Scale, and Patient Health Questionnaire-9. To improve clinical outcome, screening must be coupled with appropriate follow-up and treatment. Clinical staff should be prepared to initiate medical therapy, refer women to appropriate behavioral health resources when indicated, or both.

Women who were receiving treatment for depression before pregnancy should receive counseling concerning management options during pregnancy. Consultation with the prescribing psychiatrist is recommended regarding antidepressant medication dosing and safety.

Intimate Partner Violence

Risk assessment during pregnancy should include identification of women who are victims of intimate partner violence, which is a significant public health problem affecting millions of American women each year. Screening should occur at the first prenatal visit, at least once per trimester, and at the postpartum checkup.

Trauma, including trauma caused by intimate partner violence, is one of the most frequent causes of maternal death in the United States. The prevalence of violence during pregnancy ranges from 1% to 20%, with most studies identifying rates between 4% and 8%. There is no single profile of an abused woman. Victims come from all ages, sexual orientations, and backgrounds. The prevalence of abuse, particularly sexual abuse, may be greater in pregnant adolescents compared with pregnant adult women.

Most abused women continue to be victimized during pregnancy. Violence against women also may begin or escalate during pregnancy and affects both maternal and fetal well-being. The presence of violence between intimate partners also affects children in the household. Child abuse occurs in 33–77% of families in which there is abuse of adults. Among women who are abused, 27% demonstrate abusive behavior toward their children while living in a violent environment.

Abuse may involve threatened or actual physical, sexual, verbal, or psychologic abuse. The fundamental issues at play are power, control, and coercion. There is no clearly established set of symptoms that signal abuse. However, some of the obstetric presentations of abused women include the following:

- Unwanted pregnancy
- STIs
- Late entry into prenatal care or missed appointments
- Nonmedical or excessive prescribed substance use
- Poor weight gain and nutrition
- Multiple, repeated somatic complaints

Detection may be possible by discussing with the woman that pregnancy sometimes places increased stress on a relationship and then asking how the woman and her partner resolve their differences. In many cases, however, women will not disclose their abuse unless asked directly. Abused women usually are forthright when asked directly in a caring, nonjudgmental manner. The likelihood of disclosure increases with repeated inquiries.

Screening should be conducted in private. Translation services may be helpful in inquiring about these issues with women who have limited English proficiency. It is important to avoid using a family member or friend as an interpreter. If a woman confides that she is being abused, verbatim accounts of the abuse should be recorded in her medical record. The obstetrician–gynecologist or other obstetric care provider should inquire about her immediate safety and the safety of her children and should become familiar with local resources. Referrals to appropriate counseling, legal, and social-service advocacy programs should be made. Additionally, health care providers should be familiar with state laws that may require reporting of intimate partner violence. Child abuse is always reportable. When abuse is suspected, whether or not it is corroborated by the woman, supportive statements should be offered, and the necessity for follow-up needs be addressed. It is important to encourage women who are victims of violence, with the assistance of social services, to begin to create an escape plan, with a reliable safe haven for retreat, particularly if they believe the violence is escalating.

First-Trimester Patient Education

Patient education is an essential element of prenatal care. Topics for specialized counseling include nutrition, weight gain, exercise, dental care, nausea and vomiting, vitamin and mineral toxicity, teratogens, and air travel.

Nutrition

Both fetal and maternal outcomes can be affected by maternal nutritional status during pregnancy. Dietary counseling and intervention based on special or individual needs usually are most effectively accomplished by referral to a nutritionist or registered dietitian. Such circumstances may include diabetes, restricted dietary preferences, obesity, or having had bariatric surgery.

All women should receive information focused on a well-balanced, varied, nutritional food plan that is consistent with her access to food and food preferences. Special attention should be given to low-income and minority women who are more likely to have higher body mass index (BMI) scores, consume diets of poor nutritional quality, and get less exercise. If a woman is financially unable to meet nutritional needs, she should be referred to federal food and nutrition programs, such as the Special Supplemental Nutrition Program for Women, Infants, and Children.

The recommended dietary allowances for most vitamins and minerals increase during pregnancy (Table 6-4). The National Academy of Sciences recommends 27 mg of iron supplementation (present in most prenatal vitamins) daily because the iron content of the standard American diet and the endogenous iron stores of many American women are not sufficient to provide for the increased iron requirements of pregnancy. The U.S. Preventive Services Task Force recommends that all pregnant women be routinely screened for iron-deficiency anemia, which may be accomplished by looking for microcytosis on a complete blood count. The treatment of frank iron deficiency anemia requires dosages of 60–120 mg of elemental iron each day.

TABLE 6-4. Recommended Daily Dietary Allowances and Tolerable Upper Intake Levels* for Pregnant and Lactating Adolescents and Women

Nutrient (unit)	Pregnant			Lactating		
	14–18 years	19–30 years	31–50 years	14–18 years	19–30 years	31–50 years
Fat-soluble vitamins						
Vitamin A (micrograms/d)†	750	770	770	1,200	1,300	1,300
UL*, ‡	2,800	3,000	3,000	2,800	3,000	3,000
Vitamin D (micrograms/d)§	15	15	15	15	15	15
UL*	100	100	100	100	100	100
Vitamin E (mg/d)‖	15	15	15	19	19	19
UL*,¶	800	1,000	1,000	800	1,000	1,000
Vitamin K (micrograms/d)#	75	90	90	75	90	90
UL*	—	—	—	—	—	—
Water-soluble vitamins						
Folate (micrograms/d)**	600	600	600	500	500	500
UL*	800	1,000	1,000	800	1,000	1,000
Niacin (mg/d)††	18	18	18	17	17	17
UL*	30	35	35	30	35	35
Riboflavin (mg/d)	1.4	1.4	1.4	1.6	1.6	1.6
UL*	—	—	—	—	—	—
Thiamin (mg/d)	1.4	1.4	1.4	1.4	1.4	1.4
UL*	—	—	—	—	—	—
Vitamin B_6 (mg/d)	1.9	1.9	1.9	2	2	2
UL*	80	100	100	80	100	100
Vitamin B_{12} (micrograms/d)	2.6	2.6	2.6	2.8	2.8	2.8
UL*	—	—	—	—	—	—
Vitamin C (mg/d)	80	85	85	115	120	120
UL*	1,800	2,000	2,000	1,800	2,000	2,000
Minerals						
Calcium (mg/d)	1,300	1,000	1,000	1,300	1,000	1,000
UL*	3,000	2,500	2,500	3,000	2,500	2,500

(continued)

TABLE 6-4. Recommended Daily Dietary Allowances and Tolerable Upper Intake Levels* for Pregnant and Lactating Adolescents and Women *(continued)*

Nutrient (unit)	Pregnant 14–18 years	Pregnant 19–30 years	Pregnant 31–50 years	Lactating 14–18 years	Lactating 19–30 years	Lactating 31–50 years
***Minerals* (continued)**						
Iodine (micrograms/d)	220	220	220	290	290	290
UL*	900	1,100	1,100	900	1,100	1,100
Iron (mg/d)	27	27	27	10	9	9
UL*	45	45	45	45	45	45
Phosphorus (mg/d)	1,250	700	700	1,250	700	700
UL*	3,500	3,500	3,500	4,000	4,000	4,000
Selenium (micrograms/d)	60	60	60	70	70	70
UL*	400	400	400	400	400	400
Zinc (mg/d)	12	11	11	13	12	12
UL*	34	40	40	34	40	40

*UL = tolerable upper intake level. This is the highest level of daily nutrient intake that is likely to pose no risk of adverse effects to almost all individuals in the general population. Unless otherwise specified, the UL represents total intake from food, water, and supplements. Due to lack of suitable data, ULs could not be established for vitamin K, thiamin, riboflavin, and Vitamin B_{12}. In the absence of ULs, extra caution may be warranted in consuming levels above recommended intakes. Members of the general population should be advised not to routinely exceed the UL. The UL is not meant to apply to individuals who are treated with the nutrient under medical supervision or to individuals with predisposing conditions that modify their sensitivity to the nutrient.

†As retinol activity equivalents (RAE). 1 RAE=3.3 international units.

‡As preformed vitamin A only.

§1) Under the assumption of minimal sunlight. 2) As cholecalciferol; 1 microgram cholecalciferol=40 international units of vitamin D.

‖As α-tocopherol.

¶The ULs for vitamin E, niacin, and folate apply to synthetic forms obtained from supplements, fortified foods, or a combination of the two.

#Recommendations measured as Adequate Intake (AI) instead of Recommended Daily Dietary Allowance (RDA). An AI is set instead of an RDA if insufficient evidence is available to determine an RDA. The AI is based on observed or experimentally determined estimates of average nutrient intake by a group (or groups) of healthy people.

**As dietary folate equivalents (DFE). 1 DFE=1 microgram food folate=0.6 micrograms of folic acid from fortified food or as a supplement consumed with food=0.5 micrograms of a supplement taken on an empty stomach. In view of the evidence linking folate intake with neural tube defects in the fetus, it is recommended that all women capable of becoming pregnant consume 400 micrograms from supplements or fortified foods in addition to intake of food folate from a varied diet.

††As niacin equivalents.

Modified with permission from Institute of Medicine. Dietary Reference Intakes for Calcium and Vitamin D. Washington, DC: The National Academies Press; 2011.

Iron absorption is facilitated by or with vitamin C supplementation or ingestion between meals or at bedtime on an empty stomach.

During pregnancy, severe maternal vitamin D deficiency has been associated with biochemical evidence of disordered skeletal homeostasis in the newborn, congenital rickets, and fractures. Recent evidence suggests that vitamin D deficiency is common during pregnancy especially in high-risk groups, including vegetarians, women with limited sun exposure (eg, those who live in cold climates, reside in northern latitudes, or wear sun and winter protective clothing), and ethnic minorities, especially those with darker skin. In 2010, the Food and Nutrition Board at the Institute of Medicine (now known as the Health and Medicine Division of the National Academies of Sciences, Engineering, and Medicine) established that an adequate intake of vitamin D during pregnancy and lactation was 15 micrograms daily (or 600 international units per day) (see Table 6-4).

Most prenatal vitamins typically contain 10 micrograms (400 international units) of vitamin D per tablet. For pregnant women thought to be at increased risk of vitamin D deficiency, maternal serum 25-hydroxyvitamin D levels can be considered and should be interpreted in the context of the individual clinical circumstance. When vitamin D deficiency is identified during pregnancy, most experts agree that 25–50 micrograms (1,000–2,000 international units) per day of vitamin D is safe. Higher-dose regimens used for treatment of vitamin D deficiency have not been studied during pregnancy. Recommendations concerning routine vitamin D supplementation during pregnancy beyond that contained in a prenatal vitamin should await the completion of ongoing randomized clinical trials.

Women need to supplement their diets with folic acid before and during pregnancy (see also "Prepregnancy Nutritional Counseling" in chapter 5). Current U.S. dietary guidelines recommend that women who are pregnant consume 600 micrograms of dietary folate equivalents daily from all sources (Table 6-4).

Weight Gain

Ideally, women should have a normal BMI before pregnancy and then adjust their diets during pregnancy in order to gain a recommended amount of weight and to obtain the appropriate nutrition for both maternal and fetal benefit. Increasingly, however, women are becoming pregnant when they are obese, are gaining more weight than is necessary during pregnancy, and are retaining the weight postpartum.

TABLE 6-5. Institute of Medicine Weight Gain Recommendations for Pregnancy

Prepregnancy Weight Category	BMI* (kg)/[height (m)]^2	Recommended Total Weight Gain Range (lb)	Recommended Rates of Weight Gain† Second and Third Trimesters (Mean Range, lb/wk)
Underweight	Less than 18.5	28–40	1 (1–1.3)
Normal weight	18.5–24.9	25–35	1 (0.8–1)
Overweight	25.0–29.9	15–25	0.6 (0.5–0.7)
Obese (includes all classes)	30.0 or greater	11–20	0.5 (0.4–0.6)

*BMI, body mass index. To calculate BMI, go to www.nhlbi.nih.gov/health/educational/lose_wt/BMI/bmicalc.htm.

†Calculations assume a 1.1–4.4 lb (0.5–2 kg) weight gain in the first trimester.

Modified with permission from Institute of Medicine. Weight gain during pregnancy: reexamining the guidelines. Institute of Medicine (US) and National Research Council (US) Committee to Reexamine IOM Pregnancy Weight Guidelines. Rasmussen KM, Yaktine AL, editors. Washington, DC. The National Academies Press (US); 2009. Copyright 2009. National Academy of Sciences.

The Institute of Medicine (now known as the Health and Medicine Division of the National Academies of Sciences, Engineering, and Medicine) guidelines for maternal weight gain based on prepregnancy BMI are listed in Table 6-5. These same recommendations are made for adolescents, short women, and women of all racial and ethnic groups. Empiric recommendations for weight gain with twin gestations in women include: normal BMI: 37–54 lb; overweight women: 31–50 lb; and obese women 25–42 lb. Progress toward meeting these weight gain goals should be monitored and specific individualized counseling provided if considerable deviations are noted.

The Institute of Medicine (now known as the Health and Medicine Division of the National Academies of Sciences, Engineering, and Medicine) guidelines provide health care providers with a basis for practice. Health care providers caring for pregnant women should determine a woman's BMI at the initial prenatal visit (an online BMI calculator is available at www.nhlbi.nih.gov/health/educational/lose_wt/BMI/bmicalc.htm.) It is important to discuss appropriate weight gain, diet, and exercise, both at the initial visit and periodically throughout the pregnancy. Individualized care and clinical judgment are necessary in the management of the obese and overweight woman who wishes to gain, or is gaining, less weight than recommended but has an appropriately growing fetus. Balancing the risks of fetal growth (both large and small), obstetric complications, and maternal weight retention are essential until research provides evidence to further refine the recommendations for gestational weight gain. Postpartum and interpregnancy care should include advice and recommendations to help the woman to return to her prepregnancy weight, or lower if necessary to achieve a normal BMI, in the first year after the delivery.

Exercise

In the absence of either medical or obstetric complications, 30 minutes or more of moderate exercise per day on most, if not all, days of the week is recommended for pregnant women. A moderate exercise program as part of the treatment plan for women with gestational diabetes mellitus is recommended. Generally, participation in a wide range of recreational activities appears to be safe during pregnancy; however, each sport should be reviewed individually for its potential risk, and activities with a high risk of falling or those with a high risk of abdominal trauma should be avoided. Pregnant women also should avoid supine positions during exercise as much as possible. Recreational and competitive athletes with uncomplicated pregnancies can remain active during pregnancy and should modify their usual exercise routines as medically indicated. Pregnant competitive athletes may require close obstetric supervision. Women are advised not to take up a new strenuous sport during pregnancy, and previously inactive women and those with medical or obstetric complications should be evaluated before recommendations for physical activity participation during pregnancy are made. Additionally, a physically active woman with a history of or risk of preterm delivery or IUGR may be advised to reduce her activity in the second trimester and third trimester. Warning signs to terminate exercise while pregnant include the following:

- Chest pain
- Vaginal bleeding
- Dizziness
- Headache
- Decreased fetal movement
- Amniotic fluid leakage
- Muscle weakness

- Calf pain or swelling
- Regular uterine contractions

The following medical conditions are absolute contraindications to aerobic exercise in pregnancy:

- Hemodynamically significant heart disease
- Restrictive lung disease
- Cervical insufficiency or cerclage
- Persistent second-trimester or third-trimester bleeding
- Placenta previa confirmed after 26 weeks of gestation
- Current premature labor
- Ruptured membranes
- Preeclampsia or pregnancy-induced hypertension

Dental Care

It is important that pregnant women continue usual dental care in pregnancy, and obstetric care providers should conduct an oral health assessment during the first prenatal visit. Obstetric care providers should also be prepared to refer patients for oral health care with a written note or call, as would be the practice with referrals to any medical specialist. Dental care includes routine brushing and flossing, scheduled cleanings, and any medically needed dental work. Pregnant women should be aware that their gums bleed more easily. Physiologic changes during pregnancy may result in noticeable changes in the oral cavity. These changes include pregnancy gingivitis, benign oral gingival lesions, tooth mobility, tooth erosion, dental caries, and periodontitis (see Table 6-6). It is important to reassure women about these various changes to the gums and teeth during pregnancy and to reinforce good oral health habits to keep the gums and teeth healthy.

Caries, poor dentition, and periodontal disease may be associated with an increased risk of preterm delivery. However, patients should be reassured that prevention, diagnosis, and treatment of oral conditions, including dental X-rays (with shielding of the abdomen and thyroid) and local anesthesia (lidocaine with or without epinephrine), are safe during pregnancy. They should also be informed that conditions that require immediate treatment, such as extractions, root canals, and restoration (amalgam or composite) of untreated caries, may be managed at any time during pregnancy. Many

TABLE 6-6. Common Oral Health Conditions During Pregnancy

Pregnancy gingivitis	An increased inflammatory response to dental plaque during pregnancy causes the gingivae to swell and bleed more easily in most women. Rinsing with salt-water (ie, 1 teaspoon of salt in 1 cup of warm water) may help with the irritation. Pregnancy gingivitis typically peaks during the third trimester. Women who have gingivitis before pregnancy are more prone to exacerbation during pregnancy.
Benign oral gingival lesions (known as pyogenic granuloma, granuloma gravidarum or epulis of pregnancy)	In approximately 5% of pregnancies, a highly vascularized, hyperplastic, and often pedunculated lesion up to 2 cm in diameter may appear, usually on the anterior gingiva. These lesions may result from a heightened inflammatory response to oral pathogens and usually regress after pregnancy. Excision is rarely necessary but may be needed if there is severe pain, bleeding, or interference with mastication.
Tooth mobility	Ligaments and bone that support the teeth may temporarily loosen during pregnancy, which results in increased tooth mobility. There is normally not any tooth loss unless other complications are present.
Tooth erosion	Erosion of tooth enamel may be more common because of increased exposure to gastric acid from vomiting secondary to morning sickness, hyperemesis gravidarum, or gastric reflux during late pregnancy. Rinsing with a baking soda solution (ie, a teaspoon of baking soda dissolved in a cup of water) may help neutralize the associated acid.
Dental caries	Pregnancy may result in dental caries due to the increased acidity in the mouth, greater intake of sugary snacks and drinks secondary to pregnancy cravings, and decreased attention to prenatal oral health maintenance.
Periodontitis	Untreated gingivitis can progress to periodontitis, an inflammatory response in which a film of bacteria, known as plaque, adheres to teeth and releases bacterial toxins that create pockets of destructive infection in the gums and bones. The teeth may loosen, bone may be lost, and a bacteremia may result.

Data from Silk H, Douglass AB, Douglass JM, Silk L. Oral health during pregnancy. Am Fam Physician 2008;77:1139–44; Pirie M, Cooke I, Linden G, Irwin C. Dental manifestations of pregnancy. The Obstetrician & Gynaecologist 2007;9:21–6; Boggess KA. Maternal oral health in pregnancy. Society for Maternal–Fetal Medicine. Obstet Gynecol 2008;111:976–86; *and* Polyzos NP, Polyzos IP, Zavos A, Valachis A, Mauri D, Papanikolaou EG, et al. Obstetric outcomes after treatment of periodontal disease during pregnancy: systematic review and meta-analysis. BMJ 2010;341:c7017.

dentists will require a note from the obstetric provider stating that dental care requiring local anesthesia, antibiotics, or narcotic analgesia is not contraindicated in pregnancy.

Nausea and Vomiting

Nausea and vomiting affects more than 70% of pregnant women and can diminish the woman's quality of life. For women with prior pregnancies complicated by nausea and vomiting, it is reasonable to recommend prepregnancy and early pregnancy use of a multivitamin because studies show this reduces the risk of vomiting requiring medical attention. First-line therapy for nausea and vomiting is vitamin B_6 with or without doxylamine. Other effective nonpharmacologic treatments for mild cases include increasing protein consumption and taking powdered ginger capsules daily. For patients with vomiting secondary to morning sickness, hyperemesis gravidarum, or gastric reflux during late pregnancy, the use of antacids or rinsing with a baking soda solution (ie, 1 teaspoon of baking soda dissolved in 1 cup of water) may help neutralize the associated acid. Acupressure treatments have mixed results. Effective and safe treatments for more serious cases include antihistamine H1-receptor blockers, phenothiazines, and benzamides. Hyperemesis gravidarum, a severe form of pregnancy-associated nausea and vomiting that occurs in less than 2% of pregnancies may require more intense therapy, including hospitalization; additional medications; intravenous hydration and nutrition; and, if refractory, total parenteral nutrition.

Vitamin and Mineral Toxicity

Although vitamin A is essential, excessive vitamin A (more than 10,000 international units per day) may be associated with fetal malformations. Dietary intake of vitamin A in the United States is adequate to meet the needs of most pregnant women throughout gestation. Therefore, additional supplementation besides a prenatal vitamin during pregnancy is not recommended except in women in whom the dietary intake of vitamin A may not be adequate, such as strict vegetarians. Vitamin tablets containing 25,000 international units or more of vitamin A are available as over-the-counter preparations; however, pregnant women or those planning to become pregnant who use high doses of vitamin A supplements (and topical retinol) should be cautioned about the potential teratogenicity because excess vitamin A is associated with anomalies of bones, the urinary tract, and the central nervous system. The use of beta carotene, the precursor of vitamin A found in fruits and vegetables, has not been shown to produce vitamin A toxicity.

Excessive vitamin and mineral intake (ie, more than twice the recommended dietary allowances) should be avoided during pregnancy. For example, excess iodine is associated with congenital goiter. There also may be toxicity from excessive use of other fat-soluble vitamins (vitamin D, vitamin E, and vitamin K; see Table 6-4).

Fish provides a source of easily digestible protein with high biologic value in terms of vitamins, amino acids, and minerals. Also many fish are a uniquely rich food source of long-chain omega-3 fatty acids and long-chain polyunsaturated fatty acids. There is strong evidence suggesting that these fatty acids are important in central nervous system development and that maternal consumption benefits fetal development and provides good nutrition for the mother. Some large fish, however, are known to contain high levels of methylmercury, a known fetal teratogen.

Therefore, to gain the benefits of consuming fish while avoiding the risks of methylmercury consumption, pregnant women, women who may become pregnant, and breastfeeding mothers should be encouraged to:

- Eat two or three servings a week (8–12 ounces in total) of a variety of fish that have a low mercury content, including shrimp, pollock, tuna (light canned), tilapia, catfish, and cod (see FDA list of "best choices" available at www.fda.gov/food/foodborneillnesscontaminants/metals/ucm393070.htm.
- Eat only one serving a week (no more than 6 ounces) of some fish, such as albacore (white) tuna and fish with similar mercury concentrations to albacore (white) tuna.
- Avoid certain fish with the highest mercury concentrations, such as shark, swordfish, king mackerel, marlin, orange roughy, tilefish, and bigeye tuna.
- Check for advisories for fish caught by family and friends and where no advisories exist, limit eating those fish to one service a week and do not eat other fish that week.
- Avoid all raw and undercooked seafood.

To prevent pregnancy-related listeria infections, pregnant women should be advised to avoid eating foods with a high risk of listeria, such as hot dogs or luncheon meats unless they are steaming hot; unpasteurized soft cheeses; refrigerated paté and meat spreads; refrigerated smoked seafood; raw (unpasteurized) milk; raw and undercooked seafood, eggs, and meat;

and unwashed fresh fruits and vegetables. Maternal infection has been associated with preterm delivery and other obstetric and neonatal complications. For more information on listeriosis and its prevention during pregnancy, see "Listeriosis" in Chapter 12 and the CDC website at www.cdc.gov/listeria.

Teratogens

Major birth defects occur in 2–3% of the general population. The possible occurrence of a major birth defect is a frequent cause of anxiety among pregnant women. Many consumer inquiries concern the teratogenic potential of environmental exposures. There is little scientifically valid information to estimate risk in human pregnancy. Women need to be counseled that relatively few agents are known to cause malformations in pregnancy and that relatively few women are exposed to agents known to be associated with increased risk of fetal malformations or mental retardation. The health care provider may wish to consult with or refer such women to health care providers with special knowledge or experience in teratology and birth defects. The Organization of Teratology Information Specialists provides information on teratology issues and exposures in pregnancy (www.otispregnancy.org).

Prenatal lead exposure has known adverse effects on maternal health and infant outcomes across a wide range of maternal blood lead levels. In 2010, the CDC issued the first guidelines regarding the screening and management of pregnant and lactating women who have been exposed to lead (available at www.cdc.gov/nceh/lead/tips/pregnant.htm). Routine blood lead testing of all pregnant women is not recommended. Obstetric health care providers need to consider the possibility of lead exposure in individual pregnant women by evaluating risk factors for exposure as part of a comprehensive health risk assessment and perform blood lead testing if a single risk factor is identified. Risk assessment of lead exposure should take place at the earliest contact with pregnant or lactating women.

Although most medications are not known to be teratogens, women need to consult with their health care providers before using prescription and nonprescription medications or herbal remedies (see also "Medication Use" in Chapter 5). Health care provider and patient information about known teratogenic medications, as well as other teratogenic exposures, can be found on the Organization of Teratology Information Specialists' website. Health care providers also can refer women to the CDC's web page on medication use during pregnancy, available at www.cdc.gov/pregnancy/meds/treatingfortwo/index.html for more information on medication safety.

Many women raise questions about the methods of detecting birth defects related to drug exposure. Amniocentesis or CVS for chromosome analysis is not helpful for the diagnosis of birth defects caused by teratogens. Although obstetric ultrasonography has been the mainstay of surveillance for teratogen-induced congenital anomalies, its sensitivity varies with the experience and skill of the imager as well as the specific anatomic abnormality. However, even in expert hands, the overall sensitivity of ultrasonography in the detection of fetal anatomic anomalies is in the range of 50–70%.

Concerns frequently are expressed over the teratogenic potential of diagnostic imaging modalities used during pregnancy. The imaging modality that causes the most anxiety for both the health care provider and the woman is X-ray or ionizing radiation. Much of this anxiety is secondary to a general misperception that any radiation exposure is harmful and may result in injury to or anomaly of the fetus. Most diagnostic X-ray procedures are associated with few, if any, risks to the fetus. Exposure to less than 5 rads has not been associated with an increase in fetal anomalies or pregnancy loss. Moreover, according to the American College of Radiology, no single diagnostic X-ray procedure results in radiation exposure to a degree that would threaten the well-being of a developing preembryo, embryo, or fetus.

Concern about radiation exposure during pregnancy should not prevent medically indicated diagnostic X-ray studies when these are important for the care of the woman. When such a study is indicated, the minimal dose of radiation should be used. Because MRI does not use ionizing radiation, it may be the preferred test. Both spiral computed tomography and ventilation–perfusion scanning expose the fetus to only small amounts of radiation. However, most centers avoid the use of iodinated contrast agents in pregnancy because of the risk of neonatal hypothyroidism. Women concerned about previously performed or planned diagnostic studies need to be counseled to allay these concerns.

Most diagnostic studies in which radioisotopes are used are not hazardous to the fetus and result in low levels of radiation exposure. A typical technetium Tc-99m scan results in a fetal dose of less than 0.5 rads, and a thallium 201 scan also results in a low dose. Many of these isotopes are excreted in the urine. Therefore, women should be advised to drink plenty of fluids and to void frequently after a radionuclide study.

One important exception is the use of iodine 131 for the treatment of Graves disease. The fetal thyroid gland begins to incorporate iodine actively by the end of the first trimester. Administration of iodine 131 after this time can result in destruction of the fetal thyroid gland. Therefore, iodine 131 is contraindicated for therapeutic use during pregnancy. By comparison, there are few reports on the safety of radioisotope imaging of the maternal thyroid during pregnancy, and such studies should be undertaken only after careful consideration of the risks and benefits of the procedure.

Because significant elevation of core body temperature may be associated with fetal anomalies, pregnant women might reasonably be advised to remain in saunas for no more than 15 minutes and in hot tubs for no more than 10 minutes. As an additional precaution, it is best for women to ensure their head, arms, shoulders and upper chest are not submerged in a hot tub so there will be less surface area to absorb heat and more surface area to radiate it.

Air Travel

Occasional air travel during pregnancy is generally safe. Recent cohort studies suggest no increase in adverse pregnancy outcomes for occasional air travelers. Most commercial airlines allow pregnant women to fly up to 36 weeks of gestation. Some restrict pregnant women from international flights earlier in gestation and some require documentation of gestational age. For specific airline requirements, women should check with the individual carrier. Civilian and military aircrew members who become pregnant should check with their specific agencies for regulations or restrictions to their flying duties.

Air travel is not recommended at any time during pregnancy for women who have medical or obstetric conditions that may be exacerbated by flight or that could require emergency care. The duration of the flight also should be considered when planning travel. Pregnant women should be informed that the most common obstetric emergencies occur in the first and third trimester.

In-craft environmental conditions, such as changes in cabin pressure and low humidity, coupled with the physiologic changes of pregnancy, result in increased heart rate and blood pressure and a significant decrease in aerobic capacity. The risks associated with long hours of air travel immobilization and low cabin humidity, such as lower extremity edema and venous thrombotic events, have been the focus of attention for all air travelers. Despite the lack of evidence of such events during pregnancy, certain preventive measures can be used to minimize these risks, eg, use of support stockings and periodic movement of the lower extremities, avoidance of restrictive clothing, occasional ambulation, and maintenance of adequate hydration.

In pregnant women the seat belt should be belted low on the hipbones, between the protuberant abdomen and pelvis. Several precautions may ease discomfort for pregnant air travelers. For example, gas-producing foods or drinks should be avoided before scheduled flights because entrapped gases expand at altitude. Preventive antiemetic medication can be considered for women with increased nausea.

Antepartum Tests of Fetal Well-Being

Fetal heart rate (FHR) pattern, level of activity, and degree of muscular tone are sensitive to hypoxemia and acidemia. Redistribution of fetal blood flow in response to hypoxemia may result in diminished renal perfusion and oligohydramnios. Surveillance techniques such as cardiotocography, real-time ultrasonography, and maternal perception of fetal movement can identify the fetus that may be undergoing some degree of uteroplacental compromise. Identification of suspected fetal compromise provides the opportunity to intervene before progressive metabolic acidosis results in fetal death. However, acute, catastrophic changes in fetal status, such as those that can occur with abruptio placentae or an umbilical cord accident, are generally not predicted by tests of fetal well-being. Therefore, fetal deaths from such events are less amenable to prevention.

Although there have been no randomized clinical trials that clearly demonstrate improved perinatal outcome with the use of antepartum testing or that determine the optimal time to initiate testing, certain tests have become an integral part of the clinical care of pregnancies suspected to be at increased risk of fetal demise due to uteroplacental insufficiency. Indications for initiating antenatal testing include, but are not limited to:

Maternal conditions

- Antiphospholipid syndrome
- Cyanotic heart disease
- Systemic lupus erythematosus
- Chronic renal disease
- Insulin-treated diabetes mellitus
- Hypertensive disorders

Pregnancy-related or fetal conditions

- Pregnancy-induced hypertension
- Decreased fetal movement

- Oligohydramnios and polyhydramnios
- IUGR
- Postterm pregnancy
- Isoimmunization (moderate to severe)
- Previous fetal demise (unexplained)
- Multiple gestation (with significant growth discrepancy)
- Monochorionic diamniotic and monoamniotic multiple gestation

Antenatal Testing Strategy

Devising the appropriate antenatal testing strategy—what test to use, when to start testing, and how frequently to retest—requires balancing several considerations. The prognosis for neonatal survival, the severity of maternal disease, the risk of fetal death, and the potential for iatrogenic prematurity as a complication from false-positive test results all should be taken into account when considering antenatal testing. Antenatal testing is intended for use in pregnancies at risk of fetal demise. There are risks of false-positive test results, including unnecessary delivery of a healthy baby. As with any screening test, false-positive test results are more common in populations at low risk of the disease. Hence antepartum surveillance should be reserved for high-risk pregnancies.

In general, antepartum testing is not appropriate before a gestational age at which the health care provider is willing to intervene and should be targeted at the gestational age at which the increased risk of stillbirth is likely. Therefore, ACOG supports initiating antenatal testing at 32–34 weeks of gestation for most pregnancies with increased risk of stillbirth. However, for pregnancies with particularly high-risk conditions or multiple complicating factors, testing may begin earlier. The following tests are commonly used in clinical practice to assess fetal status and are described in detail later in this section:

- Assessment of fetal movement (eg, kick counts)
- Nonstress test (NST)
- Acoustic stimulation
- Biophysical profile (BPP)
- Modified biophysical profile (NST plus amniotic fluid index [AFI] or deepest vertical pocket of amniotic fluid)

- Contraction stress test (CST) or oxytocin challenge test
- Doppler ultrasonography of umbilical artery blood flow velocity

Repeat antenatal testing should be performed when the condition that initiated testing persists. Typically the NST, CST, and BPP are repeated at weekly intervals. However, in the presence of certain conditions, such as postterm pregnancy, IUGR, or pregnancy-induced hypertension, some investigators perform twice-weekly antenatal testing. In addition, any significant deterioration in maternal condition or new decrease in fetal activity requires fetal testing independent of time elapsed from previous testing. Usually only one antenatal testing episode is indicated when a decrease in fetal activity is noted.

A normal test is highly reassuring. The risk of a fetal death within 7 days of a reassuring testing is as follows (rates expressed per 1,000 fetuses): NST, 1.9; CST, 0.3; BPP, 0.8; modified BPP, 0.8.

Interpretation of abnormal test results should take into consideration the overall clinical picture and the possibility that the test result is falsely positive. An abnormal NST or modified BPP should be further evaluated using either a CST or full BPP. Decisions regarding serial testing or proceeding with delivery should be made in the context of the gestational age, and the maternal and fetal condition. Certain maternal conditions, such as diabetic ketoacidosis, hypoxemia, hypotension, or general anesthesia can result in abnormal test results. In these circumstances, stabilization of the maternal condition and retesting the fetus may be appropriate. If delivery is planned, in the absence of obstetric indications, an induction of labor with continuous FHR monitoring may be attempted, with a plan for cesarean delivery, if indicated.

Assessment of Fetal Movement. Women who report decreased fetal movement are at increased risk of adverse perinatal outcome. Although not all women need to perform a daily fetal movement assessment, if a woman notices a decrease in fetal activity, she should be encouraged to contact her health care provider, and further assessment should be performed. Fetal kick counting is an inexpensive test of fetal well-being, however the effectiveness in preventing stillbirth is uncertain. Neither the ideal number of kicks nor the ideal duration of daily movement count assessment has been defined. Perhaps more important than any single quantitative guideline is the mother's perception of a decrease in fetal activity relative to a previous level.

Although several counting protocols have been used, neither the optimal number of movements nor the ideal duration for counting movements has been defined. Thus, numerous protocols have been reported and appear to be acceptable. In one approach, the woman was instructed to lie on her side and count distinct fetal movements. Perception of 10 distinct movements in a period of up to 2 hours was considered reassuring. The count was discontinued after 10 movements were perceived. The mean time interval to perceive 10 movements was 20.9 (±18.1) minutes. In another approach, women were instructed to count fetal movements for 1 hour three times per week. The count was considered reassuring if it equaled or exceeded the woman's previously established baseline count. Thus, regardless of the fetal movement approach used, in the absence of a reassuring count, further fetal assessment is recommended.

Nonstress Test. A nonstress test (NST) uses FHR patterns and accelerations as an indicator of fetal well-being. Fetal heart rate accelerations occur through a link between fetal peripheral movements and a cardioregulatory center in the midbrain, which requires intact peripheral, central, and autonomic neural in-flow and out-flow pathways. These pathways mature as the fetus matures, such that criteria for accelerations differ based on gestational age.

To perform an NST, the FHR is monitored with an external transducer for at least 20 minutes. The tracing is observed for FHR accelerations. The testing can be continued for an additional 40 minutes or longer to take into account the typical fetal sleep–wake cycle. Fetal heart rate accelerations that peak at 15 beats per minute above the baseline and persist for 15 seconds are associated with an extremely low risk of fetal acidosis and, thus, are considered reassuring. If a nonstress test is performed at an early gestational age, it is more likely to be nonreactive in the absence of fetal compromise. Before 32 weeks of gestation, accelerations that peak at 10 beats per minute and persist for 10 seconds (from baseline to baseline) are as reassuring as the 15 beat criteria for those fetuses beyond 32 weeks of gestation.

The results of an NST are considered reactive if two or more FHR accelerations are detected within a 20-minute period, with or without fetal movement discernible by the mother. A nonreactive tracing is one without sufficient FHR accelerations in a 40-minute period and requires further testing for confirmation of fetal reassurance. An NST may be nonreactive for a variety of reasons, including fetal sleep-cycles, maternal ingestion of sedatives, fetal cardiac or central nervous system abnormalities, or a lack of fetal movement as an adaptive mechanism for conservation of energy and metabolism in the context of hypoxemia (detection of the latter being the specific aim of antepartum testing).

Perinatal outcomes after a reactive tracing provoked with acoustic stimulation are comparable to those associated with a spontaneously reactive NST. The use of acoustic stimulation decreases false nonreactive NSTs and reduces overall testing time. Stimulation is delivered for 1–2 seconds using a specially designed artificial larynx that is placed on the maternal abdomen. It can be repeated up to three times, each for a maximum duration of 2 seconds, to elicit FHR accelerations.

Variable decelerations may be observed in up to 50% of NSTs. Variable decelerations that are nonrepetitive and brief (less than 30 seconds) are not associated with lack of fetal well-being or the need for obstetric intervention. Repetitive variable decelerations (at least three in 20 minutes), even if mild, have been associated with an increased risk of cesarean delivery for a nonreassuring intrapartum FHR pattern. Fetal heart rate decelerations that persist for 1 minute or longer are associated with a markedly increased risk of both cesarean delivery and fetal demise. In this setting, the decision to deliver should be made with consideration of whether the benefits outweigh the potential risks of expectant management.

Contraction Stress Test. Contraction stress test (CST), formerly known as an oxytocin challenge test, involves subjecting the fetus to the physiologic stress of uterine contractions. Relative contraindications to inducing contractions for CSTs include preterm labor, pregnancies with a high risk of preterm delivery, preterm premature rupture of membranes, known placenta previa, or history of classical uterine scar.

To perform a CST, the FHR is obtained using an external transducer, and uterine contraction activity is monitored with a tocodynamometer. A baseline tracing is obtained for 10–20 minutes. If at least three contractions of 40 seconds or more are present in a 10-minute period, uterine stimulation is not necessary. If the contractions are not present, they are induced with either nipple stimulation or intravenously administered oxytocin. Intravenous infusion of low-dose oxytocin can be initiated, usually at a rate of 0.5–1 microunit per min, and increased every 15–20 minutes until an adequate contraction pattern occurs (ie, three contractions in 10 minutes).

The results of the CST can be categorized as follows:

- Negative—No late or significant variable decelerations
- Positive—Late decelerations are present following 50% or more of contractions, even if the frequency of contractions is less than three in 10 minutes
- Equivocal-Suspicious—Intermittent late decelerations or significant variable decelerations
- Equivocal—FHR decelerations that occur in the presence of contractions more frequent than every 2 minutes or lasting longer than 90 seconds
- Unsatisfactory—Fewer than three contractions within 10 minutes or an uninterpretable tracing

Oxytocin and nipple stimulation can produce tachysystole. If FHR decelerations occur in the presence of tachysystole, retesting is appropriate to ensure a correct interpretation. Equivocal testing may be repeated in 24 hours or sooner unless an intervening indication for delivery arises, or it may prompt admission for closer observation. As with all antepartum testing, the management of a positive (or nonreassuring) CST requires individualized decision making based on other parameters of fetal reassurance and gestational age.

Biophysical Profile. A biophysical profile (BPP) consists of assessment of five fetal variables. The five components of a reassuring BPP are as follows:

1. NST reactive—The probability of fetal well-being is identical with scores of 10 out of 10 and 8 out of 10
2. Fetal breathing movements—At least one or more episodes of rhythmic fetal breathing movements of 30 seconds or more within 30 minutes
3. Fetal movement—Three or more discrete body or limb movements within 30 minutes
4. Fetal tone—One or more episodes of fetal extremity extension with return to flexion, or opening or closing of a hand within 30 minutes
5. Determination of amniotic fluid volume—a single deepest vertical pocket greater than 2 cm

The combination of the aforementioned parameters accounts for both acute changes in fetal reserve (NST, breathing, flexion, and extension) as well as changes that are influenced over a more chronic time course (amniotic fluid volume and fetal tone).

A BPP is scored from 0–10 with a score of either 2 (present) or 0 (absent) being assigned to each of the five observations. Before a 0 can be given for any of the variables, the fetus must be observed for 30 minutes. A score of 8 or 10 is reassuring. A score of 6 is equivocal and a decision to retest within 12–24 hours or proceed with delivery should be made within the context of gestational age and weighed against the risk of prematurity. A score of 4 or less is abnormal and warrants further evaluation and consideration of delivery. Irrespective of the overall score, except in the setting of premature rupture of membranes, the finding of oligohydramnios may warrant consideration of delivery in term pregnancies or more frequent antepartum testing in the case of preterm gestations.

Modified Biophysical Profile. Another approach to fetal surveillance, the modified BPP, combines the use of an NST as a short-term indicator of fetal status with the assessment of amniotic fluid index (AFI) as an indicator of long-term placental function. Nonstress test changes are thought to be one of the early manifestations of fetal hypoxia, whereas amniotic fluid volume likely changes more slowly over time. Thus, the results of the modified BPP are considered normal if the NST is reactive and the amniotic fluid volume is greater than 2 cm in the deepest vertical pocket, or, if the AFI is used, it is normal. The results of the modified BPP are considered abnormal if either the NST is nonreactive or amniotic fluid volume in the deepest vertical pocket is 2 cm or less (ie, oligohydramnios are present) or the AFI is less than 5.0. The modified BPP is less cumbersome than complete BPP assessment and appears to be as predictive of fetal well-being as other approaches of biophysical fetal surveillance.

Doppler Ultrasonography of Umbilical Artery. The umbilical arteries comprise the main out-flow tract of fetal blood back to the placental bed. Vascular resistance in the placenta decreases as gestational age progresses and, more specifically, high velocity forward diastolic flow in the umbilical arteries is maintained. Umbilical artery Doppler flow ultrasonography uses these hemodynamic characteristics to assess resistance to blood flow in the placenta. Umbilical artery Doppler ultrasonography is not a screening test for detecting fetal compromise in the general population, but it can be used in conjunction with other biophysical tests in high-risk pregnancies associated with suspected IUGR. The index most commonly used to quantify the flow velocity waveform is the systolic/diastolic ratio. As placental resistance increases, the systolic/diastolic ratio increases, the end diastolic flow decreases and may become absent or reversed. Randomized studies on the utility of umbilical artery Doppler velocimetry generally have defined abnormal flow as either absent or reversed end-diastolic flow. In the fetus with IUGR, the presence of absent or reversed end-diastolic flow is generally an indication for consideration for possible delivery versus more intensive fetal monitoring. Multiple waveforms need to be assessed, and wall-filter settings need to be set low enough (typically less than 150 Hz) to avoid masking diastolic flow. Currently, there is no evidence that umbilical artery Doppler velocimetry provides information about fetal well-being in the fetus with normal growth.

Serial Doppler studies can be performed in the growth-restricted fetus and used in conjunction with other measures of fetal well-being to guide the timing of delivery. The finding of abnormal umbilical artery Doppler studies also may be used to guide the administration of corticosteroids in anticipation of delivery.

Special Populations and Considerations

All pregnant women should receive the best appropriate care. However, each of the following groups is potentially more vulnerable to poor pregnancy outcomes or barriers to health care and has unique circumstances that require additional attention.

Adolescents

Minors typically have legal rights protecting their privacy regarding the diagnosis and treatment of pregnancy. Once the gestational age is determined, a minor should be fully informed in a balanced manner about all options, including continuation of the pregnancy, either with the intent of raising the child herself or placing the child for adoption, or termination of the pregnancy. The health care provider should assess the adolescent's ability to understand the implications of the diagnosis of pregnancy and the options available.

The adolescent should be encouraged to return for visits as needed and helped to understand the importance of a timely decision. She should be encouraged to include her parents or guardian and the father of the fetus in her decisions, if appropriate. The adolescent's right to decide the outcome of her pregnancy and who should be involved should be respected. Many states have laws regarding adolescent rights, and the health care provider needs be aware of these state laws when making health care decisions.

If the adolescent chooses to continue the pregnancy, she should be referred for psychosocial support. There is an increased incidence of low birth weight, neonatal death, preterm delivery, preeclampsia, anemia, and STIs in pregnant adolescents, which necessitates more frequent monitoring. Pregnant adolescents need to be counseled about the effects of STIs on themselves and their fetuses. They need to receive repetitive reinforcement that condoms need to be used during pregnancy for STI protection. Rapid repeat pregnancy is common in adolescents. Plans for postpartum contraception should be discussed during prenatal care visits and the adolescent's contraceptive method should be provided before discharge.

Incarcerated Women

Generally, pregnant inmates are at a higher risk of poor pregnancy outcomes than the general population. Upon entry into a prison or jail, every woman of childbearing age should be assessed for pregnancy risk by inquiring about menstrual history, heterosexual activity, and contraceptive use, and tested for pregnancy, as appropriate. Incarcerated women who wish to continue their pregnancies should have access to readily available and regularly scheduled obstetric care, beginning in early pregnancy and continuing through the postpartum period. Incarcerated pregnant women also should have access to unscheduled or emergency obstetric visits on a 24-hour basis. Prenatal care in correctional facilities must reflect national standards, including visit frequency with a qualified prenatal care provider, screening and diagnostic tests, and referrals for complications.

Because of high rates of nonmedical substance use and HIV infection, prompt screening for these conditions is important. All pregnant women should be questioned about their past and present use of alcohol, tobacco, and other drugs, including the recreational use of prescription and over-the-counter medication. Nonmedical substance use can continue during incarceration despite efforts to prevent drugs from entering correctional facilities. Incarcerated pregnant women also should be screened for depression or mental stress and for postpartum depression after delivery and be appropriately treated.

Although maintaining adequate safety is critical, correctional officers do not need to routinely be present in the room while a pregnant woman is being examined or in the hospital room during labor and delivery unless requested by medical staff or the situation poses a danger to the safety of the medical staff or others. While in labor and during prenatal visits, correctional staff must respect women's privacy, especially during pelvic exams and childbirth.

Pregnant inmates must deliver at an appropriate health care facility. Delivery services for incarcerated pregnant women should be provided in a licensed hospital with facilities for high-risk pregnancies when available. It is important to avoid separating the mother from the infant to allow for the formation of maternal–child bonds. Breastfeeding should be encouraged. Because incarcerated pregnant women often have short jail or prison stays and may not give birth while incarcerated, postpartum contraceptive options, including immediate postpartum LARC, should be discussed and provided during incarceration to decrease the likelihood of an unintended pregnancy during and after release from incarceration.

The use of physical restraints on pregnant incarcerated women may not only compromise health care, but is demeaning and rarely necessary. Shackling of pregnant and postpartum women (within 6 weeks postpartum) during transportation to medical care facilities and during the receipt of health services should occur only in exceptional circumstances after a strong consideration of the health effects of restraints by the health care provider. Exceptions include when there is imminent risk of escape or harm. If restraint is needed, it should be the least restrictive possible to ensure safety and need never include restraints that interfere with leg movement or the ability of the woman to break a fall. The woman should be allowed to lie on her side, not flat on her back or stomach. Pressure must not be applied directly or indirectly to the abdomen. Correctional officers should be available and required to remove the shackles immediately upon request of medical personnel. Women should never be shackled during evaluation for labor and delivery. If restraint is used, a report should be filed by the Department of Corrections and reviewed by an independent body. There should be consequences for individuals and institutions when use of restraints was unjustified.

Homeless Women

It has been estimated that as many as 14% of individuals living in the United States have been homeless at some time, and as many as 3.5 million people (1% of the U.S. population, or 10% of the poor population) experience homelessness in a given year. Domestic and sexual violence is the leading cause of homelessness for women and families, and 20–50% of all homeless women and children become homeless as a direct result of fleeing domestic violence. Compared with women who are not homeless, homeless women are far more likely to experience violence of all sorts because of a lack of personal security when living outdoors or in shelters.

Homeless women are less likely to receive prenatal care than women who are not homeless, and adverse birth outcomes are substantially higher in homeless women compared with the general population. A Canadian study found that compared with women who are not homeless, homeless women were 2.9 times more likely to have a preterm delivery, 6.9 times more likely to give birth to an infant who weighed less than 2,000 g, and 3.3 times more likely to have a small-for-gestational-age newborn, even after adjustment for risk factors, such as maternal age, number of previous pregnancies, and smoking. In the United States, preterm birth rates and low birth weight rates in homeless women exceed national averages.

It is important for physicians to identify women within the practice who are (or are at risk of becoming) homeless by asking questions about living conditions, nutrition, substance abuse, and intimate partner violence; provide health care, including preventive care, for homeless women without bias; and not withhold treatment based on concerns about lack of adherence. Health care providers are advised to simplify medical regimens and address barriers, including transportation needs for follow-up health care visits. In addition, health care providers should inform women who are (or at risk of becoming) homeless about appropriate community resources, including local substance abuse programs, intimate partner violence services, and social service agencies.

Women With Disabilities

Physical, intellectual and developmental, sensory, and psychiatric impairments may affect the quality and availability of health care services for women. With all disabilities, consideration of the history of the disability, the number and severity of limitations, and its expected progression is critical in meeting the health care needs and concerns of women. Health care providers may be unfamiliar with the individual's specific disability and its consequences on health, sexual functioning, and reproductive potential. This information may be accessible through various means, such as consultation with rehabilitation physicians or other disability health care providers, further investigation of medical literature, disability organizations, and through discussion with the woman and her family. Many women are well informed about their disabilities and the resources available to them.

Language and educational differences between women and their health care providers are barriers to effective care. Women with disabilities may have additional challenges. Knowledge of the women's mode of communication and patience in the process are critical to ensure informed health care delivery. Women with disabilities also may need extra time allotted for their appointment. When scheduling appointments, asking a woman about the need for extra time or services in a nonjudgmental and nonstigmatizing fashion may be one way of accommodating such needs. Creativity and flexibility on the part of each staff member can go a long way in ameliorating these challenges and establishing mutually rewarding and respectful services.

Physical Disabilities

Pregnancy and parenting for women with physical disabilities may pose unique medical and social challenges but rarely are precluded by the disability itself. Few, if any, physical disabilities directly limit fertility. Health care providers have the responsibility to provide appropriate reproductive health care services to these women or arrange adequate consultation or referral. Nonbiased prepregnancy counseling for couples in which one partner has a physical disability may decrease subsequent psychosocial and medical complications of pregnancy. Screening and provision of disability-specific information, such as condition-appropriate genetic counseling and folate supplementation for women who have spina bifida, are highly desirable (see also "Prepregnancy Nutritional Counseling" in Chapter 5).

Once pregnancy occurs, the women should have early contact with their obstetrician–gynecologists or other obstetric care providers. Detailed pregnancy care plans should be developed in negotiation with managed care plans and other insurers to increase access to and use of prenatal care services, ensure appropriate postpartum hospital length of stay, and arrange postpartum home care services, if necessary. Assessment of the need for additional assistance during pregnancy to ambulate, perform safe transfers, and maintain hygiene and household activities is recommended. Regular consultation or referral may be required to achieve the optimum outcome.

Intellectual and Developmental Disabilities

In caring for pregnant women with intellectual and developmental disabilities, it is important to consider the following psychosocial factors: whether the individual lives at home or in a domiciliary care setting; whether there is a reliable caregiver present; previous history of sexual abuse; and cognitive factors, including her ability to relay a personal or family history of disease and symptoms. Genetic screening is particularly important for pregnant women with Down syndrome. First-trimester screening with serum analytes or cell-free DNA, or ultrasound examinations, or both, should be offered (see also "Antepartum Genetic Screening and Diagnosis" earlier in this chapter).

Before examination, it should be determined who will give consent for the examination and any consequential treatment. It also is important at this time to ascertain if the patient is competent to understand findings and health recommendations or whether this information should be transmitted to an identified guardian or caregiver. For women with intellectual and developmental disabilities, making materials available in pictorial formats or in simple, straightforward language can greatly facilitate communication. It often is helpful, with the woman's consent, to have a companion with whom she is familiar accompany her to the examination room. Additionally, health care providers who care for patients with intellectual and developmental disabilities may find it helpful to provide a short summary of the patient's medical problems for the patient (or guardian) to keep in her billfold along with the names of her primary medical care provider and a contact person.

Consent and Power of Attorney

Obtaining informed consent for medical treatment is an ethical requirement that is partially reflected in legal doctrines and requirements. Seeking informed consent expresses respect for the patient as an individual. It not only ensures the protection of the patient against unwanted medical treatment, but it also makes possible the patient's active involvement in her medical planning and care. Communication is necessary if informed consent is to be realized, and health care providers can and should help to find ways to facilitate communication not only in individual relations with women but also in the structured context of medical care institutions. When informed consent by the women is impossible, a surrogate decision maker should be identified to represent her wishes or best interests. In emergency situations, medical professionals may have to act according to their perceptions of the best interests of the woman; in rare instances, they may have to forgo obtaining consent because of some other overriding ethical obligation, such as protecting the public health.

An advance directive is the formal mechanism by which a woman may express her values regarding her future health status. It may take the form of a proxy directive or an instructional directive or both. Proxy directives, such as the durable power of attorney for health care, designate a surrogate to make medical decisions on behalf of the woman if she is no longer competent to express her choices. Instructional directives, such as living wills, focus on the types of life-sustaining treatment that a woman would or would not choose in various clinical circumstances, but many states limit the power of such documents and directives in pregnancy.

Although courts at times have intervened to impose treatment on a pregnant woman, currently there is general agreement that a pregnant woman who has decision-making capacity has the same right to refuse treatment as a nonpregnant woman. When a pregnant woman does not have decision-making capacity, however, legislation frequently limits her ability to refuse treatment through an advance directive. Statutes that prohibit pregnant women from exercising their right to determine or refuse current or future medical treatment are unethical.

Second-Trimester and Third-Trimester Patient Education

Important topics to discuss with women before delivery include working, childbirth education classes, choosing a newborn care provider, anticipating labor, preterm labor, breech presentation at term, trial of labor after cesarean delivery, elective delivery, cesarean delivery on maternal request, umbilical cord blood banking, breastfeeding, preparation for discharge, and neonatal interventions.

Working

A woman with an uncomplicated pregnancy usually can continue to work until the onset of labor. Women with medical or obstetric complications of pregnancy may need to make adjustments based on the nature of their activities, occupations, and specific complications. It also has been reported that pregnant women whose occupations require standing or repetitive, strenuous, physical lifting have a tendency to give birth earlier and have small-for-gestational-age infants.

A period of 4–6 weeks after delivery generally is required for a woman's physiologic condition to return to normal; however, the woman's individual circumstances should be considered when recommending resumption of full activity. It also is important for the development of children and the family unit that adequate paid parental leave be available for parents in order to participate in early childrearing. The federal Family and Medical Leave Act and state laws should be consulted to determine the family and medical leave that is available.

Childbirth Education Classes and Choosing a Newborn Care Provider

Pregnant women should be referred to appropriate educational literature and urged to attend childbirth education classes. Studies have shown that childbirth education programs can have a beneficial effect on patient experience in labor and delivery. Other family members also should be encouraged to participate in childbirth education programs. Adequate preparation of family members may benefit the mother, the newborn infants, and, ultimately, the family unit. The woman and her family members should be educated regarding hospital practices that enable women to achieve their breastfeeding intentions, such as immediate skin-to-skin contact, rooming in, feeding in response to infant cues, and avoiding pacifiers and unindicated supplementation.

Many hospitals, community agencies, and other groups offer such educational programs. The participation of physicians, certified nurse–midwives, and hospital obstetric nurses in educational programs is desirable to ensure continuity and consistency of care and information. National organizations are available for assistance as well. Integration of parenting education in prenatal education is beneficial in facilitating transition to parenthood.

Sometime during the third trimester, the pregnant woman should be encouraged to meet with a newborn care provider to discuss the importance of newborn care, including the importance of vaccines and feeding. If she has not identified a newborn care provider, she should be referred to the appropriate resources to identify her newborn care provider before delivery, if possible.

Anticipating Labor

Most women will give birth near term. As pregnancy progresses, women need to be advised when and how to contact their health care providers should symptoms of labor or membrane rupture occur. If a woman has a birth plan, she should be encouraged to review it with her health care provider before labor. A detailed discussion should take place during the third trimester regarding analgesic and anesthetic options available for labor and delivery.

Preterm Labor

Preterm labor generally is defined as regular contractions that occur before 37 weeks of gestation and is associated with changes in the cervix. Toward the end of the second trimester, signs and symptoms of preterm birth, ruptured membranes, and vaginal bleeding should be reviewed with the woman, and she should be encouraged to contact the health care provider should these symptoms occur. Women should be given a telephone number to call where assistance is available 24 hours per day. Short-term interventions to allow for steroid administration and transfer of the pregnant woman to an appropriate level of hospital for her situation are possible if a woman is seen early enough after onset of symptoms (see also “Preterm Birth” in Chapter 9).

Breech Presentation at Term

If the fetus persists in a breech presentation at 36–38 weeks of gestation, women should be offered an external cephalic version if appropriate. Contraindications to the procedure include multifetal gestation, nonreassuring fetal testing, müllerian duct anomalies, and suspected abruptio placentae or placenta previa. Relative contraindications include intrauterine growth restriction and oligohydramnios. The success rate of external cephalic version ranges from 35–86%, with an average success rate of approximately 58%. Planned cesarean delivery is the most common and safest route of delivery for singleton fetuses at term in breech presentations. However, planned vaginal delivery of a term singleton breech may be reasonable under hospital-specific protocol guidelines for both eligibility and labor management if the health care provider is experienced in vaginal breech deliveries. Before embarking on a plan for a vaginal breech delivery, women should be informed that the risk of perinatal or neonatal mortality or short-term serious neonatal morbidity might be somewhat higher than if a cesarean delivery is planned. Informed consent for vaginal delivery should be obtained and documented.

Trial of Labor After Cesarean Delivery

The enthusiasm to consider trial of labor after cesarean delivery (TOLAC) varies greatly among women, and this variation is at least partly related to the differences in the way individuals value the potential risks and benefits.

Accordingly, potential benefits and risks of both TOLAC and elective repeat cesarean delivery should be discussed and documented. Discussion should consider individual characteristics that affect the chances of vaginal birth after cesarean delivery (VBAC) and TOLAC-associated complications so that a woman can choose her intended route of delivery based on data that are personally relevant.

A discussion of VBAC early in a woman's prenatal care course, if possible, will allow the most time for her to consider options for TOLAC or elective repeat cesarean delivery. Many of the factors that are related to the chance of VBAC or uterine rupture are known early in pregnancy. If the type of previous hysterotomy is in doubt, reasonable attempts should be made to obtain the woman's medical records. Trial of labor after cesarean delivery is not contraindicated for women with one previous cesarean delivery with an unknown uterine scar type unless there is a high clinical suspicion of a previous classical uterine incision. As the pregnancy progresses, if other circumstances arise that may change the risks or benefits of TOLAC (eg, need for induction), these should be addressed. Counseling also may include consideration of intended family size and the risk of additional cesarean deliveries, with the recognition that the future reproductive plans may be uncertain or change.

Counseling also should include a discussion of the resources available to support women electing TOLAC at their intended delivery site, and whether such resources match those recommended for caring for women electing TOLAC. Available data indicate that TOLAC may be safely undertaken in both university and community hospitals and facilities with and without residency programs (levels I–IV maternal care facilities), but all facilities should be ready at all times to initiate emergency procedures to meet unexpected needs of the woman and newborn within the center, and to facilitate transport to an acute care setting when necessary. This includes the ability to begin emergency cesarean delivery within a time interval that best incorporates maternal and fetal risks and benefits with the provision of emergency care. Trial of labor after cesarean delivery should not be available at freestanding birthing centers.

After counseling, the ultimate decision to undergo TOLAC or a repeat cesarean delivery should be made by the woman in consultation with her health care provider. Global mandates for TOLAC are inappropriate because individual risk factors are not considered. Documentation of counseling and the management plan should be included in the medical record (see also "Vaginal Birth After Cesarean Delivery" in Chapter 7).

Elective Delivery

An elective delivery is a delivery that is performed without medical indication. Elective deliveries should not be undertaken before 39 weeks of gestation. If an elective delivery is planned after 39 weeks of gestation, then accuracy of the gestational age, cervical status, and consideration of any potential risks to the mother or fetus are paramount in any discussion of a nonmedically indicated delivery. Full term gestation should be confirmed using the following criteria:

- Ultrasound measurement at less than 20 weeks of gestation supports gestational age of 39 weeks or greater; there is no role for elective delivery in a woman with a suboptimally dated pregnancy
- Fetal heart tones have been documented as present for 30 weeks by Doppler ultrasonography
- It has been 36 weeks since a positive serum or urine human chorionic gonadotropin test

(See Appendix F for gestational age categories.) (See also "Induction of Labor and Cervical Ripening" in Chapter 7 for more information.)

Cesarean Delivery on Maternal Request

When a woman desires a cesarean delivery on maternal request, her health care provider should consider her specific risk factors, such as age, body mass index, accuracy of estimated gestational age, reproductive plans, personal values, and cultural context. Critical life experiences (eg, trauma, violence, poor obstetric outcomes) and anxiety about the birth process may prompt her request. If her main concern is a fear of pain in childbirth, then prenatal childbirth education, emotional support in labor, and anesthesia for childbirth should be offered (see also "Cesarean Delivery" in Chapter 7).

Umbilical Cord Blood Banking

Prospective parents may seek information regarding umbilical cord blood banking. Balanced and accurate information regarding the advantages and disadvantages of public versus private banking should be provided. Discussion might include information regarding maternal infectious disease and genetic testing, the ultimate outcome of use of poor quality units of umbilical cord blood, and a disclosure that demographic data will be maintained. The remote chance of an autologous unit being used for a child or family member should be disclosed (about 1/2,700 individuals). Directed donation of umbilical cord blood should be considered when there is a specific diagnosis of a disease known to be treatable by a hematopoietic transplant for an immediate family member. Umbilical cord blood donation should be encouraged when the umbilical cord blood is stored in a bank for public use. In cases in which a patient and family are planning donation of umbilical cord blood, families should be counseled that delayed umbilical cord clamping—recommended in vigorous term and preterm infants—may decrease the yield of cord blood obtained. However, in the absence of directed donation, the benefits to the infant of transfusion of additional blood volume at birth likely exceed the benefits of banking that volume for possible future use. Some states have passed legislation requiring physicians to inform their patients about umbilical cord blood banking options. Health care providers should consult their state medical associations for information regarding state laws.

Breastfeeding

The advice and encouragement of the obstetrician–gynecologist and other obstetric care providers are critical in assisting mothers to make an informed infant feeding decision. As when discussing any health behavior, the obstetrician–gynecologist is obligated both to ensure patient comprehension of the relevant information and to be certain that the conversation is free from coercion, pressure, or undue influence. Families should receive noncommercial, accurate, and unbiased information so that they can make informed decisions about their health care. Obstetric care providers should be aware that personal experiences with infant feeding may affect their counseling. In addition, pervasive direct-to-consumer marketing of infant formula adversely affects patient and health care provider perceptions of the risks and benefits of breastfeeding.

Beginning conversations about lactation early in prenatal care by asking the patient and her family, "What have you heard about breastfeeding?" sets the stage for a patient-centered discussion. When taking an obstetric history, health care providers should specifically ask about any breast surgeries, prior breastfeeding duration, and any previous breastfeeding difficulties. Prior problems leading to earlier-than-desired weaning should be discussed, anticipatory guidance provided, and appropriate lactation support resources identified. The breast examination can identify surgical scars indicating prior surgery as well as widely spaced, tubular breasts that may indicate insufficient glandular tissue. A breast assessment and breastfeeding history should be obtained as part of prenatal care, and identified concerns and risk factors for breastfeeding difficulties should be discussed with the woman, and communicated to the infant's health care provider either directly or as part of shared records. Health care providers should engage the patient's partner and other family members in discussions about infant feeding and address any questions and concerns. This patient-centered approach allows the health care provider, the patient, and her family to anticipate challenges, develop strategies to address them, and collaborate to develop a feeding plan that is compatible with the family's individual values, circumstances, and concerns. Obstetrician–gynecologists and other obstetric care providers should support each mother's informed decision about whether to initiate or continue breastfeeding, recognizing that she is uniquely qualified to decide whether exclusive breastfeeding, mixed feeding, or formula feeding is optimal for her and her infant (see also "Breastfeeding" in Chapter 10).

Preparation for Discharge

Prospective parents should be educated about breastfeeding, sleep safety practices, and newborn screening (see also Chapter 10). The woman's reproductive life plans should be reviewed, and commensurate methods of contraception should be discussed. Women should be encouraged to select a contraceptive method before discharge, so that appropriate supplies and counseling can be provided (see also "Reproductive Life Plan" in Chapter 5 and "Postpartum Contraception" in Chapter 8).

Neonatal Interventions

During prenatal visits, the topic of neonatal interventions should be discussed, including male circumcision, administration of vitamin K, conjunctival eye care, and hepatitis B immunization. For more information, see Chapter 10.

Bibliography

2010 Guidelines for the Prevention of Perinatal Group B Streptococcal Disease. Atlanta (GA): CDC; 2014. Available at: https://www.cdc.gov/groupbstrep/guidelines/guidelines.html. Retrieved December 16, 2016.

Adoption. Committee Opinion No. 528. American College of Obstetricians and Gynecologists. Obstet Gynecol 2012;119:1320–4.

Air travel during pregnancy. ACOG Committee Opinion No. 443. American College of Obstetricians and Gynecologists. Obstet Gynecol 2009;114:954–5.

Alcohol abuse and other substance use disorders: ethical issues in obstetric and gynecologic practice. Committee Opinion No. 633. American College of Obstetricians and Gynecologists. Obstet Gynecol 2015;125:1529–37.

Alto WA. No need for glycosuria/proteinuria screen in pregnant Women. J Fam Pract 2005;54:978–83.

American College of Medical Genetics. Technical standards and guidelines for CFTR mutation testing. 2008 ed. Bethesda (MD): ACMG; 2011. Available at: https://www.acmg.net/StaticContent/SGs/CFTR%20Mutation%20Testing.pdf. Retrieved October 26, 2016.

American College of Obstetricians and Gynecologists. Access to reproductive health care for women with disabilities. In: Special issues in women's health. Washington, DC: ACOG; 2005. p. 39–59.

American College of Obstetricians and Gynecologists. Update on seafood consumption during pregnancy. Practice Advisory. Washington, DC: American College of Obstetricians and Gynecologists; 2017. Available at: http://www.acog.org/About-ACOG/News-Room/Practice-Advisories/ACOG-Practice-Advisory-Seafood-Consumption-During-Pregnancy. Retrieved April 4, 2017.

American College of Radiology. ACR-ACOG-AIUM-SRU practice parameter for the performance of obstetrical ultrasound. ACR Resolution 17. Reston (VA): ACR; 2013. Available at: http://www.acr.org/~/media/f7bc35bd59264e7cbe648f6d1bb8b8e2.pdf. Retrieved October 28, 2016.

American College of Radiology. Practice guideline for the performance of obstetrical ultrasound. In: ACR Practice Parameters and Technical Standards 2016. Available at: https://www.acr.org/Quality-Safety/Standards-Guidelines. Retrieved September 27, 2016.

Anemia in pregnancy. ACOG Practice Bulletin No. 95. American College of Obstetricians and Gynecologists. Obstet Gynecol 2008;112:201–7.

Antepartum fetal surveillance. Practice Bulletin No. 145. American College of Obstetricians and Gynecologists. Obstet Gynecol 2014;124:182–92.

At-risk drinking and alcohol dependence: obstetric and gynecologic implications. Committee Opinion No. 496. American College of Obstetricians and Gynecologists. Obstet Gynecol 2011;118:383–8.

Briggs GG, Freeman RK. Drugs in pregnancy and lactation: a reference guide to fetal and neonatal risk. 10th ed. Philadelphia (PA): Wolters Kluwer; 2015.

Carrier screening for genetic conditions. Committee Opinion No. 691. American College of Obstetricians and Gynecologists. Obstet Gynecol 2017;129:e41–55.

Carrier screening in the age of genomic medicine. Committee Opinion No. 690. American College of Obstetricians and Gynecologists. Obstet Gynecol 2017;129: e35–40.

Castles A, Adams EK, Melvin CL, Kelsch C, Boulton ML. Effects of smoking during pregnancy. five meta-analyses. Am J Prev Med 1999;16:208–15.

Cell-free DNA screening for fetal aneuploidy. Committee Opinion No. 640. American College of Obstetricians and Gynecologists. Obstet Gynecol 2015;126:e31–7.

Cerclage for the management of cervical insufficiency. Practice Bulletin No. 142. American College of Obstetricians and Gynecologists. Obstet Gynecol 2014;123: 372–9.

Controversies concerning vitamin K and the newborn. American Academy of Pediatrics Committee on Fetus and Newborn. Pediatrics 2003;112:191–2.

Counseling about genetic testing and communication of genetic test results. Committee Opinion No. 693. American College of Obstetricians and Gynecologists. Obstet Gynecol 2017;129:e96–101.

Cuckle H, Benn P, Wright D. Down syndrome screening in the first and/or second trimester: model predicted performance using meta-analysis parameters. Semin Perinatol 2005;29:252–7.

Cuckle HS, Wald NJ, Thompson SG. Estimating a woman's risk of having a pregnancy associated with down's syndrome using her age and serum alpha-fetoprotein level. Br J Obstet Gynaecol 1987;94:387–402.

Cunniff C, Hudgins L. Prenatal genetic screening and diagnosis for pediatricians. Curr Opin Pediatr 2010;22:809–13.

Delayed umbilical cord clamping after birth. Committee Opinion No. 684. American College of Obstetricians and Gynecologists. Obstet Gynecol 2017;129:e5–10.

Dietz PM, England LJ, Shapiro-Mendoza CK, Tong VT, Farr SL, Callaghan WM. Infant morbidity and mortality attributable to prenatal smoking in the U.S. Am J Prev Med 2010;39:45–52.

External cephalic version. Practice Bulletin No. 161. American College of Obstetricians and Gynecologists. Obstet Gynecol 2016;127:e54–61.

Fiore MC, Jaen CR, Baker TB, Bailey WC, Benowitz NL, Curry SJ, et al. Treating tobacco use and dependence: 2008 update. Clinical Practice Guideline. Rockville (MD): U.S. Department of Health and Human Services; 2008. Available at: https://www.ahrq.gov/sites/default/files/wysiwyg/professionals/clinicians-providers/guidelines-recommendations/tobacco/clinicians/update/treating_tobacco_use08.pdf. Retrieved July 18, 2017.

First-trimester risk assessment for early-onset preeclampsia. Committee Opinion No. 638. American College of Obstetricians and Gynecologists. Obstet Gynecol 2015;126:e25–7.

Gestational diabetes mellitus. Practice Bulletin No. 180. American College of Obstetricians and Gynecologists. Obstet Gynecol 2017;130:e17–31.

Gribble RK, Fee SC, Berg RL. The value of routine urine dipstick screening for protein at each prenatal visit. Am J Obstet Gynecol 1995;173:214–7.

Guidelines for diagnostic imaging during pregnancy and lactation. Committee Opinion No. 656. American College of Obstetricians and Gynecologists. Obstet Gynecol 2016;127:e75–80.

Guidelines for the Identification and Management of Lead Exposure in Pregnant and Lactating Women. Atlanta (GA): CDC; 2010. Available at: https://www.cdc.gov/nceh/lead/publications/leadandpregnancy2010.pdf. Retrieved December 19, 2016.

Guttmacher Institute. Substance abuse during pregnancy. State laws and policies. New York (NY): Guttmacher Institute; 2016. Available at: https://www.guttmacher.org/state-policy/explore/substance-abuse-during-pregnancy. Retrieved October 28, 2016.

Health care for pregnant and postpartum incarcerated women and adolescent females. Committee Opinion No. 511. American College Obstetricians and Gynecologists. Obstet Gynecol 2011;118:1198–202.

Henderson JT, Whitlock EP, O'Connor E, Senger CA, Thompson JH, Rowland MG. Low-dose aspirin for prevention of morbidity and mortality from preeclampsia: a systematic evidence review for the U.S. Preventive Services Task Force. Ann Intern Med 2014;160:695–703.

Hook EB. Rates of chromosome abnormalities at different maternal ages. Obstet Gynecol 1981;58:282–5.

Ickovics JR, Kershaw TS, Westdahl C, Magriples U, Massey Z, Reynolds H, et al. Group prenatal care and perinatal outcomes: a randomized controlled trial [published erratum appears in Obstet Gynecol 2007;110:937]. Obstet Gynecol 2007;110:330–9.

Ickovics JR, Kershaw TS, Westdahl C, Rising SS, Klima C, Reynolds H, et al. Group prenatal care and preterm birth weight: results from a matched cohort study at public clinics. Obstet Gynecol 2003;102:1051–7.

Influenza vaccination during pregnancy. Committee Opinion No. 608. American College of Obstetricians and Gynecologists. Obstet Gynecol 2014;124:648–51.

Informed consent. ACOG Committee Opinion No. 439. American College of Obstetricians and Gynecologists. Obstet Gynecol 2009;114:401–8.

Intimate partner violence. Committee Opinion No. 518. American College of Obstetricians and Gynecologists. Obstet Gynecol 2012;119:412–7.

Klein JD. Adolescent pregnancy: current trends and issues. American Academy of Pediatrics Committee on Adolescence. Pediatrics 2005;116:281–6.

Lead screening during pregnancy and lactation. Committee Opinion No. 533. American College of Obstetricians and Gynecologists. Obstet Gynecol 2012;120:416–20.

LeFevre ML. Low-dose aspirin use for the prevention of morbidity and mortality from preeclampsia: U.S. Preventive Services Task Force recommendation statement. U.S. Preventive Services Task Force. Ann Intern Med 2014;161:819–26.

Malone FD, Canick JA, Ball RH, Nyberg DA, Comstock CH, Bukowski R, et al. First-trimester or second-trimester screening, or both, for Down's syndrome. First- and Second-Trimester Evaluation of Risk (FASTER) Research Consortium. N Engl J Med 2005;353:2001–11.

Management of pregnant women with presumptive exposure to Listeria monocytogenes. Committee Opinion No. 614. American College of Obstetricians and Gynecologists. Obstet Gynecol 2014;124:1241–4.

Management of suboptimally dated pregnancies. Committee Opinion No. 688. American College of Obstetricians and Gynecologists. Obstet Gynecol 2017;129: e29–32.

March of Dimes. Toward improving the outcome of pregnancy: the 90s and beyond. Committee on Perinatal Health. White Plains (NY): National Foundation—March of Dimes; 1993.

March of Dimes. Toward improving the outcome of pregnancy III: enhancing perinatal health through quality, safety and performance initiatives. Committee on Perinatal Health. White Plains (NY): National Foundation—March of Dimes; 2010.

McDonald SD, Walker MC, Ohlsson A, Murphy KE, Beyene J, Perkins SL. the effect of tobacco exposure on maternal and fetal thyroid function. Eur J Obstet Gynecol Reprod Biol 2008;140:38–42.

Methamphetamine abuse in women of reproductive age. Committee Opinion No. 479. American College of Obstetricians and Gynecologists. Obstet Gynecol 2011;117:751–5.

Methods for estimating due date. Committee Opinion No. 700. American College of Obstetricians and Gynecologists. Obstet Gynecol 2017;129:e150–4.

Microarrays and next-generation sequencing technology: the use of advanced genetic diagnostic tools in obstetrics and gynecology. Committee Opinion No. 682. American College of Obstetricians and Gynecologists. Obstet Gynecol 2016;128:e262–8.

Mode of term singleton breech delivery. ACOG Committee Opinion No. 340. American College of Obstetricians and Gynecologists. Obstet Gynecol 2006;108:235–7.

Moore ER, Anderson GC, Bergman N, Dowswell T. Early skin-to-skin contact for mothers and their healthy newborn infants. Cochrane Database of Systematic Reviews2012, Issue 5.Art. No. CD003519. DOI: 10.1002/14651858.CD003519.pub3.

Morris JK, Wald NJ, Mutton DE, Alberman E. Comparison of models of maternal age-specific risk for Down syndrome live births. Prenat Diagn 2003;23:252–8.

Murray N, Homer CS, Davis GK, Curtis J, Mangos G, Brown MA. The clinical utility of routine urinalysis in pregnancy: a prospective study. Med J Aust 2002;177:477–80.

National Institute for Health and Care Excellence. Diabetes in pregnancy: management from preconception to the postnatal period. NICE Guideline NG3. London: NICE; 2015. Available at: https://www.nice.org.uk/guidance/ng3?unlid=634501629201610123565 5. Retrieved October 26, 2016.

Nausea and vomiting of pregnancy. Practice Bulletin No. 153. American College of Obstetricians and Gynecologists. Obstet Gynecol 2015;126:e12–24.

Newborn screening and the role of the obstetrician–gynecologist. Committee Opinion No. 616. American College of Obstetricians and Gynecologists. Obstet Gynecol 2015;125:256–60.

Obesity in pregnancy. Practice Bulletin No. 156. American College of Obstetricians and Gynecologists. Obstet Gynecol 2015;126:e112–26.

Opioid abuse, dependence, and addiction in pregnancy. Committee Opinion No. 524. American College of Obstetricians and Gynecologists. Obstet Gynecol 2012;119: 1070–6.

Optimizing support for breastfeeding as part of obstetric practice. Committee Opinion No. 658. American College of Obstetricians and Gynecologists. Obstet Gynecol 2016;127:e86–92.

Oral intake during labor. ACOG Committee Opinion No. 441. American College of Obstetricians and Gynecologists. Obstet Gynecol 2009;114:714.

Otten JJ, Hellwig JP, Meyers LD, editors. DRI, Dietary Reference Intakes: the essential guide to nutrient requirements. Institute of Medicine. Washington, D.C.: National Academies Press; 2006.

Physical activity and exercise during pregnancy and the postpartum period. Committee Opinion No. 650. American College of Obstetricians and Gynecologists. Obstet Gynecol 2015;126:e135–42.

Prenatal and perinatal human immunodeficiency virus testing: expanded recommendations. Committee Opinion No: 635. American College of Obstetricians and Gynecologists. Obstet Gynecol 2015;125:1544–7.

Prenatal diagnostic testing for genetic disorders. Practice Bulletin No. 162. American College of Obstetricians and Gynecologists. Obstet Gynecol 2016;127:e108–22.

Progesterone and preterm birth prevention: translating clinical trials data into clinical practice. Society for Maternal–Fetal Medicine Publications Committee. Am J Obstet Gynecol 2012;206:376–86.

Rasmussen KM, Yaktine AL, editors. Weight gain during pregnancy: reexamining the guidelines. Institute of Medicine. Washington, DC: National Academies Press; 2009.

Ross AC, Taylor CL, Yaktine AL, Del Valle HB, editors. Dietary reference intakes: calcium vitamin D. Committee to Review Dietary Reference Intakes for Vitamin D and Calcium, Food and Nutrition Board, Institute of Medicine. Washington, D.C.: National Academies Press; 2011.

Screening and diagnosis of gestational diabetes mellitus. Committee Opinion No. 504. American College of Obstetricians and Gynecologists. Obstet Gynecol 2011;118: 751–3.

Screening for fetal aneuploidy. Practice Bulletin No. 163. American College of Obstetricians and Gynecologists. Obstet Gynecol 2016;127:e123–37.

Siu AL. Behavioral and pharmacotherapy interventions for tobacco smoking cessation in adults, including pregnant women. U.S. Preventive Services Task Force Recommendation Statement. U.S. Preventive Services Task Force. Ann Intern Med 2015;163:622–34.

Sufrin C. Pregnancy and postpartum care in correctional settings. National Commission on Correctional Health Care. Chicago (IL): National Commission on Correctional Health Care; 2014. Available at: http://www.ncchc.org/filebin/Resources/Pregnancy-and-Postpartum-Care-2014.pdf. Retrieved March 6, 2017.

Smoking cessation during pregnancy. Committee Opinion No. 471. American College of Obstetricians and Gynecologists. Obstet Gynecol 2010;116:1241–4.

Spinillo A, Nicola S, Piazzi G, Ghazal K, Colonna L, Baltaro F. Epidemiological correlates of preterm premature rupture of membranes. Int J Gynaecol Obstet 1994; 47:7–15.

Substance abuse reporting and pregnancy: the role of the obstetrician-gynecologist. Committee Opinion No. 473. American College of Obstetricians and Gynecologists. Obstet Gynecol 2011;117:200–1.

Tobacco use and women's health. Committee Opinion No. 503. American College of Obstetricians and Gynecologists. Obstet Gynecol 2011;118:746–50.

Toriello HV, Meck JM. Statement on guidance for genetic counseling in advanced paternal age. Professional Practice and Guidelines Committee. Genet Med 2008;10:457–60.

U.S. Dept. of Health and Human Services. The health consequences of smoking: 50 years of progress. A report of the Surgeon General. Atlanta (GA): U.S. Department of Health and Human Services, Centers for Disease Control and Prevention, National Center for Chronic Disease Prevention and Health Promotion, Office on Smoking and Health; 2014. Available at: http://www.surgeongeneral.gov/library/reports/50-years-of-progress/full-report.pdf. Retrieved October 26, 2016.

Ultrasound in pregnancy. Practice Bulletin No. 175. American College of Obstetricians and Gynecologists. Obstet Gynecol 2016;128:e241–56.

Umbilical cord blood banking. Committee Opinion No. 648. American College of Obstetricians and Gynecologists. Obstet Gynecol 2015;126:e127–9.

Update on immunization and pregnancy: tetanus, diphtheria, and pertussis vaccination. ACOG Committee Opinion No. 566. American College of Obstetricians and Gynecologists. Obstet Gynecol 2013;121:1411–4.

Vaginal birth after previous cesarean delivery. Practice Bulletin No. 115. American College of Obstetricians and Gynecologists. Obstet Gynecol 2010;116:450–63.

Verani JR, McGee L, Schrag SJ. Prevention of perinatal group b streptococcal disease—revised guidelines from CDC, 2010. Division of Bacterial Diseases, National Center for Immunization and Respiratory Diseases, Centers for Disease Control and Prevention. MMWR Recomm Rep 2010;59(RR-10):1–36.

Villar J, Say L, Shennan A, Lindheimer M, Duley L, Conde-Agudelo A, et al. Methodological and technical issues related to the diagnosis, screening, prevention, and treatment of pre-eclampsia and eclampsia. Int J Gynaecol Obstet 2004;85 (suppl):S28–41.

Vitamin D: screening and supplementation during pregnancy. Committee Opinion No. 495. American College of Obstetricians and Gynecologists. Obstet Gynecol 2011;118:197–8.

Wapner R, Thom E, Simpson JL, Pergament E, Silver R, Filkins K, et al. First-trimester screening for Trisomies 21 and 18. First Trimester Maternal Serum Biochemistry And Fetal Nuchal Translucency Screening (BUN) Study Group. N Engl J Med 2003;349:1405–13.

Weight gain during pregnancy. Committee Opinion No. 548. American College of Obstetricians and Gynecologists. Obstet Gynecol 2013;121:210–2.

Williams JF, Smith VC. Fetal alcohol spectrum disorders. Committee on Substance Abuse. Pediatrics 2015;136:e1395–406.

Resources

American College of Obstetricians and Gynecologists. Immunization for women. Washington, DC: American College of Obstetricians and Gynecologists; 2016. Available at: http://immunizationforwomen.org/. Retrieved December 20, 2011; October 26, 2016.

American College of Obstetricians and Gynecologists. Tobacco and nicotine cessation toolkit. Washington, DC: American College of Obstetricians and Gynecologists; 2016. Available at: http://www.acog.org/About-ACOG/ACOG-Departments/Toolkits-for-Health-Care-Providers/Tobacco-and-Nicotine-Cessation-Toolkit. Retrieved April 4, 2017.

American Psychiatric Association (APA). Arlington (VA): APA; 2011;2016. Available at: https://www.psychiatry.org/. Retrieved December 20, 2011; October 26, 2016.

CDC Recommendations on Vaccination Precautions during Breastfeeding. Atlanta (GA): CDC; 2015. Available at: https://www.cdc.gov/breastfeeding/recommendations/vaccinations.htm#modalIdString_CDCTable_0. Retrieved December 19, 2016.

Centers for Disease Control and Prevention. Listeria (Listeriosis). Atlanta, GA: CDC; 2016. Available at: https://www.cdc.gov/listeria/. Retrieved October 28, 2016.

Centers for Disease Control and Prevention. Medication use during pregnancy. Atlanta (GA): CDC; 2016. Retrieved October 31, 2016.

Centers for Disease Control and Prevention. Medications and pregnancy. Atlanta (GA): CDC; 2016. Available at: https://www.cdc.gov/pregnancy/meds/. Retrieved October 31, 2016.

Centers for Disease Control and Prevention. Vaccines and immunizations. Atlanta (GA): CDC; 2011; 2016. Available at: http://www.cdc.gov/vaccines/. Retrieved October 26, 2016.

Drugs and Lactation Database: LactMed. Bethesda (MD): National Library of Medicine; 2016. Available at: https://toxnet.nlm.nih.gov/newtoxnet/lactmed.htm. Retrieved November 7, 2016.

Fish: What Pregnant Women and Parents Should Know. Silver Spring (MD): FDA; 2015. Available at: http://www.fda.gov/food/foodborneillnesscontaminants/metals/ucm393070.htm. Retrieved December 19, 2016.

Genetests. Elmwood Park (NJ): BioReference Laboratories; 2016. Available at: https://www.genetests.org/. Retrieved December 19, 2016.

Institute for Patient- and Family-Centered Care. Bethesda (MD): IPFCC; 2011; 2016. Available at: http://www.ipfcc.org/. Retrieved September 21, 2016.

March of Dimes. Toward improving the outcome of pregnancy III: enhancing perinatal health through quality, safety and performance initiatives. Committee on Perinatal Health. White Plains (NY): National Foundation—March of Dimes; 2010.

McKusick-Nathans Institute of Genetic Medicine. Online Mendelian inheritance in man (OMIM). Baltimore (MD): Johns Hopkins University School of Medicine; 2011; 2016. Available at: http://www.omim.org/. Retrieved October 26, 2016.

National Center for Complementary and Integrative Health. National Institutes of Health. Bethesda (MD): NIH; 2016. Available at: https://nccih.nih.gov/. Retrieved October 26, 2016.

National Heart Lung and Blood Institute. Aim for a healthy weight. Calculate your body mass index. BMI Calculator. Bethesda (MD): NHLBI; 2011; 2016. Available at: http://www.nhlbi.nih.gov/health/educational/lose_wt/BMI/bmicalc.htm. Retrieved October 26, 2016.

Noninvasive Prenatal Tests (NIPT)/Cell Free DNA Screening Predictive Value Calculator. Chicago (IL): NSGC; 2016. Available at: http://www.perinatalquality.org/vendors/nsgc/nipt. Retrieved December 19, 2016.

Organization of Teratology Information Specialists. MotherToBaby fact sheets. Brentwood (TN): OTIS; 2016. Available at: http://mothertobaby.org/fact-sheets-parent/. Retrieved October 26, 2016.

TERIS: Teratogen Information System and the on-Line Version of Shepard's Catalog of Teratogenic Agents. Seattle (WA): University of Washington; 2016. Available at: http://depts.washington.edu/terisweb/teris/. Retrieved December 19, 2016.

Treating for Two: Medications and Pregnancy. Atlanta (GA): CDC; 2016. Available at: https://www.cdc.gov/pregnancy/meds/treatingfortwo/index.html. Retrieved December 19, 2016.

U.S. Department of Agriculture, United States Department of Health and Human Services. 2015—2020 dietary guidelines for Americans. 8th ed. Washington, D.C.: U.S. Dept. of Agriculture; U.S. Dept. of Health and Human Services; 2015. Available at: https://health.gov/dietaryguidelines/2015/resources/2015-2020_Dietary_Guidelines.pdf. Retrieved October 26, 2016.

Williams JF, Smith VC. Fetal alcohol spectrum disorders. Committee on Substance Abuse. Pediatrics 2015;136:e1395–406. Available at: http://pediatrics.aappublications.org/content/early/2015/10/13/peds.2015-3113?sid=22f04c16-1473-4774-b2a3-cb6b53934fd4. Retrieved April 4, 2017.

Chapter 7

Intrapartum Care of the Mother

The goal of all labor and delivery units is a safe birth for mothers and their newborn infants. At the same time, staff need to make the woman feel welcome, comfortable, and informed throughout the labor and delivery process. Ongoing risk assessment will determine appropriate care for each woman. The partner, or other primary support person, also needs to feel welcome and encouraged to participate throughout the labor and delivery experience.

Labor and delivery are normal physiologic processes that most women experience without complications. Obstetric staff can greatly enhance the birthing experience for the woman and her family by exhibiting a caring attitude and helping them understand the process. Efforts to promote healthy behavior can be as effective during labor and delivery as they are during antepartum care. Physical contact between the newborn infant and family in the delivery room is desirable and efforts to foster family interaction need to be encouraged.

Because intrapartum complications can arise, sometimes quickly and without warning, ongoing risk assessment and surveillance of the woman and her fetus are essential. A hospital, birthing center within a hospital complex, or a freestanding birthing center that meets the standards of the Accreditation Association for Ambulatory Health Care, The Joint Commission, or the American Association of Birth Centers provides the safest setting for labor, delivery, and the postpartum period if the woman's risk profile matches her delivery site. Although the American College of Obstetricians and Gynecologists (ACOG) believes that hospitals and accredited birth centers are the safest settings for birth, it respects the right of a woman to make a medically informed decision about her delivery.

A pregnant woman should be cared for at the facility that best meets her needs as well as those of her newborn infant. Hence the goal of regionalized care is for pregnant women to receive care in facilities that are prepared to provide the optimal level of care for them and their newborn infants (see "Classification System for Levels of Maternal Care" in Chapter 1).

Hospital Evaluation and Admission: General Concepts

Pregnant women may come to a hospital's labor and delivery area not only for obstetric care but also for evaluation and treatment of nonobstetric illnesses. However, some nonobstetric conditions (eg, highly transmissible infectious diseases like influenza or varicella, critical traumas, and acute chest pain) may be better treated in another area of the hospital, regardless of gestational age. Conversely, many postpartum conditions may be best addressed by labor and delivery staff. Disaster preparedness plans should include care of pregnant women. For all these reasons, coordination and communication between obstetric and emergency departments, as well as hospital ancillary services, is critical. Hospital-based obstetric units are urged to collaborate with emergency departments and hospital ancillary services, as well as emergency response systems outside of the hospital, to establish guidelines for triage of pregnant women. Obstetric departments, in conjunction with other appropriate departments, should establish written guidelines defining the appropriate unit to evaluate obstetric patients based upon criteria such as gestational age and delivery status, symptoms, medical condition, and available medical staff. Written departmental policies regarding triage of women who come to a labor and delivery area need to be reviewed periodically for compliance with appropriate regulations.

Qualified obstetric care providers need to evaluate women with medical or surgical conditions that could reasonably be expected to cause obstetric complications. Emergency departments should consider early consultation with obstetric care providers when triaging and managing pregnant patients, especially for patients beyond the first and early second trimesters. To be considered an appropriate location to evaluate and care for pregnant patients, a unit should have the ability to perform basic ultrasonography and fetal monitoring. In cases that involve a woman with a viable pregnancy who is evaluated outside of an obstetric unit, it may be necessary to bring these resources from the obstetric unit to the location of the patient. The priority of that evaluation and the site where it is best performed are determined by the woman's needs (including gestational age of the fetus) and the unit's ability to provide for those needs. The obstetric department also should establish policies for the admission of pregnant patients with nonobstetric conditions according to state regulations. Federal and state regulations address the management and treatment of patients in hospital acute care areas, including labor and delivery (see also Appendix G).

Triage

Although a separate triage area and standing orders may facilitate care for obstetric triage patients, having an available health care provider appears to best optimize patient flow and reduce length of stay. The use of certified nurse–midwives or certified midwives who provide obstetric emergency care triage services, for example, may improve efficiency, reduce length of stay, and improve screening and evaluation.

A pregnant woman who comes to the labor and delivery area should be evaluated in a timely fashion. Typical triage protocols involve an initial assessment and decision about the priority level for evaluation. In the case of the pregnant patient, this assessment may be conducted by a registered nurse, certified nurse–midwife or certified midwife, nurse practitioner, physician assistant, or physician as designated by hospital policy. Triage algorithms for obstetric acuity to asses and assign priority to obstetric patients may be useful. Women should be cared for according to the triage acuity rather than by time of arrival. The health care provider performing triage should assign the patient's acuity during the first encounter which minimally includes assessment of the following:

- Maternal vital signs
- Fetal heart rate
- Uterine contractions
- Reason for presentation (chief concern)
- Status of labor: presence of uterine contractions, vaginal bleeding, status of membranes
- Woman's perception of fetal movement
- Any high-risk medical or obstetric conditions as identified by a review of history or the woman's report

The Emergency Severity Index was designed by the Agency for Healthcare Research and Quality to triage nonpregnant adults and has been adopted by many emergency departments. Several obstetric triage acuity tools have been developed based on this model. These tools typically classify patients based on urgency of the patient's condition, often using a five-level system, and can increase the proportion of high-acuity patients seen in urgent care. Several of these tools have been tested for content validity and interrater reliability and may be used to improve quality and efficiency of care and guide allocation of resources. Hospital obstetric units are encouraged to develop triage protocols based on local conditions but informed by evidence-based decision making. Recently developed validated algorithms such as the Association of Women's Health, Obstetric and Neonatal Nurses' Maternal Fetal Triage Index (Fig. 7-1) could serve as templates for use in individual hospital units.

Triage is followed by the complete evaluation of the woman and the fetus by a health care provider with skills and training appropriate to evaluate the issues identified during triage. The responsible obstetric care provider should be informed promptly if any of the following findings are present or suspected:

- Vaginal bleeding
- Acute abdominal pain
- Temperature of 100.4°F or higher
- Abnormal maternal heart rate or respiratory rate
- Preterm labor
- Preterm premature rupture of membranes (also known as prelabor rupture of membranes)
- Hypertension
- Category II or category III fetal heart rate pattern (see also "Fetal Heart Rate Monitoring" later in this chapter)
- Signs of imminent delivery
- Inability to detect fetal heart rate

Any woman who is suspected to be in labor, has ruptured membranes, or has vaginal bleeding should be evaluated promptly in an obstetric service area. Whenever a pregnant woman is evaluated for labor, the following factors should be assessed and recorded in her permanent medical record:

- Estimated due date
- Vital signs
- Frequency and duration of uterine contractions

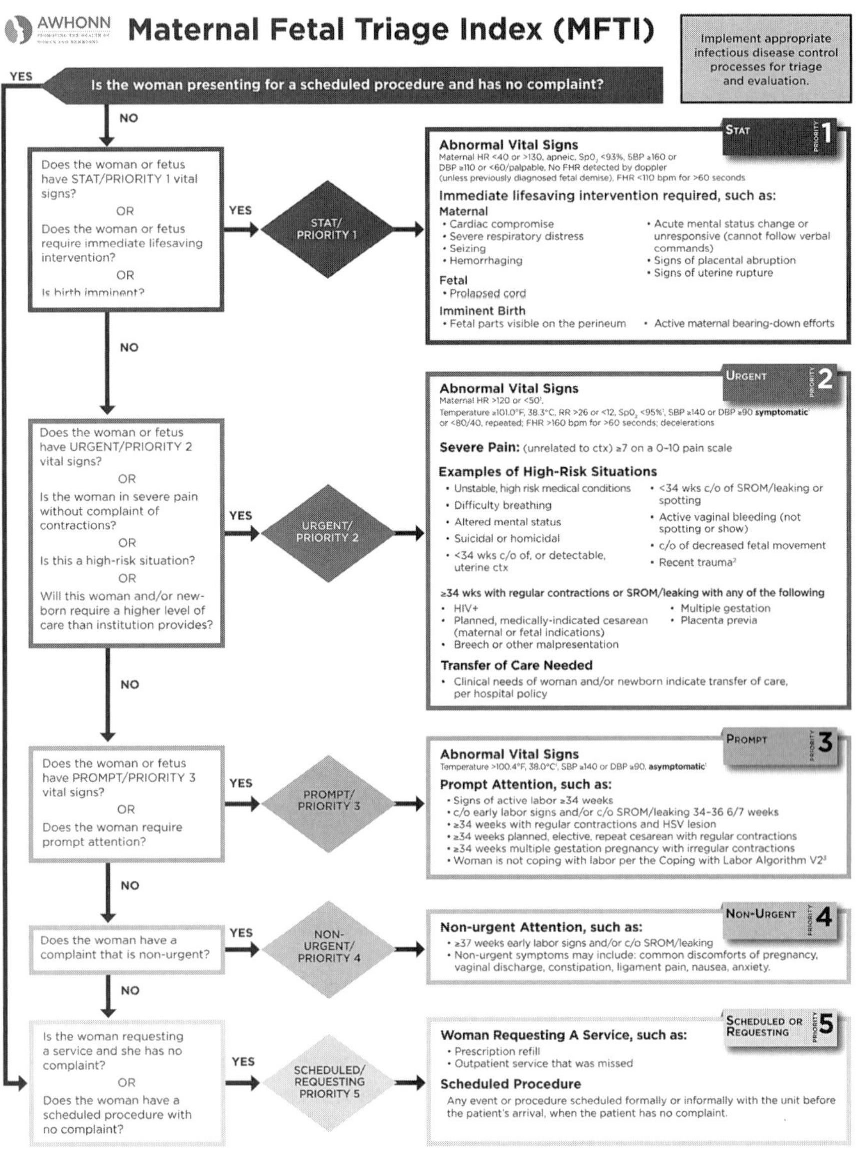

[1]High Risk and Critical Care Obstetrics, 2013
[2]Trauma may or may not include a direct assault on the abdomen. Examples are trauma from motor vehicle accidents, falls, and intimate partner violence.
[3]Coping with Labor Algorithm V2 used with permission

The MFTI is exemplary and does not include all possible patient complaints or conditions. The MFTI is designed to guide clinical decision-making but does not replace clinical judgment. Vital signs in the MFTI are suggested values. Values appropriate for the population and geographic region should be determined by each clinical team, taking into account variables such as altitude.

Figure 7-1. Maternal–fetal triage index. (Reprinted from Ruhl C, Scheich B, Onokpise B, Bingham D. Content validity testing of the maternal fetal triage index. J Obstet Gynecol Neonatal Nurs 2015;44:701–9.)

- Documentation of fetal well-being
- Cervical dilation and effacement, or cervical length, as ascertained by transvaginal ultrasonography, unless contraindicated (eg, placenta previa, preterm premature rupture of membranes)
- Fetal presentation and station of the presenting part
- Status of the membranes
- Date and time of the woman's arrival and of notification of the health care provider
- Estimation of fetal weight
- History of allergies
- Use of any medications
- Time, content, and amount of the most recent food or fluid ingestion

Admission for Labor

If the woman is in prodromal or early labor and has no complications, admission to the labor and delivery area may be deferred after initial evaluation and documentation of maternal and fetal well-being (see also Appendix G). A patient with a transmissible infection should be admitted to a site where isolation techniques can be followed according to hospital policy.

Women who have not received prenatal care, had episodic prenatal care, or who received care late in pregnancy are more likely to have sexually transmitted infections and substance use disorders. Serologic testing for hepatitis B virus surface antigen may be necessary, as described in Chapter 12. Social problems, such as poverty and family conflict, also may affect patients' health.

If no complications are detected during initial assessment in the labor and delivery area and if contraindications have been ruled out, qualified nursing personnel may perform the initial pelvic examination during or following admission. Once the results of the examination have been obtained and documented, the health care provider responsible for the woman's care in the labor and delivery area should be informed of her status and make a decision regarding her management. The timing of the health care provider's arrival in the labor area needs to be based on this information and hospital policy. If epidural, combined spinal epidural, spinal, or general anesthesia is anticipated, or if the woman may require rapid institution of an anesthetic, anesthesia personnel need to be informed of the woman's presence soon after her admission. If a preterm delivery or the delivery if a high-risk newborn infant is expected, the pediatric care provider who will assume responsibility for the infant's care needs to be informed. When the woman has been examined and instructions regarding her management have been given and noted in her medical record, all necessary consent forms should be signed and incorporated into the medical record.

By 36 weeks of gestation, preregistration for labor and delivery at a hospital should be confirmed and a copy of the prenatal medical record, including information pertaining to the woman's antepartum course (see also Appendix A), should be on file in the hospital's labor registration area. If electronic medical records are used, the electronic prenatal records need to be accessible.

At the time of a woman's admission to the labor and delivery area, pertinent information from the prenatal record should be noted in the admission records. Whether facilities use electronic medical records, paper records, or a combination of both, pertinent information about the woman's past medical and obstetric history and prenatal care that can influence intrapartum or neonatal care should be integrated into those records. Because labor and delivery is a dynamic process, all entries into a woman's medical record need to include the date and time of occurrence. Blood typing and screening tests need not be repeated if they were performed during the antepartum period and no antibodies were present. If the results of the woman's antenatal laboratory evaluation are not known and cannot be obtained, blood typing, Rh D type determination, hepatitis B virus antigen testing, and serologic testing for syphilis need to be performed before the woman is discharged. State laws governing testing of umbilical cord blood may vary. Serologic testing for human immunodeficiency virus (HIV) infection and other tests are encouraged and performed according to state law. Rapid HIV testing can be done in labor if the woman's HIV status is unknown (see also "Routine Laboratory Testing in Pregnancy" in Chapter 6 and "Human Immunodeficiency Virus" in Chapter 12). Collection of umbilical cord blood may be useful for subsequent evaluation of ABO incompatibility if the mother is type O. Policies should be developed to ensure expeditious preparation of blood products for transfusion if the patient is at increased risk of hemorrhage or if the need arises.

It is not necessary to restrict the activity of women with uncomplicated labor and delivery, or exclude people who are supportive of her. Frequent position changes during labor to enhance maternal comfort and promote optimal fetal positioning can be supported as long as adopted positions allow appropriate maternal and fetal monitoring and treatments and are not contraindicated by maternal medical or obstetric complication. During the early stages of labor, a woman, if she so desires, can get out of bed to ambulate, sit on a birth ball, or rest in a comfortable chair as long as the fetal status is reassuring. Practices such as showers during labor, placement of intravenous lines, use of fetal heart rate (FHR) monitoring, and restrictions on ambulation need to be reviewed in departmental policies and the health care providers' preferences as well as the woman's desires for comfort, privacy, and a sense of participation need to be taken into consideration. Likewise, the use of drugs for relief of pain during labor and delivery depend on the needs and desires of the woman. Some nonpharmacologic methods seem to help women cope with labor pain rather than directly mitigating the pain. Conversely, pharmacologic methods mitigate pain, but they may not relieve anxiety or suffering. Use of the coping scale in conjunction with different nonpharmacologic and pharmacologic pain management techniques can help obstetrician–gynecologists and other obstetric care providers tailor interventions to best meet the needs of each woman. The development of a birth plan that has been discussed previously with a woman's obstetrician–gynecologist or other obstetric care provider and placed in her medical record may promote her participation in and satisfaction with her care. The woman's health care team should communicate regarding all factors that may pose a risk to her, her fetus, or her newborn infant. Obstetric department policies should include recommendations for transmitting to the nursery maternal and fetal historical and laboratory data that may affect the care of the newborn infant. Any additional information that may influence neonatal care should be communicated as well. The lack of such data, perhaps because of a lack of prenatal care, also should be made known to the nursery personnel. The health care provider who will care for the newborn infant needs to be identified on the maternal medical record (see Appendix A).

Labor

The onset of true labor is established by observing progressive change in cervical dilation in the setting of regular, phasic, uterine contractions. This may require two or more cervical examinations that are separated by an adequate period of time to observe change. Women may arrive at the hospital labor and delivery area before true labor has begun. Expectant management is reasonable for women at 4–6 cm dilatation who are in latent labor if maternal and fetal status are reassuring. Care for women in latent labor may be facilitated by having an alternate unit where women can rest and be offered support techniques before admission to labor and delivery. For women who are in latent labor and are not admitted, a process of shared decision making is recommended to create a plan for self-care activities and coping techniques. An agreed-upon time for reassessment should be determined at the time of each contact. Admission during the latent phase of labor may be necessary for a variety of reasons, including pain management or maternal fatigue. When women are observed or admitted for pain or fatigue in latent labor, techniques such as education and support, oral hydration, positions of comfort, and nonpharmacologic pain management techniques such as massage or water immersion may be beneficial. A policy that allows for adequate evaluation of patients for the presence of active labor and prevents unnecessary admissions to the labor and delivery unit is advisable (see also Appendix G).

False Labor at Term

Uterine contractions in the absence of cervical change are commonly referred to as false labor. Treatment for this condition is based on individual circumstances. Women who are having uterine contractions and may not yet be in latent or active labor may be observed for evidence of cervical change in a casual, comfortable area. The woman may be discharged after observation and evaluation by appropriate hospital-designated personnel and assurance of maternal and fetal well-being (see also Appendix G).

Premature Rupture of Membranes at Term

The definition of *PROM* is rupture of membranes before the onset of labor. Membrane rupture that occurs before 37 weeks of gestation is referred to as preterm PROM (see also "Premature Rupture of Membranes" in Chapter 9). Management is influenced by gestational age and the presence of complicating factors, such as clinical infection, abruptio placentae, labor, or nonreassuring fetal status. An accurate assessment of gestational age and knowledge of the maternal, fetal, and neonatal risks are essential for appropriate evaluation, counseling, and care of patients with PROM. Membrane rupture may occur for a variety of reasons. Although membrane rupture at term can result from a normal physiologic weakening of the membranes combined with shearing forces created by uterine contractions, preterm PROM can result from a wide array of pathologic mechanisms that act individually or in concert. At term, PROM complicates approximately 8% of pregnancies and generally is followed by the prompt onset of spontaneous labor and delivery. The most significant maternal consequence of term PROM is intrauterine infection, the risk of which increases with the duration of membrane rupture.

Most cases of PROM can be diagnosed on the basis of the woman's history and physical examination. Examination should be performed in a manner that minimizes the risk of introducing infection. Because digital cervical examinations may increase the risk of infection and add little information to that available with sterile speculum examination, digital examinations generally should be avoided unless the woman appears to be in active labor or delivery seems imminent. Sterile speculum examination provides an opportunity to inspect for umbilical cord prolapse, assess cervical dilatation and effacement, and obtain cultures as appropriate.

The diagnosis of membrane rupture typically is confirmed by the visualization of amniotic fluid passing from the cervical canal and pooling in the vagina or arborization (ferning) of dried vaginal fluid, which is identified under microscopic evaluation. False-positive test results may occur in the presence of blood or semen, alkaline antiseptics, or bacterial vaginosis. Alternatively, false-negative test results may occur with prolonged membrane rupture and minimal residual fluid.

In equivocal cases, additional tests may aid in the diagnosis. Ultrasonographic examination of amniotic fluid volume may be a useful adjunct, but is not diagnostic. Fetal fibronectin is a sensitive but nonspecific test for ruptured membranes. A negative test result is strongly suggestive of intact membranes, but a positive test result is not diagnostic of PROM. Several commercially available tests for amniotic proteins are currently on the market, with high reported sensitivity for PROM. However, false-positive test result rates of 19–30% have been reported in patients with clinically intact membranes and symptoms of labor. If the diagnosis remains unclear after a full evaluation, membrane rupture can be diagnosed unequivocally with ultrasonographically guided transabdominal instillation of indigo carmine dye, followed by the passage of blue-dyed fluid into the vagina, which is documented by a stained tampon or pad. It is important to note that the maternal urine also will turn blue and should not be confused with amniotic fluid. In recent years, indigo carmine dye has been in short supply throughout the United States. In the event that indigo carmine dye is unavailable, methylene blue should never be used as a substitute because it can cause fetal harm and is contraindicated in women who are pregnant.

In all women with PROM, gestational age, fetal presentation, and fetal well-being (using FHR monitoring) should be determined. The examination should evaluate for evidence of intrauterine infection, abruptio placentae, and fetal compromise.

For women with PROM at 37 0/7 weeks of gestation or more, if spontaneous labor does not occur near the time of presentation in those who do not have contraindication to labor, labor should be induced, generally with oxytocin infusion. However, for informed women, the choice of expectant management for a period may be appropriately offered and supported if it is concordant with their individual preferences and if there are no other maternal or fetal reasons to expedite delivery. The randomized controlled trials addressing pregnancies experiencing term PROM included expectant care intervals ranging from 10 hours to 4 days. The risk of infection increases with the prolonged duration of ruptured membranes. However, the optimal duration of expectant management that maximizes the chance of spontaneous labor while minimizing the risk of infection has not been determined. Nonreassuring fetal status, clinical intraamniotic infection (also referred to as chorioamnionitis), and significant abruption placentae are contraindications to expectant management. For women who are group B streptococci positive, administration of antibiotics for group B streptococci prophylaxis should not be delayed while awaiting labor. In such cases, many patients and obstetrician–gynecologists or other obstetric care providers may prefer immediate induction. Failed induction should not be diagnosed unless the woman has been in latent phase for up to 24 hours and has had oxytocin administered for at least 12–18 hours.

Management of Labor

Ideally, every woman admitted to the labor and delivery area knows who her principal, designated health care provider will be. Members of the obstetric team need to observe the woman to follow the progress of labor, record her vital signs and the FHR characteristics in her medical record at regular intervals, and make an effort to ensure her understanding of the events that are occurring. The health care provider principally responsible for the woman's care should be kept informed of her progress and notified promptly of any concerns. When the woman is in active labor, that health care provider should be readily available (see also "Cesarean Delivery" later in this chapter).

Solid foods should be avoided in laboring women. The oral intake of moderate amounts of clear liquids may be allowed for women with uncomplicated labor. Women without complications undergoing elective cesarean delivery may have moderate amounts of clear liquids up to 2 hours before induction of anesthesia. Particulate containing fluids should be avoided. Women with risk factors for aspiration (eg, morbid obesity, diabetes, and difficult airway), or women at increased risk of operative delivery may require further restrictions of oral intake, determined on a case-by-case basis. Pregnant women are at highest risk of aspiration pneumonitis when stomach contents are greater than 25 mL and when the pH of those contents is less than 2.5. Pregnancy slows gastric emptying, and labor can delay it further. The type of aspiration pneumonitis that produces the most severe physiologic and histologic alteration is partially digested food.

Women in spontaneously progressing labor may not require routine continuous infusion of intravenous fluids. Although safe, intravenous hydration limits freedom of movement and may not be necessary. Oral hydration can be encouraged to meet hydration and caloric needs. Arguments for limiting oral intake during labor center on concerns for aspiration and its sequelae. Current guidance supports oral intake of moderate amounts of clear liquids by women in labor who do not have complications. Assessment of urinary output and the presence or absence of ketosis can be used to monitor hydration. If such monitoring indicates concern, intravenous fluids can be administered as needed. If intravenous fluids are required, the solution and the infusion rate should be determined by individual clinical need and anticipated duration of labor. Despite historic concerns regarding the use of dextrose-containing solutions and the possibility that these solutions may induce neonatal hypoglycemia, recent randomized controlled trials did not find lower umbilical cord pH values or increased rates of neonatal hypoglycemia after continuous administration of 5% dextrose in normal saline.

If intravenous fluids are required, intravenous access should ideally be secured when the active phase of labor begins. The progress of labor should be evaluated by periodic vaginal examinations, and the obstetrician–gynecologist or other obstetric care provider needs to be notified of the woman's labor progress. Sterile, water-soluble lubricants may be used to reduce discomfort during vaginal examinations. Antiseptics, such as povidone-iodine and hexachlorophene, have not been shown to decrease the risk of infections acquired during the intrapartum period. Furthermore, these agents may produce local irritation and are absorbed through maternal mucous membranes.

Evaluation of the quality of the uterine contractions and pelvic examinations should be sufficient to detect abnormalities in the progress of labor.

Vital signs need to be recorded at least every 4 hours. This frequency may be increased, particularly as active labor progresses, according to clinical signs and symptoms, and is increased in the presence of complications such as infection or preeclampsia. Documentation of the course of a woman's labor includes documentation of the woman's status, fetal status, and status of labor progress. Specific items regarding maternal status include maternal position changes, maternal vital signs, oxygen and drug administration, amniotomy or spontaneous rupture of membranes, color of amniotic fluid, use of spontaneous pushing efforts or Valsalva maneuver, and maternal use of nonpharmacologic or pharmacologic analgesic techniques. Specific items regarding fetal status include FHR, variability, accelerations, decelerations, and changes over time. Documentation of labor status includes cervical examination results including dilatation, station, and position.

Fetal Heart Rate Monitoring

Either electronic FHR monitoring or intermittent auscultation, if the woman is term and at low risk, may be used to determine fetal status during labor. Low risk in this context has been variously defined, but generally includes women who have no meconium staining, intrapartum bleeding, or abnormal or undetermined fetal test results before birth or at initial admission; no increased risk of developing fetal acidemia during labor (eg, congenital anomalies, intrauterine growth restriction); no maternal condition that may affect fetal well-being (eg, prior cesarean scar, diabetes, hypertensive disease); and no requirement for oxytocin induction or augmentation of labor.

Obstetric unit guidelines need to clearly delineate the criteria for each type of FHR monitoring and procedures to be followed for using these techniques according to the patient's condition and phase and stage of labor. The method of FHR monitoring for fetal surveillance during labor may vary depending on the risk assessment at admission, the preferences of the woman and obstetric staff, and departmental policy. To facilitate the option of intermittent auscultation, obstetrician–gynecologists and other obstetric care providers and facilities should consider adopting protocols and training staff to use a hand-held Doppler device for low-risk women who desire such monitoring during labor. In considering the relative merits of intermittent auscultation and continuous electronic FHR monitoring, patients and obstetrician–gynecologists and other obstetric care providers also should evaluate how the technical requirements of each approach may affect a woman's experience in labor; intermittent auscultation can facilitate freedom of movement, which some women find more comfortable. The effect on staffing is an additional important consideration. Guidelines, indications, and protocols for intermittent auscultation are available from the American College of Nurse–Midwives, the National Institute for Health and Care Excellence, and the Association of Women's Health, Obstetric and Neonatal Nurses.

If no risk factors are present at the time of the woman's admission, a standard approach to fetal surveillance is to determine, evaluate, and record the FHR every 30 minutes in the active phase of the first stage of labor and at least every 15 minutes in the second stage of labor. Cervical dilatation of 6 cm should be considered the threshold for the active phase of most women in labor. Thus, before 6 cm of dilatation is achieved, standards of active phase progress should not be applied.

If risk factors are present at admission or appear during labor, the following guidelines should be followed:

- During the active phase of the first stage of labor, the FHR should be determined, evaluated, and recorded at least every 15 minutes, preferably before, during, and after a uterine contraction, when intermittent auscultation is used. If continuous electronic FHR monitoring is used, the heart rate tracing should be evaluated at least every 15 minutes.
- During the second stage of labor, the FHR should be determined, evaluated, and recorded at least every 5 minutes if auscultation is used. If continuous electronic FHR monitoring is used, the tracing should be evaluated at least every 5 minutes.

Frequency of Fetal Assessment During Labor

To date, there have been no clinical trials in which investigators have examined fetal surveillance methods and frequency during the latent phase of labor. Therefore, during this phase, health care providers should use best clinical judgment when deciding the method and frequency of fetal surveillance.

Documentation

Clinical information about the mother and fetus should be documented throughout the course of labor. The nature of documentation, including style, format, and frequency interval, should be clearly delineated in each institution. Documentation should occur concurrent with assessment when using intermittent auscultation, as there is no other record of FHR monitoring data in this situation. Documentation does not necessarily need to occur at the same intervals as assessment when using continuous electronic FHR monitoring because FHR monitoring data are recorded in the tracing. For example, while evaluation of the FHR may be occurring every 15 minutes with electronic FHR monitoring, a summary note including findings of fetal status may be documented in the medical record less frequently. However, it is important that the documentation reflects the frequency of assessment and the interpretation of FHR monitoring findings. During induction or augmentation of labor with oxytocin, the FHR should be evaluated and documented before each dose increase and after each dose decrease. Summary documentation of fetal status approximately every 30 minutes indicating continuous nursing bedside attendance and evaluation is sufficient when a woman is in the active pushing phase of the second stage of labor.

The appropriate use of electronic FHR monitoring includes recording and interpreting the tracings. Concerning fetal monitor tracing characteristics need to be noted and communicated to the physician or certified nurse–midwife so that the appropriate intervention can occur. When a change in the rate or pattern has been noted, it also is important to document a subsequent return to reassuring findings. The nomenclature used to describe electronic FHR monitoring and contraction patterns should be consistent with the guidelines developed at the 2008 *Eunice Kennedy Shriver* National Institute of Child Health and Human Development Workshop. The use of this terminology applies to medical record entries and verbal communication among obstetric personnel. Uterine contractions are described as normal (five contractions or fewer in 10 minutes) or tachysystole (more than five contractions in 10 minutes) averaged over a 30-minute window. Fetal heart rate patterns are described by baseline rate, variability, accelerations, and decelerations, which can be early, late, or variable. Based on these characteristics of FHR monitoring, tracings can be categorized using a three-tier system (Box 7-1). Category I FHR tracing characteristics are normal and may be monitored in a routine manner, and no specific action is required. Category II tracing characteristics are indeterminate, requiring evaluation and continued surveillance and re-evaluation. Category III tracing results are abnormal and require prompt evaluation and management because they are predictive of abnormal fetal acid–base status at the time they are noted.

Internal FHR monitoring and internal uterine pressure monitoring may be used to gain additional information about fetal status and uterine

Box 7-1. Three-Tiered Fetal Heart Rate Interpretation System

Category I

Category I FHR tracings include all of the following:

- Baseline rate: 110–160 beats per minute
- Baseline FHR variability: moderate
- Late or variable decelerations: absent
- Early decelerations: present or absent
- Accelerations: present or absent

Category II

Category II FHR tracings include all FHR tracings not categorized as Category I or Category III. Category II tracings may represent an appreciable fraction of those encountered in clinical care. Examples of Category II FHR tracings include any of the following:

Baseline rate

- Bradycardia not accompanied by absent baseline variability
- Tachycardia

Baseline FHR variability

- Minimal baseline variability
- Absent baseline variability with no recurrent decelerations
- Marked baseline variability

Accelerations

- Absence of induced accelerations after fetal stimulation

Periodic or episodic decelerations

- Recurrent variable decelerations accompanied by minimal or moderate baseline variability
- Prolonged deceleration more than 2 minutes but less than 10 minutes
- Recurrent late decelerations with moderate baseline variability
- Variable decelerations with other characteristics, such as slow return to baseline, overshoots, or "shoulders"

Category III

Category III FHR tracings include either:

- Absent baseline FHR and any of the following:
  - — Recurrent late decelerations
  - — Recurrent variable decelerations
  - — Bradycardia
- Sinusoidal pattern

Abbreviation: FHR, fetal heart rate.

Reprinted from Macones GA, Hankins GD, Spong CY, Hauth J, Moore T. The 2008 National Institute of Child Health and Human Development Workshop report on electronic fetal monitoring: update on definitions, interpretation, and research guidelines. Obstet Gynecol 2008;112:661–6.

contractility, respectively. Relative contraindications to internal fetal monitoring include maternal HIV infection and other high-risk factors of fetal infection, including herpes simplex virus and hepatitis B virus or hepatitis C virus. Other contraindications include conditions in which the fetus is at moderate to severe risk of bleeding based on inherited conditions such as von Willebrand disease or hemophilia.

If electronic FHR monitoring is used, all FHR tracings need to be identified with the woman's name, hospital number, and the date and time of admission. All FHR tracings need to be easily retrievable from storage so that the events of labor can be studied in proper relationship to the tracings.

Induction of Labor and Cervical Ripening

The goal of induction of labor is to stimulate uterine contractions and labor before the spontaneous onset of labor. Generally, induction of labor has merit as a therapeutic option when the benefits of expeditious delivery outweigh the risks of continuing the pregnancy. The benefits of labor induction need to be weighed against the potential maternal and fetal risks associated with this procedure.

Methods used for induction of labor include administration of oxytocic agents, membrane stripping, and amniotomy. Because exogenous synthetic oxytocin commonly is administered for labor induction and augmentation, some have hypothesized that synthetic oxytocin used for these purposes may alter fetal oxytocin receptors and predispose exposed offspring to autism spectrum disorders (ASD). However, current evidence does not identify a causal relationship between labor induction or augmentation in general, or oxytocin labor induction specifically, and autism or ASD. If the cervix is unfavorable for induction, cervical ripening may be beneficial and can be considered. Cervical ripening agents facilitate the process of cervical softening, thinning, and dilating with resultant reduction in the rate of failed induction and induction-to-delivery time. Effective methods for cervical ripening include the use of mechanical cervical dilators and administration of synthetic prostaglandin E_1 and prostaglandin E_2.

Indications for induction of labor are not absolute but need to take into account maternal and fetal conditions, gestational age, cervical status, and other factors. Elective inductions are not performed before 39 weeks of gestation. The individual woman and clinical situation need to be considered in determining when induction of labor is contraindicated. Generally, the absolute contraindications to labor induction are the same as absolute contraindications for spontaneous labor and vaginal delivery.

The woman should be counseled regarding the indications for induction, the agents and methods of labor stimulation, and risks of induction. Additional requirements for cervical ripening and induction of labor include assessment of the cervix, pelvis, fetal size, and presentation. Monitoring FHR and uterine contractions is recommended for any high-risk patient in active labor.

Each hospital's department of obstetrics and gynecology should develop written guidelines for preparing and administering oxytocin solution or other agents for labor induction or augmentation. The guideline should include the indications for induction and augmentation of labor, the qualifications of personnel authorized to administer oxytocic agents and the appropriate personnel who need to be in attendance during administration of the induction agent(s). Institutional guidelines also should include descriptions of how to manage oxytoxic agents. In addition, the methods for assessment of the woman and the fetus before and during administration of these agents should be specified. A physician capable of performing a cesarean delivery should be available.

Amnioinfusion

The transcervical infusion of sterile, balanced salt solutions during labor (amnioinfusion) may be used to mitigate recurrent variable decelerations in the FHR tracing that are suspected to be caused by umbilical cord compression. Meta-analysis confirms that amnioinfusion lowers caesarean delivery rates in the setting of oligohydramnios and recurrent variable FHR decelerations. There is no proven benefit of amnioinfusion for other FHR abnormalities, such as late decelerations. Because it is possible to introduce fluid into the uterus at too rapid a rate, each obstetric unit should establish a guideline for monitoring during amnioinfusion, including limitations of the volume and infusion rate. Based on current literature, routine prophylactic amnioinfusion for the dilution of meconium-stained amniotic fluid is not recommended. However, amnioinfusion remains a reasonable approach in the treatment of repetitive variable decelerations, regardless of amniotic fluid meconium status.

Analgesia and Anesthesia

Management of discomfort and pain during labor and delivery is an essential part of good obstetric practice. Decisions regarding analgesia should be coordinated closely among the obstetrician–gynecologist or other obstetric care provider, the anesthesiologist, the patient, and skilled support personnel. Existing data suggest that administering analgesia or anesthesia during childbirth per se has no demonstrable effect on an infant's later mental and neurologic development. In the absence of a medical contraindication, maternal request is a sufficient medical indication for pain relief during labor.

Some women cope with the pain of labor by using techniques learned in childbirth preparation programs. Although specific techniques vary, classes usually seek to relieve pain through the general principles of education, support, relaxation, paced breathing, focusing, and touch. Nonpharmacologic options such as massage, immersion in water during the first stage of labor, acupuncture, relaxation, and hypnotherapy are not covered in this book, though they may be useful as adjuncts or alternatives in many cases. The staff at the bedside need to be knowledgeable about these pain management techniques and be supportive of a woman's decision to use them.

Administration of Anesthesia Services

It is the responsibility of the director of anesthesia services to determine the clinical privileges of all personnel providing anesthesia services. All anesthesia services in a given facility need to be organized under a single medical director. If obstetric analgesia (other than pudendal or local techniques) is provided by obstetricians, the director of anesthesia services should participate with a representative of the obstetric department in the formulation of procedures designed to ensure the uniform quality of anesthesia services throughout the hospital. Specific recommendations regarding these procedures are provided in the *Accreditation Manual for Hospitals* published by the Joint Commission. The directors of departments providing anesthesia services are responsible for implementing processes to monitor and evaluate the quality and appropriateness of these services in their respective departments.

Regional anesthesia in obstetrics should be initiated and maintained by health care providers who are approved through the institutional credentialing process to administer or supervise the administration of regional obstetric anesthesia. These individuals must be qualified to manage anesthetic complications. An obstetrician may administer the anesthesia if granted privileges for these procedures. However, having an anesthesia care provider provide this care permits the obstetrician to give undivided attention to the delivery. Regional anesthesia should be administered only after the woman has been examined and the fetal status and progress of labor have been evaluated by a qualified individual. A physician with obstetric privileges who has knowledge of the maternal and fetal status and the progress of labor and who approves initiation of labor anesthesia should be readily available (see also "Anesthesia for Cesarean Deliveries" later in this chapter) to deal with any obstetric complications that may arise.

Available Methods of Analgesia and Anesthesia

Available methods of obstetric analgesia and anesthesia include parenteral or systemic agents and regional, general, local, and inhaled anesthesia. The choice of technique, agent, and dosage is based on many factors, including patient preference, medical status, and contraindications. Decisions regarding analgesia should be coordinated closely among the obstetrician–gynecologist or other obstetric care provider, the anesthesiologist, the patient, and skilled support personnel.

Parenteral or Systemic Agents

Various opioid agonists and opioid agonist–antagonists are available for systemic peripartum analgesia and can be administered during labor to allow the woman to rest (see Table 7-1). In the United States, morphine, meperidine, nalbuphine, fentanyl, and remifentanil are commonly used. These drugs can be given intramuscularly or intravenously. Remifentanil is ultra short-acting and is administered only as a patient-controlled intravenous infusion.

The decision to use parenteral agents to manage labor pain should be made in collaboration with the woman after a careful discussion of the risks and benefits. Parenteral opioids have little effect on pain scores, analgesia is unreliable, and maternal side effects are common. A Cochrane review failed to identify the "ideal" parenteral opioid and concluded that although there was some pain relief in labor, it was poor; there were significant adverse effects, mostly nausea, vomiting, and drowsiness; and there was no great difference between the various agents studied.

Although regional analgesia provides superior pain relief, some women are satisfied with the level of analgesia provided by parenteral opioids when adequate doses are used. Individuals exposed to high doses of opioids are at increased risk of aspiration and respiratory arrest. Nalbuphine is a mixed agonist–antagonist and, thereby, is associated with less respiratory depression for an equianalgesic dose. The risk of maternal apneic episodes has been reported in up to 26% of women with remifentanil administered by patient-controlled intravenous analgesia. Consideration should be given to

TABLE 7-1. Opioids for Labor Analgesia

Drug	Dose and Route of Delivery	Onset	Duration	Elimination Half-life (Maternal)
Fentanyl	50–100 micrograms (every hour); Alternatively, as PCA, load 50 micrograms then 10–25 micrograms Q 10–12 minutes	2–4 minutes IV	30–60 minutes	3 hours
Morphine	2–5 mg (IV); 5–10 mg (IM)	10 minutes IV; 30 minutes IM	1–3 hours	2 hours
Nalbuphine	10–20 mg IV, SQ, or IM or IM	2–3 minutes IV; 15 minutes SQ	2–4 hours	2–5 hours
Butorphanol	1–2 mg IV or IM 30–60 minutes IM	5–10 minutes IV;	4–6 hours	2–5 hours
Remifentanil	0.15–0.5 micrograms/kg Q 2 minutes as PCA	20–90 seconds	3–4 minutes	9–10 minutes

Abbreviations: IM, intramuscular; IV, intravenous; PCA, patient-controlled analgesia; Q, every; SQ, subcutaneous.

Obstetric analgesia and anesthesia. Practice Bulletin No. 177. American College of Obstetricians and Gynecologists. Obstet Gynecol 2017;129:e73–89.

one-to-one nurse-to-patient ratios, respiratory monitoring, and supplemental oxygen when remifentanil patient-controlled intravenous analgesia is used.

All opioids cross the placenta and may have adverse effects for the fetus and newborn. This may be reflected in the loss of variability in the FHR, in neonatal respiratory depression, or in neurobehavioral changes. Caution should be used in administering these drugs in the setting of diminished FHR variability. Drug elimination is longer in the newborn than in adults, so effects may be prolonged. The use of meperidine is further complicated by the role of its active metabolite, normeperidine, which has a prolonged half-life even in the mother, and a half-life up to 72 hours in the newborn infant. The normeperidine effect cannot be antagonized by naloxone. Because of its long half-life, the use of meperidine is generally not recommended.

Regional Analgesia and Anesthesia

Regional (neuraxial) anesthesia is another option for peripartum pain relief, and several methods of administration are available: epidural, combined spinal–epidural and spinal. In obstetric patients, regional analgesia refers to a partial to complete loss of pain sensation below the T8–T10 level. In addition, varying degrees of motor blockade may be present, depending on the agents used. Low-dose neuraxial analgesia administered in early labor does not increase the rate of cesarean delivery. Thus, there seems to be little justification to withhold this form of pain relief from women in early labor until an arbitrary cervical dilation is achieved (ie, 4-cm cervical dilation). When regional anesthesia is administered during labor, the woman's vital signs need to be monitored at regular intervals.

Epidural Analgesia and Anesthesia. Epidural analgesia offers one of the most effective forms of intrapartum pain relief and is used by most women in the United States. A catheter is placed in the epidural space, allowing for a continuous infusion or intermittent injection of pain medication during labor. The medication mixture consists of a local anesthetic, often with an opioid, which allows for the use of lower concentrations of each agent and thereby minimizes the potential for adverse effects. Lower concentrations of local anesthetic predispose to less motor blockade, whereas lower concentrations of opioids result in less systemic effect for mother and fetus or newborn infant. The commonly used local anesthetics are bupivacaine and ropivacaine and are equivalent in outcome and adverse effects. The two opioids that are used are 1) fentanyl and 2) sufentanil. The advantage of epidural analgesia is that the medication may be titrated over the course of labor as needed. In addition, epidural catheters placed for labor may be dosed and used for cesarean delivery, postpartum tubal ligation, postcesarean pain control, or repair of obstetric lacerations after vaginal delivery, if needed.

Single-Injection Spinal Anesthesia. Single-injection spinal analgesia provides excellent pain relief for procedures of limited duration, such as cesarean delivery, the second stage of labor, rapidly progressing labor, and postpartum tubal ligation. A long-acting local anesthetic often is used, with or without an opioid agonist. However, because of its inability to extend the duration of action, single-injection spinal analgesia is of limited use for the management of labor. The local anesthetics commonly used include lidocaine, bupivacaine, and ropivacaine. Fentanyl, sufentanil, or morphine may be added to the mixture to improve intraoperative comfort, postoperative comfort, or both. If local anesthetic is administered into the cerebrospinal fluid, the degree of motor block is greater than with epidural. As with epidural, coadministration of opioid and local anesthetic decreases the total dose of each.

Continuous Spinal Analgesia. Continuous spinal analgesia is seldom used for labor because of concerns about postdural puncture headache, and an FDA withdrawal of spinal catheters from the market in 1991 following reports of cauda equina syndrome. In cases of inadvertent dural puncture when epidural is attempted, the planned epidural may be converted to a continuous spinal epidural by threading the catheter into the subarachnoid space for continuous infusion. Deliberate continuous spinal techniques with specially designed catheters have also occasionally been investigated for labor and results are encouraging.

Combined Spinal–Epidural Analgesia. Combined spinal–epidural offers the rapid onset of spinal analgesia combined with the ability to use the epidural catheter to prolong the duration of analgesia with a continuous epidural infusion for labor, to convert to anesthesia for cesarean delivery, or to provide postcesarean delivery pain control. In early labor, subarachnoid opioid alone (fentanyl or sufentanil) is sufficient for analgesia. As labor progresses and pain becomes more somatic, local anesthetic is required to achieve analgesia and is usually bupivacaine, although ropivacaine may be used instead. The major advantage of combined spinal–epidural over epidural analgesia is the rapid onset of analgesia because of the initial spinal component. A Cochrane review found no difference in patient mobility, labor augmentation, or cesarean delivery between traditional epidural (higher concentrations of local anesthetic) and combined spinal–epidural analgesia and less need for additional or rescue anesthesia interventions, instrumental delivery, and urinary retention with combined spinal–epidural analgesia. The same review compared combined spinal–epidural analgesia with low-dose epidural techniques, concluding that higher rates of pruritus occur with combined spinal–epidural analgesia than with epidural analgesia and found no difference for other endpoints, including mode of delivery, patient satisfaction, and neonatal outcome.

There appears to be a higher incidence of fetal bradycardia with combined spinal–epidural analgesia than with epidural analgesia alone but no increased rate of cesarean delivery for FHR abnormalities. Fetal bradycardia is attributed to intrathecal opioids and is independent of maternal hypotension. Additionally, there are reports that the epidural catheter may become dislodged with change in maternal position.

General Anesthesia

Because general anesthesia results in a loss of maternal consciousness, it requires airway management by trained anesthesia personnel. General anesthesia is uncommon for vaginal or cesarean delivery in contemporary obstetrics and is limited to emergency cesarean deliveries or scenarios in which neuraxial anesthesia cannot be undertaken or has already failed.

Airway management is more challenging in obstetric anesthesia, and the risk of difficult or failed intubation is much higher. In elective cases, awake intubation or videolaryngoscopy can be performed when a difficult airway is anticipated, and the laryngeal mask airway is an alternative to endotracheal intubation in other cases.

Local Anesthesia

Local anesthesia is another method of pain control. At the time of delivery, local anesthetics may be injected into the tissues of the perineum and the vagina to provide anesthesia for episiotomy and repair of vaginal and perineal lacerations. Local anesthetics also may be injected to perform pudendal nerve block in patients who did not receive regional anesthesia during labor. This regional block may provide adequate anesthesia for outlet operative deliveries and performance of any necessary episiotomy or repair.

Inhaled Anesthesia

Nitrous oxide is an anesthetic gas frequently used during general anesthesia and has been used for labor and postpartum laceration repair analgesia for decades, although more extensively in the United Kingdom and other countries than in the United States. Groups have called for expanded access to nitrous oxide for laboring women in the United States, as well as more research and evaluation. It is self-administered using a mouthpiece or facemask, with a mix of 50% nitrous oxide and 50% oxygen either blended from two separate gas cylinders or the hospital's piped gas supply through a small regulator, or from a single premixed cylinder. The apparatus must use a demand valve so that doses are given only when the patient inhales using the mask and scavenging equipment to limit environmental exposure to others. The analgesia provided by nitrous oxide is less effective than epidural analgesia when pain scores are the outcome of interest. Nitrous oxide use does not preclude mobility for the patient, does not require additional monitoring, and allows the laboring woman to control the effect. Another advantage is its quick termination of effect once the parturient removes the mask. It is transmitted to the placenta but is rapidly eliminated by the newborn infant once the infant begins to breathe. Maternal adverse effects include nausea, vomiting, dizziness, and drowsiness.

Anesthesia for Cesarean Deliveries

For most cesarean deliveries, properly administered regional or general anesthesia are effective and have little effect on the newborn infant. Because of potential risks associated with airway management, intubation, and the possibility of aspiration during induction of general anesthesia, regional anesthesia is usually the preferred technique and should be available in all hospitals that provide obstetric care. The advantages and disadvantages of both techniques should be discussed with the woman. In some circumstances, when the maternal evaluation indicates it can be safely performed, rapid induction of general anesthesia may be indicated. Such circumstances might include a prolapsed umbilical cord with severe fetal bradycardia or suspected uterine rupture with an abnormal FHR pattern.

Indications for Anesthesiology Consultation

Box 7-2 includes some of the most common indications for anesthesia consultation during the antenatal period or peripartum period. In many cases, a telephone consultation may be sufficient; in other cases, a face-to-face consultation will be appropriate.

When such risk factors are identified, a physician who has the credentials to provide general and regional anesthesia should be consulted in a timely manner to allow for joint development of a plan of management, including optimal location for delivery. Strategies thereby can be developed to minimize the need for emergency induction of general anesthesia in women for whom this would be hazardous. For those women with risk factors, consideration should be given to the planned placement in early labor of an intravenous line and an epidural catheter or spinal catheter with confirmation that the catheter is functional. If a woman at unusual risk of complications from anesthesia is identified (eg, prior failed intubation), strong consideration should be given to antepartum referral to allow for delivery at a hospital that can manage such anesthesia on a 24-hour basis.

Box 7-2. Common Indications for Anesthesiology Consultation

Cardiac Disease

- Congenital and acquired disorders such as repaired tetralogy of Fallot and transposition of the great vessels
- Cardiomyopathy
- Valvular disease such as aortic and mitral stenosis, tricuspid regurgitation, and pulmonary stenosis
- Pulmonary hypertension and Eisenmenger syndrome
- Rhythm abnormalities such as supraventricular tachycardia and Wolff–Parkinson–White syndrome
- Presence of an implanted pacemaker or defibrillator

Hematologic Abnormalities or Risk Factors

- Immune and gestational thrombocytopenia
- Coagulation abnormalities such as von Willebrand disease
- Current use of anticoagulant medications
- Jehovah's witness

Spinal, Muscular, and Neurologic Disease

- Structural vertebral abnormalities and prior surgeries such as vertebral fusion and rod placement
- Prior spinal cord injury
- Central nervous system problems such as known arterial–venous malformation, aneurysm, Chiari malformation, or ventriculoperitoneal shunt

Major Hepatic or Renal Disease

- Chronic renal insufficiency
- Hepatitis or cirrhosis with significantly abnormal liver function tests or coagulopathy

History of or Risk Factors for Anesthetic Complications

- Anticipated difficult airway
- Obstructive sleep apnea
- Previous difficult or failed neuraxial anesthesia
- Malignant hyperthermia
- Allergy to local anesthetics

Obstetric Complications That May Affect Anesthesia Management

- Placenta accreta
- Nonobstetric surgery during pregnancy
- Planned cesarean delivery with concurrent major abdominal procedure

(continued)

Box 7-2. Common Indications for Anesthesiology Consultation *(continued)*

Miscellaneous Medical Conditions That May Influence Anesthesia Management

- Body mass index of 50 or greater
- History of solid organ transplantation
- Myasthenia gravis
- Dwarfism
- Sickle cell anemia
- Neurofibromatosis

Special Populations

Women receiving opioid-assisted therapy who are undergoing labor should receive pain relief as if they were not taking opioids because the maintenance dosage does not provide adequate analgesia for labor. Epidural or spinal anesthesia should be offered where appropriate for management of pain in labor or for delivery. Narcotic agonist–antagonist drugs, such as butorphanol, nalbuphine, and pentazocine, should be avoided because they may precipitate acute withdrawal. Buprenorphine should not be administered to a patient who takes methadone. Pediatric staff should be notified of all narcotic-exposed infants.

In general, patients undergoing opioid maintenance treatment will require higher doses of opioids to achieve analgesia than other patients. A consultation with an anesthesiologist can be beneficial in pregnant women with substance use disorder or chronic opiate use to formulate a pain management plan tailored to the individual patient. Injectable nonsteroidal antiinflammatory agents, such as ketorolac, also are highly effective in postpartum and postcesarean delivery pain control. Daily doses of methadone or buprenorphine should be maintained during labor to prevent withdrawal, and patients should be reassured of this plan in order to reduce anxiety. Dividing the usual daily maintenance dose of buprenorphine or methadone into three or four doses every 6–8 hours may provide partial pain relief; however, additional analgesia will be required.

Other Pain Management Options

Nonpharmacologic Labor Support

Nonpharmacological support includes physical and emotional nursing interventions that support a woman who is in labor to enhance her physical comfort, confidence in her ability to give birth, and a sense of being cared for and being safe (see also "Support Persons in the Delivery Room" later in this chapter). A registered nurse or other members of the care team with licenses must supervise nonlicensed individuals performing labor support interventions (eg, a doula). Individuals must have evidence-based knowledge concerning how to perform and customize nonpharmacologic labor support interventions. Nonpharmacologic comfort and pain relief interventions include the following:

- Be in the room with the woman continuously
- Encourage the woman to labor in positions of her choice (eg, ambulating, rhythmic movement, or use of a birthing ball) and change positions frequently
- Use relaxation techniques such as guided imagery, paced breathing, touch therapy (eg, back rub, leg massage, or counter pressure), aromatherapy
- Use hydrotherapy in a tub or shower
- Apply warm or cool compresses to various parts of the woman's body
- Provide emotional support: verbally encourage, reassure, and praise the woman and provide easy to understand information about how labor is progressing and how she and her baby are doing
- Support the woman's nutritional needs
- Advocate for the woman by helping her to articulate her wishes to others

The staff at the bedside need to be knowledgeable about these comfort and pain management techniques, offer them as appropriate to all women, either in place of or as an adjunct to analgesia and anesthesia, and be supportive of a woman's decision to use them.

Immersion in Water During Labor and Delivery

Immersion in water during the first stage of labor may be associated with shorter labor and decreased use of spinal and epidural analgesia and may be offered to healthy women with uncomplicated pregnancies between 37 0/7 weeks and 41 6/7 weeks. However, there are insufficient data on which to draw conclusions regarding the relative benefits and risks of immersion in water during the second stage of labor and delivery. Therefore, until such data are available, it is recommended that birth occur on land, not in water. A woman who requests to give birth while submerged in water should be informed that the maternal and perinatal benefits and risks of this choice have not been studied sufficiently to either support or discourage her request.

Delivery

Vaginal Delivery

Vaginal delivery is associated with less risk of maternal operative and postoperative complications than nonelective cesarean delivery and results in shorter hospital stays. Vaginal delivery requires consideration of factors, such as the availability of skilled personnel for the delivery (including obstetric attendants and professionals skilled in neonatal resuscitation and anesthesia administration) and the potential need to move a woman from a labor, delivery, and recovery room to an operative suite.

The risk assessment performed on the woman's admission, the course of her labor, the fetal presentation, any abnormalities encountered during the labor process, and the anesthetic technique in use or anticipated for delivery will all have an effect on the need for other professionals. At least one obstetric nurse, preferably the woman's designated primary nurse for the labor, should be present in the delivery room throughout the delivery. Under no circumstances should an attempt be made to delay birth by physical restraint or anesthetic means.

The routine use of episiotomy is not necessary and may lead to an increase in the risk of third-degree and fourth-degree perineal lacerations and a delay in the woman's resumption of sexual activity. Episiotomy is only done for a specific medical indication. If there is need for episiotomy, mediolateral episiotomy may be preferred over midline episiotomy because of the association of midline episiotomy with increased risk of injury to the anal sphincter complex; however, limited data suggest mediolateral episiotomy may be associated with an increased likelihood of perineal pain and dyspareunia. Restrictive episiotomy use is recommended over routine episiotomy. Labor and delivery units should have a written policy outlining procedures to prevent unintentionally retained foreign objects during vaginal delivery.

Vaginal Birth After Cesarean Delivery

The term vaginal birth after cesarean delivery (VBAC) is used to denote a vaginal delivery after a trial of labor in a woman who has had a previous cesarean delivery, regardless of the outcome. Trial of labor after cesarean delivery (TOLAC) provides a woman who desires a vaginal delivery with the possibility of achieving that goal—a vaginal birth after cesarean delivery. In addition to fulfilling a woman's preference for vaginal delivery, at an individual level VBAC is associated with decreased maternal morbidity and a decreased risk of complications in future pregnancies. At a population level, VBAC also is associated with a decrease in the overall cesarean delivery rate. Although TOLAC is appropriate for many women with a history of a cesarean delivery, several factors increase the likelihood of a failed trial of labor, which compared with VBAC is associated with increased maternal and perinatal morbidity. Assessment of individual risks and the likelihood of VBAC is, therefore, important in determining the appropriate candidates for TOLAC (see also "Trial of Labor After Cesarean Delivery" in Chapter 6).

In addition to providing an option for those who want the experience of a vaginal birth, VBAC has several potential health advantages for women. Women who achieve VBAC avoid major abdominal surgery, which results in lower rates of hemorrhage, infection, and a shorter recovery period compared with elective repeat cesarean delivery. Additionally, for those considering larger families, VBAC may avoid potential future maternal consequences of multiple cesarean deliveries, such as hysterectomy; bowel or bladder injury; transfusion; infection; and abnormal placentation, such as placenta previa and placenta accreta.

Neither elective repeat cesarean delivery nor TOLAC is without maternal or neonatal risk. The risks of either approach include maternal hemorrhage, infection, operative injury, thromboembolism, hysterectomy, and death. Most maternal morbidity that occurs during TOLAC occurs when repeat cesarean delivery becomes necessary. Uterine rupture or dehiscence is the outcome associated with TOLAC that most significantly increases the chance of additional maternal and neonatal morbidity. One factor that markedly influences the chance of uterine rupture is the location of the prior incision on the uterus.

The preponderance of evidence suggests that most women with one previous cesarean delivery with a low transverse incision, or an unknown scar with no historical evidence suggesting it was a classical scar, are candidates for and should be counseled about VBAC and offered TOLAC. Conversely, those at high risk of complications (eg, those with previous classical incision or T-incision, prior uterine rupture, or extensive transfundal uterine surgery) and those in whom vaginal delivery is otherwise contraindicated are not generally candidates for planned TOLAC. Individual circumstances should be considered in all cases. Some common situations that may modify the balance of risks and benefits are listed in Box 7-3.

Because of the risks associated with TOLAC and that uterine rupture and other complications may be unpredictable, it is recommended that TOLAC be undertaken in facilities with staff immediately available to provide emergency care. It is important that health care providers and women considering TOLAC be clearly informed of potential increased levels of risk and management alternatives. After counseling, the ultimate decision to undergo TOLAC or a repeat cesarean delivery should be made by the woman in consultation with her health care provider. Documentation of counseling and the management plan should be included in the medical record.

Box 7-3. Selected Clinical Factors Associated With Trial of Labor Success After Previous Cesarean Delivery Success

Increased Probability of Success (Strong Predictors)

- Prior vaginal birth
- Spontaneous labor

Decreased Probability of Success (Other Predictors)

- Recurrent indication for initial cesarean delivery (labor dystocia)
- Increased maternal age
- Nonwhite ethnicity
- Gestational age greater than 40 weeks
- Maternal obesity
- Preeclampsia
- Short interpregnancy interval
- Increased neonatal birth weight

Vaginal birth after previous cesarean delivery. Practice Bulletin No. 115. American College of Obstetricians and Gynecologists. Obstet Gynecol 2010;116:450–63.

Operative Vaginal Delivery

Operative vaginal delivery is used to achieve or expedite safe vaginal delivery for maternal or fetal indications. Operative vaginal deliveries are accomplished by applying direct traction on the fetal skull with forceps, or by applying traction to the fetal scalp with a vacuum extractor. Forceps and vacuum extractors are acceptable and safe instruments for operative vaginal delivery. The choice of instrument in a particular situation is determined by the clinical circumstance and operator preference based on training and experience. Vacuum extraction is believed to be easier to learn and may be used when asynclitism prevents proper forceps placement. Forceps provide a more secure application and they are appropriate for rotation of the fetal head to occiput anterior or occiput posterior position. The vacuum extractor is associated with an increased incidence of neonatal cephalohematoma, retinal hemorrhage, and jaundice when compared with forceps delivery. Although cephalohematoma is more likely to occur as the duration of vacuum application increases, delivery rates and newborn outcomes do not appear to be improved with release of vacuum pressure between pulls. Forceps delivery is associated with a higher rate of third- and fourth-degree perineal tears. Routine use of episiotomy with all operative vaginal deliveries is not recommended because of concerns for poor healing and prolonged discomfort with mediolateral episiotomy and because midline episiotomy with operative vaginal delivery is associated with an increased likelihood of anal sphincter and rectal injury. Neonatal care providers should be made aware of the mode of delivery in order to observe for potential complications.

Indications. Indications for a forceps or vacuum extraction and the position and station of the vertex at the time of application of the forceps or vacuum apparatus need to be identified in a detailed operative description in the woman's medical record. No indication for operative vaginal delivery is absolute. The following indications apply when the fetal head is engaged and the cervix is fully dilated:

- Prolonged second stage of labor
  - Nulliparous women: lack of continuing progress for at least 3 hours with regional anesthesia, or at least 2 hours without regional anesthesia
  - Multiparous women: lack of continuing progress for at least 2 hours with regional anesthesia, or at least 1 hour without regional anesthesia

- Suspicion of immediate or potential fetal compromise
- Shortening of the second stage for maternal benefit

Operative Delivery Classification. Operative vaginal deliveries are classified by the station of the fetal head at application and the degree of rotation necessary for delivery. Before use of either forceps or vacuum extractor, an assessment by the operator of the factors that contribute to success and safety should be performed, including estimated fetal weight, the clinical adequacy of the maternal pelvis, the fetal station and position, and the adequacy of anesthesia. Station refers to the estimated distance, in centimeters, between the leading bony portion of the fetal head and the pelvic inlet, defined as the level of the maternal ischial spines. Engagement is clinically diagnosed when the leading bony portion of the fetal head is at or below the level of the ischial spines (station 0 or more). The method to describe station beyond the level of the ischial spines is to estimate centimeters (+1 to +5 cm) below the spines.

There are three classes of operative deliveries:

1. Outlet application—Outlet forceps or vacuum delivery follows the application of the instrument when the fetal scalp is visible at the introitus without separating the labia, the fetal skull has reached the pelvic floor, the fetal sagittal suture is in the anterior–posterior diameter or in the right or left occiput anterior or posterior position, and the fetal head is at or on the perineum. According to this definition, rotation cannot exceed 45 degrees. There is no difference in perinatal outcome when outlet operative vaginal deliveries are compared with spontaneous deliveries, and no data support the concept that rotating the head on the pelvic floor 45 degrees or less increases the rate of morbidity.
2. Low application—Low operative vaginal delivery follows the application of forceps or vacuum when the leading point of the fetal skull is at station +2 cm or more and is not on the pelvic floor. Low operative vaginal delivery applications have two subdivisions: 1) a rotation of 45 degrees or less and 2) a rotation of more than 45 degrees. Although rotation of the fetal head often accompanies the use of the vacuum extractor, the vacuum should not be used to provide a direct rotational force to the fetal scalp.
3. Midpelvic application—Midpelvic operative vaginal delivery follows the application of forceps or vacuum when the fetal head is engaged

but the leading point of the skull is above station +2 cm. Under very unusual circumstances, such as the sudden onset of severe fetal or maternal compromise, or the presence of a twin, application of forceps or vacuum above station +2 cm may be attempted while simultaneously initiating preparations for a cesarean delivery in the event that the operative vaginal delivery maneuver is unsuccessful. Neither forceps nor vacuum should be applied to an unengaged fetal presenting part or when the cervix is not completely dilated.

Requirements for Operative Vaginal Delivery. Each of the following prerequisites must be met before a forceps or vacuum delivery:

- The cervix is fully dilated and retracted
- The membranes are ruptured
- The fetal head is engaged in the pelvis
- The position of the fetal head has been determined
- The fetal weight has been estimated
- The maternal pelvis has been assessed and is thought to be adequate for vaginal delivery
- There is an adequate level of anesthesia
- The maternal bladder has been emptied
- The patient has agreed to operative vaginal delivery after being informed of the risks and benefits of the procedure
- The operator is willing to abandon the trial of operative vaginal delivery, and a back-up plan is in place in case of failure to deliver

Shoulder Dystocia

Shoulder dystocia is most often defined as a delivery that requires additional obstetric maneuvers after failure of gentle downward traction on the fetal head to effect delivery of the shoulders. Retraction of the delivered fetal head against the maternal perineum (turtle sign) may be present and may assist in the diagnosis. Shoulder dystocia is caused by the impaction of the anterior fetal shoulder behind the maternal pubis symphysis. It also can occur from impaction of the posterior fetal shoulder on the sacral promontory. Because the delivering attendant needs to determine whether ancillary maneuvers are actually necessary, the diagnosis of shoulder dystocia has a subjective component.

Elective induction of labor or elective cesarean delivery for all women suspected of carrying a fetus with macrosomia is not appropriate. Because most subsequent deliveries will not be complicated by shoulder dystocia, the benefit of universal elective cesarean delivery is questionable in women who have such a history of shoulder dystocia. In women with a history of shoulder dystocia, estimated fetal weight, gestational age, maternal glucose intolerance, and the severity of the prior neonatal injury should be evaluated and the risks and benefits of cesarean versus vaginal delivery discussed with the woman. Planned cesarean delivery to prevent shoulder dystocia may be considered for suspected fetal macrosomia with estimated fetal weights exceeding 5,000 g in women without diabetes and 4,500 g in women with diabetes.

When shoulder dystocia is recognized, as in any medical emergency, it is important that communication among all health care providers be clear, succinct, and focused on the essential issues facing the delivery team. These issues include delivery of the infant, while minimizing, if possible, hypoxic ischemic encephalopathy and additional strain on the brachial plexus beyond that generated by endogenous forces.

There is no evidence that any one maneuver is superior to another in releasing an impacted shoulder or reducing the chance of injury. However, performance of the McRoberts maneuver is a reasonable initial approach. Suprapubic pressure may be used at the same time to assist in dislodging the impacted shoulder. In contrast, fundal pressure may further worsen impaction of the shoulder and also may result in uterine rupture. Controversy exists as to whether episiotomy is necessary because shoulder dystocia typically is not caused by obstructing soft tissue. Direct fetal manipulation with either rotational maneuvers or delivery of the posterior arm also may be used. In these circumstances, performance of a proctoepisiotomy may be helpful to create more room within the posterior vagina.

In cases of severe shoulder dystocia that are not responsive to commonly used maneuvers, more aggressive approaches may be warranted. Cephalic replacement (Zavanelli maneuver) has been described for relieving catastrophic cases; however, it is associated with a significantly increased risk of fetal morbidity and mortality and maternal morbidity. Intentional fracture of the fetal clavicle may help decrease the bisacromial diameter, but it may be difficult to perform in emergent situations. It is clear that brachial plexus injury can occur regardless of the procedure or procedures used to disimpact the shoulders.

Contemporaneous documentation of the management of shoulder dystocia is recommended to record significant facts, findings, and observations about the shoulder dystocia event and its sequelae. Some clinicians use a detailed written or dictated report that includes a description of the maneuvers used, the sequence of maneuvers, and exogenous forces applied. Others use a checklist-type report that contains the critical information needed for documentation, such as ACOG's Patient Safety Checklist No. 6, *Documenting Shoulder Dystocia*.

Third Stage of Labor

Delivery of the placenta should occur spontaneously within 30 minutes. Several care practices to facilitate delivery of the placenta and prevent postpartum hemorrhage have been evaluated. The care practices that make up the practice of active management of the third stage of labor have been recommended by the World Health Organization because they lower the incidence of immediate postpartum hemorrhage.

The components of active management of the third stage of labor have included administration of a uterotonic agent with delivery of the fetal shoulder or immediately after birth, controlled umbilical cord traction to deliver the placenta, and fundal massage immediately after delivery of the placenta. Although immediate umbilical cord clamping was originally recommended in the active management of third stage labor because of concern that delayed umbilical cord clamping may increase the risk of maternal hemorrhage, recent data do not support these concerns. Therefore, ACOG now recommends delayed umbilical cord clamping for at least 30–60 seconds in vigorous term and preterm infants. However, delayed umbilical cord clamping should not interfere with active management of the third stage of labor, including the use of uterotonic agents after delivery of the newborn to minimize maternal bleeding. If the placental circulation is not intact, such as in the case of abnormal placentation, abruptio placentae, or umbilical cord avulsion, immediate cord clamping is appropriate. Similarly, maternal hemodynamic instability or the need for immediate resuscitation of the newborn on the warmer would be an indication for immediate umbilical cord clamping (Table 7-2).

In addition, studies that evaluated the individual components of active management of the third stage of labor found that routine use of a uterotonic agents has the strongest evidence for effectiveness and the least risk of adverse effects. Today the World Health Organization recommends routine use of uterotonics for all births and controlled umbilical cord traction in

TABLE 7-2. Clinical Situations in Which Immediate Umbilical Cord Clamping Should Be Considered or Care Should Be Individualized

Maternal	Hemorrhage, hemodynamic instability, or both Abnormal placentation (previa, abruption)
Fetal/neonatal	Need for immediate resuscitation Placental circulation not intact (abruption, previa, cord avulsion, IUGR with abnormal cord Doppler evaluation)

Abbreviation: IUGR, intrauterine growth restriction.

Delayed umbilical cord clamping after birth. Committee Opinion No. 684. American College of Obstetricians and Gynecologists. Obstet Gynecol 2017;129:e5–10.

settings where skilled birth attendants are available. Fundal massage is no longer a recommended practice for prevention of postpartum hemorrhage. If after 30 minutes the placenta has not delivered, it is appropriate to consider other maneuvers to remove the placenta, which include manual removal or dilation and curettage. Clinical judgment should be used to decide the type of analgesia and location of procedure. Women who have a retained placenta are at high risk of hemorrhage and should be managed accordingly.

Cesarean Delivery

In 2011, one in three women who gave birth in the United States did so by cesarean delivery. Cesarean birth can be lifesaving for the fetus, the mother, or both in certain cases. However, the rapid increase in cesarean birth rates from 1996 through 2011 without clear evidence of concomitant decreases in maternal or neonatal morbidity or mortality raises significant concern that cesarean delivery is overused. Variation in the rates of nulliparous, term, singleton, vertex cesarean births also indicates that clinical practice patterns affect the number of cesarean births performed. The most common indications for primary cesarean delivery include, in order of frequency, labor dystocia, abnormal or indeterminate (formerly, nonreassuring) FHR tracing, fetal malpresentation, multiple gestation, and suspected fetal macrosomia. Safe reduction of the rate of primary cesarean deliveries will require different approaches for each of these, as well as other, indications. For example, it may be necessary to revisit the definition of labor dystocia because recent data show that contemporary labor progresses at a rate substantially slower than what was historically taught. Additionally, improved and standardized FHR interpretation and management may have an effect. Increasing women's access to nonmedical interventions during labor, such as continuous labor and delivery support, also has been shown to reduce cesarean birth rates. External cephalic version for breech presentation and a trial of labor for women with twin gestations when the first twin is in cephalic presentation are other examples of interventions that can contribute to the safe lowering of the primary cesarean delivery rate. Recommendations for safe prevention of the primary cesarean delivery can be found in Table 7-3.

TABLE 7-3. Recommendations for the Safe Prevention of the Primary Cesarean Delivery

Recommendations	Grade of Recommendations
First stage of labor	
A prolonged latent phase (eg, greater than 20 hours in nulliparous women and greater than 14 hours in multiparous women) should not be an indication for cesarean delivery.	1B Strong recommendation, moderate-quality evidence
Slow but progressive labor in the first stage of labor should not be an indication for cesarean delivery.	1B Strong recommendation, moderate-quality evidence
Cervical dilation of 6 cm should be considered the threshold for the active phase of most women in labor. Thus, before 6 cm of dilation is achieved, standards of active phase progress should not be applied.	1B Strong recommendation, moderate-quality evidence
Cesarean delivery for active phase arrest in the first stage of labor should be reserved for women at or beyond 6 cm of dilatation with ruptured membranes who fail to progress despite 4 hours of adequate uterine activity, or at least 6 hours of oxytocin administration with inadequate uterine activity and no cervical change.	1B Strong recommendation, moderate-quality evidence
Second stage of labor	
A specific absolute maximum length of time spent in the second stage of labor beyond which all women should undergo operative delivery has not been identified.	1C Strong recommendation, low-quality evidence
Before diagnosing arrest of labor in the second stage, if the maternal and fetal conditions permit, allow for the following: • At least 2 hours of pushing in multiparous women • At least 3 hours of pushing in nulliparous women	1B Strong recommendation, moderate-quality evidence

(continued)

TABLE 7-3. Recommendations for the Safe Prevention of the Primary Cesarean Delivery *(continued)*

Recommendations	Grade of Recommendations
***Second stage of labor* (continued)** Longer durations may be appropriate on an individualized basis (eg, with the use of epidural analgesia or with fetal malposition) as long as progress is being documented.	
Operative vaginal delivery in the second stage of labor by experienced and well-trained physicians should be considered a safe, acceptable alternative to cesarean delivery. Training in, and ongoing maintenance of, practical skills related to operative vaginal delivery should be encouraged.	1B Strong recommendation, moderate-quality evidence
Manual rotation of the fetal occiput in the setting of fetal malposition in the second stage of labor is a reasonable intervention to consider before moving to operative vaginal delivery or cesarean delivery. In order to safely prevent cesarean delivery in the setting of malposition, it is important to assess the fetal position in the second stage of labor, particularly in the setting of abnormal fetal descent.	1B Strong recommendation, moderate-quality evidence
Fetal heart rate monitoring Amnioinfusion for repetitive variable fetal heart rate decelerations may safely reduce the rate of cesarean delivery.	1A Strong recommendation, high-quality evidence
Scalp stimulation can be used as a means of assessing fetal acid–base status when abnormal or indeterminate (formerly, nonreassuring) fetal heart patterns (eg, minimal variability) are present and is a safe alternative to cesarean delivery in this setting.	1C Strong recommendation, low-quality evidence
Induction of labor Before 41 0/7 weeks of gestation, induction of labor generally should be performed based on maternal and fetal medical indications. Inductions at 41 0/7 weeks of gestation and beyond should be performed to reduce the risk of cesarean delivery and the risk of perinatal morbidity and mortality.	1A Strong recommendation, high-quality evidence
Cervical ripening methods should be used when labor is induced in women with an unfavorable cervix.	1B Strong recommendation, moderate-quality evidence

(continued)

TABLE 7-3. Recommendations for the Safe Prevention of the Primary Cesarean Delivery *(continued)*

Recommendations	Grade of Recommendations
***Induction of labor* (continued)**	
If the maternal and fetal status allow, cesarean delivery for failed induction of labor in the latent phase can be avoided by allowing longer duration of the latent phase (up to 24 hours or longer) and requiring that oxytocin be administered for at least 12–18 hours after membrane rupture before deeming the induction a failure.	1B Strong recommendation, moderate-quality evidence
Fetal malpresentation	
Fetal presentation should be assessed and documented beginning at 36 0/7 weeks of gestation to allow for external cephalic version to be offered.	1C Strong recommendation, low-quality evidence
Suspected fetal macrosomia	
Cesarean delivery to avoid potential birth trauma should be limited to estimated fetal weights of at least 5,000 g in women without diabetes and at least 4,500 g in women with diabetes. The prevalence of birth weight of 5,000 g or more is rare, and patients should be counseled that estimates of fetal weight, particularly late in gestation, are imprecise.	2C Weak recommendation, low-quality evidence
Excessive maternal weight gain	
Women should be counseled about the IOM maternal weight guidelines in an attempt to avoid excessive weight gain.	1B Strong recommendation, moderate-quality evidence
Twin gestations	
Perinatal outcomes for twin gestations in which the first twin is in cephalic presentation are not improved by cesarean delivery. Thus, women with either cephalic/cephalic-presenting twins or cephalic/noncephalic presenting twins should be counseled to attempt vaginal delivery.	1B Strong recommendation, moderate-quality evidence
Other	
Individuals, organizations, and governing bodies should work to ensure that research is conducted to provide a better knowledge base to guide decisions regarding cesarean delivery and to encourage policy changes that safely lower the rate of primary cesarean delivery.	1C Strong recommendation, low-quality evidence

Abbreviation: IOM, Health and Medicine Division of the National Academies of Sciences, Engineering, and Medicine (previously known as the Institute of Medicine).

Safe prevention of the primary cesarean delivery. Obstetric Care Consensus No. 1. American College of Obstetricians and Gynecologists. Obstet Gynecol 2014;123:693–711.

All hospitals offering labor and delivery services should be equipped to perform emergency cesarean delivery. The required personnel, including nurses, anesthesia personnel, neonatal resuscitation team members, and obstetric attendants, should be in the hospital or readily available. Any hospital providing an obstetric service should have the capability of responding to an obstetric emergency. Historically, the consensus has been that hospitals need to have the capability of beginning a cesarean delivery within 30 minutes of the decision to operate. However, the scientific evidence to support this threshold is lacking. The decision-to-incision interval should be based on the timing that best incorporates maternal and fetal risks and benefits. For instance, many of these clinical scenarios will include high-risk conditions or pregnancy complications (eg, morbid obesity, eclampsia, cardiopulmonary compromise, or hemorrhage), which may require maternal stabilization or additional surgical preparation before performance of emergent cesarean delivery. Conversely, examples of indications that may mandate more expeditious delivery include hemorrhage from placenta previa, abruptio placentae, prolapse of the umbilical cord, and uterine rupture. Therefore, it is reasonable to tailor the time to delivery to local circumstances and logistics. Sterile materials and supplies needed for emergency cesarean delivery should be kept sealed but properly arranged so that the instrument table can be made ready at once for an obstetric emergency. Anesthesia services should be available in all hospitals offering laboring and delivery services, and available at all times within level II–IV facilities. The anesthesia and pediatric staff responsible for covering the labor and delivery unit should be informed in advance when a complicated delivery is anticipated and upon admission of a woman with risk factors requiring a high-acuity level of care.

For women planning a cesarean delivery at 39 weeks of gestation, whether primary or repeat, gestational age should be established based on any one of the following criteria:

- Ultrasound measurement at less than 20 weeks of gestation supports gestational age of 39 weeks or greater.
- Fetal heart tones have been documented as present for 30 weeks by Doppler ultrasonography.
- It has been 36 weeks since a positive serum or urine human chorionic gonadotropin test result.

These criteria are not intended to preclude the use of menstrual dating. If any one criterion confirms gestational age assessment in a woman who has normal menstrual cycles and no immediate antecedent use of oral contraceptives, it is appropriate to schedule delivery at 39 weeks of gestation or later on the basis of menstrual dates. Another option is to await the onset of spontaneous labor. Inductions or cesarean deliveries before 39 weeks of gestation should always have a maternal or fetal indication that warrants delivery before 39 weeks of gestation.

Cesarean delivery on maternal request is defined as a primary prelabor cesarean delivery on maternal request in the absence of any maternal or fetal indications. Potential short-term maternal benefits of planned cesarean delivery compared with a planned vaginal delivery include a decreased risk of postpartum hemorrhage and transfusion, fewer surgical complications, and a decrease in urinary incontinence during the first year after delivery. Potential risks of cesarean delivery on maternal request include greater complications in subsequent pregnancies, such as uterine rupture, placenta previa, placenta accreta, bladder and bowel injuries, and the need for hysterectomy. There are limited studies on cesarean delivery on maternal request and neonatal outcomes. The risk of respiratory morbidity is higher for elective cesarean delivery compared with vaginal delivery when delivery is earlier than 39–40 weeks of gestation. The literature on elective cesarean delivery without labor also shows an increased rate of complications related to prematurity for infants delivered by cesarean delivery before 39 weeks of gestation. Because of these potential complications, cesarean delivery on maternal request should not be performed before a gestational age of 39 weeks of gestation. Cesarean delivery on maternal request should not be motivated by the unavailability of effective pain management. Cesarean delivery on maternal request particularly is not recommended for women desiring several children, given that the risks of placenta previa, placenta accreta, and gravid hysterectomy increase with each cesarean delivery.

The decision to monitor the fetus before scheduled cesarean delivery should be individualized. Presence of fetal heart tones before surgery should be documented. However, in women requiring unscheduled cesarean delivery, fetal surveillance should continue until abdominal sterile preparation has begun. If internal FHR monitoring is in use, it should be continued until the abdominal sterile preparation is complete or longer if indicated. Given that cesarean delivery approximately doubles the risk of venous thromboembolism (although in the otherwise normal patient, the risk still remains low: approximately 1 per 1,000), placement of pneumatic compression devices before cesarean delivery is recommended for all women not already receiving thromboprophylaxis. However, cesarean delivery in the emergency setting should not be delayed because of the timing necessary to implement thromboprophylaxis (see also "Deep Vein Thrombosis and Pulmonary Embolism" in Chapter 9). When the cesarean delivery is performed for fetal indications, consideration should be given to sending the placenta for pathologic evaluation.

Updated safety bundles on obstetric hemorrhage, preeclampsia, severe hypertension, safe reduction of primary cesarean births, maternal venous thromboembolism prevention, and other safety topics are available at www.safehealthcareforeverywoman.org.

Prophylaxis Against Postcesarean Infection

The single most important risk factor for infection in the postpartum period is cesarean delivery. Antimicrobial prophylaxis is recommended for all cesarean deliveries and should be administered within 60 minutes before the start of the cesarean delivery, unless the woman is already receiving an antibiotic regimen with appropriate coverage (eg, for intraamniotic infection). When this is not possible (eg, need for emergent delivery), prophylaxis needs to be administered as soon as possible after the incision is made.

A single dose of first-generation cephalosporin is the antibiotic of choice, unless significant drug allergies are present. For women with a history of a significant penicillin or cephalosporin allergy (anaphylaxis, angioedema, respiratory distress, or urticaria), a single-dose combination of clindamycin and aminoglycoside is a reasonable alternative. For women with a mild penicillin allergy, cefazolin is the recommended agent. After a single 1-gram intravenous dose of cefazolin, a therapeutic level is maintained for approximately 3–4 hours. A higher dose may be indicated if a woman is obese. Women with lengthy surgeries or those who experience excessive blood loss need to receive an additional intraoperative dose.

Umbilical Cord Clamping After Birth

In term infants, delayed umbilical cord clamping increases hemoglobin levels at birth and improves iron stores in the first several months of life, which may have a favorable effect on developmental outcomes. In preterm infants, delayed umbilical cord clamping results in improved transitional circulation, better establishment of red blood cell volume, decreased need for blood transfusion and lower incidence of necrotizing enterocolitis and intraventricular hemorrhage. Given these benefits, delayed umbilical cord clamping for at least 30–60 seconds is recommended in vigorous term and preterm infants. There is a small increase in the incidence of jaundice requiring phototherapy in term infants undergoing delayed umbilical cord clamping. Consequently, obstetrician–gynecologists and other obstetric care providers adopting delayed umbilical cord clamping in term infants should ensure that mechanisms are in place to monitor and treat neonatal jaundice. Delayed umbilical cord clamping does not increase the risk of postpartum hemorrhage. However, when there is increased risk of hemorrhage (eg, placenta previa or abruptio placentae), the benefits of delayed umbilical cord clamping need to be balanced with the need for timely hemodynamic stabilization of the woman (Table 7-2).

The ability to provide delayed umbilical cord clamping may vary among institutions and settings; decisions in those circumstances are best made by the team caring for the mother–infant dyad. There are several situations in which data are limited and decisions regarding timing of umbilical cord clamping should be individualized (Table 7-2). For example, in cases of fetal growth restriction with abnormal umbilical artery Doppler studies or other situations in which uteroplacental perfusion or umbilical cord flow may be compromised, a discussion between neonatal and obstetric teams can help weigh the relative risks and benefits of immediate or delayed umbilical cord clamping.

In cases where directed donation of cord blood is planned for a medical reason, immediate cord clamping may increase the yield of cord blood obtained. However, in the absence of directed donation, the benefits to the infant of transfusion of additional blood volume at delivery likely exceed the benefits of banking that volume for possible future use. Families who are considering banking of umbilical cord blood should be counseled accordingly.

Multiple Gestation

The risk of perinatal mortality increases in twin pregnancies at approximately 38 weeks of gestation. Based on these data, and in the absence of large randomized trials that demonstrate a clearly optimal time for delivery, the following recommendations for timing of delivery seem reasonable for women with twin gestations:

- Women with uncomplicated dichorionic–diamniotic twin gestations can undergo delivery at 38 weeks of gestation.

- Women with uncomplicated monochorionic–diamniotic twin gestations can undergo delivery between 34 0/7 weeks and 37 6/7 weeks of gestation.
- For women with monochorionic–monoamniotic twin gestations, delivery is recommended between 32 0/7 weeks and 34 0/7 weeks of gestation.

The optimal route of delivery in women with twin gestations depends on the type of twins, fetal presentations, gestational age, and experience of the clinician performing the delivery.

Support Persons in the Delivery Room

Childbirth is a momentous family experience. Evidence suggests that, in addition to regular nursing care, continuous one-to-one emotional support provided by support personnel, such as a doula, is associated with improved outcomes for women in labor. Benefits found in randomized trials include shortened labor, decreased need for analgesia, fewer operative deliveries, and fewer reports of dissatisfaction with the experience of labor. It also may be effective to teach labor-support techniques to a friend or family member. This approach was tested in a randomized trial of 600 nulliparous, low-income, low-risk women, and the treatment resulted in significantly shorter length of labor, greater cervical dilation at the time of epidural anesthesia, and higher Apgar scores at 1 minute and 5 minutes. Continuous labor support also may be cost effective given the associated lower cesarean rate. One analysis suggested that paying for such personnel might result in substantial cost savings annually. Given these benefits and the absence of demonstrable risk, patients, obstetrician–gynecologists and other obstetric care providers, and health care organizations may want to develop programs and policies to integrate trained support personnel into the intrapartum care environment to provide continuous one-to-one emotional support to women undergoing labor.

Obstetric care providers willingly should provide opportunities for those accompanying and supporting the woman giving birth to be present. These support persons must be informed about requirements for safety and must be willing to follow the directions of the obstetric staff concerning behavior in the delivery room. They also should understand the normal events and procedures in the labor and delivery area. They must conform to the dress code required of personnel in attendance in a delivery room. The obstetrician and the patient should consent to the presence of fathers, partners, or other support persons in the delivery room. Support persons should realize that their major function is to provide psychologic support to the mother during labor and delivery.

The judgment of the obstetric staff, the individual obstetrician, the anesthesiologist, and pediatric support personnel, as well as the policies of the hospital, determines whether support persons may be present at a cesarean delivery. A written policy developed by all involved hospital staff is recommended.

Complications

Intraamniotic Infection

Intraamniotic infection, also known as chorioamnionitis, is an infection with resultant inflammation of any combination of the amniotic fluid, placenta, fetus, fetal membranes, or decidua. It is strongly associated acute neonatal morbidity, including neonatal pneumonia, meningitis, sepsis, and death. Diagnosis and treatment of intraamniotic infection is discussed further in Chapter 12.

Maternal Hemorrhage

Hemorrhage remains one of the leading causes of maternal mortality worldwide. One half of all maternal deaths occur within 24 hours of delivery and most commonly from excessive bleeding. Facilities that provide labor and delivery services need to be prepared to manage maternal hemorrhage. Proper preparation and resources to manage maternal hemorrhage in a timely manner can be lifesaving. Strategies to more accurately measure maternal blood loss by transitioning from visual estimation of blood loss to quantification of blood loss methods for every birth need to be adopted. Policies to ensure the rapid availability of blood products for transfusion in the event of hemorrhage need to be in place.

Postpartum Hemorrhage. There is no single definition of postpartum hemorrhage. Criteria of an estimated blood loss of greater than 500 mL after a vaginal delivery or 1,000 mL after cesarean delivery are often used, but the average volume of blood lost at delivery can approach these amounts. Symptoms of hypotension, pallor, and oliguria typically do not occur until blood loss is substantial. Risk factors for excessive bleeding include prolonged, augmented, or rapid labor; history of postpartum hemorrhage;

episiotomy, especially mediolateral; preeclampsia; overdistended uterus (macrosomia, twins, or hydramnios); operative delivery; Asian or Hispanic ethnicity; and intraamniotic infection. Most cases of postpartum hemorrhage occur immediately or soon after delivery. Uterine atony is the most common cause of postpartum hemorrhage. Other etiologies include retained placenta, placenta accreta, uterine rupture, uterine inversion, obstetric lacerations, retained products of conception, maternal coagulopathy, and infection. In an effort to prevent uterine atony and associated bleeding, it is routine to administer oxytocin soon after delivery.

Management may vary greatly, depending on etiology of the hemorrhage and available treatment options, and often a multidisciplinary approach is required. Less-invasive methods need to be tried initially if possible, but if unsuccessful, preservation of life may require hysterectomy. Treatment options for postpartum hemorrhage due to uterine atony include administration of uterotonics and pharmacologic agents, tamponade of the uterus, surgical techniques to control the bleeding, and embolization of pelvic arteries. Treatment of hemorrhage due to uterine rupture should be tailored to the site of uterine injury, maternal condition, and the patient's desire for future childbearing; hysterectomy may be necessary in a life-threatening situation. In the presence of previa or a history of cesarean delivery, the obstetrician–gynecologist or other obstetric care provider must have a high clinical suspicion for placenta accreta and take appropriate precautions. The extent (area, depth) of the abnormal attachment will determine the response—curettage, wedge resection, medical management, or hysterectomy; abdominal hysterectomy usually is the most definitive treatment. Manual replacement with or without uterine relaxants usually is successful for management of uterine inversion. In the unusual circumstance in which it is not, laparotomy is required.

Each obstetric unit should have and follow a hemorrhage management protocol such as those provided in the Council on Patient Safety in Women's Health Care Obstetric Hemorrhage Bundle (www.safehealthcareforeverywoman.org/patient-safety-bundles/obstetric-hemorrhage/) or the California Maternal Quality Care Collaborative hemorrhage toolkit (https://www.cmqcc.org/resources-tool-kits/ob-hemorrhage-toolkit).

Transfusion. Transfusion therapy is used to prevent or treat hemorrhagic shock and its consequences. Transfusion of blood products is necessary when the extent of blood loss is significant and ongoing, particularly if vital signs are unstable. Clinical judgment is an important determinant, given that estimates of blood loss often are inaccurate, determination of hematocrit or hemoglobin concentrations may not accurately reflect the current hematologic status, and symptoms and signs of hemorrhage may not occur until blood loss exceeds 15%. The decision to initiate and continue transfusion therapy is based on the amount of quantified maternal blood loss, the presence of continued blood loss or bleeding, and maternal response to interventions. The purpose of transfusion of blood products is to replace coagulation factors and red blood cells for oxygen-carrying capacity, not for volume replacement. To avoid dilutional coagulopathy, concurrent replacement with coagulation factors and platelets may be necessary. Each obstetric unit should have protocols and capabilities for massive transfusion process, emergency release of blood products, and management of multiple component therapy.

Obstetric Lacerations

Lacerations are common after vaginal birth. Trauma can occur on the cervix, vagina, and vulva, including the labial, periclitoral, and periurethral regions, and the perineum. Most of these lacerations do not result in adverse functional outcomes. Severe perineal lacerations, extending into or through the anal sphincter complex, although less frequent, are more commonly associated with increased risk of pelvic floor injury, fecal and urinary incontinence, pain, and sexual dysfunction with symptoms that may persist or be present many years after giving birth.

A number of different perineal management interventions have been used in the antepartum period or at the time of delivery in an effort to reduce perineal trauma, including maternal perineal massage, manual perineal support, warm compresses, different birthing positions, and delayed pushing. Perineal massage (antepartum or during the second stage of labor) is intended to decrease perineal muscular resistance and reduce the likelihood of laceration at delivery. Because application of warm perineal compresses during pushing reduces the incidence of third-degree and fourth-degree lacerations, obstetrician–gynecologists and other obstetric care providers can apply warm compresses to the perineum during pushing to reduce the risk of perineal trauma.

Diagnosis of obstetric lacerations in the setting of perineal trauma requires adequate lighting, exposure, and analgesia. If a deep perineal laceration is noted, a digital rectal examination can improve the diagnosis of obstetric and anal sphincter injuries (OASIS). For repair, the laceration apex must be identified for adequate closure and hemostasis. When complex lacerations exist or if there is excessive bleeding, better positioning, visualization, suitable lighting, and assistance may be necessary to perform the repair. Although most perineal lacerations are sutured, insufficient evidence exists to recommend surgical or nonsurgical repair of first-degree or second-degree perineal tears sustained during childbirth.

Small tears of the anterior vaginal wall and labia are relatively common, are often superficial with no bleeding, and can be left unrepaired. In the absence of bleeding or distortion of anatomy, vulvar, vaginal, or cervical lacerations usually are not repaired. There are no data on which to recommend a specific practice for closure of vulvar, vaginal, and cervical laceration. Clinical practice generally is guided by experience and expert opinion.

First-degree lacerations that do not distort anatomy and are not bleeding may not need to be repaired. Either standard suture or adhesive glue may be used to repair a hemostatic first-degree laceration or the perineal skin of a second-degree laceration. Continuous suturing of a second-degree laceration is preferred over interrupted suturing.

If the internal anal sphincter can be adequately identified, repair has been recommended either as a part of the distal portion of the reinforcing second layer of the rectal muscularis using a 3-0 polyglactin suture or separately from the external anal sphincter using a 3-0 monofilament polydioxanone suture. For full-thickness external anal sphincter lacerations, end-to-end repair or overlap repair is acceptable.

A single dose of antibiotic at the time of repair is recommended in the setting of OASIS. Stool softeners and oral laxatives should be prescribed to women who sustain OASIS, and counseling postpartum should include discussing ways to avoid constipation. Women who have a history of OASIS should be counseled that the absolute risk of a recurrent OASIS is low with a subsequent vaginal delivery; however, it is reasonable to perform a cesarean delivery based on patient request after advising of the associated risks.

Bibliography

Amnioinfusion does not prevent meconium aspiration syndrome. ACOG Committee Opinion No. 346. American College of Obstetricians and Gynecologists. Obstet Gynecol 2006;108:1053.

Approaches to limit intervention during labor and birth. Committee Opinion No. 687. American College of Obstetricians and Gynecologists. Obstet Gynecol 2017;129: e20–8.

Begley CM, Gyte GML, Devane D, McGuire W, Weeks A. Active versus expectant management for women in the third stage of labour. Cochrane Database of Systematic Reviews 2015, Issue 3. Art. No. CD007412. DOI: 10.1002/14651858.CD007412.pub4.

Cesarean delivery on maternal request. Committee Opinion No. 559. American College of Obstetricians and Gynecologists. Obstet Gynecol 2013;121:904–7.

Delayed umbilical cord clamping after birth. Committee Opinion No. 684. American College of Obstetricians and Gynecologists. Obstet Gynecol 2017;129:e5–10.

Hodnett ED, Gates S, Hofmeyr GJ, Sakala C. Continuous support for women during childbirth. Cochrane Database of Systematic Reviews2013, Issue 7.Art. No. CD003766. DOI: 10.1002/14651858.CD003766.pub5.

Hospital-based triage of obstetric patients. Committee Opinion No. 667. American College of Obstetricians and Gynecologists. Obstet Gynecol 2016;128:e16–9.

Immersion in water during labor and delivery. Committee Opinion No. 679. American College of Obstetricians and Gynecologists. Obstet Gynecol 2016;128:e231–6.

Induction of labor. ACOG Practice Bulletin No. 107. American College of Obstetricians and Gynecologists; Obstet Gynecol 2009;114:386–97.

Intermittent auscultation for intrapartum fetal heart rate surveillance: American College of Nurse-Midwives [published erratum appears in J Midwifery Womens Health 2016;61:134]. J Midwifery Womens Health 2015;60:626–32.

Intrapartum fetal heart rate monitoring: nomenclature, interpretation, and general management principles. ACOG Practice Bulletin No. 106. American College of Obstetricians and Gynecologists. Obstet Gynecol 2009;114:192–202.

Labor induction or augmentation and autism. Committee Opinion No. 597. American College of Obstetricians and Gynecologists. Obstet Gynecol 2014;123:1140–2.

Levels of maternal care. Obstetric Care Consensus No. 2. American College of Obstetricians and Gynecologists. Obstet Gynecol 2015;125:502–15.

Lyndon A, Ali LU, editors. Fetal heart monitoring: principles and practices. 5th ed. Washington, DC: Association of Women's Health, Obstetric, and Neonatal Nurses; 2015.

Macones GA, Hankins GD, Spong CY, Hauth J, Moore T. The 2008 National Institute of Child Health and Human Development Workshop report on electronic fetal monitoring: update on definitions, interpretation, and research guidelines. Obstet Gynecol 2008;112:661–6.

Magann EF, Evans S, Chauhan SP, Lanneau G, Fisk AD, Morrison JC. The length of the third stage of labor and the risk of postpartum hemorrhage. Obstet Gynecol 2005;105:290–3.

Main EK, Goffman D, Scavone BM, Low LK, Bingham D, Fontaine PL, et al. National Partnership for Maternal Safety: consensus bundle on obstetric hemorrhage. National Partnership for Maternal Safety and Council on Patient Safety in Women's Health Care [published erratum appears in Obstet Gynecol 2015;126:1111]. Obstet Gynecol 2015;126:155–62.

Management of intrapartum fetal heart rate tracings. Practice Bulletin No. 116. American College of Obstetricians and Gynecologists. Obstet Gynecol 2010;116: 1232–40.

Multifetal gestations: twin, triplet, and higher-order multifetal pregnancies. Practice Bulletin No. 169. American College of Obstetricians and Gynecologists. Obstet Gynecol 2016;128:e131–46.

National Institute for Health and Care Excellence. Intrapartum care for healthy women and babies. NICE Clinical Guideline CG190. London: NICE; 2014. Available at: https://www.nice.org.uk/guidance/cg190. Retrieved April 4, 2017.

Obstetric analgesia and anesthesia. ACOG Practice Bulletin No. 177. American College of Obstetricians and Gynecologists. Obstet Gynecol 2017;129:e73–89.

Operative vaginal delivery. Practice Bulletin No. 154. American College of Obstetricians and Gynecologists. Obstet Gynecol 2015;126:e56-65.

Oral intake during labor. ACOG Committee Opinion No. 441. American College of Obstetricians and Gynecologists. Obstet Gynecol 2009;114:714.

Placenta accreta. Committee Opinion No. 529. American College of Obstetricians and Gynecologists. Obstet Gynecol 2012;120:207–11.

Postpartum hemorrhage. ACOG Practice Bulletin No. 76. American College of Obstetricians and Gynecologists. Obstet Gynecol 2006;108:1039–47.

Premature rupture of membranes. Practice Bulletin No. 172. American College of Obstetricians and Gynecologists. Obstet Gynecol 2016;128:e165–77.

Prenatal and perinatal human immunodeficiency virus testing: expanded recommendations. Committee Opinion No. 635. American College of Obstetricians and Gynecologists. Obstet Gynecol 2015;125:1544–7.

Prevention and management of obstetric lacerations at vaginal delivery. Practice Bulletin No. 165. American College of Obstetricians and Gynecologists. Obstet Gynecol 2016;128:e1–15.

Ruhl C, Scheich B, Onokpise B, Bingham D. Content validity testing of the maternal fetal triage index. J Obstet Gynecol Neonatal Nurs 2015;44:701–9.

Safe prevention of the primary cesarean delivery. Obstetric Care Consensus No. 1. American College of Obstetricians and Gynecologists. Obstet Gynecol 2014;123: 693–711.

Shoulder Dystocia. ACOG Practice Bulletin No. 40. American College of Obstetricians and Gynecologists. Obstet Gynecol 2002;100:1045–50.

The Apgar score. Committee Opinion No. 644. American College of Obstetricians and Gynecologists. Obstet Gynecol 2015;126:e52–5.

Use of prophylactic antibiotics in labor and delivery. ACOG Practice Bulletin No. 120. American College of Obstetricians and Gynecologists. Obstet Gynecol 2011;117: 1472–83.

Vaginal birth after previous cesarean delivery. Practice Bulletin No. 115. American College of Obstetricians and Gynecologists. Obstet Gynecol 2010;116:450–63.

Wong CA, Scavone BM, Peaceman AM, McCarthy RJ, Sullivan JT, Diaz NT, et al. The risk of cesarean delivery with neuraxial analgesia given early versus late in labor. N Engl J Med 2005;352:655–65.

Resources

American College of Obstetricians and Gynecologists. Immunization for women. Washington, DC: American College of Obstetricians and Gynecologists; 2011; 2016. Available at: http://immunizationforwomen.org/. Retrieved December 20, 2011; October 26, 2016.

Council on Patient Safety in Women's Health Care. Washington, DC: CPSWHC; 2016. Available at: http://safehealthcareforeverywoman.org. Retrieved December 9, 2016.

Neurological disorders. In: Cunningham FG, Leveno KJ, Bloom SL, Spong CY, Dashe JS, Hoffman BL et al., editors. Williams obstetrics. 24th ed. New York (NY): McGraw Hill Medical; 2014. p. 1187-203.

Psychiatric disorders. In: Cunningham FG, Leveno KJ, Bloom SL, Spong CY, Dashe JS, Hoffman BL et al., editors. Williams obstetrics. 24th ed. New York (NY): McGraw Hill Medical; 2014. p. 1204–13.

Shealy KR, Li R, Benton-Davis S, Grummer-Strawn LM. The CDC guide to breastfeeding interventions. Atlanta (GA): Centers for Disease Control and Prevention; 2005. Available at: https://www.cdc.gov/breastfeeding/pdf/breastfeeding_interventions.pdf. Retrieved October 31, 2016.

World Health Organization. Active management of the third stage of labour: new WHO recommendations health to focus implementation. Geneva: WHO; 2013. Available at: http://apps.who.int/iris/bitstream/10665/119831/1/WHO_RHR_14.18_eng.pdf. Retrieved March 6, 2017.

Chapter 8

Postpartum Care of the Mother

Monitoring during the postpartum period is dictated in part by the events of the delivery, the type of anesthesia or analgesia used, and the complications identified. Pain management should be guided by guidelines established by the anesthesiologists and obstetricians in concert.

Immediate Postpartum Maternal Care

Blood pressure levels and pulse should be monitored at least every 15 minutes for 2 hours, but more frequently and for longer duration if there are complications. The woman's temperature should be taken at least every 4 hours for the first 8 hours after delivery, and at least every 8 hours subsequently.

Healthy term infants should be placed skin-to-skin with the mother immediately after birth and remain there for the first hour of life. In a meta-analysis of randomized controlled trials, skin-to-skin care in the first hour of life increased neonatal glucose concentrations, improved cardiorespiratory stability among late preterm infants, and increased breastfeeding duration by approximately 6 weeks. Evidence suggests that skin-to-skin care reduces infant stress during painful procedures, such as vitamin K injection. Skin-to-skin contact is feasible in the operating room and is associated with reduced need for formula supplementation among breastfed infants.

Nursing staff assigned to the delivery and immediate recovery of a woman should be free of other obligations. Discharge from the delivery room, which may involve recovery from an anesthetic, should be at the discretion of the woman's obstetrician–gynecologist or other obstetric care provider or the anesthesia personnel in charge.

If regional or general anesthesia was administered, the woman should be observed in an appropriately staffed and equipped hospital area until she has recovered from the anesthetic. After cesarean delivery, postanesthesia care should be similar to that given to other patients who have received similar anesthesia. Monitoring needs to include the mother and her newborn infant. The institution should ensure that a health care provider is readily available to manage anesthetic complications for the mother and her newborn infant. Discharge from the recovery area should be at the discretion of the woman's obstetric caregiver after communication with anesthesia personnel in charge. Vital signs and additional signs or events should be monitored and recorded as they occur.

Subsequent Postpartum Care

In the postpartum period, staff should facilitate a woman's learning how to care for her own general needs and those of her newborn infant. Care for the woman should be specific to her needs and vary depending on the type of delivery and any complications (eg, cesarean delivery, perineal lacerations).

The obstetric caregiver should note postpartum orders on the woman's medical record (see also "Postpartum Form" in Appendix A). If routine postpartum orders are used, they should be reviewed and modified as necessary for the particular woman and then entered into the medical record and signed by the obstetric caregiver before the woman is transferred to the postpartum unit. When a labor, delivery, and recovery room is used, the same guidelines apply.

Bed Rest, Ambulation, and Diet

It is important for the new mother to sleep, regain her strength, and recover from the effects of any analgesic or anesthetic agents that she may have received during labor. In the absence of complications, she may have a regular diet as soon as she wishes. Because early ambulation has been shown to decrease the incidence of subsequent deep vein thrombosis, the mother should be encouraged to walk as soon as she feels able to do so. However, she should not attempt to get out of bed for the first time without assistance. She may shower as soon as she wishes. It may be necessary to administer fluids intravenously for hydration. If the woman has an intravenous line in place, her fluid and hemodynamic status should be evaluated before it is removed. If blood loss is greater than usual, the woman's hemoglobin also should be assessed before discontinuing intravenous access.

Postpartum Analgesia

After vaginal delivery, analgesic medication may be necessary to relieve perineal and episiotomy pain and facilitate maternal mobility. This is best addressed by administering the medications on an as-needed basis according to postpartum orders. Orally administered analgesics often are required and usually are sufficient for relief of discomfort from episiotomy or repaired lacerations. Pain that is not relieved by such medication suggests hematoma formation and mandates a careful examination of the vulva, vagina, and rectum. Beginning 24 hours after delivery, moist heat in the form of a warm sitz bath may reduce local discomfort and promote healing.

Adequate pain control also is an important part of managing severe perineal trauma. Local treatment options include topical anesthetic sprays or creams, ice packs, baths, and rectal suppositories. A meta-analysis showed no improvement in pain control when topical anesthetics were compared with placebo. There is limited evidence to support the effectiveness of local cooling treatments, including ice packs, cold gel pads, and cold or iced baths, applied to the perineum after childbirth to relieve pain.

Although women with third-degree and fourth-degree lacerations were included in this meta-analysis, the number of women with fourth-degree lacerations was not specified. Expert opinion suggests that rectal suppositories should be used cautiously in women with a fourth-degree laceration because of the theoretical risk of poor wound healing and disruption of the repair. Nonsteroidal antiinflammatory or opiate agents can be offered for pain control, but opiates should be coupled with oral laxatives and stool softeners to help mediate the significant constipating adverse effects of these medications.

Many mothers experience considerable pain in the first 24 hours after cesarean delivery. However, spinal or epidural opiates, patient-controlled epidural or intravenous analgesia, and potent oral analgesics, provide pain relief and satisfaction. Regardless of the route of administration, opioids potentially can cause respiratory depression and decrease intestinal motility. Therefore, adequate supervision and monitoring should be ensured for all postpartum women receiving these drugs.

Urogenital Care

Women should be encouraged to void as soon as possible after delivery. Often women have difficulty voiding immediately after delivery, possibly because of trauma to the bladder or urethra during labor and delivery, regional anesthesia, or vulvar–perineal pain and swelling. In addition, the diuresis that often follows delivery can distend the bladder before the woman is aware of a sensation of a full bladder. To ensure adequate emptying of the bladder, the woman should be checked frequently during the first 24 hours after delivery, with particular attention to displacement of the uterine fundus and any indication of the presence of a fluid-filled bladder above the symphysis. Although every effort should be made to help the woman void spontaneously, catheterization may be necessary. If the woman continues to have difficulty voiding, use of an indwelling catheter is preferable to repeated catheterization.

Support for Establishing Breastfeeding

Maternity care practices affect the extent to which women are able to achieve their breastfeeding goals. Women should be provided with guidance on infant feeding cues and the role of frequent, exclusive breastfeeding in establishing a milk supply. For mothers who are separated from their infants, initiation of milk expression within 6 hours of birth is associated with improved milk production. Drops of colostrum obtained from early expression can be used for oral care of the infant as well as for initial feedings of even the smallest preterm infant. All obstetrician–gynecologists and other obstetric care providers should support women who have given birth to preterm infants to establish a full supply of milk by providing anticipatory guidance and working with hospital staff to facilitate early, frequent milk expression.

Infants whose mothers intend to breastfeed should not be supplemented with formula without the explicit agreement of the mother. Rooming-in is encouraged to enable mothers to learn to care for their infants and to allow feeding when infants show early signs of hunger. If a mother wishes to send her infant to the nursery, staff should discuss her preferences regarding bringing the infant back to the room if feeding cues are seen versus supplementing the infant with formula. This discussion should include counseling that on-demand breastfeeding without supplementation is associated with earlier onset of mature milk production.

Care of the Breasts If Breastfeeding Is Not Initiated

A woman's decision about breastfeeding determines the appropriate care of the breasts. The woman who chooses not to breastfeed should be reassured that milk production will abate over the first few days after delivery if she does not breastfeed. During the stage of engorgement, the breasts may become painful and should be supported with a well-fitting brassiere. Ice packs and analgesics can help relieve discomfort during this period. Medications for lactation cessation are discouraged. Women who do not wish to breastfeed should be encouraged to avoid nipple stimulation and should be cautioned against continued manual expression of milk.

Postpartum Immunizations

For women who previously have not received the tetanus toxoid, reduced diphtheria toxoid, and acellular pertussis (Tdap) vaccine and it was not administered during pregnancy, it should be administered immediately postpartum to the mother in order to reduce the risk of transmission to the newborn. Additionally, other family members and planned direct caregivers also should receive Tdap as previously recommended (sustained efforts at cocooning). Likewise, a woman who is identified as susceptible to rubella or varicella infection should receive the appropriate vaccine postpartum before discharge. During the flu season, women who were not vaccinated antepartum should be offered the seasonal flu vaccine before discharge. Breastfeeding is not a contraindication to receiving any of these vaccinations.

A woman who is unsensitized and Rh D-negative and who gives birth to a newborn infant who is Rh D-positive or Du-positive (ie, weak Rh positive) should receive 300 micrograms of anti-D immune globulin postpartum, ideally within 72 hours, even when anti-D immune globulin has been administered in the antepartum period. No further administration of anti-D immune globulin is necessary when the infants of Rh D-negative women are also Rh D-negative. (For more information on specific vaccinations, see Chapter 12.)

Endometritis

Postpartum endometritis is caused by a mixture of skin or vaginal flora, including organisms, such as aerobic streptococci (group B β-hemolytic streptococci and the enterococci), gram-negative aerobes (especially *Escherichia coli*), gram-negative anaerobic rods (especially *Bacteroides bivius*), and anaerobic cocci (*Peptococcus* species and *Peptostreptococcus* species). Clinically, endometritis is characterized by fever, uterine tenderness, malaise, tachycardia, abdominal pain, or foul-smelling lochia. Of these, fever is the most characteristic and may be the only sign early in the course of infection. Risk factors for postpartum endometritis include cesarean delivery, prolonged rupture of membranes, prolonged labor with multiple vaginal examinations, intrapartum fever, and lower socioeconomic status.

Management

Endometritis usually is diagnosed within a few days after delivery. A woman with postpartum fever needs to be evaluated by pertinent history, physical examination, blood count, and urine culture. Blood cultures rarely influence therapeutic decisions but could be indicated if septicemia is suspected. Cervical, vaginal, or endometrial cultures need not be routinely performed.

Principles for managing postpartum endometritis are as follows:

- Parenteral, broad-spectrum antibiotic treatment needs to be initiated according to a proven regimen and continued until the woman is afebrile. A combination of clindamycin and gentamicin, with the addition of ampicillin in refractory cases, is recommended for cost-effective therapy.
- Response usually is prompt. If fever persists beyond antibiotic treatment for 24–48 hours, a search for alternative etiologies, including pelvic abscess, wound infection, septic pelvic thrombophlebitis, inadequate antibiotic coverage, and retained placental tissue, needs to be performed.
- Because postpartum endometritis may have implications for a newborn infant, information about the mother's condition needs to be provided to the infant's health care provider.

Length of Hospital Stay

When no complications are present, the postpartum hospital stay is based upon the mother's recovery and ability to care for her infant. The length of stay may range from 48 hours for vaginal delivery to 72 hours for cesarean delivery, excluding the day of delivery, although some women may choose earlier discharge. A shorter hospital stay may be considered if the infant does not require continued hospitalization and both the mother and the obstetrician–gynecologist or other obstetric care provider desire a shortened hospital stay. Regardless of hospital stay length, the following minimal criteria should be met before discharge:

Physical exam findings and laboratory results:

- The mother has normal vital signs.
- The amount and color of lochia are appropriate for the duration of recovery.
- The uterine fundus is firm.
- Urinary output is adequate.
- Any surgical repair or wound has no evidence of infection and appears to be healing without complication.

- There are no abnormal physical or emotional findings.
- Pertinent laboratory results are available.

Maternal readiness for discharge:

- The mother is able to ambulate with ease and has adequate pain control.
- The mother is able to eat and drink without difficulty.
- The mother demonstrates readiness to care for herself and her newborn infant.

Postpartum care plan:

In collaboration with the patient, the postpartum care plan has been updated and reviewed, inclusive of the following topics:

- Care team: Family members or other support persons have been identified that are available to the mother for the weeks after discharge. The woman should receive contact information for her postpartum care team and written instructions regarding the timing of follow-up postpartum care.
- Postpartum visits: Arrangements have been made for postpartum follow-up care, with the woman receiving written instructions regarding the timing of follow-up postpartum care. Arrangement for an early postpartum visit should be made for women with high risk of complications.
- For women with hypertensive disorders, arrangements have been made to monitor blood pressure within 72 hours postpartum and to monitor again 7–10 days after delivery.
- Contraceptive plan: The woman's preferences for contraception, including immediate postpartum long-acting reversible contraceptive (LARC), have been discussed, documented, and implemented, if appropriate.
- Infant feeding: The mother's infant feeding intentions have been discussed and documented, and community resources have been provided (see Chapter 2 and Chapter 10).
- Pregnancy complications: If the pregnancy was complicated by hypertension, a blood pressure check has been scheduled within 7–10 days of birth and postpartum preeclampsia precautions reviewed. If the

pregnancy was complicated by gestational diabetes, the importance of follow-up glucose screening has been discussed.

- Mental health: The patient's risk of postpartum depression and anxiety has been assessed, and commensurate follow-up arranged.

Anticipatory guidance:

- The mother has been instructed in caring for herself and her newborn infant at home, is aware of deviations from normal, and is prepared to recognize and respond to danger signs and symptoms.
- The mother has received instructions on postpartum activity and exercises and common postpartum discomforts and relief measures.

The medical and nursing staff should be aware of potential problems associated with shortened hospital stays and should develop mechanisms to address any questions that arise after discharge. With a shortened hospital stay, a home visit or follow-up telephone call is recommended within 48 hours of discharge from an obstetrician–gynecologist or other obstetric care provider knowledgeable about maternal postpartum care. This contact should include review of major risk factors for maternal morbidity. If early discharge of the mother is being considered, there should be communication with the pediatric care provider about the safety of early discharge for the infant (see also "Hospital Discharge and Parent Education" in Chapter 10).

Because of factors, such as poverty and family conflict, a shortened obstetric hospital stay poses even greater problems for women who have had no prenatal care. Routine obstetric screening tests (eg, hemoglobin level, blood type, and Rh factor), social intervention, and additional education may be needed. Women with unidentified alcohol or drug dependence often opt for early postpartum discharge or leave the hospital against medical advice putting themselves and their infants in danger.

Postpartum Nutritional Guidelines

Postnatal dietary guidelines are similar to those established during pregnancy (see also Chapter 6). The minimal caloric requirement for adequate milk production in a woman of average size is 1,800 kcal per day. In general, an additional 500 kcal of energy daily is recommended throughout lactation. A balanced, nutritious diet will ensure the quality and the quantity of the milk produced without depletion of maternal stores. Fluid intake by the mother is governed by thirst (see also "Breastfeeding" in Chapter 10).

A vitamin–mineral supplement is not needed routinely. Mothers at nutritional risk should be given a multivitamin supplement with particular emphasis on calcium and vitamin B_{12} and vitamin D (see also Chapter 6). Iron should be administered only if the mother herself needs it.

Maternal postpartum weight loss can occur at a rate of 2 lb per month without affecting lactation. On average, a woman will retain 2 lb more than her prepregnancy weight at 1 year postpartum. Evidence supports associations between excessive gestational weight gain and postpartum weight retention. Resuming exercise activities or incorporating new exercise routines after delivery is important in supporting lifelong healthy habits. For healthy pregnant and postpartum women, the guidelines recommend at least 150 minutes per week of moderate-intensity aerobic activity (ie, equivalent to brisk walking).

Residual postpartum retention of weight gained during pregnancy that results in obesity is a concern. Special attention to lifestyle, including exercise and eating habits, will help these women return to a normal body mass index.

Postpartum Considerations

Before discharge, the mother should receive information about the following normal postpartum events:

- Changes in lochia pattern expected in the first few weeks
- Range of activities that she may reasonably undertake
- Care of the breasts, perineum, and bladder
- Dietary needs, particularly if she is breastfeeding
- Recommended amount of exercise
- "Baby blues," emotional responses, and risk of postpartum depression
- Signs of complications (eg, temperature elevation, chills, leg pains, episiotomy or wound drainage, or increased vaginal bleeding)
- Contact information for community-based lactation support
- Contact information for her postpartum care team and written instructions regarding the timing of follow-up postpartum care. When prolonged infant hospitalization is anticipated and is far from the woman's home, it is recommended that a local maternity health care provider be identified for postpartum care and support, even if delivery did not take place at a local hospital.

- For all women in the postpartum period (not just women with preeclampsia), it is suggested that instructions include information about the signs and symptoms of preeclampsia as well as the importance of prompt reporting of this information to their health care providers.

The length of convalescence that the woman can expect, based on the type of delivery, also should be discussed. For women who have had a cesarean delivery, additional precautions may be appropriate, such as wound care and minimizing lifting objects heavier than her newborn infant. Recommendations regarding when it is reasonable to drive after cesarean delivery should incorporate considerations such as use of narcotic medications, incisional discomfort with turning to check blind spots, and ability to brake for an emergency stop without hesitation. It is helpful to reinforce verbal discussions with written information.

The earliest time at which coitus may be resumed safely after childbirth is unknown. Resumption of coitus should be discussed with the mother. Risks of hemorrhage and infection are minimal approximately 2 weeks postpartum. Although a common recommendation is that sexual activity should be delayed until 6 weeks postpartum, there are no data to direct this statement. Therefore, sexual activity can resume after healing of the perineum and when bleeding has decreased, depending on resolution of contraceptive management and, most importantly, on the woman's desire and comfort.

At the time of discharge, the family should be given the name of the maternal and infant care providers to contact if questions or problems arise for either the mother or her newborn infant. Arrangements should be made for a follow-up examination and specific instructions conveyed to the woman, including when she should contact her health care provider. Specific newborn care plans should be reviewed (see Chapter 10).

Postpartum Contraception

Discussion of contraceptive options and prompt initiation of a method is a primary focus of routine antenatal and postpartum care. The benefits of child spacing include decreases in preterm delivery and perinatal mortality, and most women wish to avoid pregnancy for at least several months, if not considerably longer, after delivering a baby. In nonbreastfeeding women, ovulation may return quickly after delivery.

Contraceptive counseling should be tailored depending on whether the mother is breastfeeding because this may influence contraceptive choice. Of note, breastfeeding will only prevent ovulation when women are fully or nearly fully breastfeeding and there is continued amenorrhea. Relying on breastfeeding as a contraceptive is not recommended. Contraceptive options should be explained in detail and include nonhormonal methods (copper intrauterine devices, condoms, diaphragms) and hormonal methods (levonorgestrel-releasing intrauterine system, etonogestrel implants, medroxyprogesterone acetate injection, progestin-only pills, and combined hormonal contraceptive pills) (see Table 8-1).

TABLE 8-1. U.S. Medical Eligibility Criteria for Postpartum Initiation of Contraception*

	Timing of Initiation (U.S. MEC Category Rating[†])	
Contraceptive Type	Breastfeeding	Not Breastfeeding
Combined oral contraceptives, combined hormonal patch, combined vaginal ring	Avoid if less than 21 days postpartum (4)	Avoid if less than 21 days postpartum (4)
	Risks outweigh benefits if 21–29 days postpartum, regardless of venous thromboembolism risk (3)	Risks outweigh benefits if 21–42 days postpartum, with other risk factors for venous thromboembolism (3)
	Risks outweigh benefits if 30–42 days postpartum, with other risk factors for venous thromboembolism (3)	Benefits outweigh risks if 21–42 days postpartum, without other risk factors for venous thromboembolism (2)
	Benefits outweigh risks if 30–42 days postpartum, without other risk factors for venous thromboembolism (2)	No safety concerns if >42 days postpartum (1)
	Benefits outweigh risks if >42 days postpartum (2)	
Progestin-only pills	Any time, including immediately postpartum (1 or 2)[‡]	Any time, including immediately postpartum (1)
Injectable contraception	Any time, including immediately postpartum (1 or 2)[§]	Any time, including immediately postpartum (1)
Contraceptive implant	Any time, including immediately postpartum (1 or 2)[‖]	Any time, including immediately postpartum (1)

(continued)

TABLE 8-1. U.S. Medical Eligibility Criteria for Postpartum Initiation of Contraception* *(continued)*

	Timing of Initiation (U.S. MEC Category Rating[†])	
Contraceptive Type	Breastfeeding	Not Breastfeeding
Intrauterine devices (copper and 3-year or 5-year levonorgestrel)	Any time, including immediately postpartum (after vaginal or cesarean delivery), unless contra-indications exist[¶] (1 or 2)	Any time, including immediately postpartum (after vaginal or cesarean delivery), unless contraindica-tions exist[¶] (1 or 2)

U.S. MEC, *U.S. Medical Eligibility Criteria for Contraceptive Use*, 2016.

*Before initiation of contraception, the health care provider should confirm that the woman meets medical eligibility criteria for the chosen method (see *U.S. Medical Eligibility Criteria for Contraceptive Use,* 2016) and be reasonably certain that she is not pregnant (see *U.S. Selected Practice Recommendations for Contraceptive Use*).

[†]*U.S. Medical Eligibility Criteria for Contraceptive Use,* 2016, categories for classifying hormonal contraceptives and intrauterine devices are as follows: 1 = A condition for which there is no restriction for the use of the contraceptive method; 2 = A condition for which the advantage of using the method generally outweigh the theoretical or proven risks; 3 = A condition for which the theoretical or proven risks usually outweigh the advantages of using the method; 4 = A condition that represents an unacceptable health risk if the contraceptive method is used.

[‡]In breastfeeding women who use progestin-only oral contraceptives, very small amounts of progestin are passed into the breast milk. Two small, randomized controlled trials found no adverse effect on breastfeeding with initiation of etonogestrel implants within 48 hours postpartum. Other studies found that initiation of progestin-only pills, injectables, and implants at 6 weeks or less postpartum compared with nonhormonal use had no detrimental effect on breastfeeding outcomes or infant health, growth, and development in the first year postpartum. In general, these studies are of poor quality, lack standard definitions of breastfeeding or outcome measures, and have not included premature or ill infants.

[§]When initiated immediately postpartum, use of depot medroxyprogesterone acetate has not been found to adversely affect breastfeeding outcomes or infant development.

[||]A category 2 rating is given for less than 30 days postpartum because of theoretical concerns regarding milk production and infant growth and development. Certain women might be at risk of breastfeeding difficulties, such as women with previous breastfeeding difficulties, certain medical conditions, or certain perinatal complications and those who deliver preterm. For these women, as for all women, discussions about contraception for breastfeeding women should include information about risks, benefits, and alternatives.

[¶]Two randomized controlled trials found conflicting results on breastfeeding outcomes when levonorgestrel-intrauterine devices were initiated immediately postpartum compared with 6–8 weeks postpartum. Immediate postpartum insertion of an intrauterine device is contraindicated in cases of postpartum sepsis or septic abortion.

Data from Curtis KM, Tepper NK, Jatlaoui TC, Berry-Bibee E, Horton LG, Zapata LB, et al. U.S. medical eligibility criteria for contraceptive use, 2016. MMWR Recomm Rep 2016;65:1-103 and Curtis KM, Jatlaoui TC, Tepper NK, Zapata LB, Horton LG, Jamieson DJ, et al. U.S. selected practice recommendations for contraceptive use, 2016. MMWR Recomm Rep 2016;65:1–66.

Most postpartum women rapidly become fertile and should be encouraged to adopt a contraceptive method if they wish to avoid pregnancy. Important considerations in contraceptive counseling include method effectiveness and safety, continuation rates, prior success in contraceptive adherence, timing of initiation, and effect on breastfeeding. Ideally, contraceptive counseling takes place during the woman's antenatal visits because in the postpartum period women are typically focused on other challenges, including adapting to a new baby and breastfeeding.

The Centers for Disease Control and Prevention (CDC) have developed evidence-based medical eligibility criteria for contraceptive use (available at: www.cdc.gov/reproductivehealth/contraception/usmec.htm) that have been endorsed by the American College of Obstetricians and Gynecologists. The CDC classifies sterilization and intrauterine and implant contraception (also known as long-acting reversible contraception) as top-tier methods of contraception, based on high effectiveness, and because of their ease of adherence. These methods are first-line choices for postpartum women. Other methods of contraception include hormonal contraceptives and barrier methods.

Surgical Tubal Sterilization

Surgical tubal sterilization often can be safely performed in the immediate postpartum period. In the antepartum period, informed consent should be obtained, and women should receive counseling about the permanence and irreversibility of sterilization so that they can make a considered decision, review the benefits and risks of the procedure, and consider alternative reversible contraceptive methods.

If the woman is stable and has no acute medical problems after vaginal delivery, she may undergo tubal sterilization immediately or within the first few days postpartum. Tubal ligation at the time of cesarean delivery is safe and effective. In a patient with medical or obstetric complications during the peripartum period—including cardiovascular, respiratory, infections, or metabolic abnormalities—the woman's stability should be ensured before proceeding with tubal sterilization. Every attempt should be made to honor the woman's wishes for a postpartum tubal ligation, particularly if a subsequent pregnancy would be dangerous. Although volume and staffing in the labor and delivery department may sometimes preclude performing a tubal sterilization immediately after delivery, consideration may be given to other arrangements, such as using the main operating room. Women who did not receive their desired postpartum tubal sterilization were found to have a higher pregnancy rate postpartum than women who did not plan for any postpartum contraception.

There is only one device available in the United States and approved by the U.S. Food and Drug Administration (FDA) for hysteroscopic sterilization. This method involves placement of a metal microinsert under hysteroscopic guidance into the interstitial portion of each fallopian tube. This minimally invasive method can be performed without general anesthesia at 6–12 weeks after delivery, depending on the device used for tubal occlusion. Women choosing hysteroscopic sterilization should undergo hysterosalpingography 3 months after the procedure to confirm bilateral occlusion, and they should rely on a method of interim contraception until hysterosalpingography confirms occlusion.

Long-Acting Reversible Contraception

Intrauterine devices (IUDs) and contraceptive implants, or LARC, are the most effective reversible contraceptives. The major advantage of LARC methods compared with other reversible contraceptive methods is that they require only a single act of motivation for long-term use. In addition, return to fertility is rapid after removal of the device. According to contraceptive use guidelines from the World Health Organization and the CDC, LARC methods have few contraindications, and almost all women, including adolescents, are eligible for implants and IUDs. Both IUD and contraceptive implant use in women with a variety of characteristics and medical conditions are addressed in the document *U.S. Medical Eligibility Criteria for Contraceptive Use,* 2016 (see "Resources" in this chapter).

Intrauterine contraception is highly effective and has continuation rates approaching 80% at 1 year. Two long-acting IUDs are available in the United States. The FDA has approved use of the copper IUD for up to 10 continuous years and of the levonorgestrel IUD for 3–5 years depending on the type. Although intrauterine contraception is typically initiated at 4–6 weeks postpartum, IUDs may be safely inserted immediately postpartum (before hospital discharge) or after the delivery of the placenta (while still in the delivery room). Best practice for immediate postpartum IUD insertion is to place the IUD in the delivery room, within 10 minutes of placental separation in vaginal and cesarean births. Immediate postpartum LARC should be offered as an effective option for postpartum contraception and, optimally, women should be counseled prenatally about the option of immediate postpartum LARC (see Chapter 6). Immediate postpartum insertion is contraindicated in women in whom peripartum intraamniotic infection (also referred to as chorioamnionitis), endometritis, or postpartum sepsis is diagnosed. The copper IUD and the levonorgestrel-releasing intrauterine system may be used by breastfeeding women. Systems should be in place to ensure that women who desire LARC can receive it during the comprehensive postpartum visit if immediate postpartum placement is not undertaken.

The etonogestrel single-rod contraceptive implant is also highly effective, is FDA approved for up to 3 years of use, and has excellent continuation rates. Implants may be offered to women who are or who are not breastfeeding at any time, including immediately postpartum. Insertion during the delivery admission has been shown to reduce unintended pregnancy rates in the first year postpartum.

Hormonal Contraceptives

Because some hormonal contraceptives may affect breastfeeding, obstetric care providers should discuss the limitations and concerns of each contraceptive within the context of each woman's desire to breastfeed and her risk of unplanned pregnancy, so that she can make an autonomous and informed decision.

Short-acting hormonal contraceptives, include estrogen–progestin combination methods and progestin-only methods. Because of an increased risk of venous thromboembolism, combined hormonal contraceptives are not recommended for use by women who are less than 21 days postpartum. By 42 days postpartum, benefits generally outweigh risks for women without other risk factors for venous thromboembolism, and combined hormonal contraceptives can be used, provided they have no other contraindications to use. Between 21 days and 42 days postpartum, the individual risks and benefits should be considered before recommending estrogen–progestin combination methods.

Progestin-only methods include depot medroxyprogesterone acetate injections, progestin-only pills, and the already discussed levonorgestrel-releasing intrauterine system and etonogestrel single-rod contraceptive implant. Overall, progestin-only methods appear to have little effect on either breastfeeding success or infant growth and health. The CDC states that the advantages outweigh the risks of progestin-only contraception immediately after birth and for combined hormonal methods at 1 month postpartum. The depot medroxyprogesterone acetate injection is a highly effective method that can be initiated before hospital discharge and lasts for 3 months, but continuation rates are low. Progestin-only pills may be prescribed at discharge either for immediate initiation or, as aforementioned, subject to a waiting period in breastfeeding women.

Barrier Methods

Barrier methods are less effective at preventing pregnancy than sterilization, intrauterine devices, and hormonal methods. However, barrier methods, such as the male and female condoms, are particularly effective in preventing sexually transmitted infections. Most barrier methods may be used as soon as intercourse is resumed after delivery, although the diaphragm should not be used within 6 weeks postpartum.

Postpartum Mood Disorders

It is important to identify pregnant and postpartum women with depression because untreated perinatal depression and other mood disorders can have devastating effects on women, infants, and families. Regular contact with the health care delivery system during the perinatal period should provide an ideal circumstance for women with depression to be identified and treated. The American College of Obstetricians and Gynecologists recommends that clinicians screen patients at least once during the perinatal period for depression and anxiety symptoms (see also “Clinical Depression” in Chapter 6).

Perinatal depression, which includes major and minor depressive episodes that occur during pregnancy or in the first 12 months after delivery, is one of the most common medical complications during pregnancy and the postpartum period, affecting one in seven women. Perinatal depression and other mood disorders, such as bipolar disorder and anxiety disorders, can have devastating effects on women, infants, and families; maternal suicide exceeds hemorrhage and hypertensive disorders as a cause of maternal mortality.

Perinatal depression often goes unrecognized because changes in sleep, appetite, and libido may be attributed to normal pregnancy and postpartum changes. In addition to clinicians not recognizing symptoms of mood disorders, women may be reluctant to report changes in their mood. It is important for clinicians to ask the pregnant or postpartum patient about her mood. Newborn care appointments also may be an opportunity to ask a mother about her mood. Obstetric care providers should collaborate with their pediatric colleagues to facilitate treatment for women with mood disorders that are identified during newborn care.

Anxiety is a prominent feature of perinatal mood disorders, as is insomnia. It may be helpful to ask a woman whether she is having intrusive or frightening thoughts or is unable to sleep even when her infant is sleeping. Women with current depression or anxiety, a history of perinatal mood disorders, or risk factors for perinatal mood disorders (Box 8-1) warrant particularly close monitoring, evaluation, and assessment. These women may benefit from evidence-based psychologic and psychosocial interventions and,

Box 8-1. Risk Factors for Perinatal Depression

Depression during pregnancy:

- Maternal anxiety
- Life stress
- History of depression
- Lack of social support
- Unintended pregnancy
- Medicaid insurance
- Domestic violence
- Lower income
- Lower education
- Smoking
- Single status
- Poor relationship quality

Postpartum depression:

- Depression during pregnancy
- Anxiety during pregnancy
- Experiencing stressful life events during pregnancy or the early postpartum period
- Traumatic birth experience
- Preterm birth or infant admission to neonatal intensive care
- Low levels of social support
- Previous history of depression
- Breastfeeding problems

Data from Lancaster CA, Gold KJ, Flynn HA, Yoo H, Marcus SM, Davis MM. Risk factors for depressive symptoms during pregnancy: a systematic review [published erratum appears in Am J Obstet Gynecol 2011;205:326]. Am J Obstet Gynecol 2010;202:5–14 *and* Robertson E, Grace S, Wallington T, Stewart DE. Antenatal risk factors for postpartum depression: a synthesis of recent literature. Gen Hosp Psychiatry 2004;26:289–95.

in some cases, pharmacologic therapy to reduce the incidence and burden of perinatal depression. If there is concern that the patient suffers from mania or bipolar disorder, she should be referred to a psychiatrist before initiating medical therapy because antidepressant monotherapy may trigger mania or psychosis. Mania symptoms include inflated self-esteem or grandiosity, feeling rested after only 3 hours of sleep, or engaging in risky behavior that worry her friends and family (see also "Psychiatric Disease in Pregnancy" in Chapter 9).

Postpartum psychosis is the most severe form of mental illness and is most common in women with preexisting disorders, such as bipolar illness or, less commonly, schizophrenia. Women with postpartum psychosis show severe symptoms, such as severe anxiety, insomnia, and delusions concerning themselves, the infant, and others. This should be considered a psychiatric emergency, and the patient should be referred for immediate, often inpatient, treatment.

The postpartum period is a time of developmental adjustment for the whole family. Family members have new roles and relationships, and an effort needs to be made to assess the progress of the family's adaptation. If a family member finds it difficult to adapt, the health care team needs to arrange for sensitive, supportive assistance. This is particularly important for adolescent mothers, for whom it may be necessary to mobilize multiple resources within the community.

Postpartum Visits

All women should undergo a comprehensive postpartum visit within the first 6 weeks after birth. This visit should include a full assessment of physical, social, and emotional well-being. Early postpartum follow-up is recommended for women with hypertensive disorders of pregnancy. Early follow-up also may be beneficial for women at high risk of complications, such as postpartum depression, cesarean or perineal wound infection, lactation difficulties, or chronic conditions such as seizure disorders that require postpartum medication titration. Women with severe hypertension or severe preeclampsia on antihypertensive medication should be seen by their obstetric care providers within 72 hours of discharge and within 7–10 days of discharge if they are not receiving antihypertensive medication.

The review at the comprehensive postpartum visit should include an interval history and a physical examination to evaluate the woman's current status and her adaptation to the role of being a mother. Specific inquiries regarding breastfeeding should be made and breastfeeding goals should be discussed. Recommended anticipatory guidance at the postpartum visit includes infant feeding, expressing breast milk if returning to work or school, postpartum weight retention, sexuality, physical activity, and nutrition. Any pregnancy complications should be discussed with respect to risks for future pregnancies, and recommendations should be made to optimize maternal health during the interpregnancy period. The examination should include an evaluation of weight, blood pressure levels, breasts, and abdomen as well as a pelvic examination. Episiotomy repair and uterine involution should be evaluated and a Pap test performed, if needed. Postpartum depression screens should be conducted and appropriate referrals made in a timely manner, if needed.

The patient's desire for future children should be discussed. Methods of birth control should be reviewed if already selected, or plans should be made for initiation (see also "Postpartum Form" in Appendix A). Discussion of contraception should include anticipatory guidance about sexuality and libido after childbirth. Healing at the laceration site can cause the woman some discomfort during vaginal intercourse within the first year after delivery. In the lactating woman, the vagina often is atrophic and dry. Natural lubrication during sexual excitement may be unsatisfactory; water-based lubricants can be helpful. Furthermore, the demands of the infant alter the couple's ability to find time for physical intimacy. Health care providers should be prepared to address these issues and refer couples to appropriate resources.

All women who had gestational diabetes mellitus (GDM) should be screened at 6–12 weeks postpartum and managed appropriately. The American Diabetes Association recommends repeat glucose testing at least every 3 years for women who had GDM, but normal results on postpartum screening. Women should be encouraged to discuss their GDM history and need for regular screening with all of their health care providers. Obstetric care providers should communicate information regarding pregnancy outcome and pregnancy complications, such as gestational diabetes or preeclampsia, with a woman's other health care providers to optimize effective follow-up and screening (for more information, see also "Gestational Diabetes Diagnosis and Management" in Chapter 9).

Women with a history of tobacco, alcohol, or other substance use disorder should receive supportive guidance during the postpartum visit to prevent relapse. The emotional status of a woman whose pregnancy had an abnormal outcome also should be reviewed. Counseling should address specific issues regarding her future health and pregnancies, such as vaginal birth after cesarean or the implications of diabetes mellitus, intrauterine growth restriction, preterm birth, hypertension, fetal anomalies, or other conditions that may recur in any future pregnancy. The postpartum visit allows the obstetrician–gynecologist or other obstetric care provider to review adult immunizations, such as Tdap, rubella vaccination, and varicella vaccination for women who are susceptible and did not receive the vaccine immediately postpartum. Vaccination history should be reviewed and immunizations provided as needed.

The postpartum visit is an opportune time to begin prepregnancy counseling for women who wish to have future pregnancies (see also Chapter 5). This counseling may include risk assessment to facilitate the planning, spacing, and timing of the next pregnancy; health-promotion measures; and timely intervention to reduce medical and psychosocial risks. Systems should be in place to ensure that women who desire long-acting reversible contraception or any other form of contraception can receive it during the comprehensive postpartum visit, if immediate postpartum placement was not done earlier. Although physiologic considerations indicate that some women can return to a normal work schedule 6 weeks after delivery, attention also should be given to maternal–infant bonding and implications for breastfeeding duration.

At the conclusion of the postpartum visit, the woman and her obstetrician–gynecologist or other obstetric care provider should determine who will assume primary responsibility for her ongoing care. If responsibility is transferred to another primary care provider, the obstetrician–gynecologist or other obstetric care provider is responsible for ensuring that there is communication with the primary care provider so that he or she can understand the implications of any pregnancy complications for the woman's future health and maintain continuity of care.

Bibliography

Access to contraception. Committee Opinion No. 615. American College of Obstetricians and Gynecologists. Obstet Gynecol 2015;125:250–5.

Access to postpartum sterilization. Committee Opinion No. 530. American College of Obstetricians and Gynecologists. Obstet Gynecol 2012;120:212–5.

American College of Obstetricians and Gynecologists. Hypertension in pregnancy. Washington, DC: American College of Obstetricians and Gynecologists; 2013. Available at: http://www.acog.org/Resources-And-Publications/Task-Force-and-Work-Group-Reports/Hypertension-in-Pregnancy. Retrieved November 2, 2016.

Breastfeeding. J Obstet Gynecol Neonatal Nurs 2015;44:145–50.

Breastfeeding in underserved women: increasing initiation and continuation of breastfeeding. Committee Opinion No. 570. American College of Obstetricians and Gynecologists. Obstet Gynecol 2013;122:423–8.

Curtis KM, Tepper NK, Jatlaoui TC, Berry-Bibee E, Horton LG, Zapata LB, et al. U.S. medical eligibility criteria for contraceptive use, 2016. MMWR Recomm Rep 2016;65:1–103.

Curtis KM, Jatlaoui TC, Tepper NK, Zapata LB, Horton LG, Jamieson DJ, et al. U.S. selected practice recommendations for contraceptive use, 2016. MMWR Recomm Rep 2016;65:1–66.

Immediate postpartum long-acting reversible contraception. Committee Opinion No. 670. American College of Obstetricians and Gynecologists. Obstet Gynecol 2016;128:e32–7.

Long-acting reversible contraception: implants and intrauterine devices. Practice Bulletin No. 121. American College of Obstetricians and Gynecologists. Obstet Gynecol 2011;118:184–96.

Obstetric analgesia and anesthesia. Practice Bulletin No. 177. American College of Obstetricians and Gynecologists. Obstet Gynecol 2017;129:e73–89.

Optimizing postpartum care. Committee Opinion No. 666. American College of Obstetricians and Gynecologists. Obstet Gynecol 2016;127:e187–92.

Optimizing support for breastfeeding as part of obstetric practice. Committee Opinion No. 658. American College of Obstetricians and Gynecologists. Obstet Gynecol 2016;127:e86–92.

Postpartum hemorrhage. ACOG Practice Bulletin No. 76. American College of Obstetricians and Gynecologists. Obstet Gynecol 2006;108:1039–47.

Prevention and management of obstetric lacerations at vaginal delivery. Practice Bulletin No. 165. American College of Obstetricians and Gynecologists. Obstet Gynecol 2016;128:e1–15.

Screening for perinatal depression. Committee Opinion No. 630. American College of Obstetricians and Gynecologists. Obstet Gynecol 2015;125:1268–71.

U.S. Selected Practice Recommendations for Contraceptive Use, 2016. Recommendations and Reports / July 29, 2016 / 65(4);1–66.

Resources

American College of Obstetricians and Gynecologists. Immunization for women. Washington, DC: American College of Obstetricians and Gynecologists; 2011; 2016. Available at: http://immunizationforwomen.org. Retrieved October 26, 2016.

Neurological disorders. In: Cunningham FG, Leveno KJ, Bloom SL, Spong CY, Dashe JS, Hoffman BL et al., editors. Williams obstetrics. 24th ed. New York (NY): McGraw Hill Medical; 2014. p. 1187–203.

Psychiatric disorders. In: Cunningham FG, Leveno KJ, Bloom SL, Spong CY, Dashe JS, Hoffman BL et al., editors. Williams obstetrics. 24th ed. New York (NY): McGraw Hill Medical; 2014. p. 1204–13.

Shealy KR, Li R, Benton-Davis S, Grummer-Strawn LM. The CDC guide to breastfeeding interventions. Atlanta (GA): Centers for Disease Control and Prevention; 2005. Available at: https://www.cdc.gov/breastfeeding/pdf/breastfeeding_interventions.pdf. Retrieved October 31, 2016.

U.S Medical Eligibility Criteria for Contraceptive Use, 2016. Centers for Disease Control and Prevention, 2016. Available at http://www.acog.org/Resources-And-Publications/Endorsed-Documents. Retrieved October 26, 2016.

Chapter 9

Medical and Obstetric Complications

Certain complications before and during pregnancy and at the time of labor or delivery may require increased surveillance, monitoring, and special care of the obstetric patient (see also Appendix B and Appendix C). Complications can arise without warning, and in some cases early detection and timely intervention can improve the outcome. When there is a high risk of complications, it may be advisable to make arrangements for such care in advance. The pediatric and anesthesia services should be made aware of such patients so that appropriate medical care can be planned in advance of the delivery.

Medical Complications Before Pregnancy

Prepregnancy medical complications that typically require special antepartum and intrapartum care include antiphospholipid syndrome, asthma, inherited thrombophilias, hypertension, obesity, pregestational diabetes, and others.

Antiphospholipid Syndrome

Antiphospholipid antibodies are a diverse group of antibodies with specificity for binding to negatively charged phospholipids on cell surfaces. Antiphospholipid syndrome (APS) is an autoimmune disorder defined by the presence of characteristic clinical features and specified levels of circulating antiphospholipid antibodies. Antiphospholipid antibodies have been associated with a variety of medical problems, including arterial thrombosis, venous thrombosis, autoimmune thrombocytopenia, and fetal loss. In addition to fetal loss, several obstetric complications have been associated with antiphospholipid antibodies, including preeclampsia, intrauterine growth restriction, and preterm delivery (see also "Deep Vein Thrombosis and Pulmonary Embolism" later in this chapter).

Screening and Diagnosis

The three antiphospholipid antibodies that contribute to the diagnosis of APS are 1) lupus anticoagulant, 2) anticardiolipin, and 3) anti-β_2-glycoprotein I. The diagnosis of APS requires two positive antiphospholipid antibody test results at least 12 weeks apart. Testing for antiphospholipid antibodies should be performed in women with a prior unexplained arterial or venous thromboembolism, a new arterial or venous thromboembolism during pregnancy, or a history of venous thromboembolism who have not been tested previously. Obstetric indications for antiphospholipid antibody testing include a history of one fetal loss or three or more recurrent embryonic or fetal losses.

Management

The goals of treatment for APS during pregnancy are to improve maternal, fetal, and neonatal outcomes. Antepartum testing has been suggested because of the potential risk of fetal growth restriction and stillbirth in pregnancies of women with APS. Many experts recommend serial ultrasonographic assessment and antepartum testing in the third trimester. For women with APS who have had a thrombotic event, most experts recommend prophylactic anticoagulation with heparin throughout pregnancy and 6 weeks postpartum. After delivery, this prophylaxis can be safely accomplished with coumarin. For women with APS who have not had a thrombotic event, expert consensus suggests that clinical surveillance or prophylactic heparin use antepartum in addition to 6 weeks of postpartum anticoagulation may be warranted. For long-term management postpartum, patients with APS should be referred to a physician with expertise in treatment of the syndrome, such as an internist, hematologist, or rheumatologist. Women with APS should not use estrogen-containing contraceptives (for more information, see "Deep Vein Thrombosis and Pulmonary Embolism" later in this chapter).

Inherited Thrombophilias

Inherited thrombophilias are a group of disorders characterized by defects in one or more of the clotting factors. There is a strong association between inherited thrombophilias and venous thromboembolism, which makes detection of these mutations a logical target for prevention strategies. However, it is controversial whether there is an association between inherited thrombophilias and uteroplacental thrombosis that leads to adverse pregnancy outcomes such as fetal loss, preeclampsia, fetal growth restriction, and abruptio placentae.

Screening

Screening for thrombophilias is controversial and should be performed only if results will affect management decisions. Thrombophilia screening is not useful when treatment is indicated for other risk factors. Screening may be considered in patients with a personal history of venous thromboembolism that was associated with a nonrecurrent risk factor (eg, fractures, surgery, and prolonged immobilization) or who have a first-degree relative with a history of high-risk thrombophilia or venous thromboembolism before age 50 years in the absence of other risk factors. In other situations, thrombophilia testing is not routinely recommended. Testing for inherited thrombophilias in women who have experienced a recurrence of fetal loss, abruptio placentae, previous intrauterine growth restriction, or previous preeclampsia is not recommended. Whenever possible, laboratory testing should be performed remote (after 6 weeks) from the thrombotic event while the patient is neither pregnant nor taking anticoagulation nor hormonal therapy.

Management

The decision to not use pharmacologic therapy or to treat with thromboprophylaxis or full anticoagulation is influenced by the venous thromboembolism history, severity of inherited thrombophilia, and additional risk factors. All patients with inherited thrombophilias should undergo individualized risk assessment, which may modify management decisions.

Deep Vein Thrombosis and Pulmonary Embolism

Deep vein thrombosis (DVT) and pulmonary embolism (PE) are collectively referred to as venous thromboembolic events. Approximately 75–80% of cases of pregnancy-associated venous thromboembolic events are DVT and 20–25% are PE. Venous thromboembolism accounts for approximately 9% of all maternal deaths in the United States. Pregnant women have a fourfold to fivefold increased risk of thromboembolism compared with nonpregnant women. The most important individual risk factor for venous thromboembolism in pregnancy is a personal history of thrombosis. The next most important individual risk factor is the presence of a thrombophilia (either acquired or inherited). Other risk factors include the physiologic changes that accompany pregnancy and childbirth, medical factors (such as obesity, hemoglobinopathies, hypertension, and smoking), and pregnancy complications (including operative delivery).

Evaluation and Diagnosis

Women with a history of thrombosis who have not had a complete evaluation of possible underlying etiologies should be tested for antiphospholipid antibodies and for inherited thrombophilias. Medical records, including imaging studies from any prior venous thromboembolic event may be helpful in evaluation. When signs or symptoms suggest new onset DVT, the recommended initial diagnostic test is compression ultrasonography of the proximal veins. Ventilation–perfusion scanning and computed tomographic angiography are used to diagnose new onset PE. Both tests are associated with relatively low radiation exposure for the fetus.

Antepartum Management

Therapeutic anticoagulation is recommended for women with acute thromboembolism during the current pregnancy or those at high risk of venous thromboembolism, such as women with mechanical heart valves. Other candidates for either prophylactic or therapeutic anticoagulation during pregnancy include women with a history of thrombosis or those who are at significant risk of venous thromboembolism during pregnancy or the postpartum period, such as those with high-risk acquired or inherited thrombophilias.

Common anticoagulation medications include unfractionated heparin, low-molecular-weight heparin (LMWH), and coumarin (which is contraindicated during pregnancy). The preferred anticoagulants in pregnancy are heparin compounds. Patients with an incidentally discovered low-risk thrombophilia without a prior venous thromboembolic event can be managed antepartum with either surveillance or prophylactic LMWH or unfractionated heparin, and in the postpartum period with either LMWH and unfractionated heparin prophylaxis or with surveillance if the patient has no additional risk factors for DVT. Guidelines recommend obtaining platelet counts when initiating therapeutic unfractionated heparin therapy in order to monitor for heparin-induced thrombocytopenia.

Intrapartum Management

Women receiving either therapeutic or prophylactic anticoagulation may be converted from LMWH to the shorter half-life unfractionated heparin in the last month of pregnancy or sooner if delivery appears imminent. An alternative option may be to stop therapeutic anticoagulation and induce labor within 24 hours, if clinically appropriate. The American Society of Regional

Anesthesia and Pain Medicine guidelines recommend withholding neuraxial blockade for 10–12 hours after the most recent prophylactic dose of LMWH or 24 hours after the most recent therapeutic dose of LMWH. These guidelines support the use of neuraxial anesthesia in patients receiving dosages of 5,000 units of unfractionated heparin twice daily. If a woman goes into labor while taking unfractionated heparin, clearance can be verified by a partial thromboplastin time test. Reversal of heparin is rarely required and is not indicated with a prophylactic dose of heparin. For women in whom anticoagulation therapy has temporarily been discontinued, pneumatic compression devices are recommended.

Cesarean delivery approximately doubles the risk of venous thromboembolism, but in the otherwise normal patient, this risk is still low (approximately 1 per 1,000 patients). Given this increased risk, and based on extrapolation from perioperative data, placement of pneumatic compression devices before cesarean delivery is recommended for all women not already receiving thromboprophylaxis. For patients with additional risk factors for thromboembolism who are undergoing cesarean delivery, individual risk assessment may require thromboprophylaxis with pneumatic compression devices and unfractionated heparin or LMWH. However, cesarean delivery in the emergency setting should not be delayed because of the timing necessary to implement thromboprophylaxis.

Additional measures should be considered for certain women at particularly high risk of thrombosis at the time of delivery. Women who have antithrombin deficiency may be candidates for antithrombin concentrates peripartum. Women who have had DVT in the 2–4 weeks before giving birth may be candidates for placement of a temporary vena caval filter, with removal postpartum. Other women who may be candidates for vena caval filter placement during pregnancy include women with a recurrence of a venous thromboembolic event despite therapeutic anticoagulation.

Postpartum Management

The risk of venous thromboembolic event is higher postpartum, especially during the first week, than it is during pregnancy. Most patients who receive thromboprophylaxis during pregnancy will benefit from thromboprophylaxis postpartum, but the dose and route will vary by indication. The optimal time to restart anticoagulation postpartum is unclear. A reasonable approach to minimize bleeding complications is to restart unfractionated heparin or LMWH no sooner than 4–6 hours after vaginal delivery or 6–12 hours after cesarean delivery. When reinstitution of anticoagulation is planned postpartum, pneumatic compression devices should be left in place until the patient is ambulatory and until anticoagulation is restarted. Women who require more than 6 weeks of anticoagulation may be bridged to warfarin. Because warfarin, LMWH, and unfractionated heparin do not accumulate in breast milk and do not induce an anticoagulant effect in the infant, these anticoagulants are compatible with breastfeeding.

Anemia

The definition of *anemia* recommended by the Centers for Disease Control and Prevention is a hemoglobin (Hgb) or hematocrit (Hct) value less than the fifth percentile of the distribution of Hgb or Hct in a healthy reference population based on the stage of pregnancy. The two most common causes of anemia in pregnancy and the puerperium are iron deficiency and acute blood loss. Anemia may be classified according to the causative mechanism (decreased production, increased destruction, blood loss), red blood cell morphology (microcytic, normocytic, macrocytic), or whether it is an inherited or acquired disorder. Iron deficiency anemia during pregnancy has been associated with an increased risk of low birth weight, preterm delivery, and perinatal mortality.

Screening and Diagnosis

All pregnant women should be screened for anemia during pregnancy. Measurements of serum Hgb concentration or Hct are the primary screening tests for identifying anemia but are nonspecific for identifying iron deficiency. Normal iron indices are listed in Table 9-1. Asymptomatic women who meet the criteria for anemia (Hct levels less than 33% in the first trimester and third trimester and less than 32% in the second trimester) should be evaluated. Hemoglobin and Hct levels are lower in African American women compared with white women. Thus, for African American adults, the Health and Medicine Division of the National Academies of Sciences, Engineering, and Medicine (previously known as the Institute of Medicine) recommends lowering the cutoff levels for Hgb and Hct by 0.8 g per dL and 2%, respectively.

The initial evaluation of pregnant women with mild to moderate anemia may include a medical history, physical examination, red blood cell indices, and serum iron and ferritin concentrations. Iron deficiency anemia is defined by abnormal values for serum ferritin, transferrin saturation, and free erythrocyte protoporphyrin, along with low Hgb or Hct levels. Patients with anemia other than iron deficiency anemia should be further evaluated.

TABLE 9-1. Normal Iron Indices in Pregnancy

Test	Normal Value
Plasma iron level	40–175 micrograms/dL
Plasma total iron-binding capacity	216–400 micrograms/dL
Transferrin saturation	16–60%
Serum ferritin level	More than 10 micrograms/dL
Free erythrocyte protoporphyrin level	Less than 3 micrograms/g

Anemia in pregnancy. ACOG Practice Bulletin No. 95. American College of Obstetricians and Gynecologists. Obstet Gynecol 2008;112:201–7.

Antepartum Management

Pregnant women with iron deficiency anemia should be treated with supplemental iron, in addition to prenatal vitamins (see also "Nutrition" in Chapter 6). Failure to respond to iron therapy should prompt further investigation and may suggest an incorrect diagnosis, coexisting disease, malabsorption (sometimes caused by the use of enteric-coated tablets or concomitant use of antacids), nonadherence, or blood loss. Parenteral iron is used in the rare patient who cannot tolerate or will not take modest doses of oral iron.

Intrapartum Management

Iron supplementation decreases the prevalence of maternal anemia at delivery. Transfusions of red cells seldom are indicated unless hypovolemia from blood loss coexists or an operative delivery must be performed on a patient with anemia. Severe anemia with maternal Hgb levels less than 6 g per dL has been associated with abnormal fetal oxygenation, resulting in altered fetal heart rate patterns, reduced amniotic fluid volume, fetal cerebral vasodilatation, and fetal death. Thus, maternal transfusion should be considered for fetal indications in cases of severe anemia.

Pregestational Diabetes Mellitus

Pregestational diabetes mellitus represents one of the most challenging medical complications of pregnancy. Type 2 pregestational diabetes mellitus is most common and is characterized by peripheral insulin resistance; relative insulin deficiency; obesity; and the development of vascular, renal, and neuropathic complications. The rapidly increasing incidence of type 2 pregestational diabetes mellitus is caused, in part, by increasing obesity in the United States. In contrast to type 2 pregestational diabetes mellitus, type 1 pregestational diabetes mellitus is characterized by an autoimmune process that destroys the pancreatic β cells, leading to insulin deficiency and the need for insulin therapy.

Maternal Complications

Overall perinatal outcome is best when glucose control is achieved before pregnancy and in the absence of maternal vascular disease. Pregnancy has been associated with exacerbation of many diabetes-related complications, including diabetic retinopathy, nephropathy, and ketoacidosis. Poorly controlled pregestational diabetes mellitus leads to serious end-organ damage that may eventually become life threatening. In turn, preexisting diabetes-related end-organ disease may have deleterious effects on obstetric outcomes. The rates of spontaneous preterm labor, preeclampsia, intrauterine growth restriction, and primary cesarean delivery are all increased in women with pregestational diabetes mellitus.

Fetal and Neonatal Complications

The risk of congenital anomalies, particularly cardiac anomalies, is increased in women with preexisting diabetes. The fetus of a woman with poorly controlled diabetes is also at increased risk of fetal death and is more likely to weigh more than 4,000 g, with a disproportionate concentration of fat around the shoulders and chest, more than doubling the risk of shoulder dystocia at vaginal delivery. Neonatal consequences of poorly controlled pregestational diabetes mellitus during pregnancy include profound hypoglycemia, a higher rate of respiratory distress syndrome, polycythemia, organomegaly, electrolyte disturbances, and hyperbilirubinemia, among others. Long-term outcomes for newborns born to mothers with type 1 diabetes mellitus include obesity and carbohydrate intolerance.

Fetal Assessment

An ultrasound examination early in gestation can be used not only to demonstrate fetal viability but also to accurately date the pregnancy. Most major anomalies can be detected at 18–20 weeks of gestation by a specialized (or targeted) ultrasound examination that includes a carefully performed assessment of fetal cardiac structure, including the great vessels. A fetal echo is also warranted in the midtrimester. Periodic ultrasound examinations may be used to confirm appropriate fetal growth. Antepartum fetal monitoring is a valuable tool for monitoring the pregnancies of women with pregestational diabetes mellitus (see also "Antepartum Tests of Fetal Well-Being" in Chapter 6).

Antepartum Management

The management of diabetes in pregnancy must focus on excellent glucose control achieved by using a careful combination of diet, exercise, and insulin therapy. Patients may need to be seen every 1–2 weeks during the first two trimesters and weekly after 28–30 weeks of gestation. A registered dietitian may be of value in providing an individualized nutrition program.

Pregnancy is characterized by increased insulin resistance and reduced sensitivity to insulin action. Insulin requirements will increase throughout pregnancy, most markedly in the period between 28 weeks and 32 weeks of gestation. Most insulin used in the treatment of pregestational diabetes mellitus is biosynthetic human insulin. Short-acting or rapid-acting insulins are administered before meals to reduce glucose elevations associated with eating. Longer-acting insulins are used to restrain hepatic glucose production between meals and in the fasting state. Intermediate-acting insulin usually is given before breakfast, together with a rapid-acting or short-acting insulin, and before the evening meal or at bedtime. Frequent self-monitoring of blood glucose is essential to achieve euglycemia without significant hypoglycemia during pregnancy. Even with meticulous monitoring, hypoglycemia is more frequent in pregnancy than at other times, particularly in patients with type 1 pregestational diabetes mellitus. Patients and their families should be taught how to respond quickly and appropriately to hypoglycemia.

Intrapartum Management

Optimal timing of delivery relies on balancing the risk of fetal death with the risks of preterm birth. Early delivery may be indicated in some patients with vasculopathy, nephropathy, poor glucose control, or a prior stillbirth. If corticosteroids are administered to accelerate lung maturation, an increased insulin requirement over the next 5 days should be anticipated, and the patient's glucose levels should be closely monitored. In contrast, patients with well-controlled diabetes may be allowed to progress to their expected date of delivery as long as antenatal testing remains reassuring. Expectant management beyond the estimated due date generally is not recommended. However, to prevent traumatic birth injury, cesarean delivery may be considered if the estimated fetal weight is greater than 4,500 g. Induction of labor in a pregnancy with a fetus with suspected macrosomia has not been found to reduce birth trauma and may increase the cesarean delivery rate.

During induction of labor, maternal glycemia can be controlled with an intravenous infusion of regular insulin titrated to maintain hourly readings of blood glucose levels less than 110 mg per dL. Avoiding intrapartum maternal hyperglycemia may prevent fetal hyperglycemia and reduce the likelihood of subsequent neonatal hypoglycemia. During active labor, insulin may not be needed. Patients who are using an insulin pump may continue their basal infusion during labor.

Insulin requirements decrease rapidly after delivery. One half of the predelivery dose may be reinstituted after starting regular food intake. Breastfeeding should be encouraged, and an additional 500 kcal is required per day. Small snacks before breastfeeding may reduce the risks of hypoglycemia.

Gestational Diabetes Mellitus Diagnosis and Management

Gestational diabetes mellitus (GDM) is carbohydrate intolerance with onset or recognition during pregnancy. The prevalence of GDM varies in direct proportion to the prevalence of type 2 diabetes in a given population or ethnic group. An increased prevalence of GDM is found among Hispanic, African American, Native American, Asian, and Pacific Islander women. With the increase in obesity and sedentary lifestyle, the prevalence of diabetes mellitus among reproductive-aged women is increasing globally.

Diagnosis

All pregnant women should be screened for GDM with a laboratory-based screening test(s) using blood glucose levels. Screening is generally performed at 24–28 weeks of gestation. Early pregnancy screening for undiagnosed type 2 diabetes, preferably at the initiation of prenatal care, also is suggested in overweight and obese women with additional diabetic risk factors, including those with a prior history of GDM (see Box 9-1). If the result of early testing is negative, repeat screening for high-risk women is recommended at 24–28 weeks of gestation. The two-step approach to testing for GDM that is commonly used in the United States is based on first screening with the administration of 50-g oral glucose solution followed by a 1-hour venous glucose determination. Women whose glucose level meets or exceeds the

Box 9-1. Early Screening Strategy for Detecting Pregestational Diabetes or Early Gestational Diabetes Mellitus

Consider testing in all women who are overweight or obese (BMI [kg/m^2] >25 kg, and in Asian Americans, a BMI >23 and have one or more additional risk factors:

- Physical inactivity
- First-degree relative with diabetes
- High-risk race/ethnicity (eg, African American, Hispanic, Native American, Asian American, Pacific Islander)
- Women who have previously delivered a baby weighing 4,000 g (~9 lb) or more
- Women with previous GDM
- Hypertension (140/90 mmHg or on therapy for hypertension)
- HDL cholesterol level <35 mg/dL (0.90 mmol/L) and/or a triglyceride level >250 mg/dL (2.82 mmol/L)
- Women with polycystic ovarian syndrome
- A_{1C} ≥5.7%, IGT, or IFG on previous testing
- Other clinical conditions associated with insulin resistance (eg, prepregnancy BMI >40), acanthosis nigricans)
- History of cardiovascular disease

If pregestational/gestational diabetes mellitus is not diagnosed, blood glucose testing should be repeated at 24–28 weeks of gestation.

Abbreviations: BMI, body mass index; GDM, gestational diabetes mellitus; HDL, high-density lipoprotein; IFG, impaired fasting glucose; IGT, impaired glucose tolerance.

Adapted from American Diabetes Association. Classification and Diagnosis of Diabetes. Diabetes Care 2017;40(Suppl. 1):S11–24.

recommended screening threshold (130–140 mg per dL) undergo a 100-g, 3-hour diagnostic oral glucose tolerance test (OGTT) (see also "Routine Laboratory Testing in Pregnancy" in Chapter 6). Most commonly, women who have two or more abnormal values on the 3-hour OGTT are then given a diagnosis of GDM (see Table 9-2).

Antepartum Management

Treatment of GDM to improve glycemic control has been shown to decrease pregnancy-related morbidity, including cesarean delivery, shoulder dystocia, macrosomia, and neonatal hypoglycemia.

TABLE 9-2. Proposed Diagnostic Criteria for Gestational Diabetes Mellitus*

Status	Plasma or Serum Glucose Level Carpenter/Coustan Conversion		Plasma Level National Diabetes Data Group Conversion	
	mg/dL	mmol/L	mg/dL	mmol/L
Fasting	95	5.3	105	5.8
One hour	180	10.0	190	10.6
Two hour	155	8.6	165	9.2
Three hour	140	7.8	145	8.0

*A diagnosis generally requires that two or more thresholds be met or exceeded, though some clinicians choose to use just one elevated value.

Adapted from Classification and diagnosis of diabetes. American Diabetes Association. Diabetes Care 2017;40(suppl 1):S11–24. Available at: http://care.diabetesjournals.org/content/40/Supplement_1/S11.long. Retrieved July 17, 2017.

Nonpharmacologic Treatment

The goal of nutrition therapy in women with GDM is to achieve normoglycemia, prevent ketosis, provide adequate weight gain, and contribute to fetal well-being. The American Diabetes Association recommends nutritional counseling for all patients with GDM by a registered dietitian, if possible, with a personalized nutrition plan based on the individual's body mass index. Exercise often is recommended for individuals with diabetes, both as a way to achieve weight reduction and as a treatment to improve glucose metabolism. In women with GDM, exercise also may be able to improve glycemic control and facilitate weight loss. Therefore, a moderate exercise program as part of the treatment plan for women with GDM is recommended.

Glucose Monitoring

Once a woman with GDM begins nutrition therapy, surveillance of blood glucose levels is required to assure glycemic control. The optimal frequency of blood glucose testing in women with GDM has not been established, but the general recommendation is four-times daily glucose monitoring, performed as fasting and either 1 hour or 2 hours after each meal. Once the patient's glucose levels are well controlled by her diet, the frequency of glucose monitoring can be modified.

Medical Treatment

When target glucose levels cannot be consistently achieved through nutrition and exercise therapy, pharmacologic treatment is recommended. Insulin, which does not cross the placenta, can achieve tight metabolic control and traditionally has been added to nutrition therapy if fasting blood glucose levels are consistently greater than or equal to 95 mg per dL, if 1-hour levels are consistently greater than or equal to 140 mg per dL, or if 2-hour levels are consistently greater than or equal to 120 mg per dL. If insulin is used, the typical starting total dosage is 0.7–1.0 units per kg per day, given in divided doses. In cases in which fasting and postprandial hyperglycemia are present, a regimen of multiple injections using long-acting or intermediate-acting insulin and short-acting insulin alone or in combination is administered. However, if there are only isolated abnormal values at a specific time of day, focusing the insulin regimen to correct the specific hyperglycemia is preferred. Regardless of the starting dosage, subsequent dosage adjustments should be individualized according to the woman's monitored blood glucose levels at particular times of the day.

Fetal Surveillance

Because the increased risk of fetal demise in patients with pregestational diabetes is related to suboptimal glycemic control, women with GDM and poor glycemic control also would be expected to be at risk. Therefore, for women with GDM and poor glycemic control, fetal surveillance may be beneficial. There is no consensus regarding antepartum testing in women with well-controlled GDM. The specific antepartum test and frequency of testing may be chosen according to local practice. It is reasonable for obstetricians to assess fetal growth either by ultrasonography or by clinical examination late in the third trimester in an attempt to identify macrosomia before delivery. The specific antepartum test and frequency of testing may be chosen according to local practice, but because polyhydramnios can result from fetal hyperglycemia, it is common for clinicians to use testing that incorporates serial measures of amniotic fluid.

Intrapartum Management

Women with GDM with good glycemic control and no other complications can be managed expectantly. In most cases, women with good glycemic control who are receiving medical therapy do not require delivery before

39 weeks of gestation. Macrosomia is distinctly more common in women with GDM, and shoulder dystocia is more likely at a given fetal weight in pregnancies complicated by diabetes than in pregnancies not complicated by diabetes.

In contrast to women with well-controlled GDM, delivery before 39 weeks of gestation has been supported by expert opinion in those whose GDM is poorly controlled. However, there is lack of clear guidance about the degree of glycemic control that necessitates earlier delivery and the recommendations about timing of delivery lacks specificity as well. It appears that consideration of timing should incorporate tradeoffs between the risks of prematurity versus the ongoing risks of stillbirth. In such a setting, delivery between 37 0/7 weeks and 38 6/7 weeks of gestation may be justified, but delivery in the late preterm period from 34 0/7 weeks to 36 6/7 weeks of gestation should be reserved for those women who fail in-hospital attempts to improve glycemic control or who have abnormal antepartum testing.

Postpartum Screening

Although the carbohydrate intolerance of GDM frequently resolves after delivery, up to one third of affected women will have diabetes or impaired glucose metabolism at postpartum screening, and it has been estimated that 15–70% will develop diabetes later in life.

Postpartum screening at 4–12 weeks is recommended for all women who had GDM in order to identify women with diabetes mellitus, impaired fasting glucose levels, or impaired glucose tolerance. Either a fasting plasma glucose test or a 75-g, 2-hour oral glucose tolerance test is appropriate for diagnosing diabetes in the postpartum period. Although the fasting plasma glucose test is easier to perform, it lacks sensitivity for detecting other forms of abnormal glucose metabolism. Results of the oral glucose tolerance test can confirm an impaired fasting glucose level and impaired glucose tolerance. Women with abnormal testing results should be referred to the appropriate health care provider for follow-up. The American Diabetes Association and the American College of Obstetricians and Gynecologists (ACOG) recommend repeat testing every 1–3 years for women who had pregnancies affected by GDM and normal postpartum screening results.

For women who may have subsequent pregnancies, screening more frequently has the advantage of detecting abnormal glucose metabolism before pregnancy and provides an opportunity to ensure prepregnancy glucose control. Women should be encouraged to discuss their GDM history and need for screening with all of their health care providers.

Asthma

Asthma is a common, potentially serious medical condition that complicates approximately 4–8% of pregnancies. The condition is characterized by chronic airway inflammation, with increased airway responsiveness to a variety of stimuli, and airway obstruction that is partially or completely reversible. Severe and poorly controlled asthma may be associated with increased prematurity, need for cesarean delivery, preeclampsia, growth restriction, and maternal morbidity and mortality.

Diagnosis and Assessment

The diagnosis of asthma in a pregnant patient is the same as that for a nonpregnant patient. For patients who received a diagnosis of asthma and seek care, subjective assessment of disease status and pulmonary function tests should be performed. For pulmonary function assessment during outpatient visits, spirometry is preferable but peak expiratory flow measurement with a peak flow meter also is sufficient. Patients with worsening symptoms should be evaluated with peak flow measurement and lung auscultation. The assessment in a pregnant patient with asthma also should include the effect of any prior pregnancies on asthma severity or control because this may predict the course of the asthma during subsequent pregnancies.

Management

Management of asthma during pregnancy is important to control symptoms, prevent hypoxic episodes in the mother, and maintain oxygenation of the fetus. Optimal management of asthma during pregnancy includes objective monitoring of lung function, avoiding or controlling asthma triggers, educating patients, and individualizing pharmacologic therapy to maintain normal pulmonary function. Identifying and controlling or avoiding factors such as allergens and irritants, particularly tobacco smoke, can lead to improved maternal well-being with less need for medication. The step-care therapeutic approach uses the lowest amount of drug intervention necessary to control a patient's severity of asthma (see Box 9-2).

First-trimester ultrasound dating should be performed, if possible, to facilitate subsequent evaluations of fetal growth restriction and the risk of

Box 9-2. Step-Therapy Medical Management of Asthma During Pregnancy

Mild Intermittent Asthma

- No daily medications, albutrol as needed

Mild Persistent Asthma

- Preferred—Low-dose inhaled corticosteroid
- Alternative—Cromolyn, leukotriene receptor antagonist, or theophylline (serum level 5–12 micrograms/mL)

Moderate Persistent Asthma

- Preferred—Low-dose inhaled corticosteroid and salmeterol or medium-dose inhaled corticosteroid or (if needed) medium-dose inhaled corticosteroid and salmeterol
- Alternative—Low-dose or (if needed) medium-dose inhaled corticosteroid and either leukotriene receptor antagonist, or theophylline (serum level 5–12 micrograms/mL)

Severe Persistent Asthma

- Preferred—High-dose inhaled corticosteroid and salmeterol and (if needed) oral corticosteroid
- Alternative—High-dose inhaled corticosteroid and theophylline (serum level 5–12 micrograms/mL) and oral corticosteroid if needed

Asthma in pregnancy. ACOG Practice Bulletin No. 90. American College of Obstetricians and Gynecologists. Obstet Gynecol 2008;111:457–64.

preterm birth. In addition to the usual prenatal care and dating confirmation, serial ultrasound examinations to monitor fetal activity and growth should be considered starting at 32 weeks of gestation for women who have poorly controlled asthma, moderate-to-severe asthma, or are recovering from a severe asthma exacerbation. All patients should be instructed to be attentive to fetal activity.

Asthma medication use should not be discontinued during labor and delivery. The patient should be kept hydrated and should receive adequate analgesia in order to decrease the risk of bronchospasm. Women who are currently receiving or recently have taken systemic corticosteroids should receive intravenous administration of corticosteroids (eg, hydrocortisone 100 mg every 8 hours) during labor and for 24 hours after delivery to prevent adrenal crisis because of chronic steroid treatment. Some medications commonly used during labor and delivery, including nonselective β-blockers and carboprost (15-methyl prostaglandin $F_{2\alpha}$), may trigger bronchospasm and should be avoided. Acute asthma exacerbation usually responds to aggressive medical management; cesarean delivery is rarely needed.

Obesity

The prevalence of obesity in the United States has increased dramatically over the past 25 years. The recent National Health and Nutrition Examination Survey found that more than one third of women are obese, more than one half of pregnant women are overweight or obese, and 8% of reproductive-aged women are extremely obese.

Overweight and obese women are at increased risk of several pregnancy complications, including gestational diabetes mellitus, hypertension, preeclampsia, cesarean delivery, and postpartum weight retention. Similarly, fetuses of pregnant women who are overweight or obese are at increased risk of prematurity, stillbirth, congenital anomalies, macrosomia with possible birth injury, and childhood obesity. Additional concerns include potential intrapartum, operative, and postoperative complications and difficulties related to anesthesia management.

Antepartum Management

At the initial prenatal visit, height and weight should be recorded for all women, to allow calculation of body mass index (BMI). Recommendations for appropriate weight gain, guided by the Health and Medicine Division of the National Academies of Sciences, Engineering, and Medicine (previously known as the Institute of Medicine) recommendations (see Chapter 6), should be reviewed both at the initial visit and periodically throughout pregnancy. Nutrition consultation should be offered to all overweight or obese women, and all pregnant women should be encouraged to follow an exercise program. Nutrition and exercise counseling should continue postpartum and before attempting another pregnancy. Consideration should be given to screening for gestational diabetes upon presentation or during the first trimester, with repeat screening later in pregnancy if the initial screening result is negative. Because these patients are at increased risk of emergent cesarean delivery and anesthetic complications, anesthesiology consultation should be obtained for the obese gravida before labor or in early labor to allow adequate time to develop an anesthetic plan that addresses the availability of proper equipment for blood pressure monitoring, venous access, and the influence of comorbid conditions such as sleep apnea. Consultation with anesthesia service should be considered for obese pregnant women with obstructive sleep apnea because they are at an increased risk of hypoxemia, hypercapnia, and sudden death.

Intrapartum Management

It is important to discuss potential intrapartum complications with obese women, such as the challenges associated with anesthesia management and the increased risk of complicated and emergent cesarean delivery. Other potential problems include difficulty estimating fetal weight (even with ultrasonography) and the inability to obtain interpretable external fetal heart rate and uterine contraction patterns. If an anesthesiology consultation was not obtained antepartum, it should be conducted early in labor to allow adequate time for the development of an anesthetic plan. General anesthesia in obese pregnant women poses several challenges, and epidural or spinal anesthesia is recommended. The decision to perform cesarean delivery for obese women should be based on standard maternal and fetal indications.

Operative and postoperative complications among obese pregnant women include increased rates of excessive blood loss, operative time greater than 2 hours, wound infection, and endometritis. Antimicrobial prophylaxis is recommended for all cesarean deliveries. For obese women, consideration should be given to using a higher dose of preoperative antibiotics. Particular attention to the type and placement of the surgical incision is needed (ie, placing the incision above the panniculus adiposus). Management of surgical site infection after cesarean delivery may include antibiotics, exploration, and debridement. If the surgical site infection appears superficial and without purulent drainage, conservative therapy with antibiotics alone may be considered; however, deep surgical site infection may require wound exploration and debridement. The resulting open wound can be managed by secondary closure, secondary intention with dressings, and secondary intention using negative pressure wound therapy.

Suture closure of the subcutaneous layer after cesarean delivery in obese patients may lead to a significant reduction in the incidence of postoperative wound disruption. Because of the increased likelihood of complicated and emergent cesarean delivery, extremely obese women may require specific resources, such as additional blood products, a large operating table, and extra personnel in the delivery room.

Because of the increased risk of venous thromboembolism associated with cesarean delivery and obesity, individual risk assessment may require thromboprophylaxis with unfractionated heparin or LMWH in addition to the recommended use of pneumatic compression devices, during and after cesarean delivery (see also "Deep Vein Thrombosis and Pulmonary Embolism" earlier in this chapter).

Hypertensive Disorders of Pregnancy

Hypertensive disease occurs in approximately 12–22% of pregnancies and accounts for approximately 18% of maternal deaths in the United States. Hypertensive disorders during pregnancy should be considered in three categories: 1) gestational hypertension 2) preeclampsia–eclampsia, and 3) chronic hypertension/chronic hypertension with superimposed preeclampsia.

Gestational Hypertension

Gestational hypertension is characterized most often by new-onset blood pressure elevations after 20 weeks of gestation, often near term, in the absence of accompanying proteinuria or other signs and symptoms of preeclampsia (see following paragraph). Some women experience blood pressure elevations to the severe level with outcomes similar to women with preeclampsia. Gestational hypertension also may be a sign of future chronic hypertension.

Preeclampsia–Eclampsia

Preeclampsia is a pregnancy-specific hypertensive disease with multisystem involvement. Preeclampsia is predominantly a disorder of first pregnancies. Other risk factors include multifetal gestation, preeclampsia in a previous pregnancy, chronic hypertension, pregestational diabetes, vascular and connective tissue disease, nephropathy, antiphospholipid antibody syndrome, obesity, age of 35 years or older, and African American race. Genetic and environmental factors also play a role in the development of preeclampsia. No single screening test for preeclampsia has been found to be reliable and cost effective.

Diagnosis. Preeclampsia is a pregnancy-specific syndrome characterized by new onset hypertension and new onset proteinuria that occurs after 20 weeks of gestation. *Hypertension* is defined as either a systolic blood pressure of 140 mm Hg or higher, a diastolic blood pressure of 90 mm Hg or higher, or both. Hypertension is considered mild until diastolic or systolic levels reach or exceed 110 mm Hg or 160 mm Hg, respectively. Proteinuria is diagnosed when 24-hour excretion equals or exceeds 300 mg in 24 hours or the ratio of measured protein to creatinine in a single voided urine measures or exceeds 0.3 (termed the protein/creatinine ratio). In the absence of proteinuria, preeclampsia also may be diagnosed as hypertension associated with thrombocytopenia (platelet count less than 100,000 per microliter), impaired liver function (elevated liver transaminases to twice the normal concentration), the new development of renal insufficiency (serum creatinine greater than 1.1 mg per dL or doubling of serum creatinine), pulmonary edema, or new onset cerebral or visual disturbances.

Some clinical findings increase the risk of morbidity and mortality in the setting of preeclampsia and, when present, segregate preeclampsia into a more severe category (see Box 9-3). Eclampsia is the convulsive phase of the disorder and is among the more severe manifestations of the disease.

Antepartum Management. Treatment of preeclampsia should be directed toward balancing maternal and fetal risks. Gestational hypertension and preeclampsia without severe features may be managed expectantly, usually at home, with frequent maternal and fetal assessment. Women at risk of nonadherence or those with other logistical barriers to frequent follow-up

Box 9-3. Severe Features of Preeclampsia*

- Systolic blood pressure of 160 mm Hg or higher, or diastolic blood pressure of 100 mm Hg or higher on two occasions at least 4 hours apart while the patient is on bed rest (unless antihypertensive therapy is initiated before this time)
- Thrombocytopenia (platelet count less than 100,000/microliter)
- Impaired liver function as indicated by abnormally elevated blood concentrations of liver enzymes (to twice normal concentration), severe persistent right upper quadrant or epigastric pain unresponsive to medication and not accounted for by other diagnoses, or both
- Progressive renal insufficiency (serum creatinine concentration greater than 1.1 mg/dL or a doubling of the serum creatinine concentration in the absence of other renal disease)
- Pulmonary edema
- New-onset cerebral or visual disturbances

*Any of these findings is considered a severe feature of preeclampsia.

American College of Obstetricians and Gynecologists. Hypertension in Pregnancy. Washington, DC: American College of Obstetricians and Gynecologists; 2013. Available at: http://www.acog.org/Resources-And-Publications/Task-Force-and-Work-Group-Reports/Hypertension-in-Pregnancy. Retrieved November 2, 2016.

should be hospitalized. Antihypertensive medication is not generally recommended as long as blood pressure is consistently lower than 160 mm Hg systolic or 110 mm Hg diastolic. Ultrasonography to assess fetal growth and antenatal testing is suggested, and if evidence of fetal growth restriction is found, umbilical artery Doppler velocimetry is recommended as an adjunct antenatal test. Expectant management of women with severe preeclampsia at less than 34 weeks of gestation with stable maternal and fetal conditions is reasonable but it should only occur at facilities with adequate maternal and neonatal intensive care resources.

The timing of delivery in women with gestational hypertension and preeclampsia should be based on severity of hypertension and whether features of severe disease are present. For women with mild gestational hypertension or preeclampsia without severe features and no other indication for preterm delivery, expectant management with maternal and fetal monitoring until 37 weeks of gestation is reasonable. For women with severe preeclampsia at or beyond 34 weeks of gestation, and in those with unstable maternal–fetal conditions irrespective of gestational age, delivery is recommended soon after maternal stabilization.

Intrapartum Management. Two main goals of management of preeclampsia during labor and delivery include prevention of seizures and control of hypertension. Magnesium sulfate should be used for the prevention and treatment of seizures in women with preeclampsia with severe features or eclampsia. Magnesium sulfate may be withheld if the systolic blood pressure is lower than 160 mm Hg and diastolic blood pressure is lower than 110 mm Hg with no maternal symptoms. Acute-onset, severe systolic hypertension (greater than or equal to 160 mm Hg), diastolic hypertension (110 mm Hg or greater), or both can occur in pregnancy or in the postpartum period. Prolonged exposure to severe hypertension can cause central nervous system injury; therefore, acute-onset, severe hypertension requires antihypertensive therapy. The goal is not to normalize blood pressure, but to achieve a range of 140–150/90–100 mm Hg. Intravenous (IV) labetalol and hydralazine have long been considered first-line medications for the management of acute-onset, severe hypertension during pregnancy and in the postpartum period. Oral nifedipine also may be considered as a first-line therapy. If analgesia or anesthesia is required, regional or neuraxial analgesia or anesthesia is preferred.

Women with eclampsia require prompt intervention and should be delivered expeditiously. Once the patient is stabilized, the method of delivery should consider factors such as gestational age, fetal presentation, and the cervical examination. The decision to perform cesarean delivery should be individualized, with attention to maternal stability and the anticipated time course of worsening disease.

Chronic Hypertension/Chronic Hypertension With Superimposed Preeclampsia

Chronic hypertension in pregnancy is defined as hypertension present before pregnancy or before the 20th week of gestation. Chronic hypertension is associated with several adverse pregnancy outcomes, including premature birth, fetal growth restriction, fetal demise, abruptio placentae, and cesarean delivery. Superimposed preeclampsia is a diagnosis of preeclampsia made in a patient with preexisting hypertensive disease. Diagnostic criteria include new-onset proteinuria in a woman with chronic hypertension, a sudden increase in proteinuria if already present in early gestation, a sudden increase in hypertension, or the development of hemolysis, elevated liver enzymes, and low platelet count syndrome.

Diagnosis. Chronic hypertension during pregnancy is most commonly classified as mild to moderate (systolic blood pressure of 140–159 mm Hg or diastolic blood pressure of 90–109 mm Hg) or as severe (systolic blood pressure of 160 mm Hg or higher or diastolic blood pressure of 110 mm Hg or higher). To establish the diagnosis of hypertension, blood pressure levels that meet the criteria should be documented more than once, at least 4–6 hours apart. Chronic hypertension can be difficult to distinguish from either gestational hypertension or preeclampsia in women who present for care with hypertension late in gestation. When hypertension develops during pregnancy, typically in the third trimester, in the absence of signs or symptoms of preeclampsia, the diagnosis of gestational hypertension is appropriate. Chronic hypertension usually can be distinguished from preeclampsia because preeclampsia typically appears after 20 weeks of gestation in a woman who was normotensive before pregnancy and most frequently includes proteinuria. The acute onset of proteinuria or a sudden increase over baseline proteinuria and baseline hypertension in women with chronic hypertension should prompt the assessment for superimposed preeclampsia.

Antepartum Management. Ideally, a woman with chronic hypertension should be evaluated before pregnancy to rule out secondary (and potentially curable) hypertension and to seek out evidence of end organ damage.

Specific testing before pregnancy or early in pregnancy might include assessment of renal function, electrocardiography, echocardiography, and ophthalmologic evaluation. The choice of appropriate tests is dependent on the severity of the chronic hypertension. Evaluation of fetal growth by ultrasonography in women with chronic hypertension is warranted. If evidence of fetal growth restriction is found in women with chronic hypertension, fetoplacental assessment to include umbilical artery Doppler velocimetry as an adjunct antenatal test is recommended. Treatment with low-dose aspirin (81 mg) may reduce the risk of pre-eclampsia in this group.

Antihypertensive therapy has been shown to reduce the risk of a severe maternal hypertensive crisis but has not been shown to improve overall perinatal outcome. Acknowledging that there is limited evidence regarding the precise blood pressure for which antihypertensive is indicated during pregnancy, ACOG's Task Force on Hypertension in Pregnancy recommends initiation of antihypertensive therapy when blood pressure is persistently 160 mm Hg or greater systolic or 105 mm Hg or higher diastolic, and maintenance of blood pressure between 120 mm Hg and 160 mm Hg systolic and 80 mm Hg and 105 mm Hg diastolic. The Task Force also suggests no pharmacologic treatment for pregnant women with blood pressure less than 160 mm Hg systolic or 105 mm Hg diastolic and no evidence of end-organ damage.

Labetalol is a good option for first-line treatment of chronic hypertension in pregnancy, based on its good efficacy and low incidence of adverse effects. Calcium channel blockers or antagonists, the most well-studied of which is nifedipine, also have been used in pregnant women with chronic hypertension. Methyldopa has been used for decades to treat hypertension in pregnancy, and it appears to be safe for this indication. However, its strong association with significant maternal sedation at therapeutic doses limits its use. Prepregnancy thiazide diuretic therapy does not need to be discontinued during pregnancy. Angiotensin-converting enzyme inhibitors and angiotensin receptor blockers are contraindicated in all trimesters of pregnancy.

For women with chronic hypertension who are at a greatly increased risk of adverse pregnancy outcomes (history of early-onset preeclampsia and preterm delivery at less than 34 0/7 weeks of gestation or preeclampsia in more than one prior pregnancy), initiating the administration of daily low-dose aspirin beginning in the late first trimester is suggested. Antepartum fetal surveillance may be useful in this group of patients, beginning at 32 weeks (or earlier if growth restriction is present).

Intrapartum Management. Pregnant women with uncomplicated mild chronic hypertension generally are candidates for a vaginal delivery at term because most of them have good maternal and neonatal outcomes. Cesarean delivery should be reserved for obstetric indications. Women with hypertension during pregnancy and a prior adverse pregnancy outcome (eg, stillbirth) may be candidates for earlier delivery after documentation of fetal lung maturity. Women with severe chronic hypertension during pregnancy often either give birth prematurely or need early delivery for fetal or maternal indications. The combination of chronic hypertension and superimposed preeclampsia, particularly before term, represents a complicated situation, and the clinician should consider consultation with a subspecialist in maternal–fetal medicine. Women with severe hypertension or hypertension that is complicated by cardiovascular or renal disease may present special problems during the intrapartum period and should be collaboratively managed by the primary obstetrician and a maternal–fetal medicine subspecialist or an intensivist. Women with severe hypertension may require antihypertensive medications to treat acute elevation of blood pressure (see the "Intrapartum Management" section under "Preeclampsia–Eclampsia" earlier in this chapter). Women with chronic hypertension complicated by significant cardiovascular or renal disease require special attention to hydration status and urine output because they may be susceptible to fluid overload with resultant pulmonary edema. General anesthesia may pose a risk in pregnant women with severe hypertension or superimposed preeclampsia. Therefore, regional analgesia and anesthesia are recommended when needed.

Postpartum Management and Future Pregnancies

Early postpartum follow-up is recommended for women with hypertensive disorders of pregnancy. Early follow-up also may be beneficial for women at high risk of complications. If a woman has given birth to a preterm infant during a preeclamptic pregnancy or has had preeclampsia in more than one pregnancy, the use of low-dose aspirin in the upcoming pregnancy should be suggested.

Psychiatric Disease in Pregnancy

Approximately 500,000 pregnancies in the United States each year involve women who have psychiatric illnesses that either predate pregnancy or emerge during pregnancy and the postpartum period. Management of psychiatric disease during pregnancy requires consideration of multiple factors, including the importance of control of maternal symptoms and the potential risks of medication exposure for the fetus, including teratogenicity and neonatal withdrawal. Close collaboration with the mother's psychiatric care provider is essential. Untreated or inadequately treated maternal psychiatric illness can result in poor adherence to prenatal care, poor nutrition, increased alcohol or tobacco use, and disruption to mother–infant bonding. Multidisciplinary care involving the obstetrician, mental health care provider, and pediatrician is recommended.

All psychotropic medications studied to date cross the placenta, are present in amniotic fluid, and enter human breast milk. The major risk of teratogenesis occurs during the third through the eighth week of gestation. In general, a single medication used at a higher dose is favored over multiple medications to obtain control of symptoms. Providing women with well-referenced patient resources for online information is a reasonable option. Electronic resources for the fetal and neonatal effects of psychotropic drug therapy during pregnancy and lactation are RePROTOX (www.reprotox.org/) and TERIS (www.depts.washington.edu/terisweb/teris/). In addition, the U.S. Food and Drug Administration website (available at www.fda.gov) has information on the safety of individual medications during pregnancy. Consideration should be given to consulting an obstetrician–gynecologist or maternal–fetal medicine subspecialist before indicated psychotropic medications are stopped in a pregnant woman to discuss whether the risks of stopping the medication outweigh any possible fetal risks.

Other Medical Complications During Pregnancy

Trauma During Pregnancy

Trauma is the leading cause of nonobstetric maternal death. In industrialized nations, most cases of trauma during pregnancy result from motor vehicle crashes. Other frequent causes of trauma during pregnancy are falls and direct assaults to the abdomen. The appropriate use of safety restraint systems in automobiles, compliance with traffic laws, and early identification and intervention in suspected cases of domestic violence are all preventive measures that may reduce the likelihood of maternal and fetal morbidity and mortality. Obstetrician–gynecologists and other obstetric care providers play a central role both in the education of pregnant women on the appropriate use of seat belts while driving or riding in vehicles and in the early identification of suspected abuse.

Necessary evaluation and management of the trauma patient should not be changed because she is pregnant. Optimum management of the seriously injured pregnant woman requires an integrated effort of multiple specialties, starting with emergency medical technicians, emergency medicine physicians, trauma surgeons, and other specialists, depending on the type of injury. Obstetricians play a central role in the management of injured pregnant women. Their knowledge and expertise are vital to management decisions regarding the woman and the fetus. The obstetrician may be consulted regarding the condition of a pregnant trauma patient and her fetus or may be the primary physician caring for the patient after trauma. To improve multidisciplinary management of the trauma patient who is pregnant, hospital-based guidelines for clinical management should be established with input from multiple care providers (eg, emergency medicine physicians, obstetrician–gynecologists, trauma surgeons).

Management. The primary goal and initial efforts in managing the injured pregnant woman are evaluation and stabilization of maternal vital signs. If attention is drawn to the fetus before the woman is stabilized, serious or life-threatening maternal injuries may be overlooked, or circumstances that can compromise fetal oxygenation (eg, maternal hypoxemia, hypovolemia, or supine hypotension) may be ignored, lessening the likelihood of maternal and fetal survival.

Fetal Assessment. The use of electronic fetal cardiac and uterine activity monitoring in pregnant trauma victims at the time of fetal viability may reveal a diagnosis of abruptio placentae. Because abruption usually becomes apparent shortly after injury, monitoring should be initiated as soon as the woman is stabilized. The duration of fetal monitoring in the viable pregnancy has been debated, with most experts recommending a minimum of 2–4 hours. Monitoring should be continued and further evaluation carried out if uterine contractions, a nonreactive fetal heart rate tracing, vaginal bleeding, significant uterine tenderness or irritability, serious maternal injury, or rupture of the amniotic membranes is present. Upon discharge, the patient should be instructed to return if she develops vaginal bleeding, leakage of fluid, decreased fetal movement, or severe abdominal pain.

Fetal–Maternal Hemorrhage. Complications of fetal–maternal hemorrhage in trauma patients include fetal and neonatal anemia, fetal cardiac arrhythmias, and fetal death. There is no evidence that laboratory testing for fetal–maternal hemorrhage (eg, Kleihauer–Betke test) can predict or eliminate adverse immediate sequelae due to hemorrhage. Administration of D immune globulin at any time within the first 72 hours after fetal–maternal hemorrhage appears to provide protection from alloimmunization in the Rh(O) D-negative woman. Consideration should be given to administering 300 micrograms of Rh(O) D immune globulin to all unsensitized Rh(O) D-negative pregnant patients who have experienced abdominal trauma. Some experts recommend quantitative testing for fetal–maternal hemorrhage (eg, Kleihauer–Betke testing) in the Rh(O) D-negative woman to identify the unusual large-volume hemorrhage (ie, more than 30 mL of fetal–maternal hemorrhage), for which 300 micrograms of Rh(O) D immune globulin may be insufficient.

Critical Care in Pregnancy

Approximately 1–3% of pregnant women require critical care services in the United States each year, with the risk of death ranging from 2% to 11%. Hemorrhage and hypertension are the most common causes of intensive care unit (ICU) admission in obstetric patients. The care of any pregnant woman requiring ICU services should be managed in a facility with obstetric adult ICU and neonatal ICU capability (see also "Transfer for Critical Care" in Chapter 4). Decisions about care for a pregnant patient in the ICU should be made collaboratively with the intensivist, obstetrician, maternal–fetal medicine specialist, specialty nurses, and neonatologist. When a pregnant patient is transferred to the ICU, members of the care team should assess the anticipated course of her condition or disease, including possible complications, and set parameters for delivery, if appropriate. The plan should be clear to the medical team, to the patient's family, and to the patient herself if she is able to understand. Because the risk–benefit calculation for a given intervention may change as the pregnancy progresses, it is important to reevaluate the care plan on a regular basis. Ideally, the plan for delivery should be made long before birth is anticipated.

Patients who have undergone maternal–fetal surgery during pregnancy present unique management challenges because they are at risk of complications that occur acutely, postoperatively, for the duration of the pregnancy, and in subsequent pregnancies. Because these are highly technical procedures, maternal–fetal surgery should only be offered at facilities with the expertise, multidisciplinary teams, services, and facilities to provide the intensive care required for these patients.

Intrapartum Care. If a laboring patient requires critical care services, it is important to determine the optimal setting for her care. Factors that will affect this decision include the degree of patient instability, interventions required, staffing and expertise available, anticipated duration of ICU stay, and probability of delivery. If the fetus is previable or the maternal condition unstable, it may be appropriate to undertake vaginal delivery in the intensive care unit. Cesarean delivery in the ICU has significant disadvantages compared with procedures in a traditional operating room. Cesarean delivery in the ICU should be restricted to cases in which transport to the operating room or delivery room cannot be achieved safely or expeditiously, or to a perimortem procedure. Analgesia should still be used in the ICU setting, although assessment of pain may be more difficult in the sedated patient. Regional anesthesia is preferred but complications may preclude its use. Intravenous analgesia may be used but is less effective in treating pain (see also "Analgesia and Anesthesia" in Chapter 7).

Fetal Considerations. Fetal surveillance often is used when a patient is admitted to the ICU. Changes in fetal monitor values should prompt reassessment of maternal mean arterial pressure, acidemia, hypoxemia, or inferior vena cava compression, and every attempt should be made at intrauterine fetal resuscitation. Drugs that cross the placenta may have fetal effects; however, necessary medications should not be withheld from critically ill pregnant women because of fetal concerns. In addition, imaging studies should not be withheld out of potential concern for fetal status, although attempts should be made to limit fetal radiation exposure during diagnostic testing.

Postpartum Care. Approximately 75% of the obstetric patients admitted to the ICU are postpartum. Obstetric input in the care of the postpartum ICU patient may include evaluation of vaginal or intraabdominal bleeding, evaluation of obstetric sources of infection, duration of specific therapies (such as magnesium for eclampsia prophylaxis), feasibility of breast pumping, and compatibility of various medications with breastfeeding.

Nonobstetric Surgery in Pregnancy

When a nonobstetric surgery is performed during pregnancy, it is because it is medically indicated. A pregnant woman should never be denied indicated surgery, regardless of trimester. Elective surgery should be postponed until after delivery. If possible, nonurgent surgery should be performed in the second trimester when preterm contractions and spontaneous abortion are least likely. Obstetric consultation before nonobstetric surgery and some invasive procedures (eg, cardiac catheterization or colonoscopy) to confirm gestational age, discuss pertinent aspects of maternal physiology or anatomy, and make recommendations about fetal monitoring is highly recommended. Pregnant patients who undergo nonobstetric surgery are best managed with communication between involved services, including obstetrics, anesthesia, surgery, and nursing. Fetal heart rate monitoring may assist in maternal positioning and cardiorespiratory management, and may influence a decision to deliver the fetus. The decision to use fetal monitoring should be individualized, and its use should be based on gestational age, type of surgery, and facilities available. Ultimately, each case warrants a team approach (anesthesia and obstetric care providers, surgeons, pediatricians, and nurses) for optimal safety of the woman and the fetus.

Antepartum Hospitalization

Pregnant patients with complications who require hospitalization before the onset of labor should be admitted to a designated antepartum area, either inside or near the labor and delivery area. Obstetric patients with serious and acute complications should be assigned to an area where more intensive care and surveillance are available, such as the labor and delivery area or an intensive care unit. An obstetrician–gynecologist or a subspecialist in maternal–fetal medicine should be involved either as the primary or the consulting physician. When the pregnant patient is sufficiently recovered, she should be returned to the obstetric service, provided that her return does not jeopardize her care.

Acutely ill obstetric patients who are likely to give birth to newborn infants requiring intensive care should be cared for in specialty or subspecialty perinatal care centers, depending on the medical needs of the maternal–fetal dyad. When feasible, antepartum transfer to specialty or subspecialty perinatal care centers should be encouraged for these women (see also "Transfer for Critical Care" in Chapter 4). Written policies and procedures for the management of pregnant patients seen in the emergency department or admitted to nonobstetric services should be established and approved by the medical staff and must comply with the requirements of federal and state transfer laws. When warranted by patient volume, a high-risk antepartum care unit can provide maternal fetal medicine subspecialty and specialized nursing care and facilities for the mother and the fetus at risk. When this is not feasible, written policies are recommended that specify how the care and transfer of pregnant patients with obstetric, medical, or surgical complications will be handled and where these patients will be assigned.

Whether an obstetric patient is admitted to the antepartum unit or to a nonobstetric unit, her condition should be evaluated soon thereafter by the primary physician or appropriate consultants. The evaluation should encompass a complete review of current illnesses as well as a medical, family, and social history. The condition of the patient and the reason for admission should determine the extent of the physical examination performed and the laboratory studies obtained. A copy of the patient's current prenatal record should become part of the hospital medical record as soon as possible after admission. These policies also must comply with the requirements of federal and state transfer laws.

Pregnancy-Related Complications

Nonmedically Indicated Late-Preterm and Early-Term Deliveries

Historically, ACOG and the Society for Maternal–Fetal Medicine have advocated delaying deliveries until 39 completed weeks of gestation or beyond (for recommendations regarding the method for estimating gestational age and due date, see Chapter 6). Yet, the rate of nonmedically indicated early-term (37 0/7–38 6/7 weeks of gestation) deliveries continues to increase in the United States. In contrast, the late-preterm (34 0/7–36 6/7 weeks of gestation) birth rate, which increased 25% from 1990 to 2006, has leveled off and started a slow decrease from 9.1% in 2006 to 8.8% in 2008. Decreased rates were most rapid for late preterm births (-13%) and early term births (-14%), followed by early preterm births (-7%). The percentage of full-term births (39–40 weeks of gestation) increased by 13% during this period. There are medical indications in pregnancy for which there is evidence or expert opinion to support expedient delivery in the early-term period versus expectant management (see Table 9-3). In contrast, suspected macrosomia, well-controlled gestational diabetes, and documented pulmonary maturity with no other indication are all examples of conditions that are not indications for an early-term delivery. Implementation of formal policies regarding the timing of delivery has been found to decrease the rate of nonmedically indicated deliveries before 39 weeks of gestation and to improve neonatal outcomes.

TABLE 9-3. Recommendations for the Timing of Delivery When Conditions Complicate Pregnancy at or After 34 Weeks of Gestation

Condition	General Timing	Suggested Specific Timing
Placental/uterine issues		
Placenta previa*	Late preterm/early term	36 0/7–37 6/7 weeks of gestation
Placenta previa with suspected accreta, increta, or percreta*	Late preterm	34 0/7–35 6/7 weeks of gestation
Prior classical cesarean	Late preterm/early term	36 0/7–37 6/7 weeks of gestation
Prior myomectomy	Early term/term (individualize)	37 0/7–38 6/7 weeks of gestation
Fetal issues		
Growth restriction (singleton)		
Otherwise uncomplicated, no concurrent findings	Early term/term	38 0/7–39 6/7 weeks of gestation
Concurrent conditions (oligohydramnios, abnormal Doppler studies, maternal comorbidity [eg, preeclampsia, chronic hypertension])	Late preterm/early term	34 0/7–37 6/7 weeks of gestation
Growth restriction (twins)		
Di-Di twins with isolated growth restriction	Late preterm/early term	36 0/7–37 6/7 weeks of gestation
Di-Di twins with concurrent condition, abnormal Doppler studies, maternal comorbidity (eg, preeclampsia, chronic hypertension)	Late preterm	32 0/7–34 6/7 weeks of gestation
Mo-Di twins with isolated growth restriction	Late preterm	32 0/7–34 6/7 weeks of gestation

(continued)

TABLE 9-3. Recommendations for the Timing of Delivery When Conditions Complicate Pregnancy at or After 34 Weeks of Gestation *(continued)*

Condition	General Timing	Suggested Specific Timing
***Fetal issues* (continued)**		
Multiple gestations		
Di-Di twins	Early term	38 0/7–38 6/7 weeks of gestation
Mo-Di twins	Late preterm/early term	34 0/7–37 6/7 weeks of gestation
Oligohydramnios	Late preterm/early term	36 0/7–37 6/7 weeks of gestation
Maternal issues		
Chronic hypertension		
Controlled on no medications	Early term/term	38 0/7–39 6/7 weeks of gestation
Controlled on medications	Early term/term	37 0/7–39 6/7 weeks of gestation
Difficult to control	Late preterm/early term	36 0/7–37 6/7 weeks of gestation
Gestational hypertension	Early term	37 0/7–38 6/7 weeks of gestation
Preeclampsia—severe	Late preterm	At diagnosis after 34 0/7 weeks of gestation
Preeclampsia—mild	Early term	At diagnosis after 37 0/7 weeks of gestation
Diabetes		
Pregestational well controlled*	Late preterm, early term birth not indicated	
Pregestational with vascular complications	Early term/term	37 0/7–39 6/7 weeks of gestation
Pregestational poorly controlled	Late preterm or early term	Individualized
Gestational—well controlled on diet or medications	Late preterm, early term birth not indicated	
Gestational—poorly controlled	Late preterm or early term	Individualized

(continued)

TABLE 9-3. Recommendations for the Timing of Delivery When Conditions Complicate Pregnancy at or After 34 Weeks of Gestation *(continued)*

Condition	General Timing	Suggested Specific Timing
Obstetric issues		
Preterm PROM	Late preterm	34 weeks of gestation

Abbreviations: Di–Di, dichorionic–diamniotic; Mo–Di, monochorionic–diamniotic; PROM, premature rupture of membranes (also known as prelabor rupture of membranes).

*Uncomplicated, thus no fetal growth restriction, superimposed preeclampsia, or other complication. If these are present, then the complicating conditions take precedence and earlier delivery may be indicated.

Modified from Spong CY, Mercer BM, D'alton M, Kilpatrick S, Blackwell S, Saade G. Timing of indicated late-preterm and early-term birth. Obstet Gynecol 2011;118:323–33.

Neonatal and Infant Morbidity and Mortality

The risk of adverse outcomes is greater for newborns delivered in the early-term period (37–38 weeks of gestation) compared with newborns delivered at 39 weeks of gestation (Box 9-4). Mortality rates are higher among newborns and infants delivered during the early-term period compared with those delivered at full term. Mortality rates are also significantly higher among infants delivered at 37 weeks of gestation and 38 weeks of gestation compared with those delivered at 39 weeks of gestation (Table 9-4).

Amniocentesis

Amniocentesis for the determination of fetal lung maturity generally should not be used to guide the timing of delivery. First, if there is a clear indication for a late-preterm or early-term delivery for either maternal or newborn benefit, delivery should occur regardless of such maturity testing. Conversely, if delivery could be safely delayed in the context of an immature lung profile result, then no clear indication for a late-preterm or early-term delivery actually exists.

Medically Indicated Late-Preterm and Early-Term Deliveries

The neonatal risks of late preterm births (34 0/7–36 6/7 weeks of gestation) and early-term births (37 0/7–38 6/7 weeks of gestation) are well established. However, there are a number of maternal, fetal, and placental complications in which either a late-preterm or early-term delivery is warranted. Recently, the *Eunice Kennedy Shriver* National Institute of Child Health and Human Development and the Society for Maternal–Fetal

Box 9-4. Neonatal Morbidities Associated With Early-Term Delivery

- Respiratory distress syndrome
- Transient tachypnea of the newborn
- Ventilator use
- Pneumonia
- Respiratory failure
- Neonatal intensive care unit admission
- Hypoglycemia
- 5-minute Apgar score less than 7
- Neonatal mortality

Nonmedically indicated early-term deliveries. Committee Opinion No. 561. American College of Obstetricians and Gynecologists. Obstet Gynecol 2013;121:911–5.

TABLE 9-4. Neonatal and Infant Mortality Rates Associated With Late-Preterm and Early-Term Deliveries

Gestational Age (wk)	Neonatal Mortality Rate (Per 1,000 Live Births)	Relative Risk (95% CI)	Infant Mortality Rate (Per 1,000 Live Births)	Relative Risk (95% CI)
34*	7.1	9.5 (8.4–10.8)	11.8	5.4 (4.9–5.9)
35*	4.8	6.4 (5.6–7.2)	8.6	3.9 (3.6–4.3)
36*	2.8	3.7 (3.3–4.2)	5.7	2.6 (2.4–2.8)
37*	1.7	2.3 (2.1–2.6)	4.1	1.9 (1.8–2.0)
38*	1.0	1.4 (1.3–1.5)	2.7	1.2 (1.2–1.3)
39	0.8	1.00†	2.2	1.00†
40	0.8	1.0 (0.9–1.1)	2.1	0.9 (0.9–1.0)

*$P<.001$

†Reference group

Data from Reddy UM, Ko CW, Raju TN, Willinger M. Delivery indications at late-preterm gestations and infant mortality rates in the United States. Pediatrics 2009;124:234–40.

Medicine convened a workshop to summarize the available evidence and make recommendations regarding the timing of indicated delivery. For most conditions, recommendations are based largely on expert consensus and relevant observational studies, and management should be individualized.

There are several important principles to consider in the timing of delivery.

- Decision-making regarding timing of delivery is complex and must take into account relative maternal and newborn risks, practice environment, and patient preferences.
- Late-preterm or early-term deliveries may be warranted for maternal benefit, or newborn benefit, or both.
- The timing of these deliveries must balance the maternal and newborn risks of late-preterm and early-term delivery with the risks of further continuation of pregnancy.
- Recommendations for early delivery are dependent on accurate determination of gestational age.

Decisions regarding timing of delivery must be individualized. Amniocentesis for the determination of fetal lung maturity in well-dated pregnancies generally should not be used to guide the timing of delivery. Table 9-3 presents recommendations for the timing of delivery for a number of specific conditions. This list is not meant to be all-inclusive, but rather a compilation of indications commonly encountered in clinical practice. "General timing" describes the concept of whether a condition is appropriately managed with either a late-preterm or early-term delivery. "Suggested specific timing" refers to a more defined timing of delivery within the broader categories of late-preterm or early-term delivery. These are recommendations only and will need to be individualized and re-evaluated as new evidence becomes available.

Because of the aforementioned increase in rates of morbidity and mortality of late-preterm infants, preterm delivery should only occur when an accepted maternal or fetal indication for delivery exists. Examples may include nonreassuring fetal status or a maternal condition that is likely to be improved by delivery. Collaborative counseling by obstetric clinicians and neonatal clinicians about the outcomes of late-preterm births is warranted unless precluded by emergent conditions.

Premature Rupture of Membranes

The definition of *premature rupture of membranes* (also known as prelabor rupture of membranes) (PROM) is rupture of membranes before the onset of labor. Membrane rupture that occurs before 37 weeks of gestation is referred to as preterm PROM. Although the term PROM results from the normal physiologic process of progressive membrane weakening, preterm PROM can result from a wide array of pathologic mechanisms acting individually or in concert. Premature rupture of membranes is a complication in approximately one third of preterm births. It typically is associated with brief latency between membrane rupture and delivery, increased potential for perinatal infection, and in utero umbilical cord compression. Because of this, PROM at term and before term can lead to significant perinatal morbidity and mortality. The gestational age and fetal status at membrane rupture have significant implications in the etiology and consequences of PROM. Management may be dictated by the presence of overt intrauterine infection, advanced labor, or fetal compromise.

Diagnosis

In most cases, PROM can be diagnosed on the basis of the patient's history and physical examination. Examination should be performed in a manner that minimizes the risk of introducing infection, particularly before term. Digital examinations should be avoided unless the patient is in active labor or imminent delivery is planned. The diagnosis of membrane rupture is confirmed by the visualization of fluid passing from the cervical canal and pooling in the vagina; a basic pH test of vaginal fluid; or arborization (ferning) of dried vaginal fluid, which is identified under microscopic evaluation. (See also "Premature Rupture of Membranes at Term" in Chapter 7).

Management

An accurate assessment of gestational age and knowledge of the maternal, fetal, and neonatal risks are essential for appropriate evaluation, counseling, and care of patients with PROM. At any gestational age, a patient with evident intraamniotic infection (also referred to as chorioamnionitis), abruptio placentae, or evidence of fetal compromise is best cared for by expeditious delivery. If intraamniotic infection is diagnosed, appropriate antibiotic treatment also is indicated. In the absence of an indication for immediate delivery, swabs for diagnosis of *Chlamydia trachomatis* and *Neisseria gonorrhoeae* may be obtained from the cervix, if appropriate. Intrapartum antibiotic prophylaxis is to be administered to women with unknown culture status who are in preterm labor with significant risk of imminent delivery or who have preterm PROM, rupture of membranes for 18 or more hours, or intrapartum fever (temperature greater than or equal to 100.4°F or greater than or equal to 38°C). If time permits and a culture is performed, treatment should be altered if necessary after the culture results are determined.

Term Premature Rupture of Membranes

For women with PROM at term, labor should generally be induced at the time of presentation, generally with oxytocin infusion, to reduce the risk of intraamniotic infection. Obstetrician–gynecologists and other obstetric care providers should inform pregnant women with term PROM who are considering a period of expectant care of the potential risks associated with expectant management and the limitations of available data. For informed women, if concordant with their individual preferences and if there are no other maternal or fetal reasons to expedite delivery, the choice of expectant management for a period may be appropriately offered and supported. For women who are positive for group B streptococci (GBS), however, administration of antibiotics for GBS prophylaxis should not be delayed while awaiting labor. In such cases, many patients and obstetrician–gynecologists or other obstetric care providers may prefer immediate induction.

Fetal heart rate monitoring should be used to assess fetal status. Dating criteria should be reviewed to assign gestational age. Group B streptococci prophylaxis should be given based on prior culture results or intrapartum risk factors if cultures have not been previously performed. When the decision to deliver is made, GBS prophylaxis should be given based on prior culture results or risk factors if cultures have not been previously performed.

Preterm Premature Rupture of Membranes

At 34 0/7 weeks of gestation or greater, delivery is recommended for all women with ruptured membranes. Patients with PROM before 34 0/7 weeks of gestation should be managed expectantly if no maternal or fetal contraindications exist. A single course of corticosteroids is recommended for pregnant women between 24 0/7 weeks and 34 0/7 weeks of gestation, and may be considered for pregnant women as early as 23 0/7 weeks of gestation who are at risk of preterm delivery within 7 days. To reduce maternal and neonatal infections and gestational-age dependent morbidity, a 7-day course of therapy with a combination of intravenous ampicillin and erythromycin followed by oral amoxicillin and erythromycin is recommended during expectant management of women with preterm PROM who are less than 34 0/7 weeks of gestation. Women with preterm PROM before 32 0/7 weeks of gestation who are thought to be at risk of imminent delivery should be considered candidates for fetal neuroprotective treatment with magnesium sulfate. Women with preterm PROM who have fetuses and viable fetuses and who are candidates for intrapartum GBS prophylaxis should receive intrapartum GBS prophylaxis to prevent vertical transmission regardless of earlier treatments. In the setting of ruptured membranes with active labor, therapeutic tocolysis has not been shown to prolong latency or improve neonatal outcomes. Therefore, therapeutic tocolysis is not recommended. The outpatient management of a woman with preterm PROM with a viable fetus has not been sufficiently studied to establish safety and, therefore, is not recommended. Recent data indicate that administration of betamethasone in the late preterm period between 34 0/7 weeks and 36 6/7 weeks of gestation reduces respiratory morbidity in newborns. Although subgroup analysis was not done, approximately 20% of study patients had preterm PROM. It is assumed that patients with preterm PROM will benefit from betamethasone in the late preterm period, but because the study design excluded patients who had received corticosteroids earlier in the pregnancy, it is unknown whether there is any benefit to a second course of betamethasone in the late preterm period in these patients.

Preterm Birth

Preterm birth is defined as birth before 37/0 weeks of gestation. Spontaneous preterm birth includes birth that follows preterm labor, preterm spontaneous rupture of membranes, and cervical insufficiency, but does not include indicated preterm delivery for maternal or fetal conditions. Preterm birth is the leading cause of neonatal mortality and one of the most common reasons for antenatal hospitalization. The preterm birth rate (birth at less than 37 completed weeks of gestation per 100 total births) decreased 8% from 2007 to 2014. Decreases in birth rates for early-preterm birth (earlier than 34 weeks of gestation) and late-preterm birth (34 0/7–36 6/7 weeks of gestation) contributed to the overall decrease in the preterm birth rate between 2008 (10.4%) and 2014 (9.6%). The pathophysiologic events that trigger preterm parturition are largely unknown but may include decidual hemorrhage (abruption), mechanical factors (uterine overdistention or cervical incompetence), hormonal changes (perhaps mediated by fetal or maternal stress), infection, and inflammation.

Risk Factor Identification and Management

One of the strongest clinical risk factors for preterm birth is a prior preterm birth. Maternal history of preterm birth is commonly reported to confer a 1.5-fold to 2-fold increased risk in a subsequent pregnancy. *Short cervical length* measured by transvaginal ultrasonography, commonly defined as less than 25 mm, has been associated with an increased risk of preterm birth. The shorter the cervical length, the greater the risk of preterm birth. Additional proposed risk factors for preterm birth include aspects of obstetric and gynecologic history, demographic characteristics, current pregnancy complications, and behavioral factors. However, data are inconsistent about whether these factors are actually causative for preterm birth.

Screening Tests

Transvaginal cervical ultrasonography has been shown to be a reliable and reproducible way to assess the length of the cervix when performed by trained operators. Until recently, routine cervical length evaluation in women at low risk of preterm delivery was not advocated because, like other factors associated with a potentially higher preterm birth risk, no effective treatments were available to reduce that risk. However, recent randomized trials have demonstrated a lower risk of preterm birth and decreased neonatal morbidity when vaginal progesterone was given to asymptomatic women with a cervical length of 10–20 mm at 19–23 6/7 weeks of gestation. Studies of other specific tests and monitoring modalities, such as fetal fibronectin screening, bacterial vaginosis testing, and home uterine activity monitoring have not demonstrated improved perinatal outcomes and they are not recommended as screening strategies.

Interventions

Women With Spontaneous Prior Preterm Birth. A woman with a singleton gestation and a prior spontaneous preterm singleton birth should be offered progesterone supplementation starting at 16–24 weeks of gestation to reduce the risk of recurrent spontaneous preterm birth. Available evidence also suggests that cerclage placement is associated with significant decreases in recurrent preterm birth for women with a current singleton pregnancy, prior spontaneous preterm birth at less than 34 weeks of gestation, and short cervical length (less than 25 mm) before 24 weeks of gestation. Insufficient evidence exists to assess whether progesterone and cerclage together have an additive effect in reducing the risk of preterm birth in women at high risk of preterm birth.

Women Without Prior Spontaneous Preterm Birth. Vaginal progesterone is recommended as a management option to reduce the risk of preterm birth in asymptomatic women with a singleton gestation without a prior preterm birth who have an incidentally identified very short cervical length (less than or equal to 20 mm before or at 24 weeks of gestation). In contrast, cerclage placement in otherwise asymptomatic women with a cervical length less than 25 mm detected between 16 weeks of gestation and 24 weeks of gestation does not appear to reduce the risk of preterm birth in this population.

Diagnosis of Preterm Labor

Identifying women with preterm labor who ultimately will give birth preterm is difficult. Regular preterm contractions are common; however, these contractions do not reliably predict which women will have subsequent progressive cervical change. Approximately 30% of preterm labor spontaneously resolves, and 50% of patients hospitalized for preterm labor actually give birth at term. The diagnosis of preterm labor is generally based upon clinical criteria of regular uterine contractions accompanied by cervical dilation, and effacement, presentation, or both, with regular contractions and at least 2 cm dilatation.

Patients with suspected preterm labor should be examined and observed for 1–2 hours, have their uterine activity monitored, and undergo serial cervical examinations to document the presence or absence of cervical change. Knowledge of fetal fibronectin status or cervical length may help health care providers reduce use of unnecessary resources, but the positive predictive value of a positive fetal fibronectin test result or a short cervix alone is poor and should not be used exclusively to direct management in the setting of acute symptoms. Because preterm labor often is associated with urinary tract infections, a dipstick or a microscopic examination of urine and urine culture may be helpful. Ultrasound examination also may be considered to confirm gestational age, to estimate fetal weight in order to receive appropriate counseling from pediatrics, and to assess the presence of any congenital anomalies.

Management of Preterm Labor

Interventions to reduce the likelihood of delivery should be reserved for a woman likely to give birth and who is at a gestational age of which delay in delivery will provide benefit to the newborn. Proposed pharmacologic interventions to prolong pregnancy include tocolytic drugs to inhibit uterine contractions and antibiotics to treat intrauterine bacterial infection. Therapeutic agents associated with improved neonatal outcomes include antenatal corticosteroids for fetal maturation and magnesium sulfate for neuroprotection.

Tocolytic Drugs. Evidence supports the use of first-line tocolytic treatment with β-adrenergic agonist therapy, calcium channel blockers, or nonsteroidal antiinflammatory drugs for short-term prolongation of pregnancy (up to 48 hours) to allow for the administration of antenatal steroids. Tocolysis is not recommended beyond 34 weeks of gestation, and is generally not recommended before 24 weeks of gestation but may be considered based on individual circumstances at 23 weeks of gestation. Maintenance therapy with tocolytics has been ineffective for preventing preterm birth and improving neonatal outcomes and, therefore, is not recommended for this purpose. Tocolysis is contraindicated when the maternal and fetal risks of prolonging pregnancy or the risks associated with these drugs are greater than the risks associated with preterm birth.

Antibiotics. Antibiotic treatment of women with preterm labor and intact membranes has been shown to have no effect on pregnancy prolongation or on the improvement of newborn outcomes. Indeed, the combination of amoxicillin–clavulanic acid in the setting of preterm labor may worsen long-term outcomes for the offspring. Thus, although data specific to the periviable period are not available, broad-spectrum antibiotic treatment to prolong pregnancy during expectant management of periviable preterm PROM generally is recommended at 24 weeks of gestation and beyond. Conversely, there are inadequate data to help obstetrician–gynecologists and other obstetric care providers balance any potential efficacy at earlier gestational ages against potential risks. In the setting of preterm labor with intact membranes, because of the lack of evidence of benefit and the potential risks, antibiotic treatment to prolong pregnancy is not recommended.

This recommendation is distinct from recommendations for antibiotic use for preterm premature rupture of membranes (see "Premature Rupture of Membranes" earlier in this chapter) and group B streptococci carrier status (see also "Bacterial Infections" in Chapter 12).

Antenatal Corticosteroids. For women at risk of preterm birth, enhancement of fetal pulmonary function with the use of antenatal steroids lessens the prevalence and severity of neonatal respiratory distress syndrome and its sequelae. A single course of corticosteroids (betamethasone or dexamethasone) is recommended for pregnant women between 24 0/7 weeks and 33 6/7 weeks of gestation, including those with ruptured membranes and multiple gestations, and may be considered for pregnant women starting at 23 weeks of gestation, who are at risk of preterm delivery within 7 days, irrespective of membrane status. Administration of corticosteroids for pregnant women during the periviable period who are at risk of preterm delivery within 7 days is linked to a family's decision regarding resuscitation and should be considered in that context. Sparse data exist on the efficacy of corticosteroid use before fetal age of viability, and such use is not recommended. Administration of betamethasone may be considered in pregnant women between 34 0/7 weeks and 36 6/7 weeks of gestation at imminent risk of preterm birth within 7 days, and who have not received a previous course of antenatal corticosteroids. Regularly scheduled repeat courses or serial courses (more than two) are not recommended. A single repeat course of antenatal corticosteroids should be considered in women who are less than 34 weeks of gestation, who have an imminent risk of preterm delivery within the next 7 days, and whose prior course of antenatal corticosteroids was administered more than 14 days previously. Rescue course antenatal corticosteroids could be provided as early as 7 days from the prior dose, if indicated by the clinical scenario. A single course of antenatal corticosteroids should be administered to women with PROM before 32 weeks of gestation to reduce the risks of respiratory distress syndrome, perinatal mortality, and other morbidities. Whether to administer a repeat or rescue course of corticosteroids with preterm PROM is controversial, and there is insufficient evidence to make a recommendation to do so.

Magnesium Sulfate. Short-term (usually less than 48 hours) use of magnesium sulfate in obstetric care include use for prevention and treatment of seizures in women with preeclampsia or eclampsia; fetal neuroprotection before anticipated early preterm (less than 32 weeks of gestation) delivery;

and short-term prolongation of pregnancy (up to 48 hours) to allow for the administration of antenatal corticosteroids in pregnant women who are at risk of preterm delivery within 7 days (see "Tocolytic Drugs" earlier in this chapter). Hospitals electing to use magnesium sulfate for fetal neuroprotection should develop uniform and specific guidelines regarding inclusion criteria, treatment regimens, concurrent tocolysis, and monitoring in accordance with one of the larger trials. The use of magnesium sulfate for inhibition of acute preterm labor has not been demonstrated to achieve significant pregnancy prolongation.

Bibliography

American College of Obstetricians and Gynecologists. Hypertension in pregnancy. Washington, DC: American College of Obstetricians and Gynecologists; 2013. Available at: http://www.acog.org/Resources-And-Publications/Task-Force-and-Work-Group-Reports/Hypertension-in-Pregnancy. Retrieved November 2, 2016.

American College of Obstetricians and Gynecologists. Prevention of Rh D alloimmunization. ACOG Practice Bulletin 4. Washington, DC: ACOG; 1999.

Anemia in pregnancy. ACOG Practice Bulletin No. 95. American College of Obstetricians and Gynecologists. Obstet Gynecol 2008;112:201–7.

Antenatal corticosteroid therapy for fetal maturation. Committee Opinion No. 677. American College of Obstetricians and Gynecologists. Obstet Gynecol 2016;128: e187–94.

Antiphospholipid syndrome. Practice Bulletin No. 132. American College of Obstetricians and Gynecologists. Obstet Gynecol 2012;120:1514–21.

Asthma in pregnancy. ACOG Practice Bulletin No. 90. American College of Obstetricians and Gynecologists. Obstet Gynecol 2008;111:457–64.

Classification and diagnosis of diabetes. American Diabetes Association [published erratum appears in Diabetes Care 2016;39:1653]. Diabetes Care 2016;39(suppl):S13–22.

Critical care in pregnancy. Practice Bulletin No. 170. American College of Obstetricians and Gynecologists. Obstet Gynecol 2016;128:e147–54.

Emergent therapy for acute-onset, severe hypertension during pregnancy and the postpartum period. Committee Opinion No. 692. American College of Obstetricians and Gynecologists. Obstet Gynecol 2017;129:e90–5.

Flegal KM, Carroll MD, Ogden CL, Curtin LR. Prevalence and trends in obesity among us adults, 1999-2008. JAMA 2010;303:235–41.

Fryar CD, Carroll MD, Ogden CL. Prevalence of overweight, obesity, and extreme obesity among adults aged 20 and over: United States, 1960-1962 through 2013-2014. Hyattsville (MD): National Center for Health Statistics; 2016. Available at: http://www.cdc.gov/nchs/data/hestat/obesity_adult_13_14/obesity_adult_13_14.pdf. Retrieved November 2, 2016.

Genetics and molecular diagnostic testing. Technology Assessment No. 11. American College of Obstetricians and Gynecologists. Obstet Gynecol 2014;123:394–413.

Gestational diabetes mellitus. Practice Bulletin No. 137. American College of Obstetricians and Gynecologists. Obstet Gynecol 2013;122:406–16.

Inherited thrombophilias in pregnancy. Practice Bulletin No. 138. American College of Obstetricians and Gynecologists. Obstet Gynecol 2013;122:706–17.

Kim SY, Dietz PM, England L, Morrow B, Callaghan WM. Trends in pre-pregnancy obesity in nine states, 1993-2003. Obesity (Silver Spring) 2007;15:986–93.

Magnesium sulfate before anticipated preterm birth for neuroprotection. Committee Opinion No. 455. American College of Obstetricians and Gynecologists. Obstet Gynecol 2010;115:669–71.

Magnesium sulfate use in obstetrics. Committee Opinion No. 652. American College of Obstetricians and Gynecologists. Obstet Gynecol 2016;127:e52–3.

Management of alloimmunization during pregnancy. ACOG Practice Bulletin No. 75. American College of Obstetricians and Gynecologists. Obstet Gynecol 2006;108: 457–64.

Management of preterm labor. Practice Bulletin No. 171. American College of Obstetricians and Gynecologists. Obstet Gynecol 2016;128:e155–64.

Medically indicated late-preterm and early-term deliveries. Committee Opinion No. 560. American College of Obstetricians and Gynecologists. Obstet Gynecol 2013;121:908–10.

Nonmedically indicated early-term deliveries. Committee Opinion No. 561. American College of Obstetricians and Gynecologists. Obstet Gynecol 2013;121:911–5.

Obesity in pregnancy. Practice Bulletin No. 156. American College of Obstetricians and Gynecologists. Obstet Gynecol 2015;126:e112–26.

Optimizing postpartum care. Committee Opinion No. 666. American College of Obstetricians and Gynecologists. Obstet Gynecol 2016;127:e187–92.

Placenta accreta. Committee Opinion No. 529. American College of Obstetricians and Gynecologists. Obstet Gynecol 2012;120:207–11.

Postpartum hemorrhage. ACOG Practice Bulletin No. 76. American College of Obstetricians and Gynecologists. Obstet Gynecol 2006;108:1039–47.

Prediction and prevention of preterm birth. Practice Bulletin No. 130. American College of Obstetricians and Gynecologists. Obstet Gynecol 2012;120:964–73.

Pregestational diabetes mellitus. ACOG Practice Bulletin No. 60. American College of Obstetricians and Gynecologists. Obstet Gynecol 2005;105:675–85.

Premature rupture of membranes. Practice Bulletin No. 172. American College of Obstetricians and Gynecologists. Obstet Gynecol 2016;128:e165–77.

Safe prevention of the primary cesarean delivery. Obstetric Care Consensus No. 1. American College of Obstetricians and Gynecologists. Obstet Gynecol 2014;123: 693–711.

Spong CY, Mercer BM, D'alton M, Kilpatrick S, Blackwell S, Saade G. Timing of indicated late-preterm and early-term birth. Obstet Gynecol 2011;118:323–33.

Thromboembolism in pregnancy. Practice Bulletin No. 123. American College of Obstetricians and Gynecologists. Obstet Gynecol 2011;118:718–29.

Thyroid disease in pregnancy. Practice Bulletin No. 148. American College of Obstetricians and Gynecologists. Obstet Gynecol 2015;125:996–1005.

Use of prophylactic antibiotics in labor and delivery. Practice Bulletin No. 120. American College of Obstetricians and Gynecologists. Obstet Gynecol 2011;117: 1472–83.

Use of psychiatric medications during pregnancy and lactation. ACOG Practice Bulletin No. 92. American College of Obstetricians and Gynecologists. Obstet Gynecol 2008;111:1001–20.

Warnes CA, Williams RG, Bashore TM, Child JS, Connolly HM, Dearani JA, et al. ACC/AHA 2008 guidelines for the management of adults with congenital heart disease: a report of the American College of Cardiology/American Heart Association Task Force on Practice Guidelines (Writing Committee to Develop Guidelines on the Management of Adults with Congenital Heart Disease). Developed in Collaboration with the American Society of Echocardiography, Heart Rhythm Society, International Society for Adult Congenital Heart Disease, Society for Cardiovascular Angiography and Interventions, and Society of Thoracic Surgeons. J Am Coll Cardiol 2008;52: e143–263.

Resources

American College of Obstetricians and Gynecologists District II. Maternal safety bundle for severe hypertension in pregnancy. Albany (NY): American College of Obstetricians and Gynecologists District II; 2015. Available at: http://www.acog.org/-/media/Districts/District-II/Public/SMI/v2/HTNSlideSetNov2015Updated.pdf?dmc=1&ts=20170404T1856202381. Retrieved April 4, 2017.

REPROTOX: an information system developed by the Reproductive Toxicology Center for its members [After Login]. Washington, DC: The Reproductive Toxicology Center; 2016. Available at: http://www.reprotox.org. Retrieved November 2, 2016.

TERIS: Teratogen Information System and the on-Line Version of Shepard's Catalog of Teratogenic Agents. Seattle (WA): University of Washingon; 2016. Available at: http://depts.washington.edu/terisweb/teris/. Retrieved December 19, 2016.

U.S. Food and Drug Administration. Silver Spring (MD): FDA; 2016. Available at: http://www.fda.gov. Retrieved November 2, 2016.

Chapter 10

Care of the Newborn

All newborn infants should be cared for by a team of expert physicians and other trained health care providers in the context of a family-centered environment. Individuals trained in neonatal resuscitation are present in the delivery room and are ready to perform timely resuscitation, if needed. At birth, infants are quickly stabilized and assessed to determine the level of care required. All infants undergo an identification process, and copies of maternal and newborn medical records are transferred from the obstetric to the neonatal care teams.

Term (37 0/7–41 6/7 weeks of gestational age) and late-preterm infants (34 0/7–36 6/7 weeks of gestational age) are closely observed during the transition period, the first 4–8 hours after birth. Infants who are healthy and stable should remain with their mothers during this period. If possible, an infant should be placed naked on his or her mother's chest and allowed to breastfeed. The infant should be kept warm and assessed by a detailed clinical examination that includes intrauterine growth status, evaluation for gestational age, and a comprehensive risk assessment for neonatal conditions that require additional monitoring or intervention.

Neonatal nutrition is ideally provided through breastfeeding. Initiation of breastfeeding should take place soon after birth, with continued monitoring of the breastfed newborn until discharge and thereafter by the newborn care provider. There are limited contraindications to breastfeeding. In the event breastfeeding is disrupted, breast milk should be collected and stored. Breast emptying will help to establish and preserve the milk supply even when the baby is unable to directly breastfeed. Banked, pasteurized donor milk may serve as an alternative, when available, but this is a scarce and expensive resource, usually reserved for preterm infants.

The advice and encouragement of health care providers are critical in assisting women to make an informed infant feeding decision. As when discussing any health behavior, the health care provider is obligated to assess patient comprehension of the relevant information and to be certain that the conversation is free from coercion, pressure, or undue influence. Families should receive noncommercial, accurate, and unbiased information so that they can make informed decisions about their health care. Health care providers should be aware that their own personal experiences with infant feeding may affect their counseling. In addition, pervasive direct-to-consumer marketing of infant formula adversely affects patient and health care provider perception of the risks and benefits of breastfeeding. Health care providers must themselves be knowledgeable about the benefits of breastfeeding for mothers and infants.

Preventive newborn care includes attention to hygiene; hepatitis immunization; and screening for genetic and metabolic conditions, hearing impairment, critical congenital heart disease, risk of hyperbilirubinemia, and developmental hip dysplasia. Targeted assessment of glucose homeostasis and possible sepsis are implemented on a discretionary basis, depending on individualized risk.

Delivery Room Care

Approximately 10% of term and late-preterm infants require some assistance to begin breathing that includes stimulation at birth; less than 1% will need extensive resuscitative measures. Although the vast majority do not require intervention to make the transition from intrauterine to extrauterine life, because of the large total number of births a sizable number of babies will require some degree of resuscitation. Recognition and immediate resuscitation of a distressed newborn infant requires an organized plan of action that includes the immediate availability of proper equipment and on-site qualified personnel. Anticipated newborn problems should be thoroughly communicated by the obstetric care provider to the responsible lead member of the resuscitation team.

Neonatal Resuscitation Management Plan

Assessment and resuscitation of the infant at delivery should be provided in accordance with the principles of the American Heart Association and the American Academy of Pediatrics (AAP) Neonatal Resuscitation Program®. Although the guidelines for neonatal resuscitation focus on delivery room resuscitation, most of the principles are applicable throughout the neonatal period and early infancy. Each hospital should have policies and procedures addressing the care and resuscitation of the newborn infant, including the qualifications of physicians and other health care practitioners who provide this care. A program should be in place that ensures the competency of these individuals, as well as their periodic credentialing. At every delivery, there should be at least one individual whose primary responsibility is the infant and who is capable of initiating resuscitation, including positive pressure ventilation. This individual may be a physician, advanced practice neonatal nurse, nurse anesthetist, nursery nurse, physician assistant, respiratory therapist, certified nurse–midwife, or a labor and delivery nurse. If additional risk factors are present that increase the likelihood of the need for resuscitation, at least two qualified people should be present solely to manage the baby. The number and qualifications of personnel will vary depending upon the anticipated risk, the number of babies, and the hospital setting. A qualified team with full resuscitation skills, including tracheal intubation, chest compressions, emergency vascular access and medication administration, should be identified and immediately available for every resuscitation.

The provision of services and equipment for resuscitation should be planned jointly by the medical and nursing directors of the departments involved in resuscitation of the newborn infant, usually the departments of obstetrics, pediatrics, and anesthesia. A physician, usually a pediatrician, should be designated to assume primary responsibility for initiating, supervising, and reviewing the plan for management of infants requiring resuscitation in the delivery room. The following issues should be considered in this plan:

- A prioritized list should be developed of known or anticipated maternal and fetal complications that would require routine, urgent, or emergent delivery. Individual(s) qualified in all aspects of newborn resuscitation should be present.
- The capabilities of individuals qualified to perform neonatal resuscitation should include the following:
  - Ability to rapidly and accurately evaluate the newborn condition
  - Ability and authority to seek additional personnel and experts for immediate participation in newborn resuscitation
  - Knowledge of the pathogenesis of risk factors predisposing for the need for resuscitation (eg, hypoxia, maternal medication, hypovolemia, trauma, anomalies, infections, and preterm birth), as well as specific indications for resuscitation

- — Skills in airway management, including bag and mask ventilation, use of a laryngeal mask airway, laryngoscopy, endotracheal intubation and suctioning of the airway, chest compressions, emergency administration of drugs and fluids, establishing emergency umbilical venous or intraosseous needle access, and maintenance of thermal stability
- — Although not required, skill in the recognition and decompression of a tension pneumothorax by needle aspiration is desirable

- Procedures should be developed and policies should be in place to ensure the readiness of equipment and personnel and to provide for periodic review and evaluation of the effectiveness of the system.
- Contingency plans should be created for multiple births, unusual and life-threatening maternal complications, and other unusual circumstances.
- Guidelines should be developed for documentation of the resuscitation, including the personnel involved, interventions, medications, the time of each intervention or medication, and the response of the infant.
- Procedures should be developed and delineated for transfer of responsibility for care of the newborn.

Steps in Delivery Room Management

At birth, the neonatal care team implements a sequence of steps to quickly assess and stabilize the infant in order to institute the appropriate intensity of newborn care. With careful consideration of risk factors, most infants who will need resuscitation can be identified before birth, although some infants without any apparent risk factors will require resuscitation. If the need for resuscitation is anticipated, additional skilled personnel should be recruited and the necessary equipment prepared for immediate use.

Assessment

All infants should have a rapid assessment immediately after birth. Infants who are at risk of requiring interventions should have the initial steps of newborn care performed at a radiant warmer. These infants can be identified by asking three questions:

1. Is the baby term (equal to or greater than 37 0/7 weeks of gestational age)?
2. Does the baby have good muscle tone?

3. Is the baby breathing or crying?

If the answers to these questions are "yes," the infant should remain with the mother for the initial steps of newborn care. Observation of breathing, activity, and color should be ongoing.

If the answer to any of these questions is "no," the infant should receive one or more of the following categories of action in sequence (see Fig. 10-1 for a detailed treatment algorithm):

- Initial steps in stabilization (provide warmth, position to open the airway, clear airway if necessary, dry, stimulate breathing)
- Positive pressure ventilation, oxygen saturation monitoring, and supplemental oxygen, as needed
- Chest compressions
- Administration of epinephrine, or volume expansion, or both

Approximately 60 seconds are allotted for a rapid assessment, completing the initial steps of newborn care, evaluating the baby's heart rate, and beginning positive pressure ventilation if required (see Fig. 10-1). The decision to progress beyond the initial steps is determined by simultaneous assessment of two vital characteristics: 1) respirations (apnea, gasping, labored or unlabored breathing) and 2) heart rate (whether greater than or less than 100 beats per minute). Initial assessment of the heart rate should be performed using a stethoscope. Auscultation along the left side of the chest is the most accurate physical examination method of determining a newborn's heart rate. Although pulsations may be felt at the umbilical cord base, palpation is less accurate and may underestimate the true heart rate. If the heart rate cannot be determined by physical examination and the infant is not vigorous, another team member should quickly connect a pulse oximetry sensor or electrocardiogram leads to the baby in order to evaluate the heart rate. If positive pressure ventilation is needed, assessment should consist of simultaneous evaluation of three vital characteristics: 1) heart rate, 2) respirations, and 3) the state of oxygenation (the latter determined by a pulse oximeter). The most sensitive indicator of a successful response to each step is an increase in heart rate (see also "Initial Steps of Newborn Care").

Initial Steps of Newborn Care

Maintenance of Body Temperature. Immediately after delivery, the vigorous term infant should be placed skin-to-skin with the mother and dried. Then both mother and infant should be covered with a warm, dry blanket.

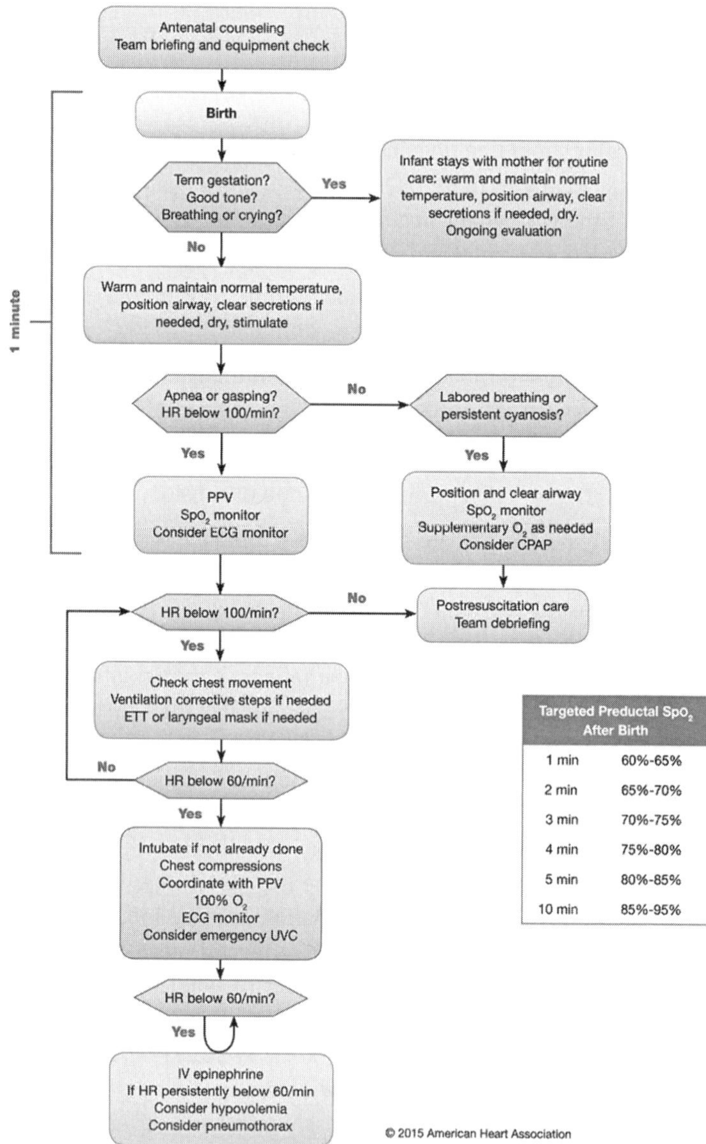

Targeted Preductal SpO_2 After Birth	
1 min	60%-65%
2 min	65%-70%
3 min	70%-75%
4 min	75%-80%
5 min	80%-85%
10 min	85%-95%

Figure 10-1. Neonatal resuscitation algorithm. Abbreviations: CPAP, continuous positive airway pressure; ECG, electrocardiogram; ETT, endotracheal tube; HR, heart rate; IV, intravenous; PPV, positive pressure ventilation; SpO_2, blood oxygen saturation; UVC, umbilical venous catheter. (Reprinted with permission from Wyckoff MH, Aziz K, Escobedo MB, Kapadia VS, Kattwinkel J, Perlman JM, et al. Part 13: neonatal resuscitation: 2015 American Heart Association guidelines update for cardiopulmonary resuscitation and emergency cardiovascular care (reprint). Pediatrics 2015;136(suppl):S196–218. Copyright 2015 American Heart Association.)

Infants born preterm, those without good muscle tone, and those who are not breathing or crying should be placed under a preheated radiant warmer. The radiant warmer will reduce heat loss and allow easy access to the infant during resuscitation procedures. Preterm infants less than 32 weeks of gestation are likely to become hypothermic despite the use of traditional techniques for decreasing heat loss. For this reason, additional warming techniques are recommended (eg, prewarming the delivery room to 26°C [78.8°F], covering the infant in plastic wrapping [food or medical grade, heat-resistant plastic], placing the infant on an exothermic mattress). The infant's temperature must be monitored closely because overheating has been described when plastic wrap is used in combination with an exothermic mattress. The goal should be an axillary temperature of approximately 36.5°C (97.7°F).

Clearing the Airway. When the newborn infant is *vigorous*, defined as strong respiratory effort and good muscle tone, routine oral or nasopharyngeal suctioning is not necessary. Suctioning of the airway immediately after birth (including suctioning with a bulb syringe) should not be performed unless the infant has an obvious airway obstruction that interferes with spontaneous breathing or requires positive pressure ventilation. If necessary, the mouth should be suctioned before the nose so there is nothing to aspirate if the newborn gasps when the nose is suctioned. Vigorous or deep suctioning of the posterior pharynx should be avoided because this may produce significant reflex bradycardia and may damage the oral mucosa, leading to interference with suckling because of pain. When meconium is present in amniotic fluid, evidence does not support routine intrapartum oropharyngeal or nasopharyngeal suctioning, as these interventions do not prevent or alter the course of meconium aspiration syndrome. If an infant is born through meconium-stained amniotic fluid and has depressed respirations or poor muscle tone, the infant should be placed under the radiant warmer and the initial steps of newborn care as aforementioned performed. If the baby is not breathing or the heart rate is less than 100 beats per minute (bpm) after the initial steps are completed, positive pressure ventilation should be initiated.

Positioning. Infants should be placed on their backs, with the neck slightly extended. This position (known as the sniffing position) readily aligns the posterior pharynx, larynx, and trachea for optimal air entry. The infant's mouth and nose may be wiped with a towel or suctioned gently to remove excess mucus or blood (see also "Clearing the Airway" earlier in this section).

Stimulation. Drying provides enough tactile stimulation for most infants; however, if the infant does not have adequate respirations, briefly rubbing the back, trunk, or extremities may stimulate spontaneous respirations. If the infant does not respond to brief additional stimulation, positive pressure ventilation should be initiated. Prolonged stimulation of an apneic infant is not effective and delays the initiation of effective ventilation.

Administration of Supplemental Oxygen. The goal of resuscitation is to achieve a heart rate of at least 100 bpm and a preductal oxygen saturation value in the interquartile range for each minute after birth as measured in healthy term babies after vaginal birth at sea level (see Fig. 10-1). Among infants born greater than or equal to 35 weeks of gestation, published data indicate that positive pressure ventilation should be initiated with air (21% oxygen). Among infants born at less than 35 weeks of gestation, positive pressure should be initiated with an oxygen concentration between 21% and 30%. The oxygen concentration should be titrated, as needed to achieve an SpO_2 in the target range. It is recommended that oximetry be used when resuscitation is anticipated, supplemental oxygen is administered, positive pressure is administered for more than a few breaths, or when cyanosis persists. Hyperoxemia and hypoxemia should be avoided. If blended oxygen is not available, resuscitation should be initiated with air.

Ventilation. The normal newborn infant breathes within seconds of birth and usually has established regular respirations within 1 minute after birth. An infant who is apneic or is gasping or whose heart rate is less than 100 bpm requires positive pressure ventilation, which can be administered with a self- or flow-inflating bag or a T-piece resuscitator. Inflation and aeration of the infant's lungs is the single most effective intervention during neonatal resuscitation. For most infants, positive pressure ventilation is the only resuscitation maneuver required to establish regular respirations. Effective ventilation almost always results in improved heart rate. If the heart rate does not increase and there is no chest movement with ventilation, it is likely that the lungs are not being inflated and aerated. In this case, corrective steps, such as adjusting the mask, repositioning the head, opening the mouth, suctioning the oropharynx, increasing the pressure used to deliver breaths, or insertion of an alternative airway should be performed.

Endotracheal intubation may be performed at various points during resuscitation, depending on the clinical circumstances. Indications for intubation include the following:

- Poor response to ventilation with mask and bag or T-piece resuscitator
- The need to enhance coordination of ventilation and chest compressions when chest compressions are necessary
- Direct tracheal suction if the airway is obstructed by thick secretions

Other possible indications for intubation include the need for surfactant administration, and suspected or known congenital diaphragmatic hernia. The skill of the resuscitator also may affect the timing of intubation. Individuals not adept at intubation should obtain assistance and focus on providing effective positive pressure ventilation with a mask rather than using valuable time attempting to intubate.

Exhaled carbon dioxide detection is the recommended method to confirm endotracheal tube placement; however, critically ill infants with poor cardiac output and poor or absent pulmonary blood flow may not exhale sufficient carbon dioxide to be detected reliably and, thus, may give false-negative test results. As with bag and mask ventilation, effective assisted ventilation with an endotracheal tube should result in an increased heart rate. If the heart rate does not improve, esophageal intubation should be suspected.

Chest Compressions. If the heart rate does not increase above 60 bpm after at least 30 seconds of effective ventilation, chest compressions should be instituted while coordinated ventilation is continued using 100% oxygen. The two-thumb encircling hand technique is recommended. There should be a 3:1 ratio of compressions to ventilations, with approximately 90 compressions and 30 ventilations per minute. Pulse oximetry may not detect the infant's pulse; therefore, heart rate monitoring by ECG is recommended if chest compressions are required. If the heart rate does not increase after 45–60 seconds of effective chest compressions, endotracheal intubation (if not already done) should be performed and epinephrine, preferably by the intravenous or intraosseous route, should be administered.

Medications. The use of medications during newborn resuscitation rarely is necessary. It should be considered only after effective ventilation and chest compressions have been established but the heart rate remains low. A list of drugs and volume expanders for resuscitation, with appropriate dosages, should be readily available, preferably in a prominent place in the resuscitation area. Neonatal Resuscitation Program reference charts that provide this information, as well as a flow diagram of the resuscitation procedure, are available from AAP for use in the delivery room and on code carts.

- Epinephrine—Epinephrine is indicated when the heart rate remains less than 60 bpm, despite adequate ventilation and chest compressions. The recommended dose is 0.1–0.3 mL per kg of a 1:10,000 solution (equal to 0.01–0.03 mg per kg) given as rapidly as possible through an emergently placed umbilical venous catheter or intraosseous needle. The efficacy of endotracheal epinephrine is unproven, and use of this route results in lower and unpredictable blood levels that may not be effective. Health care providers may choose to give epinephrine through the endotracheal tube while the umbilical venous catheter is being placed. If this route is used, administration of a higher dose (0.05–0.1 mg per kg, or 0.5–1 mL per kg of a 1:10,000 preparation) may be considered, but the safety and efficacy of this practice have not been evaluated. The higher dose should not be administered intravenously.
- Volume expanders—Routine volume expansion is not recommended during or after resuscitation. Volume expansion should be considered when an infant is not responding to resuscitation and blood loss is known or suspected. Normal saline (or type O Rh-negative packed red blood cells if fetal anemia is known or suspected) is recommended for volume expansion in the delivery room. The recommended initial dose is 10 mL per kg given over a span of 5–10 minutes through an emergently placed umbilical venous catheter or intraosseous needle, which may need to be repeated. Rapid infusion of large fluid volumes should be avoided in preterm infants.
- Naloxone—Administration of naloxone is not recommended as part of initial resuscitative efforts for infants with respiratory depression associated with maternal narcotic analgesia. Adequate support of ventilation should be sufficient to restore normal heart rate and oxygenation.

Apgar Score

The Apgar score is useful for conveying information about the infant's overall status and response to resuscitation. However, resuscitation must be initiated before the 1-minute score is assigned. Therefore, the Apgar score is not used to determine the need for initial resuscitation, what resuscitation steps are necessary, or when to use them. The score is reported at 1 minute and 5 minutes after birth for all infants, and at 5-minute intervals thereafter until

20 minutes for infants with a score less than 7. When an infant has an Apgar score of 5 or less at 5 minutes, umbilical artery blood gas from a clamped section of the umbilical cord should be obtained, if possible. Submitting the placenta for pathologic examination may be valuable. The AAP Committee on Fetus and Newborn has recommended the use of an expanded Apgar Scoring System (Fig. 10-2) that documents the assistance the infant is receiving at the time of assignment of the score.

Assessment of the Newborn in the Delivery Room

Immediately after delivery, the newborn infant must be assessed for individual needs to determine the best location for care. An infant with known or anticipated medical needs may be admitted to the special care nursery or neonatal intensive care unit (NICU) in the birth hospital or transferred to a hospital that provides the appropriate level of care (see also “Levels of Neonatal Care” in Chapter 1 and “Transport Procedure” in Chapter 4).

A healthy-appearing newborn infant should remain with the mother. If the infant’s condition is stable and the infant does not require further intervention, immediate and sustained skin-to-skin contact between the mother and her infant should be provided. Early, sustained skin-to-skin contact improves neonatal temperature stability and increases neonatal glucose levels. For mothers who have chosen to breastfeed, evidence from randomized controlled trials shows that skin-to-skin contact increases duration of breastfeeding by approximately 42 days. The nursing staff in the labor, delivery, recovery, and postpartum areas should be trained in assessing and recognizing problems in the newborn and in assessing and assisting with breastfeeding. In most circumstances, the baby can be transported safely with the mother from the delivery to postpartum area.

Infants who require intervention in the delivery room are at risk of developing subsequent complications. Such infants, and infants at risk of developing neonatal abstinence syndrome (see Chapter 11), should be evaluated frequently during the immediate neonatal period. These infants should be managed in an area where frequent vital signs can be obtained and the nursing staff is familiar with the signs and symptoms of an infant who is in distress. Some of these infants may require transport to another hospital for a higher level of care.

Immediate plans for the newborn infant should be discussed with the parents or other support person(s), preferably before leaving the delivery room.

Apgar Score

Gestational age:_______________weeks

Sign	0	1	2	1 min	5 min	10 min	15 min	20 min
Color	Blue or Pale	Acrocyanotic	Completely Pink					
Heart rate	Absent	Less than 100 min	Greater than 100 min					
Reflex irritability	No response	Grimace	Cry or active withdrawal					
Muscle tone	Limp	Some flexion	Active motion					
Respiration	Absent	Weak cry, hypoventilation	Good, crying					
			Total					

Comments:

Resuscitation					
Min	1	5	10	15	20
Oxygen					
PPV/NCPAP					
ETT					
Chest compressions					
Epinephrine					

Figure 10-2. Expanded Apgar score form. Record the score in the appropriate place at specific time intervals. The additional resuscitative measures (if appropriate) are recorded at the same time that the score is reported using a check mark in the appropriate box. Use the comment box to list other factors, including maternal medications, or the response to resuscitation, or both between the recorded times of scoring. Abbreviations: ETT, endotracheal tube; PPV/NCPAP, positive-pressure ventilation/nasal continuous positive airway pressure. (The Apgar score. Committee Opinion No. 644. American College of Obstetricians and Gynecologists. Obstet Gynecol 2015;126:e52–5.)

Whenever possible, the parents should have the opportunity to see, touch, and hold the infant before transfer to a nursery or before transfer to another facility. The physician or other health care provider delivering the infant also should be advised of the status and plans for the infant, including potential transfer or admission to a special care nursery or NICU.

Noninitiation or Withdrawal of Intensive Care for High-Risk Infants

Parents should be active participants in the decision-making process concerning the treatment of severely ill infants. This approach requires honest and open communication. Ongoing evaluation of the condition and prognosis of the high-risk infant is essential, and the physician, as the spokesperson for the health care team, must convey this information accurately and openly to the parents of the infant.

Compassionate and Comfort Care

Compassionate care to ensure comfort must be provided to all infants, including those for whom intensive care is not being provided. The decision to initiate or continue intensive care should be based only on the judgment that the infant will benefit from the intensive care. It is inappropriate for life-prolonging treatment to be continued when the condition is incompatible with life or when the treatment is judged to be harmful, of no benefit, or futile.

In formulating a plan of care for periviable newborn infants, clinicians should discuss with parents whether their goal is optimizing survival or minimizing suffering. The approach to antenatal and postdelivery care may differ dramatically depending on parental preferences regarding resuscitation.

A recommendation regarding assessment for resuscitation is not meant to indicate that resuscitation should always be either undertaken or deferred, or that every possible intervention need be offered. A stepwise approach concordant with neonatal circumstances and condition and with parental wishes is appropriate. Care should be reevaluated regularly and potentially redirected based on the evolution of the clinical situation. Assessment at birth, for example, may include confirmation that comfort measures are most appropriate.

A decision to proceed with resuscitation always should be informed by individual circumstances, including specific clinical issues (for example, estimated fetal weight and the most precise estimate of gestational age), family values and wishes, and ongoing evaluation of fetal or neonatal condition. In some cases, decisions will be informed by local institutional policy and relevant laws, of which obstetrician–gynecologists and other obstetric care providers should be aware. Accordingly, the guidelines offer recommendations with regard to the gestational ages at which assessment for resuscitation rather than resuscitation itself should be undertaken. Such assessment is meant in most cases to refer to that provided by neonatologists or other pediatric care providers, separate from that offered by obstetrician–gynecologists and other obstetric care providers.

A decision not to undertake resuscitation of a liveborn infant should not be seen as a decision to provide no care, but rather a decision to redirect care to comfort measures. Whenever nonresuscitation is considered an option, a qualified individual should be involved and present in the delivery room to manage this complex situation. Whenever possible, this individual should be a neonatologist. Comfort care should be provided for all infants for whom resuscitation is not initiated or is not successful.

Parent Counseling Regarding Resuscitation of Extremely Low-Gestational-Age Infants

Whether to initiate resuscitation of an infant born at an extremely low gestational age is a difficult decision because the consequences of this decision are either the inevitable death of the infant or the uncertainties of providing intensive care for an unknown length of time with an uncertain outcome. Each hospital that provides obstetric care should have a comprehensive and consistent approach to counseling parents and decision making. Parents should be provided the most accurate prognostic data available to help them make decisions. These predictions should not be based on gestational age alone but should include all relevant information affecting the prognosis. It is not possible to develop specific criteria for when the initiation of resuscitation should or should not be offered. Rather, the following general guidelines are suggested when discussing this situation with parents.

- If the health care providers involved believe that there is no chance of survival, resuscitation is not indicated and should not be initiated.
- If the health care providers consider a good outcome to be very unlikely, then parents should be given the choice of whether resuscitation should be initiated, and their preference should be respected.

- When the health care providers' judgment is that a good outcome is reasonably likely, resuscitation should be initiated and the decision to continue intensive care should be continually re-evaluated together with the parents.

Infant Identification

Strict guidelines are necessary to prevent the possibility of a newborn infant being accidently switched in the hospital. Human error continues to be the major cause of this, and establishing procedures with multiple checks or electronic matching systems minimizes this risk. Infant identification procedures should begin in the delivery room with matching bands for the infant and the mother. The nurse in the delivery room should be responsible for preparing and securely fastening these identification bands on the infant and the mother while the infant is still in the delivery room. These identical bands should indicate the mother's admission number, the infant's sex, the date and time of birth, and other information specified in hospital policy. Inclusion of the mother's first name on the infant's identification band can reduce wrong-patient errors (eg, Doe, BB Jane). Footprinting and fingerprinting alone are not adequate methods of patient identification. The birth records and identification bands should be checked and verified for accuracy before the infant leaves the delivery room. Policies and procedures requiring personnel to match identification bands each time the infant is taken to the mother while in the hospital and at discharge will minimize errors. If the condition of the infant does not allow placement of identification bands (eg, extreme preterm birth), the identification bands should accompany the infant and should be placed on the incubator or warmer. In these instances, the identification bands should be attached to the infant as soon as is practical.

With multiple births, each of the newborn infants should be identified according designations assigned to each fetus by the mother's obstetric care providers (if possible) or according to birth order (eg, A, B, C or 1, 2, 3). In the latter instance, the birth order may or may not correlate with the number assigned to the fetus in utero. In either case, fetal and neonatal identifiers must be explicitly correlated, particularly in the setting of prenatal diagnosis of significant anomalies in one or more of the fetuses. The corresponding umbilical cords should be identified according to hospital policy (eg, use of different number of clamps). This will ensure that umbilical cord blood specimens will be labeled correctly and can be correlated with the correct newborn infant. All umbilical cord blood samples must be labeled with an indication that these are samples of the infant's umbilical cord blood and not that of the mother.

Communication of Information

Care of the newborn infant is aided by effective communication of information about the mother and her fetus to the pediatrician or other health care provider. With an uncomplicated pregnancy, labor, and delivery, the information on the medical record accompanying the infant may be sufficient. The obstetric staff should record the following information, which also should be available on a medical record that accompanies the infant during any transfer of responsibility for care:

- The mother's name, medical record number, blood type, serologic test result, rubella status, hepatitis B test result, and human immunodeficiency virus (HIV) status
- Other maternal test results, if obtained, that are relevant to neonatal care, such as colonization with group B streptococci or intrapartum maternal antibiotic therapy (including type and number of doses of antibiotics)
- Maternal illness potentially affecting the fetus, evidence of intraamniotic infection (also referred to as chorioamnionitis), and maternal medications (including tocolytics and corticosteroids)
- Any history of nonmedical substance use or any other known high-risk circumstances, such as unstable housing, adolescent mother, maternal psychiatric disease, domestic violence, or history of previous child abuse or neglect
- Complications of pregnancy associated with abnormal fetal growth, fetal anomalies, or abnormal results from tests of fetal well-being and the corresponding interpretation
- Information regarding the labor (eg, duration) and delivery (eg, method), complications of labor, duration of rupture of amniotic membranes, presence or absence of meconium in amniotic fluid, and need for resuscitation
- Situations in which lactation may be compromised, such as history of breast surgery, trauma, or previous lactation failure, or contraindicated

due to specific infections (eg, HIV) or medication (consult LactMed: www.toxnet.nlm.nih.gov/newtoxnet/lactmed.htm)

The obstetric staff should communicate problems before and after delivery in a timely manner to the physician or other health care provider who will be caring for the newborn infant. For some high-risk pregnancies, a neonatal consultation during the antepartum period may be helpful in obstetric management and can assist the parents in understanding what to expect for their newborn infant. This is of particular importance when fetal anomalies are significant or the delivery of a preterm infant is expected.

Assessment of the Newborn Infant

Initial Assessment

A detailed clinical examination and assessment of the infant is performed by the clinical care team soon after birth and includes the following: evaluation of airway patency and skin color; auscultation of the heart and lungs; ascertainment of anal patency; assessment of muscle tone, level of consciousness, response to handling; measurement of vital signs (ie, body temperature, heart rate, and respiratory rate); and measurement of head circumference, body length, and body weight. Each newborn infant should be weighed shortly after birth and daily thereafter. The newborn infant must be kept warm during weighing. The scale pan should be covered with clean paper before each newborn infant is weighed. Additional targeted evaluations may include assessment of capillary refill, blood pressure, oxygen saturation, and need for supplemental oxygen.

Assessment of Intrauterine Growth

Gestational age can be estimated from the results of an ultrasound examination before 20 weeks of gestation or the mother's menstrual history (see also "Determining Gestational Age" in Chapter 6) and from the nursery assessment of gestational age (Fig. 10-3). Gestational age should be assigned after all nursing, pediatric, and obstetric data have been assessed. Any marked discrepancy between the presumed duration of pregnancy by obstetric assessment and the physical and neurologic findings in the newborn infant should be documented on the medical record. Growth parameters should be plotted on a birth weight–gestational age record appropriate for the community. Determination of gestational age and its relationship to weight should

Neuromuscular maturity

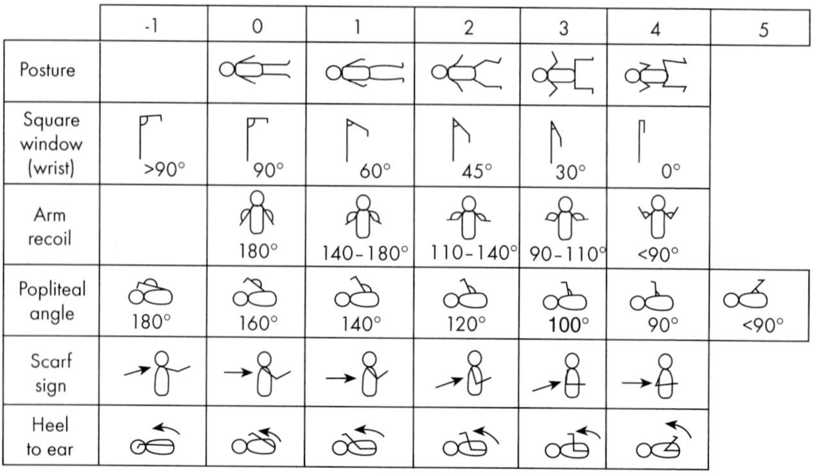

	-1	0	1	2	3	4	5
Posture							
Square window (wrist)	>90°	90°	60°	45°	30°	0°	
Arm recoil		180°	140–180°	110–140°	90–110°	<90°	
Popliteal angle	180°	160°	140°	120°	100°	90°	<90°
Scarf sign							
Heel to ear							

Physical maturity

Skin	Sticky, friable, transparent	Gelatinous, red, translucent	Smooth, pink, visible veins	Superficial peeling or rash or both, few veins	Cracking, pale areas, rare veins	Parchment, deep cracking, no vessels	Leathery, cracked, wrinkled
Lanugo	None	Sparse	Abundant	Thinning	Bald areas	Mostly bald	
Plantar surface	Heel–toe 40–50 mm:-1 <40 mm:-2	<50 mm, no crease	Faint red marks	Anterior transverse crease only	Creases on anterior 2/3	Creases over entire sole	
Breast	Impercep-tible	Barely perceptible	Flat areola–no bud	Stripped areola 1–2 mm bud	Raised areola 3–4 mm bud	Full areola 5–10 mm bud	
Eye/ear	Lids fused loosely (-1), tightly (-2)	Lids open, pinna flat, stays folded	Slightly curved pinna; soft; slow recoil	Well-curved pinna, soft but ready recoil	Formed and firm, instant recoil	Thick cartilage, ear stiff	
Genitals male	Scrotum flat, smooth	Scrotum empty, faint rugae	Testes in upper canal rare rugae	Testes descending, few rugae	Testes down, good rugae	Testes pendulous, deep rugae	
Genitals female	Clitoris prominent, labia flat	Prominent clitoris, small labia minora	Prominent clitoris, enlarging minora	Majora & minora equally prominent	Majora large, minora small	Majora cover clitoris & minora	

Maturity rating

Score	Weeks
-10	20
-5	22
0	24
5	26
10	28
15	30
20	32
25	34
30	36
35	38
40	40
45	42
50	44

Figure 10-3. The expanded new Ballard Score includes extremely preterm infants and has been refined to improve accuracy in more mature infants. (Reprinted with permission from Ballard JL, Khoury JC, Wedig K, Wang L, Eilers-Walsman BL, Lipp R. New Ballard score, expanded to include extremely premature infants. J Pediatr 1991;119:417–23.)

be used to identify infants at risk of postnatal complications. For example, infants who are either large or small for their gestational ages are at increased risk of alterations of glucose homeostasis, and appropriate tests (eg, serum glucose screen) are indicated.

Assessment of Late-Preterm Status

Infants born at 34 0/7–36 6/7 weeks of gestation are referred to as late-preterm. Late-preterm infants are physiologically immature and have limited compensatory responses to the extrauterine environment compared with term infants. Late-preterm infants are at a greater risk of acute as well as long-term morbidity and mortality than are term infants. During the birth hospitalization, temperature instability, hypoglycemia, respiratory distress, apnea, hyperbilirubinemia, and feeding difficulties are more likely to be diagnosed in late-preterm infants than term infants. During the first month after birth, late-preterm infants are more likely than term infants to be rehospitalized for hyperbilirubinemia requiring phototherapy, feeding difficulties, dehydration, suspected sepsis, parenteral antibiotic treatment, apneic events, and poor weight gain.

Risk factors that have been identified for rehospitalization or neonatal morbidity in late-preterm infants include being the first-born, being suboptimally breastfed at discharge, having a mother who had labor and delivery complications, being a recipient of public insurance at delivery, and being of Asian or Pacific Island descent. Collaborative counseling before delivery by obstetric and neonatal care providers about the outcomes of late-preterm births is warranted unless precluded by emergent conditions. In addition, discharge criteria, which recognize the specific vulnerabilities of these infants, must be met before discharge home.

Risk Assessment for Neonatal Conditions

No later than 2 hours after birth, the clinical care team should evaluate the infant's status and assess risk of neonatal illness and complications (see also "Initial Assessment" earlier in this section). Risks can be assessed through the history as documented on the antepartum and intrapartum records, as well as from the gestational age assessment and growth parameter determination. If the infant's health care provider is not present at the delivery, he or she should be notified of the admission and of the status of the infant within a time frame established by institutional policy.

Nursery policies should delineate those conditions (eg, low birth weight or small for gestational age) that require specific actions by nurses or immediate notification of the infant's health care provider, as defined by institutional policy. Clinical conditions, such as suspected maternal infection or Apgar scores less than 7 at 5 minutes or more, are associated with increased risk of neonatal illness and should prompt immediate notification of the infant's health care provider. The obstetrician should be notified of the infant's status in a timely manner, particularly if problems or complications arise.

If immediate attention is not indicated, the infant's health care provider should examine the apparently normal infant within 24 hours after birth and within 24 hours before discharge from the hospital. This may be accomplished with at least one physical examination, ideally in the mother's room. The results of the examination should be recorded on the newborn infant's medical record and discussed with the parents. The health care provider should be made aware of any deviation or variance in the infant's transition, postpartum stabilization, or risk status.

Transitional Care

After the initial evaluation of the newborn infant's condition, a care plan should be established, and the infant should be carefully observed during the subsequent stabilization–transition period (the first 2–24 hours after birth). If the infant is healthy and stable, the care plan should facilitate ongoing contact between the mother and the infant (eg, rooming-in together) during this period. Temperature, heart rate, skin color, peripheral circulation, respiration, level of consciousness, tone, and activity should be monitored and recorded at least once every 30 minutes until the infant's condition has remained stable for 2 hours. Rooming-in for the mother and her infant is optimal because it allows unrestricted contact and feeding. Mothers should be assessed (ie, fall assessment) for impairment from fatigue or intrapartum drugs and the baby should be moved to a separate sleep surface (eg, sidecar or bassinet) if the mother appears tired, sleepy, or impaired.

Clinical care includes the following: conjunctival (eye) care as required by state law, administration of vitamin K, care of the skin, care of the umbilical cord, male circumcision (if chosen by the parents) and care of the circumcision site, and provision for appropriate clothing. Skin-to-skin care or breastfeeding during painful procedures, such as vitamin K administration and heel sticks, is recommended to reduce infant distress. Hospital staff can easily assess the infant's status in the mother's room, provided that the infant is unwrapped and lighting is adequate. The infant should be observed for any signs of illness or variations from normal behavior (as listed in Box 10-1). Knowledge and understanding of the processes of newborn transition allow for early detection of newborn disorders. For example, meconium is typically passed within the first 24 hours after birth. If a term infant has not passed meconium by 48 hours after birth, the lower gastrointestinal tract may be obstructed. Urine is normally passed within the first 12 hours after birth. Failure to void within the first 24 hours may indicate genitourinary obstruction or abnormality. The infant's health care provider should be informed to determine if the clinical event requires immediate medical attention.

Box 10-1. Potential Signs of Neonatal Illness

- Temperature instability
- Change in activity, including refusal of feedings
- Unusual skin color (pallor, jaundice, plethora, mottling)
- Abnormal cardiac or respiratory rate and rhythm
- Abdominal distention or bilious vomiting and gastric aspirate
- Excessive lethargy, sleepiness, or hypotonicity
- Jitteriness, irritability, or abnormal movements
- Delayed (more than 24 hours) or abnormal stools
- Delayed voiding (more than 12 hours)
- Weight change that is greater than expected

Conjunctival (Eye) Care

In many states, prophylaxis against gonococcal ophthalmia neonatorum is mandated by law or regulation for all newborn infants, including those born by cesarean delivery. Antimicrobial ophthalmic prophylaxis soon after delivery is recommended for all newborn infants but should be delayed until after the initial breastfeeding in the delivery room. A variety of topical agents appear to be equally efficacious, but only erythromycin ophthalmic ointment is currently commercially available in the United States. Application of a 1-cm ribbon of sterile ophthalmic ointment containing erythromycin (0.5%) in each lower conjunctival sac is recommended. Care should be taken to ensure that the agent reaches all parts of the conjunctival sac. The eyes should not be irrigated with saline or distilled water after application of any of these agents; however, after 1 minute, excess ointment can be wiped away with sterile cotton. Topical agents are not effective against *Chlamydia trachomatis* (see also "Chlamydial Infection" in Chapter 12).

Gonococcal ophthalmia or disseminated gonococcal infection can occur in infants born to women with gonococcal disease. Single-dose systemic antibiotic therapy (1 dose of ceftriaxone 25–50 mg per kg, intravenously or intramuscularly, not to exceed 125 mg) is effective as treatment for gonococcal ophthalmia and as prophylaxis for disseminated disease (see also "Gonorrhea" in Chapter 12).

Administration of Vitamin K

Every newborn infant should receive a single parenteral dose of natural vitamin K_1 oxide (phytonadione) (0.5–1 mg) to prevent vitamin K-dependent hemorrhagic disease of the newborn. This dose should be administered shortly after birth but delayed until after the first breastfeeding in the delivery room. Oral administration of vitamin K is not as effective as parenteral administration for the prevention of late hemorrhagic disease.

Skin Care

Skin care, including bathing, may be important for the health and appearance of the individual newborn infant and for infection control within the nursery. Removal of blood and secretions from the skin after delivery may minimize the risk of infection with potentially contaminating microorganisms, such as hepatitis B virus, herpes simplex virus, and HIV. In the absence of maternal infection risk factors, such as HIV, the first bath should be postponed at least until breastfeeding has been initiated and the infant's thermal stability is ensured because bathing can be associated with significant heat loss. In a preintervention and postintervention study, bathing 12 hours after birth was associated with higher rates of exclusive breastfeeding. The medical and nursing services of each hospital should develop guidelines regarding the time of the first bath, measures to protect against excessive heat loss, circumstances and methods of skin cleansing, and the roles of personnel and parents. The effects on the newborn's skin should be considered in selecting skin care techniques. Whole-body bathing may not be necessary. Sterile cotton sponges (not gauze) soaked with warm water may be used to remove blood and meconium from the infant's face, head, and body. Alternatively, the infant can be cleansed with a mild, nonmedicated soap and then rinsed with water. After washing by either method, the infant should be dried well, with particular attention to drying the head to minimize heat loss.

For the remainder of the infant's stay in the hospital, local skin care of the buttocks and perianal regions with warm water and cotton, a mild soap and water, or baby wipes at diaper changes should be adequate. Ideally, agents used on the infant's skin should be dispensed in single-use containers, or each infant should have a personal dispenser.

Umbilical Cord Care

The umbilical cord should be kept clean and dry. Antiseptics, including alcohol, triple dye, and chlorhexidine, have no advantage over dry umbilical cord care in reducing the incidence of omphalitis in developed countries, although these agents may reduce neonatal morbidity and mortality in low-resource settings.

Circumcision

Existing scientific evidence indicates that the preventive health benefits of elective circumcision of newborn male infants outweigh the risks of this procedure. Benefits include significant reductions in the risk of urinary tract infection in the first year and, subsequently, in the risk of heterosexual acquisition of HIV and other sexually transmitted infections. Although health benefits are not great enough to recommend routine circumcision for all newborn male infants, the benefits of circumcision are sufficient to justify access to this procedure for families choosing it and to warrant third-party payment for circumcision. There are no data indicating that the circumcision of newborn male infants who may have been exposed to herpes simplex virus at birth should be postponed. It may be prudent, however, to delay circumcision for approximately 1 month for those at the highest risk of disease (eg, male infants delivered vaginally by women with active genital lesions).

The exact incidence of complications after circumcision is not known, but data indicate that the rate is low and that the most common complications are local infection and bleeding. To make an informed choice, the parents of all male newborn infants should be given accurate and unbiased information on circumcision and be given an opportunity to discuss this decision with a medical care provider. Parents will need to weigh medical information in the context of their own religious, ethical, and cultural beliefs and practices, as it is the parents who must ultimately decide whether circumcision is in the best interests of their male child. Information sheets for parents about circumcision are available through AAP.

Analgesia should be provided if circumcision is performed. Swaddling, sucrose by mouth, and acetaminophen administration may reduce the stress response but are not sufficient for the operative pain and cannot be recommended as the sole method of analgesia. Although local anesthesia and combination preparations of lidocaine and prilocaine provide some anesthesia benefit, ring blocks and dorsal penile blocks have been proved to be more effective. Postprocedure care of the circumcised newborn male infant should include cleaning and protecting the site from infection and irritation. With each diaper change, the penis should be cleaned and petroleum jelly can be placed over the surgical site. The jelly can be placed on a bandage or clean gauze pad and applied directly on the penis or placed on the diaper in the area with which the penis comes into contact. The petroleum jelly is not necessary for healing, but it keeps the surgical site from sticking to the diaper and causing irritation and bleeding when the diaper is removed. A postprocedure care regimen such as this is recommended for approximately 4–7 days after circumcision.

If the family decides against circumcision, gentle washing of the genital area while bathing is sufficient for normal hygiene of the uncircumcised penis. Because of physiologic adhesions, the foreskin usually does not retract fully for several years and should not be forcibly retracted.

Clothing

Once thermal stability has been established, most newborn infants require only a cotton shirt or gown without buttons in addition to a soft diaper. A supply of soft, clean cotton clothing, bed pads, sheets, and blankets should be kept at the bedside. Nontoxic dyes should be used to label clothing, blankets, or other items used in the care of newborn infants. A cap prevents excessive heat loss from the head of newborn infants.

Neonatal Nutrition

Breastfeeding

There are diverse and important advantages to infants, mothers, families, and society for breastfeeding and the use of human milk for infant feeding. These include health, nutritional, immunologic, developmental, psychological, social, economic, and environmental benefits. Human milk feeding supports optimal growth and development of the infant while decreasing the risk of a variety of acute and chronic diseases. Prenatal counseling and education regarding methods of newborn feeding may allow correction of misperceptions about feeding methods. Even mothers who are initially undecided or hesitant to breastfeed usually can do so successfully with appropriate counseling, education, and knowledgeable support, including that of a certified lactation consultant. Formula feeding should not be portrayed as equivalent to human milk feeding. If the mother chooses not to breastfeed after these interventions have been implemented, she should be supported in her decision.

Initiation of Breastfeeding

Support of successful breastfeeding begins during pregnancy. Prenatal care should include discussion of prior breastfeeding experience, feeding plans, and breast care. Ascertainment of a history of breast surgery, trauma, or prior lactation failure is important because these situations may present special challenges to successful breastfeeding.

The integration of breastfeeding into the total care of the newborn infant in the first months of life should be discussed. The mother should be offered the opportunity and be encouraged to breastfeed her infant as soon as possible after delivery. A healthy newborn infant is capable of latching on to the breast without specific assistance within the first hour after birth, and breastfeeding should be initiated within the first postnatal hour unless medically contraindicated. Appropriately triaged healthy term infants should be placed in direct skin-to skin contact with their mothers and allowed to attempt breastfeeding immediately after birth and should remain there, with frequent assessments by hospital personnel. Care should be taken to monitor the infant's nose to avoid positions that obstruct breathing, which may lead to sudden collapse. Skin-to-skin care should be encouraged throughout the postpartum stay, whenever possible.

Rooming-in with the mother facilitates breastfeeding. From the time of delivery to discharge from the hospital, the healthy mother and her healthy infant should be together continuously. The mother should be encouraged to offer the breast whenever the infant shows early signs of hunger (eg, increased alertness, increased physical activity, mouthing, or rooting), not to wait until the infant cries.

When awake, the newborn infant should be encouraged to feed frequently (8–12 breastfeedings every 24 hours) until satiety to help stimulate milk production. Scheduling specific times for feedings is not encouraged. In the early weeks after birth, an infant may need to be aroused to feed if 4 hours have elapsed since the last nursing. This is especially true for a late-preterm infant. Usually, it is practical to alternate the breast used to initiate the feeding and to equalize the time spent at each breast over the day. When satisfied, the infant will fall asleep or detach, although some infants may fall asleep before consuming sufficient nutrition and should be stimulated to continue feeding.

Supplemental feedings including water, glucose water, formula, and other fluids should not be given to the breastfeeding infant unless ordered by the health care provider after documentation of a medical indication. Supplementation of the breastfed infant is best accomplished with expressed human milk or formula, and water or glucose water is almost never indicated. Intermittent bottle-feeding of a breastfed newborn infant may lessen the success of breastfeeding. If the infant's appetite is partially satisfied by supplements, the infant will take less from the breast, and milk production will be diminished.

Monitoring the Breastfed Newborn

During the newborn hospitalization, trained caregivers should use a standardized evaluation tool, such as the LATCH (Latch, Audible swallowing, nipple Type, Comfort, Help) score to assess breastfeeding. The mother should be encouraged to record the time of each feeding, as well as the infant's urine and stool output, during the early days of breastfeeding to facilitate assessment of her infant's milk intake.

A pediatrician or other knowledgeable and experienced health care professional should see the newborn infant at 3–5 days of age or within 48 hours of discharge. A second ambulatory visit should be scheduled when the infant is 2–3 weeks of age, unless indicated earlier, to monitor progress. The initial visit should include measurement of the infant's weight, a physical examination (especially for jaundice and hydration), questions about maternal history of breast problems (including pain or engorgement), assessment of the infant's elimination patterns (expect three to five urine eliminations and three to four stool eliminations per day by 3–5 days of age, and four to six urine eliminations and three to six stool eliminations per day by 5–7 days of age), and documentation of the transition in stools from meconium to yellow around 3–4 days after birth. If the infant is breastfeeding, a caregiver knowledgeable in breastfeeding, latch, swallowing, and infant satiety should observe an actual feeding and document successful performance of these tasks in the medical record.

Tracking an infant's weight provides a useful assessment of adequacy of breast milk intake. Weight can be plotted on hour-specific curves for vaginal or cesarean delivery (Fig. 10-4; www.newbornweight.org) to assist with determining when a term infant requires a careful evaluation of the feeding techniques being used and the adequacy of breastfeeding. Some mothers may experience a delay in lactogenesis, such as that associated with primiparity, maternal obesity, diabetes, hypertensive disorders of pregnancy, cesarean delivery, or retained placental fragments. If unrecognized, delayed lactogenesis may lead to significant dehydration in the infant, hypernatremia, and hyperbilirubinemia. First-time breastfeeding mothers are most likely to have difficulty in recognizing delayed lactogenesis and its associated signs and consequences. Excessive or prolonged infant weight loss should prompt a thorough evaluation by the pediatric care provider, obstetric care provider, or both (with a certified lactation consultant as needed); close monitoring of the infant; and consideration of supplementation with infant formula. Although previous literature suggested that failure to regain birth weight by 10 days required further evaluation, a very large population-based study found that only about one half of infants had regained their birth weight by that time. Plotting the infant's weight change from birth weight on the appropriate graph (Fig. 10-5) can provide guidance on the need for further evaluation. Although delayed onset of lactogenesis is relatively common, true failure of lactogenesis occurs far less frequently, and with support, breastfeeding can usually be established. Exclusive breastfeeding is the ideal nutrition and is almost always sufficient to support optimal growth and development for the healthy term infant for approximately 6 months after delivery. In families with a strong history of allergy, breastfeeding is likely to be especially

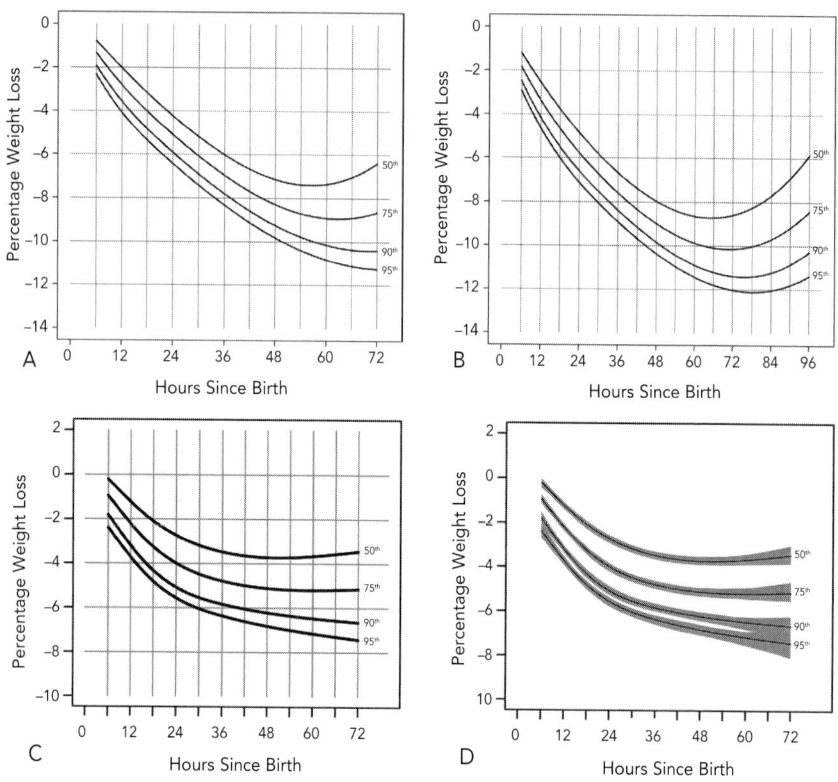

Figure 10-4. Estimated percentile curves for percent weight loss by time after birth for vaginal deliveries (**A** and **C**) or for cesarean deliveries (**B** and **D**) for breastfed (**A** and **B**) and formula-fed (**C** and **D**) infants. An online calculator for these graphs is available at https://www.newbornweight.org. (Adapted, with permission, from Flaherman VJ, Schaefer EW, Kuzniewicz MW, Li SX, Walsh EM, Paul IM. Early weight loss nomograms for exclusively breastfed newborns. Pediatrics 2015;135:e16–23 *and* Miller JR, Flaherman VJ, Schaefer EW, Kuzniewicz MW, Li SX, Walsh EM, et al. Early weight loss nomograms for formula fed newborns. Hosp Pediatr 2015;5:263–8.)

beneficial. Infants weaned before the age of 12 months should not receive cow's milk feedings; instead, they should receive iron-fortified infant formula.

Contraindications to Breastfeeding

Contraindications to breastfeeding include certain maternal infectious diseases and medications. A mother with active herpes simplex virus infection may breastfeed her infant if she has no vesicular lesions in the breast area, as long as she observes careful hand hygiene. A mother who has herpes simplex lesions on a breast should not breastfeed her infant on that breast until the lesions are cleared. Endometritis or mastitis that is being treated with antibiotics is not a contraindication to breastfeeding.

Despite the demonstrated benefits of breastfeeding, there are some situations in which breastfeeding is not in the best interest of the infant. These include the newborn infant with classic galactosemia, who must be fed nonlactose-based formula, the newborn infant whose mother is positive for human T-cell lymphotropic virus type I or II, and the newborn infant whose mother uses nonmedical drugs. In situations where maternal breast milk confers specific medical advantages (ie, very-low-birth-weight infants), the clinician must weigh the risks and benefits of formula versus maternal milk, which may be contaminated by nonmedical drugs (eg, tetrahydrocannabinol). In the United States and other developed countries where formula is safe and readily available, women infected with HIV should not breastfeed their infants (see also Chapter 10). Mothers who have received certain radioactive materials should not breastfeed as long as there is radioactivity in the milk, and mothers who are receiving antimetabolites or chemotherapy should not breastfeed until the medication has cleared from the milk. Rarely, a specific vaccine, such as live-attenuated rabies, is contraindicated during

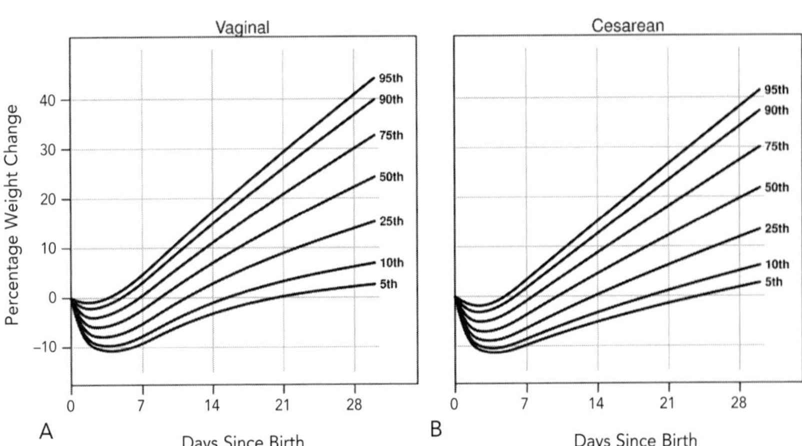

Figure 10-5. Estimated percentile curves of percentage weight change by time after birth. **A**, Vaginal delivery. **B**, Cesarean delivery. (Reprinted with permission from Paul IM, Schaefer EW, Miller JR, Kuzniewicz MW, Li SX, Walsh EM, et al. Weight change nomograms for the first month after birth. Pediatrics 2016;138:e20162625.)

breastfeeding. For up to date information on vaccinations and breastfeeding, see www.cdc.gov/breastfeeding/recommendations/vaccinations.htm.

Conditions That Are Not Contraindications to Breastfeeding

Maternal medication-assisted recovery with methadone or buprenorphine is not a contraindication to breastfeeding. Certain maternal conditions have been shown to be compatible with breastfeeding, including positive test results for hepatitis B surface antigen (HBsAg), if the infant receives hepatitis B vaccine and hepatitis B immune globulin (breastfeeding need not be delayed while waiting for the administration of hepatitis B vaccine and hepatitis B immune globulin); positive test results for hepatitis C (either hepatitis C virus antibody or hepatitis C virus-RNA-positive blood) because there have been no reported cases of transmission through human milk; uncomplicated maternal fever or intraamniotic infection; and seropositivity (not recent conversions) for cytomegalovirus (CMV), if the infant is term. Preterm infants born to women who become seropositive for CMV during lactation can develop a sepsis-like syndrome from CMV excretion in human milk (and all maternal mucosal surfaces). Pasteurization of milk inactivates CMV, and freezing milk at -20°C (-4°F) decreases viral titers but does not eliminate CMV reliably. However, the benefits of human milk for preterm infants are thought to outweigh the risk of acquiring the CMV sepsis-like syndrome.

Most medications are safe for use during breastfeeding. Health care providers should consult lactation pharmacology resources, such as LactMed (www.toxnet.nlm.nih.gov/newtoxnet/lactmed.htm), for up-to-date information on individual medications because inappropriate advice often can lead women to discontinue breastfeeding unnecessarily. Information about drug safety in pregnancy should not be extrapolated to breastfeeding, as the physiology of the placenta and breast are not the same. For example, warfarin crosses the placenta and can cause embryopathy, but minimal amounts enter breast milk, so it is considered to be safe during lactation. Counseling regarding medication use during lactation should address the risks of drug exposure through breast milk and the risks of interrupting lactation. There are few drugs that are absolute contraindications to breastfeeding. The mother should discuss the use of these medications with her health care provider and infant's health care provider if she wishes to continue breastfeeding. It must be determined whether the drug therapy is needed, whether a safer drug is available, and whether an infant's drug exposure can be minimized by having the woman take the medication after feedings. If the drug presents a risk to the infant, the infant should be carefully monitored to detect any adverse effects, and consideration should be given to measuring blood concentrations. Breastfeeding mothers may use oral contraceptives once lactation has been established but it is preferred that these be low-dose estrogen or progestin-only pills to limit the effect on milk production (see also "Postpartum Contraception" in Chapter 8).

Human Milk Storage

There are many situations in which a mother might be separated from her infant, necessitating her to express and store her milk. A mother who is in school or employed outside of the home can maintain exclusive human milk feeding by providing expressed milk to be given in her absence; therefore, it is important to encourage and support mothers in providing their infants with expressed milk. All mothers who provide milk for their infants should be instructed in the proper techniques of milk collection and storage to minimize bacterial contamination. Careful hand hygiene is critical before handling the breast, the equipment, or the milk. Previous practices of washing the breast and discarding the first expressed milk did not result in a decrease in bacterial colonization of the milk and, therefore, are not necessary. Although manual expression, when performed correctly, yields relatively uncontaminated milk, many women prefer to use a breast pump. All parts of the pump that are in contact with the milk should be washed carefully with hot, soapy water, and rinsed and dried thoroughly after each use.

The Academy of Breastfeeding Medicine recommends that fresh expressed milk be stored in sterile glass or plastic containers or plastic bags that are free of bisphenol A and made specifically for human milk storage. According to the Academy of Breastfeeding Medicine, milk that is refrigerated (at or below 4°C [39°F]) should optimally be used within 72 hours, although 5–8 days is acceptable under very clean conditions (Table 10-1). Frozen milk should optimally be stored for up to 6 months, although 12 months is acceptable. Frozen milk should be thawed quickly (usually by holding the container under warm running water or setting it in a container of warm water), using precautions to avoid contamination from the water, or thawed gradually in the refrigerator at or below 4°C (39°F). Human milk should not be defrosted in extremely hot water or in a microwave oven. The very high temperatures that may be reached with these methods can destroy valuable components of the milk and may result in thermal injury to the infant. Previously frozen milk thawed for 24 hours should not be left at room temperatures for more

TABLE 10-1. Breast Milk Storage Guidelines

Location of Storage	Temperature	Maximum Recommended Storage Duration
Room Temperature	16–29°C (60–85°F)	3–4 hours optimal 6–8 hours acceptable under very clean conditions
Refrigerator	4°C (39°F) or below	5–8 days under very clean conditions
Freezer	below −17°C (0°F)	6 months optimal 12 months acceptable

Reprinted with permission from ABM clinical protocol #8: human milk storage information for home use for full-term infants (original protocol March 2004; revision #1 March 2010). Academy of Breastfeeding Medicine Protocol Committee [published erratum appears in Breastfeed Med 2011;6:159]. Breastfeed Med 2010;5:127–30.

than a few hours because of its reduced ability to inhibit bacterial growth. Whether thawed breast milk can be safely refrozen is uncertain. When using human milk in neonatal care units, it is essential to have policies and procedures for storing the milk, appropriately identifying the milk, and checking the milk before giving it to an infant (see also "Milk and Formula Preparation Areas" in Chapter 2).

Banked Donor Milk

Banked human milk may be a suitable alternative for infants whose mothers are unable or unwilling to provide their own milk. Accredited human milk banks in North America follow national guidelines for quality control of screening and testing of donors and pasteurize all milk before distribution. Human milk from other sources, such as friends or the internet, is not recommended because of concerns about infectious disease transmission, adulteration (eg, with cow milk or water), or drug or allergen content. Information on the suitability of milk donations is available from the Human Milk Banking Association of America at www.hmbana.org/donate-milk.

Use of Formula Milk Preparations

If a mother chooses not to breastfeed or is medically unable to breastfeed her infant, the infant may be prescribed a standard infant formula. Fresh cow's milk should not be given for the first 12 months. The health care provider caring for the infant should direct the selection of milk formula. Appropriate hospital committees and the director of the newborn nursery should review the components of marketed formula-milk preparations before their use. Direct marketing and distribution of formula packages should be discouraged for all newborn infants.

Many hospitals use prepared formula units with separate nipples that allow for ready attachment to the bottles just before use. These need not be refrigerated and may be stored in a convenient, clean, cool area. The sterile cap should be kept on the nipple until the infant is ready to be fed. If there is a special area where nipples are uncapped and placed on the bottle, it should be kept very clean and should be used only for formula preparation, donor human milk, or expressed milk handling. Alternatively, nipples may be uncapped and attached to bottles at the mother's bedside just before feeding. The formula and nipple unit should be used as soon as possible, certainly within 4 hours after the bottle is uncapped, and then discarded. Particular attention is needed to maintain hygiene and safety, prevent cross-contamination of oral feeding units, and ensure correct identification of the infant.

Vitamin and Mineral Supplementation

Vitamin D

The vitamin D content of human milk is low, and rickets can occur in deeply pigmented breastfed infants or in those with inadequate exposure to sunlight. Adequate exposure to sunlight is difficult to guarantee and supplementation at the recommended dose is safe. To prevent rickets and vitamin D deficiency in healthy infants, a vitamin D intake of at least 400 international units per day has been recommended. Breastfed and partially breastfed infants should be supplemented with 400 international units per day of vitamin D beginning in the first several days after birth. Alternatively, maternal supplementation with 6,400 international units of vitamin D in breastfeeding women provides adequate vitamin D in the breast milk for the infant. Current recommendations for preterm infants include higher intake of vitamin D: 400–1,000 international units per kg per day. Formula fed infants do not need vitamin D supplementation unless they are consistently ingesting less than 1 liter per day of vitamin D fortified formula. Fluoride supplementation for breastfed and bottle-fed infants can begin at age 6 months.

Iron

The iron content of human milk is low; however, the bioavailability is high. Approximately 50% of the iron in breast milk is absorbed by infants who are breastfed exclusively. Breastfed and partially breastfed infants who receive human milk for more than one half their daily feedings should be given supplemental elemental iron (1 mg per kg per day) starting at 6 months of age. Preterm infants may have variable body iron stores at time of hospital discharge; consequently, preterm infants should receive at least 2 mg per kg per day of supplemental iron. Formula-fed infants should be placed on iron-containing milk formulas that contain 12 mg of elemental iron per liter. Term infants consuming commercial milk formulas do not need vitamin and mineral supplementation for the first 6 months of life.

Preventive Care

Immunization

Hepatitis B

Each hospital should establish procedures to assess the newborn's status regarding hepatitis exposure and timely, appropriate intervention and immunization (see also "Hepatitis B Virus" in Chapter 12). Early hepatitis B immunization is recommended for all medically stable infants with birth weights greater than 2 kg. If the mother is hepatitis B surface antigen (HBsAg)-negative, all medically stable infants weighing more than 2,000 g at birth should receive the first dose of vaccine within 24 hours of birth. Infants with birth weights less than 2,000 g born to HBsAg-negative mothers should receive the hepatitis B vaccine at 1 month of age or at hospital discharge (whichever is first).

If the mother is HBsAg-positive, hepatitis B immune globulin and hepatitis B vaccine should be administered to all infants, regardless of birth weight, at different sites within 12 hours of birth. Detailed information regarding treatment of all infants, including those whose mother's HBsAg status is positive or unknown, is presented in Chapter 12, with a flow diagram in Figure 12-1 (for more information, see also "Hepatitis B Virus" in Chapter 12).

Other Vaccines

Neonatal intensive care units should implement guidelines for immunization of term and preterm infants who require prolonged hospital stays. Preterm infants should begin the immunization series at the usual chronologic age of 2 months, unless otherwise indicated for a specific vaccine or disease process (see also "Immunization of Hospitalized Infants" in Chapter 11).

Palivizumab should be administered for respiratory syncytial virus prophylaxis when indicated (see also "Respiratory Syncytial Virus" in Chapter 12). Maternal immunity is the only effective strategy for influenza protection in newborn infants because the vaccine is not approved for use in infants younger than 6 months.

Newborn Screening

Newborn screening programs are mandated, state-based public health programs that provide infants in the United States with presymptomatic testing and necessary follow-up care for a variety of medical conditions. The goal of these essential public health programs is to decrease morbidity and mortality by screening for disorders for which early intervention will improve health outcomes. Newborn screening programs test infants for various congenital disorders, including metabolic conditions, endocrinopathies, hemoglobinopathies, cystic fibrosis, hearing loss and, more recently, severe combined immunodeficiency and related T-cell lymphocyte deficiencies, and critical congenital heart disease. Most of the disorders screened through these programs have no clinical findings at birth.

Newborn Blood Spot Screening

Almost all states have adopted the 2010 Recommended Uniform Screening Panel suggested by the U.S. Secretary of Health and Human Services' Advisory Committee on Heritable Disorders in Newborns and Children. The list of recommended conditions for newborn screening is continually being evaluated. For an updated list, see the Secretary's Advisory Committee on Heritable Disorders in Newborns and Children website (www.hrsa.gov/advisorycommittees/mchbadvisory/heritabledisorders/). Although the newborn screening program in most states includes the Recommended Uniform Screening Panel, there is some variability from state to state. The selection of an individual state's screening panel is influenced by the disease prevalence within the state, detection rates, and cost considerations. The National Newborn Screening and Global Resource Center maintains a current list of conditions screened for in each state (www.genes-r-us.uthscsa.edu/resources/consumer/statemap.htm).

Newborn blood spot screening programs are developed and managed on the state level and operate through collaborations between public health programs, laboratories, hospitals, pediatricians, subspecialists, and specialty diagnostic centers.

A comprehensive screening program includes the following components:

- Education of parents and practitioners about newborn screening and their participation in the activity
- Reliable acquisition and transportation of adequate specimens
- Reliable and prompt performance of screening tests
- Prompt retrieval and follow-up of individuals with test results that are out of range
- Appropriate further testing of individuals with out-of-range test results to establish accurate diagnoses
- Appropriate intervention, treatment, and follow-up of affected individuals
- Education, genetic counseling, and psychosocial support for families with affected newborns

Every birthing facility should establish routines to ensure that all newborn infants are screened in accordance with state law. States test newborn infants primarily through blood samples collected from heel pricks that are placed on a special filter paper. Umbilical cord blood is never an appropriate specimen because it will be inaccurate for detection of disorders in which metabolite accumulation occurs after birth and after the initiation of feeding. Newborn screening blood specimens are ideally collected between 24 hours and 48 hours of age and sent to the designated state newborn screening laboratory as soon as possible. If the initial specimen is obtained before the infant is 24 hours old, most states recommend that a second specimen be obtained to decrease the probability of false-negative test results for disorders with metabolite accumulation (eg, phenylketonuria) or false-positive test results (eg, hypothyroidism) as a consequence of early testing. Some states also mandate, or strongly recommend, that an additional newborn screening blood specimen be collected on all infants at 10–14 days of age, in order to reduce the chance of missed identification of infants with clinically significant disorders. Regardless of the screening test results, diagnostic testing should be performed if clinically indicated, as some affected infants will not be identified because of individual or biologic variations, very early discharge, or administrative or laboratory error.

An adequate dried blood specimen must be provided to the laboratory for accurate testing. Limitations for obtaining an adequate specimen include infants who receive a transfusion or total parenteral nutrition, are sick, or are preterm. The Clinical and Laboratory Standards Institute recommends that screening of preterm and sick newborn infants be performed on admission to the NICU, at 48–72 hours of age, and again either at 28 days of age or discharge (whichever is sooner). For these infants, nurseries should develop protocols that comply with state regulations.

The responsibility for transmitting the screening test results to the health care providers should rest with the authority or agency that performed the test. However, primary care providers must develop policies and procedures to ensure that newborn screening is conducted, that results are transmitted to them in a timely fashion, and that the information is documented in the medical record. Primary care providers also must develop strategies to employ should these systems fail.

In order to respond appropriately, primary care providers require immediate access to clinical and diagnostic information and guidance. The American College of Medical Genetics and Genomics ACT sheets and confirmatory algorithms for the various disorders included in newborn screening panels are a valuable source of such guidance. The ACT sheets describe the short-term actions a health professional should consider in communicating with the family and determining the appropriate steps in the follow-up of the infant that has screened positive for a particular disorder. The ACT sheets are available online at www.acmg.net/ACMG/Publications/ACT_Sheets_and_Confirmatory_Algorithms/ACMG/Publications/ACT_Sheets_and_Confirmatory_Algorithms/ACT_sheets_Homepage.aspx?hkey=6d43e3d3-71fd-49f4-88d5-7197238f9f33.

Hearing Screening

The prevalence of newborn hearing loss is approximately 1–2 per 1,000 live births, with an incidence of 1 per 1,000 in the normal newborn nursery population and 20–40 per 1,000 in the newborn intensive care unit population. In accordance with the recommendations of the AAP Task Force on Improving the Effectiveness of Newborn Hearing Screening, Diagnosis, and Intervention and the Joint Committee on Infant Hearing, the hearing of all infants should be screened by 1 month of age. Every hospital with an obstetric service and all children's hospitals that accept newborn infants should develop and implement a universal newborn hearing screening protocol to ensure that all infants are screened in accordance with jurisdictional guidelines. Screening should be performed with a physiologic measure, using an automated auditory brainstem response device, an otoacoustic emission device, or a combination of the two. Every effort should be made to complete screening before discharge from the hospital. Many programs use a two-step screening protocol, in which all infants have an initial screening test. If they pass the screening test, no further testing is done. However, if they fail the first screening test, a repeat screening test is performed before discharge. Other screening protocols include a return visit after hospital discharge for outpatient hearing screening.

All infants who fail the newborn hearing screening test should receive complete diagnostic testing by a qualified pediatric audiologist by no later than 3 months of age, with intervention provided no later than 6 months of age from health care and education professionals with expertise in hearing loss and deafness in infants and young children. Tracking and close follow-up by the state Early Hearing Detection and Intervention programs are essential to ensure that children receive appropriate evaluation and intervention.

Because children may develop progressive or late-onset hearing loss, all infants should receive ongoing surveillance of communicative development beginning at 2 months of age during well-child visits in the medical home and should be re-evaluated periodically throughout childhood with objective measures of hearing (see the AAP Recommendations for Preventive Pediatric Health Care [Periodicity Schedule], www.aap.org/en-us/Documents/periodicity_schedule.pdf).

Glucose Homeostasis Screening

Blood glucose concentrations as low as 30 mg per dL are common in healthy newborns at 1–2 hours after birth. These low concentrations usually are transient, asymptomatic, and considered part of normal adaptation to postnatal life. Clinically significant neonatal hypoglycemia reflects an imbalance between supply and use of glucose and alternative fuels and may result from a multitude of disturbed regulatory mechanisms. Current evidence does not support a specific concentration of glucose that can discriminate normal from abnormal or that can predict acute or chronic irreversible neurologic damage. Early identification of at-risk infants and institution of measures to screen for and treat low glucose values in these infants are recommended as a pragmatic approach. The following section describes the screening for neonatal hypoglycemia in at-risk late preterm and term infants. Management of neonatal hypoglycemia is discussed in Chapter 11.

Risk Factors and Clinical Signs. Healthy term newborns born after an entirely normal pregnancy and delivery do not need routine screening and monitoring of blood glucose. Blood glucose concentration should only be measured in term infants who are known to be at risk or who have clinical manifestations. Neonatal hypoglycemia occurs most commonly in infants who are small for gestational age, infants born to mothers who have diabetes, and late preterm infants. Whether otherwise healthy infants who are large for gestational age are at increased risk is uncertain; however, because it is difficult to exclude maternal hyperglycemia or diabetes, these infants also are considered at risk.

The clinical signs of neonatal hypoglycemia are not specific and include a wide range of manifestations that are common in sick newborns, including jitteriness, cyanosis, seizures, apneic episodes, tachypnea, weak or high-pitched cry, floppiness or lethargy, poor feeding, and eye rolling. It is important to screen for other possible underlying disorders (eg, infection). Coma and seizures may occur with prolonged severe neonatal hypoglycemia, such as plasma or blood glucose concentrations lower than 10 mg per dL, and with repetitive hypoglycemia. Because avoidance and treatment of cerebral energy deficiency is the principal concern, greatest attention should be paid to neurologic signs.

When to Screen. Plasma or blood glucose concentration should be measured as soon as possible (minutes, not hours) in any infant who manifests clinical signs compatible with a low blood glucose concentration. At-risk infants should be fed by 1 hour of age and screened 30 minutes after the feeding. Glucose screening should continue until 12 hours of age for infants born to mothers with diabetes and those who are large for gestational age, and until 24 hours of age for late preterm and small-for-gestational-age infants. At-risk asymptomatic infants should be fed every 2–3 hours and screened before each feeding. The target plasma glucose concentration is greater than or equal to 45 mg per dL before feedings. Management of infants who do not achieve target glucose levels is discussed in Chapter 11.

Screening Methods. When neonatal hypoglycemia is suspected, the plasma or blood glucose concentration must be determined immediately by using an enzymatic method (eg, glucose oxidase, hexokinase, or dehydrogenase method). Although a laboratory determination is the most accurate method of measuring the glucose concentration, the results may not be available quickly enough for rapid diagnosis of neonatal hypoglycemia, delaying treatment. Bedside reagent test-strip glucose analyzers can be used if the test is performed carefully and the health care provider is aware of the limited accuracy of these devices. Because of limitations of rapid bedside methods, the glucose concentration must be confirmed by laboratory testing ordered stat. Treatment of suspected neonatal hypoglycemia should not be postponed while waiting for laboratory confirmation (for information on management, see also "Hypoglycemia" in Chapter 11).

Hyperbilirubinemia Screening

Jaundice occurs in most newborn infants. Most jaundice is benign, but because of the potential toxicity of bilirubin, infants must be monitored to identify those who might develop severe hyperbilirubinemia and, in rare cases, acute or chronic bilirubin encephalopathy. Based on a consensus of expert opinion and review of available evidence, universal predischarge bilirubin screening is recommended. This can be accomplished by measuring the total serum bilirubin level (ideally at the time of routine metabolic screening) or the transcutaneous bilirubin level and plotting the result on an hour-specific nomogram to determine the risk of subsequent hyperbilirubinemia that will require treatment (Fig. 10-6). If an infant is discharged before 24 hours postnatal age, the bilirubin should be rechecked within 48 hours.

Each nursery should develop policies and procedures for hyperbilirubinemia screening. These policies should consider the following elements:

- Promotion and support of successful breastfeeding
- Protocols for identification and evaluation of hyperbilirubinemia
- Provision for measurement of the total serum bilirubin or transcutaneous bilirubin concentration in infants who are jaundiced in the first 24 hours
- Recognition that visual estimation of the degree of jaundice can lead to errors, especially in darkly pigmented infants
- Interpretation of all bilirubin levels according to the infant's age in hours (Fig. 10-6)
- Recognition that infants born at less than 38 weeks of gestational age, especially those who are breastfed, are at higher risk of developing hyperbilirubinemia and require closer surveillance and monitoring
- Performance of a systematic assessment on all infants before discharge for the risk of severe hyperbilirubinemia (Box 10-2)

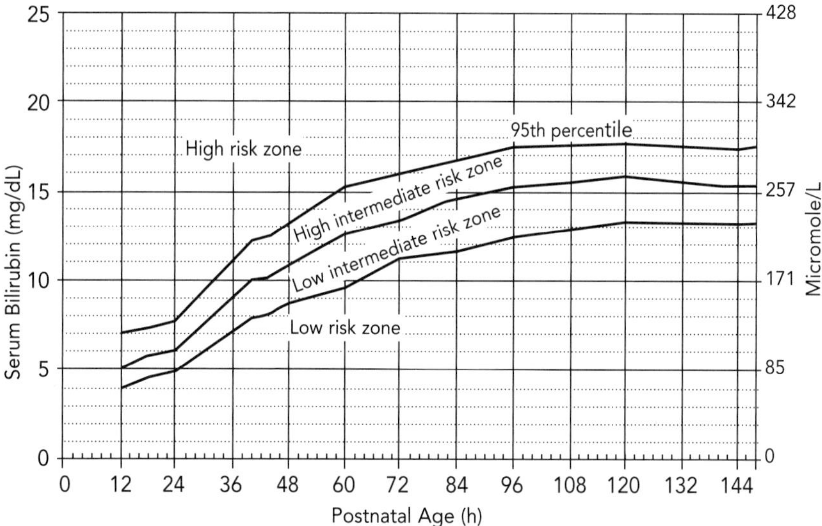

Figure 10-6. Nomogram for risk of developing severe hyperbilirubinemia derived from 2,840 well newborns at 36 or more weeks of gestational age with birth weight of 2,000 g or more or 35 or more weeks of gestational age and birth weight of 2,500 g or more based on the hour-specific serum bilirubin values. (Management of hyperbilirubinemia in the newborn infant 35 or more weeks of gestation. American Academy of Pediatrics Subcommittee on Hyperbilirubinemia [Published Erratum Appears in Pediatrics 2004;114:1138]. Pediatrics 2004;114:297–316.)

- Provision of written and verbal information to parents about newborn jaundice
- Provision of appropriate follow-up based on the time of discharge and the risk assessment
- Treatment, when indicated, with phototherapy or exchange transfusion (see also "Hyperbilirubinemia" in Chapter 11).

Developmental Dysplasia of the Hip Screening

Developmental dysplasia of the hip (DDH) refers to the condition in which the femoral head has an abnormal relationship to the acetabulum. Developmental dysplasia of the hip includes frank dislocation (luxation), partial dislocation (subluxation), instability wherein the femoral head comes in and out of the socket, and an array of radiographic abnormalities that reflect inadequate formation of the acetabulum. The term developmental

Box 10-2. Major Risk Factors for Development of Severe Hyperbilirubinemia in Infants of 35 or More Weeks of Gestation (in Approximate Order of Importance)

- Predischarge total serum bilirubin or transcutaneous concentration in the high-risk zone
- Jaundice observed in the first 24 hours
- Blood group incompatibility with positive direct antiglobulin test, other known hemolytic disease (eg, glucose-6-phosphate dehydrogenase deficiency), elevated end-tidal carbon monoxide corrected for ambient carbon monoxide
- Gestational age 35–36 weeks
- Previous sibling received phototherapy
- Cephalohematoma or significant bruising
- Exclusive breastfeeding, particularly if nursing is not going well and weight loss is excessive
- East Asian race*

*Race as defined by mother's description.

Modified from Management of hyperbilirubinemia in the newborn infant 35 or more weeks of gestation. American Academy of Pediatrics Subcommittee on Hyperbilirubinemia [Published Erratum Appears in Pediatrics 2004;114:1138]. Pediatrics 2004;114:297–316.

more accurately reflects the biologic features of hip dysplasia than does the term congenital because not every dislocated hip is detectable at birth, and hips continue to dislocate throughout the first year of life.

Health care providers should screen all newborn infants for DDH by physical examination and identification of risk factors. The two maneuvers for assessing hip stability in the newborn are the Ortolani and Barlow tests. The Ortolani test elicits the sensation of the dislocated hip reducing, and the Barlow test detects the unstable hip dislocating from the acetabulum. The Ortolani maneuver, in which a subluxated or dislocated femoral head is reduced into the acetabulum with gentle hip abduction by the examiner, is the most important clinical test for detecting newborn hip dysplasia. The Barlow test has no proven predictive value for future hip dislocation. The AAP recommends that if the Barlow test is performed, it be done by gently adducting the hip while palpating for the head falling out the back of the acetabulum and that no posterior-directed force be applied. One can think of the Barlow and Ortolani tests as a continuous smooth gentle maneuver starting with the hip flexed and adducted, with gentle anterior pressure on the trochanter while the hip is abducted to feel whether the hip is locating into the socket, followed by gently adducting the hip and relieving the anterior pressure on the trochanter while sensing whether the hip slips out the back. The examiner should not attempt to forcefully dislocate the femoral head (see video available at www.aap.org/en-us/about-the-aap/Committees-Councils-Sections/Section-on-Orthopaedics/Pages/Policy.aspx). "Hip clicks" without the sensation of instability are clinically insignificant. Evidence strongly supports screening for and treatment of hip dislocation (positive Ortolani test result) and initially observing milder early forms of dysplasia and instability (positive Barlow test result).

Universal newborn screening by ultrasonography is not recommended. Risk factors for DDH are female sex, breech position, or a positive family history. Health care providers should follow a process of care that will minimize the likelihood of late diagnosis of hip dislocation. In the newborn infant, this includes the following:

- Examine the hips of all infants using the Ortolani and Barlow tests.
- Determine the presence of risk factors: breech position, positive family history, and female sex.
- If there are no risk factors and the physical examination is negative, examine the infant's hips according to the AAP periodicity schedule and follow up until the child is walking.
- If the Ortolani test result is positive, refer the newborn to an orthopedist.
- If the Ortolani test result is equivocal, repeat the examination in 2 weeks; depending on the findings at 2 weeks, follow up, refer to an orthopedist, or obtain ultrasonography.
- If the Ortolani test result is negative or equivocal and risk factors are present, consider repeat examination in 2 weeks, referral to an orthopedist, or age-appropriate imaging.

Cyanotic Congenital Heart Disease Screening

In 2011, the U.S. Secretary of Health and Human Services recommended that screening with pulse oximetry for critical congenital heart disease be added to the Recommended Uniform Screening Panel. A detailed description of issues related to implementing screening has been published by AAP.

The publication includes a detailed screening algorithm developed by the Secretary's Advisory Committee on Heritable Disorders in Newborns and Children and also provides detailed recommendation regarding necessary equipment, personnel and training, and appropriate management of a positive screening result (see "Resources").

Infant Safety

Visiting Policies

The father, partner, or support person should be encouraged to remain with the mother throughout the intrapartum and postpartum periods. Flexible and liberal visiting policies for families are encouraged. Some institutions offer sibling classes to prepare other children in the family for the event of childbirth. Contact with the mother and newborn infant in the hospital helps prepare siblings for the new family member and is reassuring for younger children. The presence of siblings may be appropriate in labor, at delivery, or in the postpartum period, as local policy permits. The children must be accompanied by an adult to help them understand what is occurring and to remove them if circumstances demand.

Physical contact of siblings with newborn infants is a topic of ongoing concern because of the possible transmission of viral infectious diseases. If siblings are allowed to have direct contact with the infant, the visit may take place in the mother's private room or, if the mother is not in a private room, in a special sibling visitation area. Thorough hand hygiene, as practiced at the institution, should be required before physical contact with the infant. Parents should share the responsibility of preventing the exposure of their newborn infant to a sibling with a contagious illness by providing accurate information about illness or exposures. Contact of the newborn infant with children other than siblings should be avoided.

An institution that allows sibling visitation should have clearly defined, written policies and procedures that are based on currently available information. Basic guidelines for sibling visits that may serve as the basis for policy formulation are listed as follows:

- Sibling visits should be encouraged for healthy and ill newborn infants.
- Before the visit, a member of the hospital staff should interview the parents to assess the current health of each sibling visitor. Children

with fever or symptoms of an acute illness, such as upper respiratory infection or gastroenteritis, should not be allowed to visit. Children who have been exposed recently to a known communicable disease (eg, chickenpox) should not be allowed to visit.

- Children should be prepared in advance for their visit.
- Children should only visit their siblings.
- Children should practice hand hygiene according to the unit guidelines before patient contact.
- Throughout the visit, parents or another responsible adult should supervise sibling activity.

Infant Security

The threat of infant abduction requires that hospitals have active programs to prevent such an event. Infant abduction can best be minimized by policies that include educating staff about the risk factors for abduction, educating families about safe procedures for handing over their infant, and controlling access to the postpartum area. Each institution should develop a newborn security system to protect the physical safety of newborn infants, families, and staff, which may include the use of electronic sensor devices. When the newborn infant is rooming-in, families should be instructed to hand over their infants only to an individual with a picture identification badge, and they should question why and where their infants are being taken. Access to the labor and delivery and postpartum areas should be controlled. All neonatal care units should be designed to minimize the risk of newborn abduction while maintaining a family-friendly atmosphere. Policies and procedures for visitation, transfer, and discharge of newborn infants should include identification and verification of the infant and designated attendants and visitors. Security drills are helpful to maintain staff competence in carrying out these procedures.

Hospital Discharge and Parent Education

Discharge of Healthy Newborn Infants

The hospital stay of a mother and her newborn infant should be long enough to allow identification of problems and to ensure that the mother is sufficiently recovered and prepared to care for herself and her newborn infant at home. Many neonatal cardiopulmonary problems related to the transition from the intrauterine to the extrauterine environment become apparent during the first 12 hours after birth. Other neonatal problems, such as jaundice, ductal-dependent cardiac lesions, and gastrointestinal obstruction, may require a longer period of observation by skilled and experienced personnel. Breastfeeding adequacy should be evaluated by a trained health care provider and documented before discharge. The length of stay should be based on the unique characteristics of each mother–infant dyad, including the health of the mother, the health and stability of the newborn infant, the ability and confidence of the mother to care for herself and her infant, the adequacy of support systems at home, and access to appropriate follow-up care. Input from the mother and her obstetric care provider and nursing staff should be considered before a decision to discharge a newborn infant is made, and all efforts should be made to keep a mother and her infant together to encourage on-demand breastfeeding.

The timing of discharge from the hospital should be the decision of the health care provider caring for the mother and her infant in consultation with the family, and should not be based on arbitrary policies established by third-party payers. A shortened hospital stay (less than 48 hours after delivery) for healthy, term newborn infants can be accommodated but is not appropriate for every mother and infant. If possible, institutions should develop guidelines through their professional staff in collaboration with appropriate community agencies, including third-party payers, to establish hospital-stay programs for mothers and their healthy, term newborn infants. State and local public health agencies also should be involved in the oversight of existing hospital-stay programs for quality assurance and monitoring. Obstetric care, newborn nursery care, and follow-up care should be considered independent services to be paid as separate packages and not as part of a global fee for maternity-newborn labor and delivery services. Adoption of standardized processes, such as predischarge checklists, may facilitate more uniform implementation of these recommendations across the full spectrum of health care settings where care for newborn infants is provided.

The following minimum criteria should be met before a newborn infant is discharged from the hospital after an uncomplicated pregnancy, labor, and delivery.

- Clinical course and physical examination reveal no abnormalities that require continued hospitalization.

- The infant's vital signs are documented as being within normal ranges, with appropriate variations based on physiologic state, and stable for the 12 hours preceding discharge. These ranges include an axillary temperature of 36.5–37.4°C (97.7–99.3°F), measured properly in an open crib with appropriate clothing, a respiratory rate below 60 bpm and no other signs of respiratory distress, and an awake heart rate of 100–190 bpm. Heart rates as low as 70 bpm while sleeping quietly, without signs of circulatory compromise and responding appropriately to activity, are also acceptable. Sustained heart rates near or above the upper end of this range may require further evaluation.
- The infant has urinated regularly and passed at least one stool spontaneously.
- The infant has completed at least two successful feedings. If the infant is breastfeeding, a caregiver knowledgeable in breastfeeding, latch, swallowing, and infant satiety should observe an actual feeding and document successful performance of these tasks in the medical record. If the infant is bottle-feeding, document that the infant is able to coordinate sucking, swallowing, and breathing while feeding.
- The mother has received adequate information about breastfeeding or formula-feeding before discharge.
- There is no evidence of excessive bleeding at the circumcision site.
- The clinical significance of jaundice, if present before discharge, has been determined, and appropriate management, follow-up plans, or both have been instituted as recommended in the AAP clinical practice guidelines for management of hyperbilirubinemia.
- The infant has been adequately evaluated and monitored for sepsis on the basis of maternal risk factors and in accordance with current guidelines for management of newborns with suspected or proven early-onset sepsis.
- Maternal and infant laboratory tests are available and have been reviewed, including the following:
  - Maternal syphilis, HBsAg, and HIV status.
  - Umbilical cord or newborn blood type and direct Coombs test result, if clinically indicated.

- Initial hepatitis B vaccine has been administered as indicated by the infant's risk status and according to the current immunization schedule.
- If the mother has not previously been vaccinated, she should receive tetanus toxoid, reduced diphtheria toxoid, and acellular pertussis (Tdap) vaccine immediately after the baby is born. Other adolescents and adults who will have or anticipate having close contact with the infant should be encouraged to receive a single dose of Tdap at least 2 weeks before contact, if they have not previously received Tdap. If a mother who gives birth during the flu season has not been previously immunized, she also should receive an influenza vaccination.
- Newborn metabolic, hearing, and pulse oximetry screenings have been completed per hospital protocol and state regulations. If screening metabolic tests were performed before 24 hours of milk feeding, a system for repeating the test during the follow-up visit must be in place in accordance with local or state policy.
- The mother's knowledge, ability, and confidence to provide adequate care for her infant are documented by the fact that training and information has been received in the following areas:
  - — The importance and benefits of breastfeeding for mother and infant
  - — Appropriate urination and stooling frequency for the infant
  - — Umbilical cord, skin, and newborn genital care, as well as temperature assessment and measurement with a thermometer
  - — Signs of illness and common infant problems, particularly jaundice
  - — Infant safety, such as use of an appropriate car safety seat, supine positioning for sleeping, maintaining a smoke-free environment, and sleeping in proximity but not bed sharing
  - — Swaddling techniques that allow the legs to bend up and out at the hips. This position allows for natural development of the hip joints. A useful video can be found at www.hipdysplasia.org/developmental-dysplasia-of-the-hip/hip-healthy-swaddling/
  - — Hand hygiene, especially as a way to reduce infection
- A car safety seat appropriate for the infant's maturity and medical condition that meets Federal Motor Vehicle Safety Standard 213 has been obtained and is available before hospital discharge, and the mother has demonstrated appropriate infant positioning and use to trained hospital personnel.

- Family members or other support persons, including health care providers who are familiar with newborn care and are knowledgeable about lactation and the recognition of jaundice and dehydration, are available to the mother and infant after discharge. Each family should have a telephone number and other resources to contact for lactation assistance.
- A health care provider-directed source of continuing health care (medical home) for the mother and infant has been identified. A telephone number and instructions to follow in the event of a complication or emergency have been provided. The mother should know how to reach the medical home and should have scheduled the infant's first visit, if possible, or know how to do so.
- Family, environmental, and social risk factors have been assessed, and the mother and her other family members have been educated about safe home environment. When the following or other risk factors are present, discharge should be delayed until they are resolved or a plan to safeguard the infant is in place. This plan may involve discussions with social services or state agencies such as child protective services, or both. These risk factors may include, but are not limited to the following:
  - Untreated parental use of nonmedical substances or positive urine toxicology results in the mother or newborn infant consistent with maternal use of drugs or substance use disorder
  - History of child abuse or neglect by any anticipated care provider
  - Mental illness in a parent or another person in the home
  - Lack of social support, particularly for single, first-time mothers
  - No fixed home
  - History of domestic violence, particularly during this pregnancy
  - Adolescent mother, particularly if other aforementioned-listed conditions apply
  - Barriers to adequate follow-up care for the infant, such as lack of transportation to medical care services, lack of easy access to telephone communication, and non–English-speaking parents

Discharge of Late-Preterm Infants

The timing of discharge for late-preterm infants is individualized and depends on the infant's competency in thermoregulation and feeding, as well as absence of medical illness and social risk factors similar to term infants. Late-preterm infants are not expected to achieve these competencies before at least 48 hours postnatal age. In addition to meeting the aforementioned criteria outlined for term infants, late-preterm infants should not be discharged until there has been the following:

- Accurate determination of gestational age.
- Demonstration of 24 hours of successful feeding by breast or bottle, and the ability to coordinate sucking, swallowing, and breathing with feeding. An infant with weight loss greater than 2–3% of birth weight per day or a maximum of 7% of birth weight should be assessed for dehydration before discharge.
- A formal evaluation of feeding, with observation of position, latch, and milk transfer at least twice daily after birth.
- A follow-up visit scheduled for 24–48 hours after discharge. Additional visits may be needed to ensure a pattern of appropriate weight gain.
- Documentation that the infant has undergone a car safety seat study to observe for apnea, bradycardia, or oxygen desaturation (see also "Safe Transportation of Late-Preterm and Low-Birth-Weight Infants" later in this chapter and "Hospital Discharge of High-Risk Infants" in Chapter 11).

Parent Education and Psychosocial Factors

The short duration of a newborn infant's hospital stay limits the opportunity for parent education. Although nurses are excellent sources of patient education, they have many responsibilities and cannot be expected to provide comprehensive, individualized education for parents. Other methods of education that can be used include prenatal classes, audiovisual materials, printed materials at appropriate literacy levels, and online education programs. Audiovisual materials that have been reviewed and approved by the obstetric and pediatric staff, printed materials, and education by a variety of hospital personnel (eg, postpartum and nursery nurses, registered dietitians and nutritionists, lactation specialists, and physical and occupational therapists) can be helpful to parents. Many educational resources are available on the internet; for example, the AAP website has a parent education site (www.aap.org), and many individual hospitals have their own websites. Other beneficial activities are group or individual educational sessions held regularly during the postpartum period to teach and discuss patient self-care, including exercises and self-examination of the breasts; parent–infant relationships; care of the newborn infant, including bathing and feeding; and child growth and development. Family planning techniques appropriate to the patient's needs and desires also should be explained in detail (see also "Postpartum Considerations" in Chapter 8).

The educational activities should include information explaining the rapid changes in physiology that occur in the newborn infant. Parents should be familiar with normal and abnormal changes in wake–sleep patterns, temperature, respiration, voiding, stooling, and the appearance of the skin, including jaundice. They also should observe and become familiar with the behavior, temperament, and neurologic capabilities of the infant. Awareness of newborn cardiopulmonary resuscitation techniques also may be helpful.

Parent education should include instruction on breastfeeding. Mothers often seek breastfeeding assistance from their health care professionals, who should be able to provide advice that is correct and up-to-date. Before discharge, mothers should be provided with sources for outpatient lactation support.

During the postpartum hospital stay, when the mother is most likely to be uncomfortable, health care personnel can provide her with professional assistance and help her anticipate how she may feel once she is home. The mother may be unsure of the normal physical changes that occur after delivery and of her ability to care for the infant. The mother should be evaluated when she is with her infant to identify any problems she is having so that appropriate instructions can be provided before and after discharge. Prenatal instructions given to prepare the family for the newborn infant's care at home also should be reinforced.

Both in-hospital and community agencies often are available to assist the family. Information on public and private groups that provide services to families with newborn infants, and the circumstances under which these organizations may be asked for such assistance, should be available in the hospital. Information may be obtained from the following sources:

- The in-hospital social services department, as an integral part of the interdisciplinary effort to coordinate hospital and discharge activities, to obtain public or private assistance, and to render psychosocial support
- Home care services, for home visits to assess the parents' child-rearing skills, the home environment, the mother's emotional stability, and

the infant's status and development (under the health care provider's direction, home care nurses may administer drugs or provide other types of therapy)

- Groups that lend support and provide education on infant feeding, parenting, and other concerns

Safe Sleep Position and Sudden Infant Death Syndrome

In the United States, sudden infant death syndrome (SIDS) is a leading cause of mortality for infants between 1 month and 12 months of age. Several modifiable risk factors have been identified, including prone sleeping position, soft sleep surfaces, loose bedding, second-hand smoke exposure, overheating the infant, formula feeding, and bed sharing. Decreases in deaths caused by SIDS have been documented in countries where parents have changed from placing infants in prone positions to back positions for sleeping. Healthy infants should not be placed in the prone or side position for sleeping. Supine positioning (lying wholly on the back) carries the lowest risk of SIDS and is preferred; the side and prone positions confer similarly high risk of SIDS and should not be used. All caregivers, baby sitters, and child-care centers should have this emphasized to them by the parent. "Tummy time" should be encouraged when the infant is awake and supervised. Breastfeeding, and in particular, exclusive breastfeeding, is a protective factor against SIDS. Parents can further reduce their baby's risk of SIDS by not smoking when pregnant and not allowing smoking in the home or around the infant after the infant is born. Parents should be educated about this during their hospital stay. Additionally, parents should be instructed to avoid excessively loose or soft bedding materials, which can occlude the infant's airway or cover the infant's head or face. Overheating may be an independent risk factor or may be associated with the use of additional clothing or blankets. Infants should sleep on a firm surface, with no additional bedding or other materials (such as crib 'bumpers'). The use of a pacifier during sleep is protective and can be used in infants not being directly breastfed as early as desired. Pacifier use should be delayed in breastfed infants until breastfeeding has been well established.

Sleeping on a shared surface (bed sharing) is of concern because it is associated with an increased risk of SIDS. There is also increased risk of suffocation, overlaying, entrapment, wedging, falling, or strangulation. The risks of suffocation or entrapment are extremely high on a couch or a chair, and these surfaces should never be used for infant sleep. It is less hazardous to fall asleep with an infant on an adult bed that is free of loose or soft bedding materials than on a sofa or armchair. This information should be shared with families, because parents may inadvertently fall asleep during nocturnal feeding. Proponents of bed sharing propose that breastfeeding, especially nocturnal breastfeeding, is enhanced, and some mothers will choose to co-sleep. However, a meta-analysis found that among breastfed infants in a household without smoking or alcohol, the risk of SIDS increases from 0.08 per 1,000 live births with room sharing to 0.23 per 1,000 live births with bed sharing. The risk is higher for formula fed infants and markedly increased when the bed sharing parent is a smoker or has consumed alcohol or nonmedical or sedating drugs before bed sharing, or when the mother smoked during pregnancy. The risk is also greater when the infant sleeps on the same surface with children or other adults besides the parents. The Task Force on Sudden Infant Death Syndrome recommends that the infant sleep in the same room as the caregiver for the first year (or at least the first 6 months) as this decreases the risk of SIDS and is safer than bed sharing or sleeping in a separate room.

Infants with gastroesophageal reflux should be placed supine for sleep, as the risk of SIDS outweighs the benefit of prone or side positioning for reflux. Prone positioning for sleep should only be considered in infants with upper airway disorders if the risk of death from gastroesophageal reflux is greater than the risk of SIDS. Preterm infants in the NICU unit should be placed supine as soon as clinical status has stabilized, as far in advance of discharge as possible.

Cardiorespiratory monitoring has not been demonstrated to decrease the incidence of SIDS, and home cardiorespiratory monitoring should not be prescribed to prevent SIDS. Serious adverse effects to the infant because of supine positioning have not been reported. There has been an increase in the diagnosis of cranial asymmetry or positional plagiocephaly temporally related to the Back to Sleep national campaign positioning recommendation. This can be minimized by alternating the supine head position during sleep and by encouraging "tummy time" for awake playtime and when under direct observation by the caregiver. Upright "cuddle time" should be encouraged, and spending excessive time in car-seat carriers and rockers or bouncers in which pressure is applied to the occiput should be avoided.

Safe Transportation of Late-Preterm and Low-Birth-Weight Infants

Proper selection and use of car safety seats or car beds are important for ensuring that preterm and low-birth-weight infants are transported as safely as possible. The increased frequency of oxygen desaturation or episodes of apnea or bradycardia experienced by preterm and low-birth-weight infants positioned in car safety seats may expose them to an increased risk of cardiorespiratory events and adverse neurodevelopmental outcomes. It is suggested that preterm infants should have a period of observation of 90–120 minutes (longer, if time for travel home will exceed this amount) in a car safety seat before hospital discharge to detect complications such as apnea, bradycardia, and oxygen desaturation. Educating parents about the proper positioning of preterm and low-birth-weight infants in car safety seats is important for minimizing the risk of respiratory compromise. Car seats should only be used for travel, with observation when possible. Extended periods in car safety seats should be avoided for vulnerable infants.

Follow-up Care

The physical and psychosocial status of the mother and her infant should be monitored after discharge. The mother needs personalized care during the postpartum period to facilitate the development of a healthy mother–infant relationship and a sense of maternal confidence. Support and reassurance should be provided as the mother masters and adapts to her maternal role. Encouraging participation in the infant's care by the other parent or other close support person can not only provide additional support to the mother but also enhance the relationship between the newborn and the family. Parents and caregivers should be educated about the dangers of shaking an infant. Specifically, shaken baby syndrome results from forcefully shaking an infant, often because of frustration or anger because the child will not stop crying.

For newborn infants discharged before 48 hours after delivery, an appointment should be made for the infant to be examined by a health care practitioner within 48 hours of discharge. If this cannot be ensured, discharge should be deferred until a mechanism for follow-up is identified. The follow-up visit can take place in a home, clinic, or hospital outpatient setting as long as the health care professional who examines the infant is competent in newborn assessment and the results of the follow-up visit are reported to the infant's primary care provider or his or her designee on the day of the visit. The purpose of the follow-up visit is to do the following:

- Promote establishment of a relationship with the medical home by verifying the plan for health care maintenance, including a method for obtaining emergency services, preventive care and immunizations, periodic evaluations and physical examinations, and necessary screenings.
- Weigh the infant; assess the infant's general health, hydration, and degree of jaundice; and identify any new problems.
- Review feeding patterns and technique; encourage and support breastfeeding by observation of the adequacy of position, latch, and swallowing.
- Obtain a history of stool and urine patterns.
- Provide or make a referral for skilled lactation support as needed, particularly if the foregoing evaluations are not reassuring.
- Assess the quality of mother–infant attachment and details of infant behavior.
- Reinforce maternal or family education in infant care, particularly regarding feeding and sleep position, avoidance of co-sleeping, and appropriate use of car safety seats.
- Review results of outstanding laboratory tests, such as newborn metabolic screens, performed before discharge.
- Perform screenings in accordance with state regulations and other tests, such as bilirubin, as clinically indicated.
- Assess for parental well-being with a focus on screening for maternal postpartum depression.

The postpartum period is a time of developmental adjustment for the whole family. Family members have new roles and relationships, and an effort should be made to assess the progress of the family's adaptation. If a family member finds it difficult to assume the new role, the health care team should arrange for sensitive, supportive assistance. This is particularly important for adolescent mothers, for whom it may be necessary to mobilize multiple resources within the community. The frequency of follow-up visits for the well infant varies with patient, locale, and community practices. The intervals should be consistent with the AAP's guidelines on preventive health care. Regular follow-up visits and good records of development should be maintained. Health care providers who provide follow-up care to women and infants should assess the following physical, social, and psychological factors associated with child abuse:

- Preterm birth
- Neonatal illness with long periods of hospitalization, especially in neonatal intensive care units
- Single parenthood
- Adolescent motherhood
- Closely spaced pregnancies
- Infrequent family visits to hospitalized infants
- Substance use

Infants and parents with such a history or with other factors associated with child abuse require closer follow-up than does the average family. The interaction of the parents, especially the mother, with the infant, should be evaluated periodically. The infant or child who fails to thrive may be a victim of neglect or abuse, and a causal relationship between neglect and failure to thrive should be considered. In every state, providers of health care to children are legally obligated to report suspected child abuse by calling statewide hotlines, local child protective services, or law enforcement agencies.

Adoption

Health care for infants who are to be adopted should focus on the needs of the child, the adoptive family, and the birth parents. These infants may have acute and long-term medical, psychological, and developmental problems because of their genetic, emotional, cultural, psychosocial, or medical backgrounds. The health care provider should perform a careful medical assessment of the infant and should counsel the adopting family appropriately. Just as a birth family cannot be certain that its biologic child will be healthy, an adoptive family cannot be guaranteed that an adopted child will not have future health problems. Most adopted children, even those from high-risk backgrounds, are healthy. Those with certain disorders and special problems, however, also can be adopted successfully. The risks should be defined and explained carefully to the family so that problems can be anticipated and addressed expediently.

The health care provider's role is not to judge the advisability of a proposed adoption but to apprise the prospective parents clearly and honestly of any special health needs detected at examination or anticipated in the future. Health care providers evaluating a newborn infant for adoption should obtain as extensive history as possible from the birth parents and enter these data into the formal medical record. There may never again be a comparable opportunity to obtain this information. If the health care provider is unable to interview the parents personally, an adoption agency social worker who is trained to do a skilled genetic and medical interview should obtain a complete prenatal and postpartum history. The prenatal history should include information on the birth parents' lifestyle that may affect the fetus at birth or later in development. Health care providers and adoption agency social workers should be trained to obtain lifestyle information in a manner that is sensitive to psychological and cultural issues. Such information includes parental use of alcohol or other drugs, and a history of sexual practices that increase the risk of sexually transmitted diseases in both birth parents. After reviewing whatever history is available, the health care provider should examine the adopted child carefully and perform metabolic, genetic, and other assessments as indicated.

Health care providers must be careful with language they use when dealing with the adoptive family. This is an adoptive family, not only an adopted child. The term "parent" applies to the parents in the adoptive family; the birth parents are those who conceived the child. "Real" or "natural" parent are terms that should be eliminated, as they may imply a temporary or less-than-genuine relationship between adoptive families and their children. The health care provider should be aware of state laws regarding adoption procedures. Hospital nurseries should have policies regarding the handling of adoptions in accordance with these laws. Policies should reflect sensitivity toward the adoptive family and the birth parents. Although adoption is generally an elective decision initiated by the birth parent(s), the birth parents often need support with their decision and with adjusting to the separation from their infant.

Bibliography

ABM Clinical Protocol #8: human milk storage information for home use for full-term infants (Original Protocol March 2004; Revision #1 March 2010). Academy of Breastfeeding Medicine Protocol Committee [published erratum appears in Breastfeed Med 2011;6:159]. Breastfeed Med 2010;5:127–30.

Adamkin DH. Postnatal glucose homeostasis in late-preterm and term infants. Committee on Fetus and Newborn. Pediatrics 2011;127:575–9.

American Academy of Pediatrics. Recommendations for preventive pediatric health care. Elk Grove Village (IL): AAP; 2016. Available at: https://www.aap.org/en-us/Documents/periodicity_schedule.pdf. Retrieved November 2, 2016.

American Academy of Pediatrics, American Heart Association. Textbook of neonatal resuscitation. 7th ed. Elk Grove Village (IL): AAP; Dallas (TX): AHA; 2016.

Ballard JL, Khoury JC, Wedig K, Wang L, Eilers-Walsman BL, Lipp R. New Ballard score, expanded to include extremely premature infants. J Pediatr 1991;119:417–23.

Barfield WD. Standard terminology for fetal, infant, and perinatal deaths. Committee on Fetus and Newborn. Pediatrics 2016;137.

Bell EF. Noninitiation or withdrawal of intensive care for high-risk newborns. American Academy of Pediatrics Committee on Fetus and Newborn. Pediatrics 2007;119:401–3.

Benitz WE. Hospital stay for healthy term newborn infants. Committee on Fetus and Newborn, American Academy of Pediatrics. Pediatrics 2015;135:948–53.

Best D. Technical report--secondhand and prenatal tobacco smoke exposure. American Academy of Pediatrics Committee on Environmental Health, Committee on Native American Child Health, Committee on Adolescence. Pediatrics 2009;124:e1017–44.

Bhutani VK. Phototherapy to prevent severe neonatal hyperbilirubinemia in the newborn infant 35 or more weeks of gestation. Committee on Fetus and Newborn, American Academy of Pediatrics. Pediatrics 2011;128:e1046–52.

Borchers D. Families and adoption: the pediatrician's role in supporting communication. American Academy of Pediatrics Committee on Early Childhood, Adoption, and Dependent Care. Pediatrics 2003;112:1437–41.

Breastfeeding and the use of human milk. Section on Breastfeeding. Pediatrics 2012;129:e827–41.

Breastfeeding in underserved women: increasing initiation and continuation of breastfeeding. Committee Opinion No. 570. American College of Obstetricians and Gynecologists. Obstet Gynecol 2013;122:423–8.

Bull MJ, Engle WA. Safe transportation of preterm and low birth weight infants at hospital discharge. Committee on Injury, Violence, and Poison Prevention and Committee on Fetus and Newborn, American Academy of Pediatrics. Pediatrics 2009;123:1424–9.

Circumcision Policy Statement. American Academy of Pediatrics Task Force on Circumcision. Pediatrics 2012;130:585–6.

Cohen GJ. The prenatal visit. Committee on Psychosocial Aspects of Child and Family Health. Pediatrics 2009;124:1227–32.

Controversies concerning vitamin K and the newborn. American Academy of Pediatrics Committee on Fetus and Newborn. Pediatrics 2003;112:191–2.

Cummings J. Antenatal counseling regarding resuscitation and intensive care before 25 weeks of gestation. Committee on Fetus and Newborn. Pediatrics 2015;136: 588–95.

Domellof M, Braegger C, Campoy C, Colomb V, Decsi T, Fewtrell M, et al. Iron requirements of infants and toddlers. ESPGHAN Committee on Nutrition. J Pediatr Gastroenterol Nutr 2014;58:119–29.

Engle WA, Tomashek KM, Wallman C. "Late-preterm" infants: a population at risk. Committee on Fetus and Newborn, American Academy of Pediatrics [published erratum appears in Pediatrics 2008;121:451]. Pediatrics 2007;120:1390–401.

Farber HJ, Nelson KE, Groner JA, Walley SC. Public policy to protect children from tobacco, nicotine, and tobacco smoke. Section on Tobacco Control. Pediatrics 2015;136:998-1007. Nelson KE. Clinical practice policy to protect children from tobacco, nicotine, and tobacco smoke. Section on Tobacco Control. Pediatrics 2015;136:1008–17.

Feldman-Winter L, Goldsmith JP. Safe sleep and skin-to-skin care in the neonatal period for healthy term newborns. Committee on Fetus and Newborn and Task Force on Sudden Infant Death Syndrome. Pediatrics 2016;138:10.1542/peds.2016,1889. Epub 2016 Aug 22.

Fetal growth restriction. Practice Bulletin No. 134. American College of Obstetricians and Gynecologists. Obstet Gynecol 2013;121:1122–33.

Flaherman VJ, Schaefer EW, Kuzniewicz MW, Li SX, Walsh EM, Paul IM. Early weight loss nomograms for exclusively breastfed newborns. Pediatrics 2015;135: e16–23.

Genetics and molecular diagnostic testing. Technology Assessment No. 11. American College of Obstetricians and Gynecologists. Obstet Gynecol 2014;123:394–413.

Havens PL, Mofenson LM. Evaluation and management of the infant exposed to HIV-1 in the United States. American Academy of Pediatrics Committee on Pediatric AIDS [published erratum appears in Pediatrics 2012;130:1183-4]. Pediatrics 2009;123:175–87.

Hollis BW, Wagner CL, Howard CR, Ebeling M, Shary JR, Smith PG, et al. Maternal versus infant vitamin D supplementation during lactation: a randomized controlled trial. Pediatrics 2015;136:625–34.

Hudak ML, Tan RC. Neonatal drug withdrawal. Committee on Drugs, Committee on Fetus and Newborn American Academy of Pediatrics [published erratum appears in Pediatrics 2014;133:937]. Pediatrics 2012;129:e540–60.

Ip S, Chung M, Kulig J, O'Brien R, Sege R, Glicken S, et al. An evidence-based review of important issues concerning neonatal hyperbilirubinemia. American Academy of Pediatrics Subcommittee on Hyperbilirubinemia. Pediatrics 2004;114:e130–53.

Kaye CI, Accurso F, La Franchi S, Lane PA, Hope N, Sonya P, et al. Newborn screening fact sheets. Committee on Genetics. Pediatrics 2006;118:e934–63.

Lee PA, Houk CP, Ahmed SF, Hughes IA. Consensus statement on management of intersex disorders. International Consensus Conference on Intersex Organized by the Lawson Wilkins Pediatric Endocrine Society and the European Society for Paediatric Endocrinology. Pediatrics 2006;118:e488–500.

Levels of neonatal care. American Academy of Pediatrics Committee on Fetus and Newborn. Pediatrics 2012;130:587–97.

Mahle WT, Martin GR, Beekman RH 3rd, Morrow WR. Endorsement of Health and Human Services recommendation for pulse oximetry screening for critical congenital heart disease. Section on Cardiology and Cardiac Surgery Executive Committee. Pediatrics 2012;129:190–2.

Management of hyperbilirubinemia in the newborn infant 35 or more weeks of gestation. American Academy of Pediatrics Subcommittee on Hyperbilirubinemia [Published Erratum Appears in Pediatrics 2004;114:1138]. Pediatrics 2004;114:297-316.

Markenson D, Reynolds S. The pediatrician and disaster preparedness. American Academy of Pediatrics Committee on Pediatric Emergency Medicine Task Force on Terrorism. Pediatrics 2006;117:e340–62.

Miller JR, Flaherman VJ, Schaefer EW, Kuzniewicz MW, Li SX, Walsh EM, et al. Early weight loss nomograms for formula fed newborns. Hosp Pediatr 2015;5:263–8.

Moon RY. SIDS and other sleep-related infant deaths: evidence base for 2016 updated recommendations for a safe infant sleeping environment. Task Force on Sudden Infant Death Syndrome. Pediatrics 2016;138:e20162940.

Muse C, Harrison J, Yoshinaga-Itano C, Grimes A, Brookhouser PE, Epstein S, et al. Supplement to the JCIH 2007 position statement: principles and guidelines for early intervention after confirmation that a child is deaf or hard of hearing. Joint Committee on Infant Hearing of the American Academy of Pediatrics. Pediatrics 2013;131:e1324–49.

Newborn screening and the role of the obstetrician-gynecologist. Committee Opinion No. 616. American College of Obstetricians and Gynecologists. Obstet Gynecol 2015;125:256–60.

Newborn screening expands: recommendations for pediatricians and medical homes—implications for the system. American Academy of Pediatrics Newborn Screening Authoring Committee. Pediatrics 2008;121:192–217.

Optimizing support for breastfeeding as part of obstetric practice. Committee Opinion No. 658. American College of Obstetricians and Gynecologists. Obstet Gynecol 2016;127:e86–92.

Patient- and family-centered care and the pediatrician's role. Committee on Hospital Care and Institute for Patient- and Family-Centered Care. Pediatrics 2012; 129: 394–404.

Periviable birth. Obstetric Care Consensus No. 4. American College of Obstetricians and Gynecologists. Obstet Gynecol 2016;127:e157–69.

Prevention and management of procedural pain in the neonate: an update. Committee on Fetus and Newborn and Section on Anesthesiology and Pain Medicine. Pediatrics 2016;137:e20154271.

Sachs HC. The transfer of drugs and therapeutics into human breast milk: an update on selected topics. Committee on Drugs. Pediatrics 2013;132:e796–809.

Shaw BA, Segal LS. Evaluation and referral for developmental dysplasia of the hip in infants. Section on Orthopaedics. Pediatrics 2016;138:e20163107.

Slutzah M, Codipilly CN, Potak D, Clark RM, Schanler RJ. Refrigerator storage of expressed human milk in the neonatal intensive care unit. J Pediatr 2010;156:26–8.

The Apgar score. Committee Opinion No. 644. American College of Obstetricians and Gynecologists. Obstet Gynecol 2015;126:e52–5.

Tobacco use: a pediatric disease. Committee on Environmental Health, Committee on Substance Abuse, Committee on Adolescence, and Committee on Native American Child Health [published erratum appears in Pediatrics 2010;125:861]. Pediatrics 2009;124:1474–87.

Update on immunization and pregnancy: tetanus, diphtheria, and pertussis vaccination. ACOG Committee Opinion No. 566. American College of Obstetricians and Gynecologists. Obstet Gynecol 2013;121:1411–4.

Verani JR, McGee L, Schrag SJ. Prevention of perinatal group B streptococcal disease—revised guidelines from CDC, 2010. Division of Bacterial Diseases, National Center for Immunization and Respiratory Diseases, Centers for Disease Control and Prevention (CDC). MMWR Recomm Rep 2010;59(RR-10):1–36.

Wagner CL, Greer FR. Prevention of rickets and vitamin d deficiency in infants, children, and adolescents. American Academy of Pediatrics Section on Breastfeeding, American Academy of Pediatrics Committee on Nutrition [published erratum appears in Pediatrics 2009;123:197]. Pediatrics 2008;122:1142–52.

Wallman C. Advanced practice in neonatal nursing. Committee on Fetus and Newborn. Pediatrics 2009;123:1606–7.

Wyckoff MH, Aziz K, Escobedo MB, Kapadia VS, Kattwinkel J, Perlman JM, et al. Part 13: neonatal resuscitation: 2015 American Heart Association guidelines update for cardiopulmonary resuscitation and emergency cardiovascular care (reprint). Pediatrics 2015;136(suppl):S196–218.

Year 2007 position statement: principles and guidelines for early hearing detection and intervention programs. American Academy of Pediatrics, Joint Committee on Infant Hearing. Pediatrics 2007;120:898–921.

Ziegler EE, Nelson SE, Jeter JM. Iron supplementation of breastfed infants from an early age. Am J Clin Nutr 2009;89:525–32.

Resources

American Academy of Pediatrics. Breastfeeding Initiatives. Elk Grove Village (IL): AAP; 2016. Available at: http://www2.aap.org/breastfeeding/index.html. Retrieved November 7, 2016.

American Academy of Pediatrics. Safe and healthy beginnings: a resource toolkit for hospitals and physicians offices [CD-Rom]. Elk Grove Village (IL): AAP; 2009.

American College of Medical Genetics. Newborn screening ACT sheets and confirmatory algorithms. Bethesda (MD): ACMG; 2011. Available at: https://www.ncbi.nlm.nih.gov/books/NBK55827/. Retrieved November 7, 2016.

Drugs and Lactation Database: LactMed. Bethesda (MD): National Library of Medicine; 2016. Available at: https://toxnet.nlm.nih.gov/newtoxnet/lactmed.htm. Retrieved November 7, 2016.

National Newborn Screening and Global Resource Center. Newborn screening. Austin (TX): NNSGRC; 2016. Available at: http://genes-r-us.uthscsa.edu/resources/consumer/statemap.htm. Retrieved November 7, 2016.

U.S. Department of Health and Human Services. Secretary's Advisory Committee on Heritable Disorders in Newborns and Children: recommendations and responses from the HHS Secretary. Washington, DC: DHHS; 2015. Available at: http://www.hrsa.gov/advisorycommittees/mchbadvisory/heritabledisorders/recommendations/index.html. Retrieved November 7, 2016.

Chapter 11

Neonatal Complications and Management of High-Risk Infants

This chapter highlights some of the common complications encountered in the care of high-risk infants and, whenever possible, provides an evidence-based approach to management.

Neonatal Complications

Anemia of Prematurity

Anemia of prematurity results from multiple factors and varies with the degree of immaturity, illness, postnatal age, and nutrition. Current evidence indicates that most cases of anemia that occur in the first 2–3 weeks after delivery mainly result from the volume of blood samples obtained for clinical management. During growth, the balance of oxidative substrate (polyunsaturated free fatty acids), antioxidants (eg, vitamin E) and pro-oxidants (eg, iron) in the diet may play a role in red blood cell survival. As growth accelerates with advancing postnatal age, depletion of iron stores begins to affect erythropoiesis. Adding to these factors is the very-low-birth-weight infant's limited capacity to increase erythropoietin production in response to anemia, which further decreases red blood cell production and increases the likelihood of dilutional anemia from an expanding blood volume as the infant gains weight.

A multipronged approach to decreasing the need for red blood cell transfusion is recommended, especially in very-low-birth-weight infants. This approach includes delaying cord clamping, limiting blood sampling, using noninvasive monitoring, optimizing nutrition, and adhering to a protocol with strict indications for transfusion. Delaying umbilical cord clamping in the preterm infant until 30–60 seconds after birth is associated with neonatal benefits, including decreased mortality, higher blood pressure and blood volume, less need for blood transfusion after birth, fewer brain hemorrhages, and a lower risk of necrotizing enterocolitis. It is important to note that the timing of umbilical cord clamping should not be altered for the purpose of collecting umbilical cord blood for banking.

Randomized clinical trials have shown that adherence to protocols with strict indications for transfusion reduces both the volume of blood transfused and donor exposure; however, an appropriate threshold for transfusion remains uncertain. An ongoing multicenter randomized controlled trial comparing two different criteria for red blood cell transfusion in preterm infants may provide additional information on this topic. Use of erythropoietin stimulating agents, whether administered early in the neonatal course or several weeks after birth, have been associated with a reduction in the number of transfusions needed; however, only early use has been associated with a reduction in donor exposure. Because the reductions are small, they are likely of limited clinical importance, and the routine use of erythropoietin stimulating agents in preterm infants is not recommended. In some situations, such as the birth of a very preterm infant to parents who are Jehovah's Witnesses, routine use may be preferred.

Apnea

Apnea of prematurity can persist beyond 36 weeks' postmenstrual age, particularly in extremely preterm infants and in those with bronchopulmonary dysplasia (BPD). Neurologic immaturity of respiratory control is hypothesized to be a common underlying mechanism. Persistent apnea often is associated with inadequate oral feeding, which may be the only issue precluding discharge to home. In the absence of objective measurements that clearly identify infants at risk of clinically significant cardiorespiratory instability, clinicians have used the empiric approach of requiring an event-free interval before discharge to home. The precise number of days without apnea or bradycardia has not been determined, but the most frequent interval used is 5–7 consecutive days after discontinuing methylxanthine therapy. The use of home cardiorespiratory monitors should not be used to justify discharge of infants who are still at risk of apnea solely because of immature respiratory control.

Although preterm infants have a higher incidence of sudden infant death syndrome (SIDS) than term infants, no correlation between apnea of prematurity and SIDS has been established. In addition, formal analyses of breathing patterns (ie, pneumograms) are of no value in predicting SIDS or in identifying infants who should receive cardiorespiratory monitoring. Home cardiorespiratory monitoring may be useful for some infants who are technology dependent (see also "Hospital Discharge of High-Risk Infants" later in this chapter).

Brain Injury

Hemorrhagic and Periventricular White Matter Brain Injury

Infants born at 32 weeks of gestational age or less or who have a birth weight of 1,500 g or less are at highest risk of hemorrhagic and other brain injuries. Both the incidence and severity increase with decreasing gestational age. The vulnerability of the preterm infant arises from immaturity of the developing brain and may be compounded by attenuated autoregulation of cerebral blood flow during frequent periods of physiologic instability associated with prematurity. Periventricular–intraventricular hemorrhage, the most frequent hemorrhagic lesion, ranges from a small germinal matrix hemorrhage to varying amounts of intraventricular blood to massive intraparenchymal hemorrhage or hemorrhagic infarction. Most periventricular–intraventricular hemorrhages occur in the first 72 hours after birth. Posthemorrhagic hydrocephalus secondary to intraventricular hemorrhage often is apparent within 2–4 weeks after delivery, but can develop later. Periventricular leukomalacia is the most frequent white matter lesion identified. Residual lesions after brain injury include minimal to extensive cystic lesions in the periventricular white matter and ventriculomegaly secondary to diffuse cerebral atrophy. Porencephaly may develop after severe, localized ischemic or hemorrhagic infarction. These lesions evolve over the course of several weeks.

Screening and Follow-up. Portable bedside cranial ultrasonography is the most frequent imaging modality used to diagnose and monitor the evolution of brain injury. There can be great variability in interpretation. The quality of the images is affected by the type of equipment used and the expertise of the ultrasonographer. It is recommended that each center establish a protocol for screening cranial ultrasound examinations in infants who are at risk. The initial screening study should be performed between 7 and 14 postnatal days. Follow-up studies should be based on the clinical course and the initial findings. Although cranial ultrasonography is useful in diagnosing and monitoring the development of posthemorrhagic hydrocephalus, it is not useful for the prediction of neurodevelopmental outcomes. Studies of the utility of magnetic resonance imaging (MRI) in predicting neurodevelopmental outcome are ongoing; however, to date routine use of MRI for all preterm infants who are at risk is not recommended.

Prevention. Antenatal corticosteroids decrease the incidence and severity of periventricular–intraventricular hemorrhage. Prophylactic indomethacin given shortly after birth may decrease the frequency of severe periventricular–intraventricular hemorrhage; however, it does not lower the risk of poor neurodevelopmental outcome in early childhood. To date, no other postnatal intervention consistently prevents either periventricular–intraventricular hemorrhage or other brain lesions.

Neonatal Encephalopathy

Neonatal encephalopathy can be a neurologically devastating or fatal condition. Previous therapeutic interventions to ameliorate this condition have failed to provide benefit; however, randomized trials of selective head cooling or whole-body cooling have demonstrated that mild hypothermia consistently results in a significant improvement in survival without major neurodevelopmental impairment. The components of a hypothermia regimen include the criteria for inclusion, the timing of initiation, the duration and the depth of cooling, and the method used (see Table 11-1 for criteria for inclusion). The usefulness of amplitude-integrated electroencephalography as an entry criterion is not yet clear. Both selective head cooling and whole-body cooling target a core temperature of 33–34°C (91.4–93.2°F) for a duration of 72 hours. Cooling infants with mild encephalopathy or those less than 35 weeks of gestational age cannot be recommended because there are insufficient data to evaluate the risks and benefits for these infants.

Although inducing hypothermia is technologically straightforward, the critically ill nature of the infant requires a full range of specialty and subspecialty support available only at a level III or level IV neonatal intensive care unit (NICU). In addition, at this time, the unknown risks of overshooting the desired temperature and other adverse events under uncontrolled circumstances outweigh the possible benefits of instituting active cooling at the referring hospital. A recent randomized controlled trial demonstrated that active cooling using a servo-regulated cooling device provided more predictable temperature management during neonatal transport than does either passive cooling (turning the radiant warmer or incubator off) or active cooling (ice or gel packs) for outborn infants with neonatal encephalopathy.

TABLE 11-1. Therapeutic Hypothermia Criteria for Inclusion

Clinical Trial	Entry Criteria
CoolCap	Gestational age ≥36 weeks and ≤6 hours of age AND Apgar score ≤5 at 10 minutes after birth OR Continued need for resuscitation at 10 minutes after birth OR pH <7.00 or base deficit ≥16 mmol/L or more on an umbilical cord blood sample or an arterial or venous blood sample obtained within 60 minutes of birth AND Moderate or severe encephalopathy on clinical examination AND Moderately or severely abnormal background of at least 20 minutes' duration or seizure activity on amplitude integrated electroencephalogram (aEEG) after one hour of age
Whole-Body Cooling	Gestational age ≥36 weeks and ≤6 hours of age AND pH ≤7.00 or base deficit ≥16 mmol/L in an umbilical cord blood sample or any blood sample obtained within the first hour after birth* AND Moderate or severe encephalopathy on clinical examination
TOBY	Gestational age ≥36 weeks and ≤6 hours of age AND Apgar score ≤5 at 10 minutes after birth OR Continued need for resuscitation 10 minutes after birth OR pH <7.00 or base deficit ≥16 mmol/L on umbilical cord or arterial or capillary blood sample obtained within 60 minutes of birth AND Moderate or severe encephalopathy on clinical examination AND Abnormal background activity of at least 30 minutes' duration or seizures on amplitude integrated-electroencephalogram (aEEG)

*If blood gas is not available or pH is between 7.01 and 7.15 or base deficit is between 10 and 15.9 mmol/L on blood sample obtained within the first hour of birth, two additional criteria are needed: a history of an acute perinatal event (eg, cord prolapse, fetal heart rate decelerations) and either the need for assisted ventilation at birth and continued for 10 minutes or an Apgar score of 5 or less at 10 minutes after birth.

Reprinted from Committee on Fetus and Newborn. Hypothermia and Neonatal Encephalopathy. Pediatrics 2014;133:1149.

Data from the *Eunice Kennedy Shriver* National Institute of Child Health and Human Development whole-body hypothermia trial demonstrated that hyperthermia was clearly associated with worsened outcomes. It is not known whether hyperthermia itself causes worse outcomes or whether infants destined to have worse outcomes also have hyperthermia as a manifestation of their disease. However, it seems prudent to take steps to avoid abnormally high temperatures in infants with neonatal encephalopathy. Such steps may include turning off the radiant warmer if the infant's temperature is greater than 37.5°C (99.5°F) and giving a tepid bath for a persistent temperature above 38°C (100.4°F).

Ongoing and proposed trials of hypothermia may clarify issues, such as the benefit of hypothermia initiated after 6 hours of age, the utility of adjuvant therapies, and whether amplitude-integrated electroencephalography is a useful tool in predicting neurodevelopmental outcome. In the interim, practitioners should institute therapeutic hypothermia using a regimen similar to those used in published trials and only at institutions with practitioners who are trained in its use.

Hyperbilirubinemia

Bilirubin interferes with many cellular processes and functions. The ultimate fate of a cell in which bilirubin accumulates depends on the concentration and the duration of exposure. The most important toxicity is permanent damage to the cells of the brain stem and basal ganglia (ie, bilirubin-induced neurologic damage [BIND]); BIND is called "kernicterus" when seen at autopsy. The main host protection against BIND is extracellular albumin, which binds the toxic isomer of bilirubin tightly, preventing its entry into living cells.

Other protective mechanisms exist (eg, blood–brain barrier, P-glycoprotein) but they are not nearly as important as extracellular albumin. If the relationship between bilirubin and albumin were simple, the ratio of the two concentrations in plasma would provide a simple measure of risk. However, other factors reduce the amount of albumin available for bilirubin binding, the most important being molecules that compete for binding sites on albumin. These include free fatty acids, common antibacterial agents, antibiotics, analgesics, diuretics, and circulating products of rapid hemolysis. In addition, prematurity and hypoxia–ischemia may add to the susceptibility of an infant to bilirubin toxicity. Nevertheless, BIND is largely preventable with appropriate supervision of infants in the first week after birth, routine assessments of risk, and prompt treatment.

For the purposes of clinical evaluation of jaundice, risk assessment, and treatment decisions, this chapter will divide infants into three groups: 1) term and late-preterm infants (at 35 weeks or more of gestational age); 2) preterm infants with a birth weight of 1,000 g or more; and 3) extremely-low-birth-weight infants (less than 1,000 g birth weight).

Term and Late-Preterm Infants Without Added Risk Factors

There are few data on which to base treatment for term or late-preterm infants who do not have hemolytic disease or other risk factors and who have total bilirubin concentrations of less than 20 mg per dL (342 micromoles per liter). Follow-up data for apparently healthy term infants with bilirubin concentrations as high as 25 mg per dL (428 micromoles per liter) show no apparent neurologic sequelae. However, historical data and subsequent studies have shown that a total serum bilirubin concentration greater than 30 mg per dL (513 micromoles per liter) carries a decidedly higher risk of permanent neurologic impairment. The current American Academy of Pediatrics (AAP) guidelines for phototherapy and exchange transfusion (see Fig. 11-1 and Fig. 11-2) for infants born at 35 weeks of gestation or greater are based on limited evidence and a consensus of expert opinions.

Term and Late-Preterm Infants With Hemolysis and Other Risk Factors

A direct association between severe hemolysis with a rapid increase in unconjugated hyperbilirubinemia, bilirubin encephalopathy, and kernicterus has been demonstrated in infants with erythroblastosis fetalis. Survivors may manifest serious sequelae, including athetoid cerebral palsy, hearing loss, paralysis of upward gaze, and dentoalveolar dysplasia. Although no specific total serum bilirubin threshold for neurotoxicity has been established, clinical observations of term infants without hemolytic disease indicate that clinical bilirubin encephalopathy is unlikely at unconjugated bilirubin concentrations of less than 20 mg per dL (342 micromoles per liter). However, total serum bilirubin concentration alone has been found to be an inadequate predictor of individual risk. Measures of free (unbound) bilirubin or reserve albumin binding capacity identify infants at risk more accurately, but these measures are not widely available.

The Bhutani nomogram demonstrates that the 95th percentile rate of increase in the first few days after birth is 0.25 mg per dL per h. Any rate

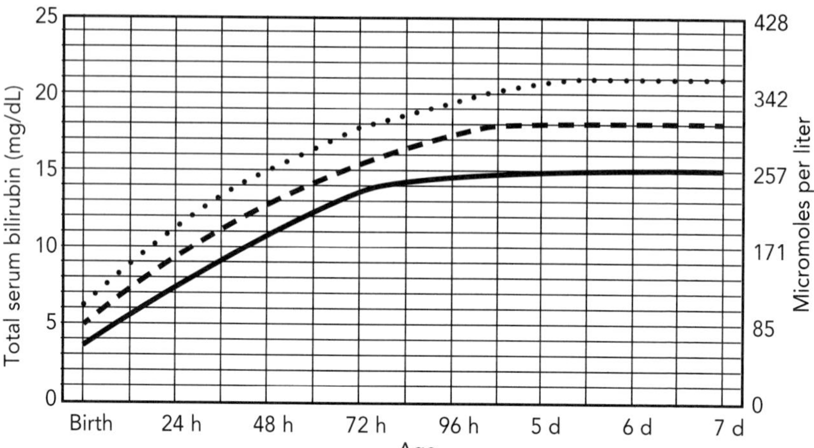

• • • Infants at lower risk (equal to or greater than 38 wk of gestation and well)
— — Infants at medium risk (equal to or greater than 38 wk of gestation with risk factors or
—— 35–37 6/7 wk of gestation and well)
Infants at higher risk (35–37 6/7 wk of gestation with risk factors)

Figure 11-1. Guidelines for phototherapy in hospitalized infants at 35 weeks of gestation or older. These guidelines are based on limited evidence, and the levels shown are approximations. The guidelines refer to the use of intensive phototherapy, which should be used when the total serum bilirubin level exceeds the line indicated for each category. Infants are designated as "higher risk" because of the potential negative effects of the conditions listed on albumin binding of bilirubin, the blood–brain barrier, and the susceptibility of the brain cells to damage by bilirubin. Use total bilirubin. Do not subtract direct reacting or conjugated bilirubin. Risk factors are isoimmune hemolytic disease, G6PD deficiency, asphyxia, significant lethargy, temperature instability, sepsis, acidosis, or albumin less than 3 g/dL (if measured). For well infants 35–37 6/7 weeks of gestation, total serum bilirubin levels can be adjusted for intervention around the medium risk line. It is an option to intervene at lower total serum bilirubin levels for infants closer to 35 weeks of gestation and at higher total serum bilirubin levels for those closer to 37 6/7 weeks of gestation. It is an option to provide conventional phototherapy in the hospital or at home with total serum bilirubin levels 2–3 mg/dL (35–50 micromoles per liter) below those shown, but home phototherapy should not be used in any infant with risk factors. (Management of hyperbilirubinemia in the newborn infant 35 or more weeks of gestation. American Academy of Pediatrics Subcommittee on Hyperbilirubinemia [published erratum appears in Pediatrics 2004;114:1138]. Pediatrics 2004;114:297–316.)

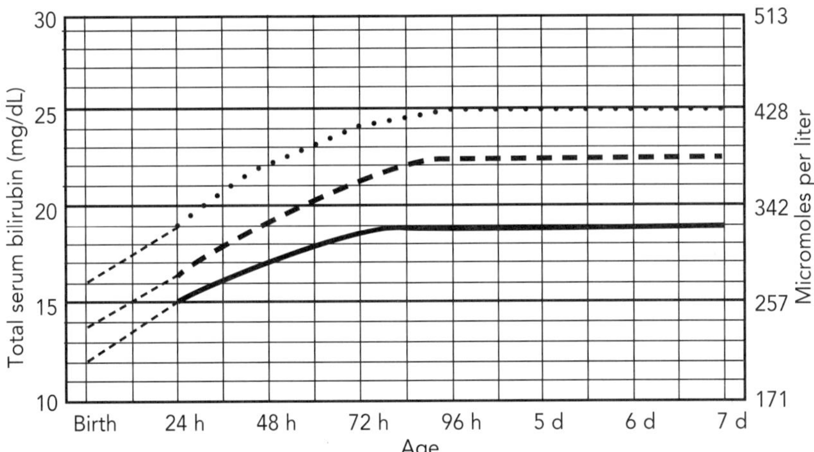

. . . Infants at lower risk (equal to or greater than 38 wk of gestation and well)
– – Infants at medium risk (equal to or greater than 38 wk of gestation with risk factors or
35–37 6/7 wk of gestation and well)
—— Infants at higher risk (35–37 6/7 wk of gestation with risk factors)

Figure 11-2. Guidelines for exchange transfusion in infants at 35 weeks of gestation or older. These suggested levels represent a consensus of most of the committee but are based on limited evidence, and the levels shown are approximations. During birth hospitalization, exchange transfusion is recommended if the total serum bilirubin level increases to these levels despite intensive phototherapy. For readmitted infants, if the total serum bilirubin level is above the exchange level, repeat total serum bilirubin measurement every 2–3 hours and consider exchange if the total serum bilirubin level remains above the levels indicated after intensive phototherapy for 6 hours. The dashed lines for the first 24 hours indicate uncertainty because of a wide range of clinical circumstances and a range of responses to phototherapy. Immediate exchange transfusion is recommended if the infant shows signs of acute bilirubin encephalopathy (hypertonia, arching, retrocollis, opisthotonos, fever, or high pitched cry) or if the total serum bilirubin level is equal to or greater than 5 mg/dL (85 micromoles per liter) above these lines. Risk factors are isoimmune hemolytic disease, G6PD deficiency, asphyxia, significant lethargy, temperature instability, sepsis, and acidosis. Measure serum albumin level and calculate bilirubin/albumin ratio. Use total bilirubin. Do not subtract direct reacting or conjugated bilirubin. If the infant is well and at 35–37 6/7 weeks of gestation (medium risk), total serum bilirubin levels for exchange can be individualized based on actual gestational age. (Management of hyperbilirubinemia in the newborn infant 35 or more weeks of gestation. American Academy of Pediatrics Subcommittee on Hyperbilirubinemia [published erratum appears in Pediatrics 2004;114:1138]. Pediatrics 2004;114:297–316.)

of increase in bilirubin concentration above this rate provides presumptive evidence of a hemolytic process and should prompt lowering the threshold for treatment by 3–5 mg per dL depending on severity. Visible jaundice during the first 24 hours after birth is also indicative of excessive hemolysis but it is not reliably seen.

Preterm Infants

Susceptibility to bilirubin toxicity increases as gestational age decreases. A recent report found that the average bilirubin binding capacity of preterm infants increased by 0.93 mg per dL for each week of gestation. Coincidently, albumin concentration increases by approximately 0.11 g per dL per week of gestation. These data provide a rationale for lowering the treatment threshold by approximately 1 mg per dL for each week of gestational age less than 37 weeks.

Extremely-Low-Birth-Weight Infants

The neurodevelopmental effects of aggressive phototherapy versus conservative phototherapy were compared in a large multicenter trial. Aggressive phototherapy was started at study entry and continued for total bilirubin values exceeding 5 mg per dL during the first postnatal week and values greater than 7 mg per dL during the second week. Conservative phototherapy was started at 8 mg per dL for infants with birth weights of 501–750 g and at 10 mg per dL for infants with birth weights of 751–1,000 g. Exchange transfusion was performed if phototherapy failed to bring the bilirubin below 13 mg per dL for the lower birth weight group and 15 mg per dL for the higher birth weight cohort. Aggressive phototherapy did not significantly reduce the rate of death or neurodevelopmental impairment at 18–22 months corrected age (52% versus 55%). Although aggressive phototherapy did significantly reduce the frequency of neurodevelopmental impairment in survivors (26% versus 30%), this reduction was offset by an increased mortality rate in infants weighing 501–750 g at birth (39% versus 34%). Thus, when to initiate phototherapy in the extremely-low-birth-weight infant remains uncertain.

Breastfeeding and Hyperbilirubinemia

Frequent breastfeeding (8–12 breastfeedings every 24 hours) decreases the incidence of hyperbilirubinemia. Supplementing with water or dextrose-water does not ameliorate jaundice and cannot be recommended. Breastfeeding can significantly affect the incidence and duration of unconjugated hyperbilirubinemia compared with formula feeding, in two ways:

1. Inadequate intake—This condition is more common with a first-time breastfeeding mother, cesarean birth, maternal diabetes, or with a late preterm infant. Early hospital discharge (less than 24 hours of age) is an additional risk factor. Inadequate milk intake can result in excessive weight loss over the initial 7–14 days of age, marked hyperbilirubinemia, and, rarely, bilirubin encephalopathy or death. Caloric deprivation and increased enterohepatic circulation of bilirubin are more likely responsible for this result than dehydration. Education and breastfeeding support of the mother, together with early and close follow-up after hospital discharge to evaluate the feeding process and the infant's health, are essential to prevent adverse outcomes. If inadequate milk intake persists, infants should be evaluated, rehydrated if needed, and supplemented with mother's milk, if available, or infant formula.
2. Breast milk jaundice—This condition is characterized by a persistence of physiologic jaundice beyond the first week of age. Breastfed infants commonly have serum bilirubin concentrations greater than 5 mg per dL (85.5 micromoles per liter) for several weeks after delivery. This persistent, mild unconjugated hyperbilirubinemia is caused by a variably identified factor in human milk that promotes an increase in intestinal absorption of bilirubin in combination with mutations of the uridine diphosphate-glucuronidase gene. Infants with jaundice that persists beyond 2 weeks of age should be monitored to ensure that the jaundice is not cholestatic in nature, the concentration of bilirubin is not increasing, and other pathologic causes for jaundice are not present.

If the serum unconjugated bilirubin concentration in a breastfed, term, healthy infant is increasing and exceeds 20 mg per dL (171 micromoles per liter), the physician has several options:

- Phototherapy and assessment of the mother–infant dyad during breastfeeding.
- Phototherapy with continued breastfeeding plus supplementation with mother's expressed breast milk, if available, or infant formula. Supplementation with formula is recommended only if the mother's milk supply is insufficient.

- Substitution of infant formula for breast milk for 24 hours. The bilirubin concentration should decrease at least 4 mg per dL. Mother's milk production should be supported during this time, and breastfeeding resumed thereafter.

Dehydration and Hyperbilirubinemia

Most infants readmitted to hospital with hyperbilirubinemia are not dehydrated, and phototherapy or exchange transfusion should not be delayed for rehydration. The infant should be sent directly to the service that can perform an exchange transfusion, if needed. Clinical assessment and the serum sodium concentration will indicate whether rehydration is needed or not.

Clinical Assessment

Newborn nurseries and newborn infant health care providers should have standard protocols to monitor all infants for the development of jaundice (see also "Hyperbilirubinemia Screening" in Chapter 10). Noninvasive transcutaneous bilirubin measurement devices can provide a valid estimate of the total serum bilirubin concentration of less than 15 mg per dL (257 micromoles per liter) in the majority of infants.

Laboratory Evaluation

A transcutaneous or serum measurement of bilirubin concentration should be performed whenever jaundice is observed. The need for and timing of a repeat transcutaneous bilirubin measurement or total serum bilirubin measurement will depend on the age of the infant and the progression of the hyperbilirubinemia. When serum bilirubin values exceed 15 mg per dL, measurement of serum albumin concentrations should be obtained.

Risk Assessment

Every newborn infant should undergo a risk assessment for developing hyperbilirubinemia before discharge to home. Estimating bilirubin concentration by observing the extent of clinical jaundice can be misleading and should not be used for assessing risk. The 2004 AAP guideline recommends a predischarge bilirubin measurement or assessment of clinical risk factors to evaluate the risk of severe hyperbilirubinemia (see Box 10-2 "Major Risk Factors for Development of Severe Hyperbilirubinemia in Infants of 35 or More Weeks of Gestation" in Chapter 10). A subsequent consensus opinion of experts strongly recommended that a predischarge measurement of transcutaneous or serum bilirubin be performed on all newborn infants. If the transcutaneous or serum bilirubin concentration is measured, the value obtained should be interpreted in light of the infant's age in hours (see Fig. 11-1) to estimate risk for severe hyperbilirubinemia. A structured approach to management and follow-up of infants at risk of developing hyperbilirubinemia is recommended and should include the predischarge bilirubin measurement, the infant's gestational age, and other risk factors for hyperbilirubinemia.

Follow-up

All institutions with obstetric–newborn services should provide written and verbal information to families at the time of discharge, including an explanation of jaundice, the need to monitor infants for jaundice, and advice on how monitoring should be done. (A bilingual example of a parent information handout is available at: www.healthychildren.org/English/ages-stages/baby/Pages/Jaundice.aspx).

All infants should be examined by a qualified health care professional at 3–5 days postnatal age or within 48 hours of discharge to home to assess the infant's well-being and the presence or absence of jaundice. The timing and location of this assessment will be determined by the length of stay in the nursery, risk zone assigned according to the hour-specific bilirubin concentration (see Fig. 11-1) and the presence or absence of risk factors for hyperbilirubinemia.

The follow-up assessment should include the infant's weight and percent change from birth weight (compared to the appropriate standard for breastfed or formula fed infants), adequacy of intake, the pattern of voiding and stooling, and the presence or absence of jaundice (see Fig. 10-4 and Fig. 10-5 in Chapter 10). The predischarge risk zone and clinical risk factors should be used to determine the need for a bilirubin measurement. Jaundice that persists beyond 2 weeks requires further investigation, including measurement of total and direct serum bilirubin concentrations. A concentration of direct reacting or conjugated serum bilirubin higher than 1 mg per dL should prompt further investigation for cholestasis.

Treatment

Treatment for neonatal hyperbilirubinemia includes phototherapy and exchange transfusion.

Phototherapy. Several devices for delivering phototherapy are available. The efficacy of phototherapy is influenced by the energy output (irradiance) in the blue spectrum (measured in microwatts per centimeter squared), the spectrum of the light source, and the surface area of the infant exposed to the light source. The irradiance of a unit should be monitored. More effective phototherapy can be achieved by using blue lights, decreasing the distance of the source from the infant, and increasing the surface area exposed to the lights. The infant's temperature should be monitored while phototherapy is being applied. Phototherapy may be provided in the mother's hospital room to facilitate breastfeeding. Interrupting phototherapy for feedings or family visits will not reduce effectiveness significantly.

Phototherapy has many biologic effects; however, it is undetermined if there are lasting adverse effects in the human infant. Experiments in animals have documented retinal damage from phototherapy; therefore, the infant's eyes should be covered with opaque patches during exposure to phototherapy light. Eye patches should be monitored for placement because they can obstruct the nares or cause corneal abrasions if improperly placed. Periodic inspection of the eyes and skin under the patches is advisable.

Guidelines may be developed by each institution to define criteria for infants who are eligible for home phototherapy. Home care requires appropriate follow-up and supervision by a health care professional capable of obtaining blood samples for the measurement of serum bilirubin concentration when clinically indicated. If the serum bilirubin concentration does not decrease in response to home phototherapy, admission to the hospital may be indicated for more intensive phototherapy and for further investigation for an underlying cause.

Exchange Transfusion. Guidelines for initiation of phototherapy and exchange transfusion are shown in Figure 11-1 and Figure 11-2. For example, a 33-week apparently healthy infant with no evidence of hemolysis and an albumin concentration of 3.0 g per dL would be started on phototherapy at 15 mg per dL and receive an exchange transfusion at 20 mg per dL. If the same infant had hemolytic disease, she or he would be treated at lower thresholds. Infants with hyperbilirubinemia and symptoms consistent with BIND have recovered without long-term neurodevelopmental damage when treated promptly with exchange transfusion.

Computer and smartphone-based programs are available for interpreting the hour-specific bilirubin concentration and for treatment thresholds. They include several such as BiliTool and BiliCalc based on previously published AAP guidelines.

Hypoglycemia

Neonatal hypoglycemia occurs most commonly in infants who are small for gestational age, infants born to mothers with diabetes, and preterm infants (see also "Glucose Homeostasis Screening" in Chapter 10). Routine screening and monitoring of blood glucose concentrations is not needed in healthy term newborns after an entirely normal pregnancy and delivery. Blood glucose concentrations should only be measured in term infants who are known to be at risk (infants who are small for gestational age, infants who are large for gestational age, infants who were born to mothers who have diabetes, and late preterm infants) or who have clinical manifestations. The definition of a plasma glucose concentration at which intervention is indicated needs to be tailored to the clinical situation and the particular characteristics of a given infant. Because severe, prolonged, symptomatic hypoglycemia may result in neuronal injury, prompt intervention is necessary for infants who manifest clinical signs and symptoms.

Guidelines for initiating treatment in asymptomatic infants are less clear. Figure 11-3 depicts a guideline for the screening and management of neonatal hypoglycemia in asymptomatic late-preterm infants and asymptomatic term infants who are born to mothers with diabetes, small for gestational age, or large for gestational age. The figure is divided into two periods (birth to 4 hours and 4–24 hours) and accounts for the changing values of glucose that occur over the first 12 hours after birth. The recommended values for intervention are intended to provide a margin of safety over concentrations of glucose associated with clinical signs. The recommendations also provide a range of values over which the physician can decide to refeed or provide intravenous glucose. At-risk infants should be fed by 1 hour of age and screened 30 minutes after the feeding. Gavage feeding may be considered in infants who are not suckling well.

Glucose screening should continue until 12 hours of age for infants born to mothers with diabetes and those who are large for gestational age. Late-preterm infants and infants who are small for gestational age require glucose monitoring for at least 24 hours after birth, especially if regular feedings are not yet established. It is recommended that the at-risk asymptomatic infant who has glucose concentrations of less than 25 mg per dL (birth to 4 hours of age) or less than 35 mg per dL (4–24 hours of age) be refed and that the glucose value be rechecked 1 hour after refeeding. Subsequent concentrations lower than 25 mg per dL (birth to 4 hours of age), or lower than 35 mg per dL

(4–24 hours of age), after attempts to refeed, necessitate treatment with an intravenous bolus of 2 mL per kg $D_{10}W$ (200 mg per kg), an intravenous infusion of $D_{10}W$ at 5–8 mg per kg per minute (80–100 mL per kg per day), or both. If it is not possible to maintain blood glucose concentrations of greater than 45 mg per dL after 24 hours of an intravenous glucose infusion, consideration should be given to the possibility of hyperinsulinemic hypoglycemia. A blood sample should be sent for measurement of insulin along with a glucose concentration at the time when a bedside blood glucose concentration is less than 40 mg per dL, and a pediatric endocrinologist should be consulted. Similarly, infants who require continuous intravenous infusion for more than 48 hours to maintain a glucose level greater than 45 mg per dL need further evaluation.

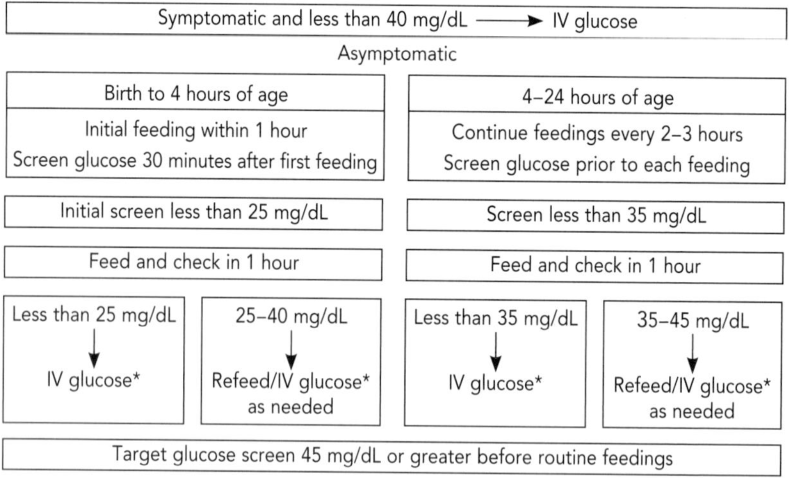

Figure 11-3. Screening and management of postnatal glucose homeostasis in late preterm (34–36 6/7 weeks of gestation) infants, small-for-gestational-age infants, infants who were born to mothers with diabetes, and large-for-gestational-age infants. Screen late preterm and small-for-gestational-age infants every 0–24 hours and infants who are born to mothers with diabetes and large-for-gestational-age infants who are 34 or more weeks of gestation, every 0–12 hours. Abbreviation: IV, intravenous. *Glucose dose is 200 mg per kg ($D_{10}W$ at mL per kg) and/or IV infusion at 5–8 mg per kg per min (80–100 mL per kg per d). Achieve plasma glucose level of 40–50 mg per dL. (Adamkin DH. Postnatal glucose homeostasis in late-preterm and term infants. American Academy of Pediatrics Committee on Fetus and Newborn. Pediatrics 2011;127:575–9.)

Neonatal Drug Withdrawal

Maternal use of certain drugs during pregnancy can result in neonatal neurobehavioral signs that may be transient (ie, hours if due to acute drug toxicity), prolonged (days to weeks if due to withdrawal) or sustained (months to years if due to a lasting drug effect). In addition, hospitalized infants who are treated with opioids or benzodiazepines to provide analgesia or sedation may be at risk of manifesting signs of withdrawal. Signs characteristic of neonatal withdrawal have been attributed to intrauterine exposure to a variety of drugs (Table 11-2). Other drugs cause signs in infants because of

TABLE 11-2. Maternal Nonnarcotic Drugs That Cause Neonatal Psychomotor Behavior Consistent With Withdrawal

Drug	Signs	Onset of Signs
Alcohol[1,2]	Hyperactivity, crying, irritability, poor suck, tremors, seizures, poor sleeping pattern, hyperphagia, diaphoresis; onset of signs at birth	3–12 hours
Barbiturates[3,4]	Irritability, severe tremors, hyperacusis, excessive crying, vasomotor instability, diarrhea, restlessness, increased tone, hyperphagia, vomiting, disturbed sleep; onset first 24 hours of life or as late as 10–14 days of age	1–14 days
Caffeine[5]	Jitteriness, vomiting, bradycardia, tachypnea	At birth
Chlordiazepoxide[6]	Irritability, tremors; signs may start at 21 days	Days to weeks
Clomipramine[7]	Hypothermia, cyanosis, tremors; onset 12 hours of age	
Diazepam[8]	Hypotonia, poor suck, hypothermia, apnea, hypertonia, hyperreflexia, tremors, vomiting, hyperactivity, tachypnea (mother receiving multiple drug therapy)	Hours to weeks
Ethchlorvynol[9]	Lethargy, jitteriness, hyperphagia, irritability, poor suck, hypotonia (mother receiving multiple drug therapy)	
Glutethimide[10]	Increased tone, tremors, opisthotonos, high-pitched cry, hyperactivity, irritability, colic	
Hydroxyzine[11]	Tremors, irritability, hyperactivity, jitteriness, shrill cry, myoclonic jerks, hypotonia, increased respiratory and heart rates, feeding problems, clonic movements (mother receiving multiple drug therapy)	

(continued)

TABLE 11-2. Maternal Nonnarcotic Drugs That Cause Neonatal Psychomotor Behavior Consistent With Withdrawal *(continued)*

Drug	Signs	Onset of Signs
Meprobamate[12]	Irritability, tremors, poor sleep patterns, abdominal pain	
Selective serotonin reuptake inhibitors[13–16]	Crying, irritability, tremors, poor suck, feeding difficulty, hypertonia, tachypnea, sleep disturbance, hypoglycemia, seizures	Hours to days

1. Pierog S, Chandavasu O, Wexler I. Withdrawal symptoms in infants with the fetal alcohol syndrome. J Pediatr 1977;90(4):630–3.
2. Nichols MM. Acute alcohol withdrawal syndrome in a newborn. Am J Dis Child 1967; 113(6):714–5.
3. Bleyer WA, Marshall RE. Barbiturate withdrawal syndrome in a passively addicted infant. JAMA 1972;221(2):185–6.
4. Desmond MM, Schwanecke RP, Wilson GS, Yasunaga S, Burgdorff I. Maternal barbiturate utilization and neonatal withdrawal symptomatology. J Pediatr 1972;80(2):190–7.
5. McGowan JD, Altman RE, Kanto WP Jr. Neonatal withdrawal symptoms after chronic maternal ingestion of caffeine. South Med J 1988;81(9):1092–4.
6. Athinarayanan P, Pierog SH, Nigam SK, Glass L. Chloriazepoxide withdrawal in the neonate. Am J Obstet Gynecol 1976;124(2):212–3.
7. Musa AB, Smith CS. Neonatal effects of maternal clomipramine therapy. Arch Dis Child 1979;54(5):405.
8. Rementería JL, Bhatt K. Withdrawal symptoms in neonates from intrauterine exposure to diazepam J Pediatr 1977;90(1):123–6.
9. Rumack BH, Walravens PA. Neonatal withdrawal following maternal ingestion of ethchlorvynol (Placidyl) Pediatrics 1973;52(5):714–6.
10. Reveri M, Pyati SP, Pildes RS. Neonatal withdrawal symptoms associated with glutethimide (Doriden) addiction in the mother during pregnancy. Clin Pediatr 1977;16(5):424–5.
11. van Baar AL, Fleury P, Soepatmi S, Ultee CA, Wesselman PJ. Neonatal behavior after drug dependent pregnancy. Arch Dis Child 1989;64(2):235–40.
12. Desmond MM, Rudolph AJ, Hill RM, Claghorn JL, Dreesen PR, Burgdorff I. Behavioral alterations in infants born to mothers on psychoactive medication during pregnancy. In: Farrell G, ed. Congenital Mental Retardation. Austin, TX: University of Texas Press; 1969:235–44.
13. Dahl ML, Olhager E, Ahlner J. Paroxetine withdrawal syndrome in a neonate. Br J Psychiatry 1997;171:391–2.
14. Sanz EJ, De-las-Cuevas C, Kiuru A, Bate A, Edwards R. Selective serotonin reuptake inhibitors in pregnant women and neonatal withdrawal syndrome: a database analysis. Lancet 2005;365(9458):482–7.
15. Chambers CD, Johnson KA, Dick LM, Felix RJ, Jones KL. Birth outcomes in pregnant women taking fluoxetine. N Engl J Med 1996;335(14):1010–5.
16. Haddad PM, Pal BR, Clarke P, Wieck A, Sridhiran S. Neonatal symptoms following maternal paroxetine treatment: serotonin toxicity or paroxetine discontinuation syndrome? J Psychopharmacol 2005;19(5):554–7.

Modified from Neonatal drug withdrawal. American Academy of Pediatrics Committee on Drugs, Committee on Fetus and Newborn. Pediatrics 2012;129:e540–60.

acute toxicity. Chronic in utero exposure to a drug (eg, alcohol) can lead to permanent phenotypical and neurodevelopmental behavioral abnormalities consistent with drug effect. In the newborn, signs of withdrawal worsen as drug levels decrease, whereas signs of acute toxicity abate with drug elimination. Clinically important neonatal withdrawal most commonly results from intrauterine opioid exposure. The constellation of clinical findings associated with opioid withdrawal has been termed "neonatal abstinence syndrome" (NAS). The national incidence of NAS has climbed from 1.2 to 5.8 per 1,000 live births between 2000 and 2012 but geographic variation is significant. A number of factors have driven this escalation, including increased use of prescription opioids. Withdrawal signs will develop in as many as 55–94% of infants exposed to certain opioids (eg, heroin or methadone) in utero, but the likelihood of withdrawal decreases to less than 5% with exposure to low-dose short-acting prescription opioids. Neonatal withdrawal signs also have been described in infants exposed antenatally to benzodiazepines, barbiturates, nicotine, and alcohol.

Because fetal drug exposure often is unrecognized in the immediate newborn period, affected infants may be discharged to homes where they are at increased risk of a variety of medical and social problems, including abuse and neglect. Women who use nonmedical substances are at increased risk of hepatitis (especially hepatitis C), human immunodeficiency virus (HIV) infection, herpes, and syphilis, each of which can have significant adverse effects on the fetus and newborn. In addition, these women may have received little or no prenatal care, further increasing risks for the infant.

The specific effect of drug exposure on the fetus and newborn will vary depending on the substance(s) ingested, the time course and amounts of doses received, and individual susceptibility. Nonmedical drugs that have been reported to have adverse effects on nursing infants include cocaine, methamphetamine, heroin, marijuana, and phencyclidine. Breastfeeding women should be counseled about the potential adverse effects of continued use of nonmedical substances on the newborn infant. A mother who has documented adherence to a treatment protocol and has no other contraindication to breastfeeding should be encouraged to breastfeed.

Screening and Testing

Because prenatal screening fails to identify a proportion of women with nonmedical substance use, clinicians have used the presence of maternal or infant characteristics known to be associated with drug use in pregnancy as indications for direct testing. Typically, infant urine or meconium samples are tested for a variety of drugs and substances. Infant characteristics that may be associated with maternal drug use include prematurity; unexplained intrauterine growth restriction; neurobehavioral abnormalities; and atypical vascular incidents, such as cerebrovascular accidents, myocardial infarction, and necrotizing enterocolitis in otherwise healthy full-term infants. The legal implications of testing a newborn who does not have clinical signs compatible with intrauterine drug exposure and the need for maternal consent to perform the test may vary among the states. Hospitals and physicians should carefully craft policies and procedures in consideration of state laws.

The duration of urinary excretion of most drugs is relatively short, and a neonatal urine sample that is positive for drug exposure may only address drug exposure in the hours immediately before the sample was collected. Thus, a urine sample may be falsely negative in the setting of significant intrauterine drug exposure. Testing a meconium sample for intrauterine drug exposure results in fewer false-negative test results but does not inform about recent exposure. For any test, the clinician should be knowledgeable about what drugs are analyzed and what thresholds are used to report a positive result. Additional assessment of infants of mothers with substance use disorders may include testing for hepatitis B, hepatitis C, HIV, and other sexually transmitted infections.

The likelihood, time of onset, and severity of NAS varies as a function of opioid exposure and other co-factors. Infants exposed exclusively to heroin, a short acting opioid, typically develop signs of NAS within the first 24 hours after birth in contrast to infants exposed to methadone or buprenorphine who may not develop signs of NAS until 7 days of age. Infants born to mothers on a low-dose prescription opioid with a short half-life are unlikely to develop NAS if they are still asymptomatic at 2–3 days of age. Buprenorphine exposure is associated with a lower incidence and a lesser severity of NAS than methadone exposure; however, severe NAS has been reported in individual buprenorphine-exposed infants. Maternal smoking, treatment with selective serotonin reuptake inhibitors, and benzodiazepine therapy increase the likelihood of clinically significant NAS. Emerging evidence suggests that both single nucleotide polymorphisms of certain genes (eg, mu opioid receptor 1 [OPRM1], catechol-*O*-methyltransferase [COMT]) and epigenetic influences (eg, methylation of the promoter gene for OPRM1) are associated with a higher incidence and greater severity of NAS. Infants born before 35 weeks of gestation have a lower likelihood of developing NAS than full-term infants.

There are insufficient data to evaluate the effects of maternal marijuana use on infants who are breastfed, and in the absence of such data, marijuana use among women who are breastfeeding their infants should be discouraged.

In-Hospital Treatment

Health care providers should be trained to recognize signs of neonatal withdrawal (Box 11-1), and drug withdrawal should be considered in the differential diagnosis of newborn infants who manifest the typical signs. Each

Box 11-1. Clinical Features of Neonatal Narcotic Abstinence Syndrome

Neurologic Excitability

- Tremors
- Irritability
- Increased wakefulness
- High-pitched crying
- Increased muscle tone
- Hyperactive deep tendon reflexes
- Exaggerated Moro reflex
- Seizures
- Frequent yawning and sneezing

Gastrointestinal Dysfunction

- Poor feeding
- Uncoordinated and constant sucking
- Vomiting
- Diarrhea
- Dehydration
- Poor weight gain

Autonomic Signs

- Increased sweating
- Nasal stuffiness
- Fever
- Mottling
- Temperature instability

Reprinted from Hudak ML, Tan RC. Neonatal drug withdrawal. Committee on Drugs, Committee on Fetus and Newborn American Academy of Pediatrics [published erratum appears in Pediatrics 2014;133:937]. Pediatrics 2012;129:e540–60.

nursery should develop an evidence-based written policy to assess and treat an infant with NAS.

The goals of treating infants with signs of drug withdrawal are to achieve consistent weight gain, establish a normal sleep–wake cycle, and encourage social interaction. Families should be encouraged to visit and care for their infants, and mothers should be supported in their effort to breastfeed their infants, if appropriate. Promotion of parental care and breastfeeding are important to the degree possible. Beyond intrinsic health benefits, breastfeeding has been linked to reductions in length of stay and a lower cumulative dose of opioid treatment.

The initial treatment of infants with confirmed intrauterine drug exposure who have no or minimal signs of withdrawal should include supportive measures such as minimizing environmental stimuli (eg, sound and light); swaddling to prevent motor hyperactivity and to facilitate oral feeding; offering frequent small feedings of hypercaloric formula (24 calories per ounce) if needed; padding the elbows, knees, and other pressure points to prevent skin excoriation; and liberally applying barrier treatments to prevent diaper dermatitis.

Although the optimal criteria for initiation of pharmacologic therapy are unknown, most institutions use the modified Finnegan Neonatal Abstinence Scoring Tool (Fig. 11-4) to decide when to treat an infant with pharmacologic therapy. The ability to score the severity of signs of withdrawal with minimal interobserver variability enables decisions about the institution of pharmacologic therapy to be more objective and allows a quantitative approach to increasing or decreasing dosages.

Seizures have been reported to occur in as many as 2–11% of infants with withdrawal and warrant pharmacologic therapy. Excessive vomiting or diarrhea, dehydration, or poor weight gain may be indications for treatment, even in the absence of high total withdrawal scores.

Primary treatment with the same class of drug as the agent causing withdrawal is successful in most cases. In the United States, oral morphine solution and methadone are the most commonly used opioids. Phenobarbital and clonidine also have been used both as initial and adjunctive treatments. Although there are no data defining an optimal treatment protocol, preliminary evidence suggests that methadone therapy shortens the length of hospital stay and reduces the total amount of postnatal opioid exposure compared with oral morphine. If pharmacologic treatment is deemed necessary, initial dosages can be tailored to the severity of the signs of withdrawal. In most cases, maintenance doses of 0.2–0.3 mg per kg per day of oral morphine (divided every 3–4 hours) or methadone (divided every 8–12 hours) can be initiated with higher initial doses used for more severe signs of withdrawal (see Table 11-3). Because methadone has a longer half-life than morphine (12–24 hours versus 3–4 hours) a loading dose of 0.4–0.5 mg per kg may be appropriate. Barring exigencies, clinicians should wait 12–24 hours to reach steady-state drug levels before increasing the dose. Infants who are not responsive to maximal doses of opioid therapy can be treated adjunctively with clonidine or phenobarbital. Once an infant has responded to treatment, the opioid dose can be weaned 10–20% every 1–2 days based on average withdrawal scores. Adjunctive therapy can be weaned once the opioid is discontinued. Opioid weaning can continue even if Finnegan scores are in the higher range of normal. Developing and adhering to a treatment protocol likely has a greater effect on reducing length of stay than does the choice of a particular drug.

Physicians should be aware that the severity of withdrawal signs, including seizures, after intrauterine drug exposure has not been associated with an increased risk of poor neurodevelopmental outcome. Furthermore, although treatment of NAS will alleviate signs of withdrawal, there is no evidence that treatment results in improved neurodevelopmental outcome.

Discharge and Follow-up Care

Documentation of in utero nonmedical substance exposure and alcohol use by the mother may preclude early discharge after birth. Social work assessment is critical to plan appropriately for discharge and subsequent follow-up care. Because of the highly variable prenatal circumstances of infants with NAS, referral to child protective services should not occur reflexively but may be made if there is a legitimate concern about the future well-being of the infant.

A number of reports from centers in the United States and across the world have described experiences with home discharge of infants who are being treated for NAS with subsequent tapering of medication in the outpatient setting. At this point, there are insufficient data to evaluate fully the safety and efficacy of this strategy compared with treatment in the hospital. Although no study has reported an increase in complications or a higher rate of rehospitalization for infants treated in the outpatient setting compared with those treated in the hospital, some studies have documented a longer duration of treatment and a higher total dose of medication associated with outpatient

System	Signs and Symptoms	Score			
Central nervous system disturbnces	Excessive high pitched (or other) cry	2			
	Continuous high pitched (or other) cry	3			
	Sleeps less than1 hour after feeding	3			
	Sleeps less than 2 hours after feeding	2			
	Sleeps less than 3 hours after feeding	1			
	Hyperactive moro reflex	2			
	Markedly hyperactive moro reflex	3			
	Mild tremors disturbed	1			
	Moderate-severe tremors disturbed	2			
	Mild tremors undisturbed	3			
	Moderate-severe tremors undisturbed	4			
	Increased muscle tone	2			
	Excoriation (specific area)	1			
	Myoclonic jerks	3			
	Generalized convulsions	5			
Metabolic/vasomotor/respiratory disturbances	Sweating	1			
	Fever 100.4-101°F (38-38.3°C)	1			
	Fever more than 101°F (38.3°C)	2			
	Frequent yawning (more than 3-4 times/interval)	1			
	Mottling	1			
	Nasal stuffiness	1			
	Sneezing (more than 3-4 times/interval)	1			
	Nasal flaring	2			
	Respiratory rate more than 60/min	1			
	Respiratory rate more than 60/min with retractions	2			
Gastrointestinal disturbances	Excessive sucking	1			
	Poor feeding	2			
	Regurgitation	2			
	Projectile vomiting	3			
	Loose stools	2			
	Watery stools	3			
	Total score				
	Initials of scorer				

Figure 11-4. Modified Finnegan Neonatal Abstinence Scoring Tool. (Adapted from Finnegan LP. Neonatal abstinence syndrome. In: Nelson NM, editor. Current therapy in neonatal-perinatal medicine. 2nd ed. Toronto: B.C.Decker; 1990. p. 314–20.)

PM

Comments

Daily Weight

management. At a minimum, careful screening of potential families by social workers and the availability of comprehensive resources to ensure outpatient follow-up are essential components of an outpatient treatment program.

TABLE 11-3. Drugs Used to Treat Infants with Neonatal Opioid Withdrawal

Drug	Initial Dose	Increment	Maximum dose	Comments
Primary therapy				
Oral morphine	Maintenance dose 0.2–0.3 mg/kg/d Divided every 3–4 hours	0.08–0.16 mg/kg/d	1.2 mg/kg/d	With moderate signs of NAS, start at 0.24 mg/kg/d (0.03 mg/kg every 3 hours or 0.04 mg/kg every 4 hours) If signs of NAS are not sufficiently relieved after initial dose, may give additional dose of 0.03–0.04 mg/kg to achieve adequate level
Oral methadone*	Maintenance dose 0.2–0.3 mg/kg/d Divided every 6–12 hours	0.1–0.2 mg/kg/day	0.5–0.6 mg/kg/d	Because of prolonged time for methadone to reach steady state level, consider loading with 0.2 mg/kg followed by institution of maintenance dose in 6–12 hours
Adjunctive therapy				
Oral clonidine	0.5–1 micrograms every 6 hours		1 microgram every 4 hours	If signs of NAS are controlled with opioid plus clonidine, wean opioid first and then wean clonidine
Oral phenobarbital	Loading dose 10–20 mg/kg Maintenance dose 5 mg/kg/d Divided every 12 hours			Caution that effect of phenobarbital is heightened by systemic opioids

Abbreviation: NAS, neonatal abstinence syndrome.

*Ward RM, Drover DR, Hammer GB, Stemland CJ, Kern S, Tristani-Firouzi M, et al. The pharmacokinetics of methadone and its metabolites in neonates, infants, and children. Paediatr Anaesth 2014;24:591–601.

Long-term effects on learning and school performance, behavioral problems, and emotional instability of infants exposed to nonmedical drugs, alcohol, and tobacco in utero remain major concerns. Drug exposure during development may have long-lasting effects on behavioral and cognitive outcomes. These effects also may result from environmental factors that place drug-exposed infants at high risk of physical, sexual, and emotional abuse, neglect, and developmental delay. Prenatal exposure to opioids does not preclude normal development. Multidisciplinary long-term follow-up should include medical, developmental, and social support. In general, a coordinated multidisciplinary approach without criminal sanctions has the best chance of helping infants and families. The separation of parents from their children solely based on substance use disorders, either suspected or confirmed, is discouraged.

Management of Acquired Opioid and Benzodiazepine Dependency

One of the cornerstones in caring for critically ill infants is to provide adequate and safe analgesia, sedation, amnesia, and anxiolysis using both pharmacologic and nonpharmacologic measures. Pharmacologic treatment typically includes medications in the opioid and benzodiazepine drug classes. If these drugs cannot safely be discontinued within a few days, physical dependence on one or both of these classes of medication can develop, and infants often manifest signs and symptoms of withdrawal upon acute dosage reduction or cessation of therapy. Infants who undergo complex surgery, who require prolonged medical intensive care for conditions such as respiratory failure or persistent pulmonary hypertension, or who are supported with extracorporeal membrane oxygenation (ECMO) therapy are among those at greatest risk of acquired drug dependency. Infants cared for in intensive care units who have developed tolerance to opioids and benzodiazepines because of an extended duration of intravenous treatment can be converted to an equivalent regimen of oral methadone and lorazepam. Doses may be increased as necessary to achieve patient comfort. These medications can then be reduced by 10–20% every 1–2 days based on the clinical response and the serial assessments using a standardized abstinence instrument.

Respiratory Complications

Oxygen Therapy

Studies conducted in the 1950s indicated that prolonged unmonitored oxygen therapy was associated with increased rates of retinopathy of prematurity

(ROP). This discovery led to widespread restriction of oxygen therapy, associated with a marked decrease in ROP but an increase in cerebral palsy and mortality. Current practice recommends supplemental oxygen as needed, based on objective monitoring of oxygenation. Clinical assessment of physical signs to determine the amount of supplemental oxygen needed may be useful for short periods, emergencies, or abrupt clinical changes, but should not be the basis for ongoing supplemental oxygen therapy.

Supplemental oxygen can be delivered through endotracheal tube, mask, oxygen hood, nasal prongs, or cannula. Except in emergency situations, supplemental oxygen should be warmed and humidified, and the concentration or flow should be monitored and regulated. Orders for oxygen therapy should include desired ambient concentration, and flow, if applicable. The concentration and flow rate of oxygen should be checked routinely. Orders should be written to adjust the fraction of inspired oxygen (FIO_2) or flow within a stated range to maintain oxygen saturation within specified limits. There should be institutional guidelines for ordering, delivering, and documenting oxygen therapy and monitoring. Oxygen analyzers should be calibrated in accordance with manufacturers' recommendations.

An important development in the care of infants who require oxygen therapy is the ability to monitor oxygenation continuously with noninvasive techniques. The pulse oximeter measures the percentage of arterial hemoglobin saturated with oxygen. For oxygen saturations less than or equal to 95%, pulse oximetry will closely predict PaO_2 (particularly if adjustments are made for the presence of fetal hemoglobin), and it is an excellent continuous monitor of oxygenation; however, at saturations greater than 95%, the PaO_2 may be unacceptably high. Transcutaneous monitoring of PaO_2 will give more accurate estimates of PaO_2 especially at higher oxygen saturations, but is technically more challenging to use. Because the heated membrane of the transcutaneous oxygen-monitoring device may cause burns, oxygenation monitoring by pulse oximetry has become the clinical standard.

Continuous measurement of pulse oximetry combined with periodic measurement of PaO_2 in samples from an umbilical or peripheral artery catheter is the most complete method of monitoring oxygen therapy. In infants whose conditions are unstable, noninvasive measurements should be correlated with PaO_2 as often as every 8–24 hours. More frequent analyses of arterial blood gas may be indicated for the assessment of pH and $PaCO_2$. In infants whose condition is stable, correlation with arterial blood gas samples may be performed when clinically indicated.

In the absence of an indwelling arterial catheter, arterialized capillary sampling provides reasonable estimates of arterial pH and $Paco_2$ if perfusion to the extremity is not compromised. Although Pao_2 is not accurately estimated in arterialized capillary samples, the combined use of continuous oxygen saturation monitoring and intermittent capillary arterialized blood gases can guide oxygen therapy. In this circumstance, oxygen saturation should not be allowed to remain above 95%, as previously described, particularly in preterm infants at risk of ROP.

The use of either pulse oximetry or transcutaneous oxygen measurement may shorten the time required to determine optimum inspired oxygen concentration and ventilator settings in the acute care setting. Both measurements are also useful in monitoring oxygen therapy in infants who are recovering from respiratory distress or who require long-term supplemental oxygen. Pulse oximetry is particularly advantageous for long-term monitoring of oxygen therapy because transcutaneous oxygen measurements underestimate oxygenation in older infants with BPD.

In consideration of the current, but incomplete, understanding of the effects of oxygen administration, the following recommendations are offered:

- Supplemental oxygen should be used for specific indications, such as cyanosis, low Pao_2, or low oxygen saturation.
- For infants who require oxygen therapy for acute care, measurements of blood pH and $Paco_2$ should accompany measurements of Pao_2. In addition, a record of blood gas measurements, noninvasive measurements of oxygenation, details of the oxygen delivery system (eg, ventilator, continuous positive airway pressure, nasal cannula, hood, mask, settings), and ambient oxygen concentrations ($F{\rm IO}_2$, liter of flow per minute, or both) should be maintained.
- The optimal range for oxygen saturation and Pao_2 that balances tissue metabolism, growth and development, and toxicity has not been elucidated for preterm infants receiving supplemental oxygen. Data from cohort studies suggest that lower saturation ranges may decrease severe ROP. Meta-analyses of five randomized controlled trials (RCTs) confirmed that a target saturation range of 85–89%, compared with a target range of 91–95%, was associated with a decrease in severe ROP, but was also associated with an increase in necrotizing enterocolitis and death before discharge; however, one meta-analysis noted that the quality of evidence for the estimate of mortality was low and that rates

of disability or death at 24 months were no different. These trials also underscored the fact that, even with careful monitoring, oxygen saturation and Pao_2 often fluctuate outside specified ranges, particularly in infants with cardiopulmonary disease.

- Regular and periodic measurement (every 1–4 hours) and recording of the concentration of oxygen delivered to the infant receiving supplemental oxygen is recommended.
- Except for an emergency situation, air–oxygen mixtures should be warmed and humidified before being administered to infants.

Respiratory Distress Syndrome

Respiratory distress syndrome (RDS) is associated with surfactant deficiency and typically occurs in preterm infants, but may occasionally be seen in term infants, particularly in the setting of maternal diabetes. Multiple randomized controlled trials have demonstrated the benefits of surfactant replacement therapy, including reduction in the severity of RDS, decrease in pulmonary complications (eg, air leak), and improvement in survival. Surfactant therapy does not change the incidence of BPD in infants born at less than 30 weeks of gestation, but does reduce the incidence of BPD in infants born at or beyond 30 weeks of gestation. Surfactant therapy has no effect on coexisting morbidities, such as necrotizing enterocolitis, nosocomial infection, patent ductus arteriosus, and intraventricular hemorrhage. Long-term outcome of treated infants has shown possible improvement in pulmonary function studies, but has not shown beneficial or adverse effects on growth and neurodevelopment.

Antenatal corticosteroid administration stimulates structural and functional maturation of the fetal lung and, like postnatal surfactant replacement, improves survival and reduces the incidence of RDS. Antenatal corticosteroids and postnatal surfactant replacement have additive effects. Therefore, both antenatal steroid administration to women at risk of preterm delivery and postnatal surfactant administration to infants at high risk of RDS are important treatments to optimize outcomes for preterm infants (see also Chapter 9).

Surfactant replacement has been proved efficacious for infants with respiratory distress associated with primary surfactant deficiency and should be administered to these infants as soon as possible after intubation. Preterm infants born at less than 30 weeks of gestation are at high risk of primary surfactant deficiency. Prophylactic surfactant given soon after birth may reduce mortality and morbidity in such infants, particularly for those without exposure to antenatal steroids; however, randomized controlled trials that compared early continuous positive airway pressure administration with early surfactant therapy have shown similar rates of death or BPD. Thus, early continuous positive airway pressure appears to be a reasonable alternative to prophylactic surfactant therapy. Rescue surfactant also may be efficacious and should be considered for infants with hypoxic respiratory failure attributable to secondary surfactant deficiency (eg, meconium aspiration, sepsis or pneumonia, pulmonary hemorrhage).

Both animal-derived (natural) and synthetic surfactant preparations have shown efficacy for the treatment of respiratory distress due to surfactant deficiency. Animal-derived products from bovine and porcine sources are similar in efficacy and have not been associated with long-term immunologic or infectious complications. Synthetic surfactant preparations contain recombinant surfactant proteins or peptides that mimic the function of surfactant-associated proteins and have been shown to be as effective as animal-derived surfactants.

Infants receiving surfactant replacement therapy often have associated multisystem organ dysfunction that requires specialized care. Caring for these infants in nurseries that do not have the full range of required capabilities may affect overall outcome adversely. Therefore, infants with respiratory failure requiring surfactant therapy should be managed in NICUs that have the expertise to provide comprehensive care for sick newborns.

In view of the documented efficacy of surfactant replacement therapy, the following recommendations should be incorporated into neonatal care systems:

- Surfactant should be administered by experienced clinical staff with the technical and clinical expertise to respond to rapid changes in lung volume and lung compliance and complications of surfactant instillation into the airway.
- Surfactant replacement therapy should be directed by physicians who are trained in the respiratory management of sick newborns, have knowledge and experience in mechanical ventilation, and are capable of managing multisystem disorders in sick newborns.
- Nursing and respiratory therapy personnel who are experienced in the management of sick newborns, including the use of mechanical ventilation, should be available when surfactant therapy is administered.

- The equipment necessary for managing and monitoring the condition of sick newborns, including that needed for mechanical ventilation, should be available when surfactant therapy is administered.
- The radiology and laboratory support necessary to manage a broad range of needs of sick newborns should be immediately available in facilities where surfactant therapy is prescribed.
- At institutions that do not meet these requirements, when timely transfer of a high-risk newborn to an appropriate institution cannot be achieved, surfactant therapy may be given by clinical staff skilled in endotracheal intubation and surfactant administration, under physician direction. Newborns who have received surfactant should be transferred from such institutions as soon as feasible to a center with appropriate facilities and trained staff to care for multisystem morbidity in sick newborns.

Hypoxic Cardiorespiratory Failure

Hypoxic cardiorespiratory failure in term or late-preterm infants may result from diverse conditions, such as primary persistent pulmonary hypertension, RDS, aspiration of meconium, pneumonia, sepsis, or congenital diaphragmatic hernia. Hypoxemia, hypercarbia, and acidosis generally are reversible with conventional therapies, such as administration of oxygen, continuous positive airway pressure, mechanical ventilation, and supportive care. Additionally, inotropic agents, intravascular volume expansion, and antibiotics may be indicated.

Term and late-preterm infants who do not respond to conventional interventions may benefit from rescue therapies targeting specific physiologic abnormalities that may accompany hypoxic respiratory failure, such as surfactant replacement for primary or secondary surfactant deficiency or inhaled nitric oxide for pulmonary hypertension. In small, randomized trials involving infants with meconium aspiration syndrome, persistent pulmonary hypertension, and sepsis, surfactant replacement reduced mortality and the need for ECMO without an increase in morbidity. Randomized clinical trials have demonstrated that inhaled nitric oxide, a selective pulmonary vasodilator, improves oxygenation and reduces the need for ECMO in term and late-preterm infants. Response to inhaled nitric oxide is optimized when the lungs are adequately recruited; if conventional mechanical ventilation is not successful in this regard, high-frequency ventilation may be useful.

It is essential that newborns with hypoxic cardiorespiratory failure receive care in institutions that have appropriately skilled personnel—including physicians, nurses, and respiratory therapists who are qualified to use multiple modes of ventilation—and readily accessible radiologic, echocardiographic, and laboratory support. Newborns who are not responding to conventional therapies should be transferred in a timely manner to the appropriate level NICU capable of providing rescue therapies, such as inhaled nitric oxide or ECMO.

Nitric Oxide Use in Preterm Infants. The use of inhaled nitric oxide in preterm infants with acute hypoxic respiratory failure appears to be of little clinical benefit in the large randomized controlled trials thus far reported. Until new trials report significant beneficial results, the general use of inhaled nitric oxide in preterm infants with acute hypoxic respiratory failure should be limited to patients in clinical research protocols. Individual preterm infants with documented pulmonary hypertension may respond to inhaled nitric oxide.

Extracorporeal Membrane Oxygenation. Extracorporeal membrane oxygenation refers to prolonged (days to weeks) cardiopulmonary bypass for infants with hypoxic respiratory or cardiac failure who are unresponsive to less invasive therapies. Lung rest during ECMO allows pulmonary and cardiac recovery with reduced risk of secondary injury from exposure to high oxygen and ventilator support. Extracorporeal membrane oxygenation is highly invasive and accompanied by risks associated with systemic anticoagulation, mechanical complications, and the cannulation procedures.

Criteria for initiating or transferring for ECMO are complex because numerous factors, including gestational age, weight, diagnosis, severity of cardiorespiratory failure, clinical course, presence of complications, postnatal age, proximity of an ECMO center, risk of transport, and parental preferences all must be considered. In general, however, a late-preterm or term infant with respiratory failure who is deteriorating and has an oxygenation index greater than 25 on conventional mechanical ventilation (oxygenation index = [mean airway pressure/Pao_2] × Fio_2 × 100) has a moderately high risk of requiring ECMO. Consultation and possible transfer to an ECMO center is advised when the oxygenation index reaches 25. Newborns with oxygenation index calculations greater than 35 on conventional mechanical ventilation are at high risk of death without ECMO. Contraindications to ECMO may include gestational age less than 34–35 weeks, birth weight less than 2,000 g, profound hypoxic–ischemic encephalopathy, large intracranial hemorrhage, congenital anomalies associated with grave prognosis, or irreversible pulmonary or cardiac disorder.

Improved survival without an increase in morbidity has been demonstrated in clinical trials for infants receiving ECMO. Medical complications may include BPD, feeding problems, gastroesophageal reflux, and slow growth. Significant neurologic abnormality, developmental delay, or neurocognitive disability occurred in approximately 15% of ECMO survivors evaluated at 5 years of age. Complications, such as seizures; hearing loss; visual disturbances; learning disability; and social, attention, and behavioral problems are seen in many neonatal patients with complex medical courses, including those treated with inhaled nitric oxide and ECMO. Because of the risk of these adverse outcomes and the emergence of subtle disabilities during the school-age and adolescent years, it is recommended that surviving infants who have been treated with rescue therapies such as ECMO be monitored by developmental specialists throughout childhood.

Bronchopulmonary Dysplasia/Chronic Lung Disease

Bronchopulmonary dysplasia, or chronic lung disease, complicates the recovery of many preterm infants with RDS and infants of any gestational age with severe pulmonary insufficiency or hypoplasia. Classic BPD is characterized pathologically by alveolar and airway destruction, inflammation, and fibrosis, which results in emphysema, atelectasis, bronchial and bronchiolar mucosal hyperplasia and metaplasia, interstitial fibrosis, narrowed airways, excess mucus accumulation, interstitial edema, lymphatic dilation, pulmonary vascular smooth muscle hypertrophy, and reduction in capillary bed size. With advances in care, such as antenatal corticosteroids and postnatal surfactant, many extremely preterm infants have mild initial lung disease but still develop BPD. This new BPD is characterized by alveolar and capillary simplification, and likely results from a complex interaction of antenatal and postnatal factors superimposed on an arrest of lung development due to extremely preterm birth. Infants with severe BPD may develop pulmonary hypertension or cor pulmonale, or may die from acute bronchospasm or infection.

Bronchopulmonary dysplasia has been variably defined as the need for oxygen at 28 days postnatal age or at 36 weeks of postmenstrual age, with or without clinical and radiographic abnormalities. Because oxygen often is administered according to inconsistent, subjective criteria, it is a challenge to compare outcomes across NICUs. To reduce variability in reporting, improve comparability among different NICUs, and develop research priorities, specific diagnostic definitions were created at a consensus workshop sponsored by the National Heart, Lung, and Blood Institute (Table 11-4). In conjunction with this set of definitions, a physiologic definition of BPD has been introduced (ie, the need for supplemental oxygen to maintain an oxygen saturation level at or above 90%). Infants receiving supplemental oxygen of 0.30 FIO_2 or less at 36 weeks of postmenstrual age who are not on positive pressure ventilation should have an oxygen reduction test performed to determine whether supplemental oxygen is necessary to maintain the saturation level at or above 90%. Infants who are receiving positive pressure ventilation, continuous positive airway pressure, or oxygen supplementation greater than 0.30 FIO_2 at 36 weeks of postmenstrual age (or 56 days postnatal age for infants born at or beyond 32 weeks of gestation) are considered to have BPD without verification by an oxygen reduction test. Although infants receiving nasal cannula oxygen or high flow were not

TABLE 11-4. Definition of Bronchopulmonary Dysplasia

	Gestational Age	
Assessment	Less Than 32 Weeks	32 Weeks or Older
Time point of assessment	36 wk PMA or discharge to home, whichever comes first	more than 28 d but less than 56 d postnatal age or discharge to home, whichever comes first
	Treatment with oxygen greater than 21% for at least 28 d plus:	Treatment with oxygen more than 21% for at least 28 d plus:
Mild BPD	Breathing room air at 36 wk PMA or discharge, whichever comes first	Breathing room air by 56 d postnatal age or discharge, whichever comes first
Moderate BPD	Need for less than 30% oxygen at 36 wk PMA or discharge, whichever comes first	Need for less than 30% oxygen at 56 d postnatal age or discharge, whichever comes first
Severe BPD	Need for 30% or greater oxygen or positive pressure (PPV or NCPAP), or both, at 36 wk PMA or discharge, whichever comes first	Need for 30% or greater oxygen or positive pressure (PPV or NCPAP), or both, at 56 d PMA postnatal age or discharge, whichever comes first

Abbreviations: BPD, bronchopulmonary dysplasia; NCPAP, nasal continuous positive airway pressure; PMA, postmenstrual age; PPV, positive-pressure ventilation.

Modified from Jobe AH, Bancalari E. Bronchopulmonary dysplasia. Am J Respir Crit Care Med 2001;163:1723–9.

specifically addressed in this workshop, a room air challenge at 36 weeks of postnatal age could be considered in these infants as well, particularly if the gas flow rate is below their body weight in kg (high-flow cannula), or effective oxygen delivery is less than 30% (low-flow cannula). Regardless, the designation of BPD by these criteria may not be strongly predictive of long-term pulmonary morbidity.

Therapeutic Approaches. Multiple pharmacologic interventions and respiratory support strategies have been proposed to decrease development of BPD in sick infants, but few are supported by controlled clinical trials of appropriate size and design:

- Antenatal administration of corticosteroids decreases the incidence of RDS and, thereby, decreases the population at risk.
- Surfactant replacement has decreased the incidence of BPD in infants born at or beyond 30 weeks of gestation but not in infants born at less than 30 weeks of gestation.
- Caffeine supplementation started within the first 10 days of life in babies weighing 500–1,250 g at birth has been associated with a significantly decreased incidence of BPD and improved neurodevelopmental outcomes at 18–21 months of corrected age, although this improvement was not statistically significant at 5 years.
- Vitamin A supplementation has been shown to significantly decrease the risk of BPD in mechanically ventilated, extremely-low-birth-weight infants.
- Postnatal corticosteroids:
  - — Postnatal dexamethasone given in the first postnatal week to very-low-birth-weight infants facilitates extubation and decreases BPD; however, its benefits are outweighed by numerous documented adverse effects, particularly possible compromise of neurodevelopment. Therefore, the routine use of systemic dexamethasone in the first postnatal week for the prevention and treatment of chronic lung disease in very-low-birth-weight infants is not recommended.
  - — After the first week of life, dexamethasone may be beneficial, but also carries risks. Given the limitations of current evidence, dexamethasone should be reserved for infants who cannot be weaned from mechanical ventilation, and the dose and duration of treatment should be minimized. Parents should be fully informed about

the known short-term risks and long-term risks and consent to treatment.

- — Low-dose hydrocortisone given in the first postnatal week appears to increase survival without BPD; long-term results from the most recent randomized controlled trials showed no significant adverse effects at 2 years.
- — Inhaled corticosteroids have not been shown to decrease BPD.

- Early use of inhaled nitric oxide appears to be of little clinical benefit; however, one large randomized trial of nitric oxide treatment initiated between 7 and 21 days and continued for 24 days was reported to increase survival without BPD and without adverse effects on growth or neurodevelopment at 2 years of age.
- Assisted ventilation strategies that avoid hyperinflation are desirable, but strong supportive evidence for most specific individual ventilation strategies are lacking; a meta-analysis of five studies, including 413 infants, suggested that volume-targeted ventilation may reduce BPD compared with pressure-limited ventilation.
- Continuous positive airway pressure beginning in the delivery room has not been proved to reduce the incidence of BPD.
- Permissive hypercapnia (ie, accepting higher $Paco_2$ levels than previously was customary) has been suggested, but controlled studies in neonates have not demonstrated a reduction in risk of BPD.
- High-frequency ventilation using various modalities and strategies has not been found to be consistently efficacious.
- The use of synchronized ventilation and short inspiratory times seems reasonable but the effects on BPD have not been demonstrated in large randomized trials.

Other modalities directed at specific antecedents of inflammatory injury have included antioxidants (vitamin E and superoxide dismutase) and erythromycin (prophylaxis or treatment for *Ureaplasma* colonization). None of these can be recommended at this time because of either safety issues (erythromycin) or unconfirmed efficacy (vitamin E supplementation beyond that required to prevent vitamin E deficiency is not beneficial); superoxide dismutase and other antioxidant medications have not been studied adequately. High volumes of fluid intake in the first week are associated with persistence of a patent ductus arteriosus and the development of BPD. Diuretics may acutely improve pulmonary function and decrease oxygen requirement, but their effectiveness in decreasing BPD is unsubstantiated in clinical trials.

Treatment. Treatment of developing or established BPD is primarily pragmatic, and includes oxygen supplementation, careful attention to optimize nutrition and growth, and appropriate immunizations. The optimal oxygen saturation range is unknown, but oxygen supplementation has been shown to improve growth and decrease the likelihood of progression to pulmonary hypertension. Growth failure is well recognized to accompany severe BPD, and energy expenditure has been shown to be significantly higher in these infants. In addition, inadequate nutrition impairs lung healing. Therefore, although not supported by controlled trials, provision of calories, minerals, and protein to sustain a growth rate comparable with non-BPD gestational age peers seems a logical approach. Immunoprophylaxis for respiratory syncytial virus and influenza has reduced the posthospitalization morbidity of infants with BPD. Infants born to mothers who have received the influenza vaccine during pregnancy have been shown to have less influenza disease during their first months of life. Infants should receive all immunizations in accordance with AAP recommendations (see also "Immunization" in Chapter 10).

Retinopathy of Prematurity

Myriad factors, including but not limited to hyperoxia, likely contribute to the pathogenesis of ROP. Prematurity; low birth weight; multiple gestation; severity of illness; prolonged ventilatory support (especially when accompanied by episodes of hypoxia and hypercapnia); and clinical conditions, including acidosis, shock, sepsis, apnea, anemia, chronic lung disease, intraventricular hemorrhage, patent ductus arteriosus, and vitamin E deficiency also have been associated with retinopathy of prematurity.

To date, a safe level of Pao_2 in relation to ROP has not been established, perhaps because multiple other factors, such as those listed previously play a part in its pathogenesis. Retinopathy of prematurity has occurred in preterm infants who have never received supplemental oxygen therapy and in infants with cyanotic congenital heart disease in whom Pao_2 levels never exceeded 50 mm Hg. Conversely, ROP has not developed in some preterm infants after prolonged periods of hyperoxemia. Data have demonstrated no additional progression of active prethreshold ROP when supplemental oxygen was administered at pulse oximetry saturations between 96% and 99%. Further, continuous monitoring of transcutaneous oxygen tension has not resulted in a decrease in the incidence of ROP when compared with intermittent transcutaneous monitoring. On the basis of published data, the following statements regarding ROP and oxygen use are warranted:

- ROP is not preventable in some infants, especially extremely premature infants.
- Many factors other than hyperoxia contribute to the pathogenesis of ROP.
- Transient hyperoxemia alone cannot be considered sufficient to cause ROP.
- Strict adherence to existing guidelines for supplemental oxygen therapy will not completely prevent ophthalmologic complications or adverse effects.

Screening and Initial Examination

An ophthalmologist with sufficient knowledge and experience in ROP and the use of binocular indirect ophthalmoscopy should examine the retinas of all preterm infants born at 30 weeks of gestation or less or weighing less than 1,500 g at birth, as well as selected infants weighing 1,500–2,000 g at birth with an unstable clinical course and who are thought to be at risk by their attending physicians. Sterile instruments should be used to examine each infant in order to avoid possible cross contamination of infectious agents. Pretreatment of the eyes with a topical anesthetic agent, such as proparacaine, may minimize the discomfort and systemic effect of this examination. Consideration also may be given to the use of nonpharmacologic pain management interventions, such as pacifiers and oral sucrose. Transient sequelae such as apnea or feeding intolerance are occasionally noted after the use of atropine-like agents for eye examination.

Table 11-5 presents a suggested schedule for timing of initial eye examinations based on postmenstrual age and chronologic (postnatal) age. This schedule was designed to detect ROP before it progresses to retinal detachment and to allow for earlier intervention, while minimizing the number of potentially traumatic examinations. The timing of follow-up examinations is best determined from the findings of the first examination, using the International Classification of Retinopathy of Prematurity (see also "Treatment and Follow-up Care" later in this section). One examination is sufficient only if it unequivocally shows the retina to be fully vascularized in each eye.

Digital photographic retinal image capture with remote interpretation is a developing approach to ROP screening. However, outcome trial data comparing large-scale operational photoscreening systems with remote interpretation to binocular indirect ophthalmoscopy have not been published. Off-site photo interpretation requires close collaboration among neonatologists, imaging staff, and ophthalmologists. Specific responsibilities of each individual must be carefully delineated in a written protocol in advance so that repeat imaging, confirmatory examinations, and required treatments can be performed without delay.

TABLE 11-5. Timing of First Eye Examination Based on Gestational Age at Birth*

Gestational Age at Birth (wk)	Age at Initial Examination (wk)	
	Postmenstrual	Chronologic
22†	31	9
23†	31	8
24	31	7
25	31	6
26	31	5
27	31	4
28	32	4
29	33	4
30	34	4
Older gestational age, high-risk factors‡		4

*Shown is a schedule for detecting prethreshold retinopathy of prematurity with 99% confidence, usually before any required treatment.

†This guideline should be considered tentative rather than evidence-based for infants with a gestational age of 22–23 weeks because of the small number of survivors in these age categories.

‡Consider timing based on severity of comorbidities.

Reprinted from Fierson WM. Screening examination of premature infants for retinopathy of prematurity. American Academy of Pediatrics Section on Ophthalmology, American Academy of Ophthalmology, American Association for Pediatric Ophthalmology and Strabismus, American Association of Certified Orthoptists. Pediatrics 2013;131:189–95. Available at: http://pediatrics.aappublications.org/content/131/1/189. Retrieved December 19, 2016.

Treatment and Follow-up Care

If intervention is considered necessary, it generally should be performed within 72 hours of the diagnosis, if possible, to minimize the risk of retinal detachment. The retinal findings requiring strong consideration of ablative treatment are as follows:

- Zone I retinopathy of prematurity: any stage with plus disease
- Zone I retinopathy of prematurity: stage 3, no plus disease
- Zone II: stage 2 or 3 with plus disease

Published data indicate that intravitreal bevacizumab monotherapy, as compared with conventional laser therapy, in infants with stage 3+ retinopathy of prematurity has a significant benefit for zone I disease but not zone II disease. However, the number of infants treated was small and there remain unanswered questions involving dosage, timing, safety, visual outcomes, and other long-term ocular and systemic effects. Until additional data are available, laser photocoagulation remains the standard of care for most cases of ROP requiring treatment.

If hospital discharge or transfer to another neonatal unit or hospital is contemplated before retinal maturation into zone III has taken place or if the infant has been treated by ablation for ROP and is not yet fully healed, the availability of an appropriate follow-up ophthalmologic examination by an experienced ophthalmologist must be ensured, and specific arrangement for that examination must be made before such discharge or transfer occurs. Responsibility for examination and follow-up of infants at risk of ROP must be carefully defined by each NICU. Unit-specific criteria for screening and follow-up examinations should be established by consultation and agreement between neonatology and ophthalmology services. These criteria should be recorded and should automatically trigger ophthalmologic examinations.

Management of High-Risk Infants

Nutritional Needs of Preterm Infants

Optimal nutrition is critical in the management of preterm infants. There is no standard for the precise nutritional needs of preterm infants comparable with the human milk standard for term infants. Present recommendations are designed to provide nutrients to approximate the rate of growth and composition of weight gain for a normal fetus of the same postmenstrual age and to maintain normal concentrations of blood and tissue nutrients. Acute illness and organ system immaturity can make provision of optimal nutrition challenging, particularly for the sickest and most immature infants, yet inadequate nutrition during this period may have life-long consequences. A combined approach with both parenteral and enteral nutrition is needed to optimize early nutritional support in preterm infants.

Parenteral Nutrition

Parenteral nutrition should be initiated as soon as possible after birth for infants who weigh less than 1,500 g. (Table 11-6). A "starter" or "stock" amino acid solution can be used to supply 2–3 g per kg of protein immediately after birth. The high incidence of respiratory and other morbidities, combined with intestinal immaturity, may necessitate slow advancement of the volume of enteral feedings. Parenteral nutrition can supplement the gradually increasing enteral feedings so that total intake by both routes meets

TABLE 11-6. Recommendations for Early Parenteral and Enteral Nutrition for Extremely-Low-Birth-Weight and Very-Low-Birth-Weight Infants

Parenteral	Day 0*	Day 1–2	Day 3
Amino Acids	≥2 g/kg/d	≥3.5 g/kg/d	3.5–4.0 g/kg/d
Lipid	≥2 g/kg/d	3.0–4.0 g/kg/d	3.0–4.0 g/kg/d
Total Energy	60–80 kcal/kg/d	80–100 kcal/kg/d	≥100 kcal/kg/d

*first 24 hours after birth

Enteral	Extremely Low Birth Weight	Very Low Birth Weight
Preferred substrate	Human milk	Human milk
First feeding	6–48 hrs	6–48 hrs
Initial feeding (MEF)	10–15 mL/kg/d	20–25 mL/ kg/d
Duration of MEF	1–4 days	1–4 days
Rate of advancement	15–25 mL/kg/d	20–30 mL/ kg/d
HM fortification	Before 100 mL/kg/d	Before 100 mL/kg/d
Target protein intake	4.0–4.5 g/kg/d	3.5–4.0 g/kg/d
Target energy intake	110–130 kcal/kg/d	110–130 kcal/kg/d

Abbreviations: HM, human milk; MEF, minimal enteral feeding. Modified from Senterre T. Practice of enteral nutrition in very low birth weight and extremely low birth weight infants. World Rev Nutr Diet 2014;110:201–14 and Embleton ND, Simmer K. Practice of parenteral nutrition in VLBW and ELBW infants. World Rev Nutr Diet 2014:110:177–89.

the infant's nutritional needs. For very-low-birth-weight and extremely-low-birth-weight infants, recommended intakes include 3.5–4.0 g per kg per day of protein, 3–4 g per kg per day of lipid, and total energy intake of 90–100 kcal per kg.

Enteral Nutrition

Enteral nutrition with human milk, optimally mother's expressed colostrum, should be initiated as soon as possible after birth (see Table 11-7). Mothers should be assisted to begin expressing milk within 6 hours of delivery and supported to establish a milk supply (see Chapter 8). A reasonable strategy is to provide 10–20 mL per kg per day of minimal enteral feeding within 48 hours of birth. The duration of minimal enteral feeding is variable, typically between 1 and 4 days with subsequent advances in enteral volume of

TABLE 11-7. Enteral Intake Recommendations for Enterally Fed Very-Low-Birth-Weight Infants

	Consensus Recommendations		
Element	Less than 1,000 g/ 100 kcal	1,000–1,500 g/kg per day	1,000–1,500 g/ 100 kcal
Water/fluids, mL	107–169	135–190	104–173
Energy, kcal	100	110–130	100
Protein, g	2.5–3.4	3.4–4.2	2.6–3.8
Carbohydrate, g	6.0–15.4	7–17	5.4–15.5
Fat, g	4.1–6.5	5.3–7.2	4.1–6.5
Linoleic acid, mg	467–1,292	600–1,440	462–1,309
Linoleate: linolenate (C18:2–C18:3)	5–15	5–15	5–15
Docosahexaenoic acid, mg	≥16	≥18	≥16
Arachidonic acid, mg	≥22	≥24	≥22
Vitamin A, IU	467–1,154	700–1,500	538–1,364
Vitamin D, IU	100–308	150–400	115–364
Vitamin E, IU	4.0–9.2	6–12	4.6–10.9
Vitamin K_1, micrograms	5.3–7.7	8–10	6.2–9.1
Ascorbate, mg	12.0–18.5	18–24	13.8–21.8
Thiamine, micrograms	120–185	180–240	138–218

Modified from Koletzko B, Poindexter B, Uauy R. Recommended nutrient intake levels for stable, fully enterally fed very low birth weight infants. World Rev Nutr Diet 2014;110:297–9.

15–25 mL per kg per day. Although the optimal strategy of initiation and advancement of enteral nutrition remains undefined, several studies suggest that having a standardized feeding protocol shortens the time to reach full enteral feedings, decreases duration of parenteral nutrition, and improves growth outcomes. Historically, enteral feedings have been delayed in the small, preterm infant because of extreme immaturity, significant respiratory or other morbidity, and a perceived increased risk of necrotizing enterocolitis. However, evidence indicates that early introduction of trophic feeding or priming feeding is safe, well tolerated, and associated with significant benefits. The actual route of enteral feeding (eg, nasogastric, orogastric, gastrostomy, transpyloric, or oral) is determined on the basis of gestational age, clinical condition, and oromotor integrity (ability to coordinate sucking, swallowing, and breathing).

Human milk has a number of special features that make its use desirable in feeding preterm infants. Fresh or properly stored refrigerated human milk contains immunologic and antimicrobial factors that are protective against infection. Fat digestion is facilitated by the lipase and the triglycerides found in human milk. However, human milk does not provide adequate protein, calcium, phosphorus, sodium, trace metals, and some vitamins to meet the tissue and bone growth needs of the very-low-birth-weight infant. Despite these deficiencies, efforts should be made to feed all very-low-birth-weight infants human milk (either from mother or donor) unless contraindicated. Human milk fortifiers designed to correct these deficiencies are available commercially and can enhance growth and bone mineralization in very-low-birth-weight infants when added to human milk.

Preterm infants who weigh more than 2,000 g at birth generally achieve adequate growth when fed their mother's milk, postdischarge formula, or a regular term-infant formula containing 67 kcal per dL. However, calcium and phosphorus retention rates are slower than fetal accretion rates. These infants may require vitamin supplementation during the period when the volume of formula or human milk ingested does not provide the recommended daily vitamin intake, particularly of vitamin D (see Table 11-7 and "Breastfeeding" in Chapter 10).

Special formulas for very-low-birth-weight infants (preterm formulas) contain additional protein, easily absorbed carbohydrates (glucose polymers and lactose), and easily digested and absorbed lipids (15–50% medium-chain triglycerides). The calcium and phosphorus contents are high to achieve a bone mineralization rate equivalent to the fetal rate. The sodium content also is high, reflecting the increased sodium requirement of preterm infants. Trace metals and vitamins have been added to meet the increased needs of the very-low-birth-weight infant. The use of formulas for preterm infants, compared with the use of formulas intended for term infants, has been shown to contribute to weight gain and a bone mineralization rate closer to that of the reference fetus and improved long-term growth and development. Also, improved neurodevelopmental outcome is seen in preterm infants fed preterm formulas or human milk versus term formula. Formulas containing long-chain polyunsaturated fatty acids may confer vision and neurodevelopmental benefits, although study results are conflicting. Formulas supplemented with docosahexaenoic acid and arachidonic acid are now available and appear safe.

Nutrient Enhancement for Preterm Infants After Discharge

The need for enhanced nutritional support for the preterm infant does not end at the time of hospital discharge. Goals of postdischarge nutritional support include promotion of human milk feeding while meeting nutrient requirements to achieve optimal growth and neurodevelopmental outcomes. In many cases, maintaining optimal growth (including need for catch-up growth) necessitates ongoing fortification of human milk or nutrient-enriched formula. Although specialized formulas containing increased protein, energy, and minerals are available, the evidence supporting their efficacy is limited. Considering the paucity of data on what to feed preterm infants after hospital discharge, it may be reasonable to provide small, preterm infants (born at or before 34 weeks of gestation, with a birth weight less than or equal to 1,800 g) and infants with other morbidities (eg, BPD) specialized formulas after hospital discharge to promote catch-up growth, acquisition of lean body mass, and improved bone mineralization. For infants receiving human milk, the ongoing use of a human milk fortifier may be needed to maintain adequate growth.

Pain Prevention and Management

Pain consists of the perception of painful stimuli (nociception) and the psychologic response to painful stimuli (anxiety). Studies measuring a variety of physiologic factors, including oxygen saturation, β-endorphin, glucose, cortisol, and epinephrine concentrations, confirm that infants of all gestational ages have a nociceptive response to pain stimuli. Observations of infant behavior suggest that anxiety also is a component of the infantile pain response, but its character, intensity, and duration remain undetermined. Therefore, the significance of anxiety in the newborn remains unknown.

The prevention of pain is important not only because it is an ethical expectation, but also because repeated painful exposures can have long-term deleterious consequences, including altered pain sensitivity and permanent neuroanatomic and behavioral abnormalities. Measures for assessing pain in the newborn have been developed and validated. Every health care facility caring for newborns should implement an effective pain-prevention and stress-reduction program that includes strategies to achieve the following goals:

- Routinely assessing pain throughout the infant's hospitalization
- Minimizing the number of painful procedures performed
- Effectively using nonpharmacologic and pharmacologic therapies for the prevention of pain associated with routine minor procedures
- Eliminating pain associated with surgery and other major procedures

Validated pain assessment tools must be used in a consistent manner, and caregivers should be trained to assess pain in newborn infants. Any unnecessary noxious stimuli (including acoustic, visual, tactile, and vestibular) should be avoided, when possible. Simple comfort measures, such as swaddling, nonnutritive sucking, skin-to-skin contact, breastfeeding, sensorial stimulation, and developmentally appropriate positioning (eg, facilitated tuck position), should be used whenever possible for minor procedures. Oral administration of sucrose or glucose reduces pain associated with painful procedures. These environmental and nonpharmacologic interventions should be provided as baseline measures to prevent, reduce, or eliminate stress and pain. Because of concerns of potential adverse neurodevelopmental outcomes when used in preterm infants, sucrose and glucose should be ordered and tracked as medications. Evidence-based protocols should be developed and implemented in nurseries, and more research needs to be conducted in order to better understand the effects of sucrose use for analgesia.

The risks and benefits of pharmacologic pain management techniques must be considered on an individualized basis. Pharmacokinetic and pharmacodynamic properties and efficacy of these drugs vary in the newborn; to the extent possible, agents whose properties have been studied in the newborn should be used. It is important to remember that sedatives and anxiolytics do not provide analgesia. Agents known to compromise cardiorespiratory function should be administered only by individuals experienced in airway management and in settings with the capacity for continuous cardiorespiratory monitoring and cardiorespiratory support. Caution should be exercised when considering medications for which data in newborn infants are sparse or nonexistent.

Intraoperative and Postoperative Pain Management

Pain is an inevitable consequence of surgery at any age. A health care facility providing surgery for infants should have an established protocol for pain management. Although it is considered unethical to perform surgery in the newborn without anesthesia, the appropriate levels of anesthesia for various surgical procedures have not been well investigated. The use of paralytic agents without analgesia during surgery is unacceptable. For major surgical procedures, general anesthesia by inhalation of anesthetic gases, intravenous administration of narcotic agents, or regional techniques can be safe and effective. Specially trained anesthesia providers should administer anesthesia for surgical procedures for all newborns, and the choice of technique and agent should be based on a comprehensive assessment of the infant, efficacy and safety of the drug, and the technical requirements of the procedure.

The use of analgesic agents is important in the immediate postoperative period and should be continued as required. Continuous or bolus infusions of opioids and continuous caudal or epidural blockade can be used to provide a steady course of pain relief, but both require careful management and continuous monitoring of cardiorespiratory and hemodynamic status. Acetaminophen can be used as an adjunct to regional anesthetics or opioids, but there are inadequate data on pharmacokinetics at gestational ages less than 28 weeks to permit calculation of appropriate doses.

Pain Management for Other Invasive Procedures

Intercostal Drain Placement and Removal. Insertion of a chest drain is a painful procedure. Because there have been no prospective trials of analgesia for this procedure to date, recommendations based on general principles include slow infiltration of the skin with a local anesthetic and systemic analgesia with a rapidly acting opioid. Removal of the chest drain also can be very painful, and the administration of a short-acting, rapid-onset systemic analgesic agent should be considered for this procedure.

Retinal Examination. Retinal examinations are painful. Although there are insufficient data to make specific recommendations, a reasonable approach would be administration of oral sucrose and a topical anesthetic. Nonpharmacologic measures, such as swaddling or nonnutritive sucking, should be used in conjunction with these agents.

Circumcision. For information on pain management during circumcision, see "Circumcision" in Chapter 10.

Intubation. The experience of being intubated is unpleasant and painful. Except for emergent intubation during resuscitation, and perhaps for infants with upper airway anomalies, premedication should be used for all endotracheal intubations in newborns. Medications with rapid onset and short duration of action are preferable, and the following principles should be observed:

- Rapid-acting analgesics should be given.
- Atropine-like agents and rapid-onset muscle relaxants should be considered.
- Use of hypnotics or sedatives without analgesics should be avoided.
- A muscle relaxant without an analgesic should not be used.
- When intravenous access is not available, alternative routes, including intranasal administration, can be considered.

Topical Anesthetics for Minor Invasive Procedures

Topical anesthetics, such as a mixture of lidocaine and prilocaine, can effectively reduce pain associated with minor invasive procedures, such as lumbar puncture and intravenous catheter insertion, if the agent is applied for a sufficient length of time before the procedure (at least 30 minutes). Repeated use should be limited to avoid the risk of methemoglobinemia. These agents are not effective for heel-stick blood draws because the pain from heel sticks is primarily from squeezing the heel rather than from the lancet.

Medication for Infants Receiving Mechanical Ventilation

The routine use of continuous analgesic or sedative agents for mechanically ventilated infants has not been shown to be helpful and may be harmful; therefore, this practice cannot be recommended. Use of analgesic and anxiolytic agents for amelioration of the discomfort associated with prolonged endotracheal intubation in newborns should be undertaken only after careful consideration of the observed response of the individual infant and the adverse effects of the commonly used agents. Cochrane reviews have concluded that if sedation is required, morphine sulfate is safer than midazolam.

Concepts that must be remembered when considering medication for intubated infants include the following:

- Chronic use of opioids, sedatives, or hypnotics may lead to tolerance, dependency, and withdrawal.
- Effects of chronic sedation on neurodevelopmental outcome are unknown.
- Opioids, sedatives, and hypnotics may cause respiratory and cardiovascular depression.
- Combined treatment with a sedative or hypnotic and an opioid requires a decreased dosage of each.
- Agitation in the chronically ventilated infant may indicate the need to confirm airway patency and position, adjust ventilatory settings, or reduce noxious environmental stimuli.

Radiation Risk

Computed tomography (CT) is a valuable imaging modality; however, it entails an obligatory radiation exposure far in excess of many other common radiographic procedures. Compared with adults, infants have an increased risk of cancer from radiation exposure for the following three reasons: 1) growing and developing tissues are more sensitive to radiation effects; 2) the oncogenic effect of radiation has a long latent period; and 3) radiation exposure from a fixed set of CT parameters results in a dose that is relatively higher for an infant's smaller cross-sectional area compared with an adult.

The amount of radiation that CT provides depends on many factors, especially the protocols used and the equipment settings. The radiologist has the responsibility to create protocols and adjust scanning techniques on the basis of special considerations of neonatal patients. If the same settings are used for both newborns and adults, newborns will receive an unnecessary and excessive amount of radiation. The radiologist can assist by suggesting alternative imaging techniques, such as MRI or ultrasonography when suitable, by using a low-dose technique, and by limiting the number of times (phases) the infant is scanned for an individual examination.

Surgical Procedures in the Neonatal Intensive Care Unit

Infants in the NICU often require surgical procedures during hospitalization. Transport of an acutely ill infant to the operating room is associated with a number of risks, including hypothermia, acute hemodynamic changes, and dislodgement of intravenous catheters or the endotracheal tube. For this reason, many centers perform selected surgical procedures (eg, laser ablation or central venous access) within the NICU. Published studies indicate that this approach can be safe and effective and may result in improved outcomes.

If surgical procedures are performed within the NICU, there must be adequate lighting and work space, as well as ongoing monitoring and anesthetic management. Personnel should wear appropriate operating room attire, and strict sterile techniques must be used. Hospitals should develop policies governing all surgical procedures performed within the NICU, including anesthetic management and infection control. Such policies should be developed in conjunction with the institutional operating room committee to ensure that all appropriate guidelines are met.

Immunization of Hospitalized Infants

Guidelines for immunization of both preterm and term infants who require prolonged hospital stays should be implemented in each NICU. Medically stable preterm infants should begin the immunization series at the usual chronological age of 6–8 weeks, unless otherwise indicated. Some very-low-birth-weight infants have been found to have a reduced immune response when the usual timing of immunizations is followed. Additional studies are needed to define the optimal immunization schedule for this group of infants. Vaccine doses should not be reduced for very-low-birth-weight infants or preterm infants. Term infants who remain in the hospital at 6–8 weeks of age should receive vaccines according to the schedule recommended by the Centers for Disease Control and Prevention Advisory Committee on Immunization Practices and included in the AAP Redbook. Rotavirus vaccine, which is a live virus vaccine, should generally not be administered until discharge and not be given to patients with severe combined immunodeficiency or a history of intussusception. A recent revision of the palivizumab guidelines has restricted the indications for administration during respiratory syncytial virus season to premature infants less than 29 weeks of gestation and those with chronic lung disease who require supplemental oxygen for more than 28 days. Immunization recommendations and vaccine safety information are frequently updated and can be verified from the Centers for Disease Control and Prevention Advisory Committee on Immunization Practices web page at www.cdc.gov/vaccines/acip/ (see also "Immunization" in Chapter 10).

Death of a Newborn

Loss of a pregnancy or death of a newborn touches every aspect of a family's life. The intense emotions of grieving can be confusing and overwhelming. Every effort should be made to determine the cause of the loss, to understand the family's grief responses, and to facilitate healthy coping and adjustment. Efforts to obtain organs for donation are strongly encouraged although frequently organs are not suitable for transplant.

In-Hospital Support and Counseling

Bereavement counseling support is important for family members to adjust to their loss and to continue with their lives. Counseling should be tailored to the specific circumstances surrounding the infant's death; should be sensitive to specific ethical, cultural, religious, and family considerations; and should be provided by specific staff within the hospital. The period after a neonatal death is challenging because of the continuing grief, the tasks of informing relatives and friends, and the need to make final arrangements.

The time in the hospital before and after the newborn has died is the only opportunity that parents have to create memories of the newborn and the experience of being a parent. Therefore, involvement of the parents in as much of the bedside care of even critically ill infants as is commensurate with safety and their needs is of major importance. Whether a neonatal death is expected or unexpected, specific management procedures can be useful in facilitating parental adjustment to the loss:

- Offer the parents, and extended family if desired, an opportunity to see, hold, and spend time with the infant both before and immediately after the death. The use of a private room away from the activity of the NICU is often helpful.
- Facilitate involvement of the family with a member of the clergy or a spiritual adviser of their choice in order to prepare the family for the death and to provide ongoing support.

- Encourage the family to name the infant, if they have not done so previously, because it is easier to connect memories to a name.
- Collect and retain pictures and remembrances of the infant (eg, identification tags, footprints, a lock of hair, birth and death certificates, height and weight records, a receiving blanket for the infant, plaster molds of the hands and feet). Even if the parents initially say that they do not want these mementos, they frequently ask for them days, weeks, or months later.
- Provide information about options for burial, cremation, funerals, or memorial services. Encourage both parents to take an active part in making these arrangements.
- Provide information regarding lactation to women who are breast feeding to help them determine how and when to terminate their breast milk supply. Mothers may wish to donate stored and pumped milk to a milk bank.
- Visit the parents daily while the mother is in the hospital, listen to them sympathetically, and give them information as it becomes available.
- Provide reliable, preliminary information from the appropriate medical professionals concerning the cause and circumstances of death.
- Be aware that the staff's potential reactions—a sense of guilt, failure, and uncertainty—may cause them to avoid the parents, thereby impeding discussion of the deceased infant with the family. The grief of caregivers, like that of parents and family, should be addressed and supported.
- Ensure that the parents have access to support from their families and friends. Relaxation of visiting rules can be helpful to allow the parents to gain the support of the extended family. Anticipate with parents the difficulties they may have in sharing information about the loss with other children, family, and friends. Provide information and suggestions on how they might handle difficult situations or times and information on the availability of support groups.
- Explain the grieving process so that the parents understand the usual reactions. Parents frequently demonstrate reactions of acute grief, such as somatic disturbances, a preoccupation with the newborn's appearance or probable future appearance, guilt, hostility, and loss of ability to function. Mourning should be allowed and encouraged to proceed.

- Encourage the parents to communicate their thoughts and feelings openly with one another. Help them understand and accept the differences in how each of them experiences grief noting that normative grief is expected to be one to two years and that individuals progress through the process at different rates and intensities.
- Provide written materials to the parents. Although there is no substitute for a multidisciplinary group of professionals carefully organized to provide support, written materials can provide concrete information about specific procedures, such as autopsy and funeral arrangements, as well as guidance on long-term issues, such as grief, marital stress, explanations for young children, and consideration of another pregnancy. These materials can be designed by the individual hospital or obtained through various associations.

Because families may come from a distance and may not be well acquainted with the attending physicians, it is especially important that referral centers providing neonatal care designate a member of the team to be an advocate for the family during the hospital stay and after discharge. The designated individual also should be responsible for documenting the management and follow-up of each death. Too often families are lost to follow-up when physicians, nurses, and families avoid sharing the sadness of bereavement.

Determining Cause of Death

When a neonatal death occurs, a special effort should be made to determine the cause of death. This process is helpful for several reasons:

- It helps the family to understand the medical reasons for the death.
- It provides a basis for counseling the family about future pregnancies, including family planning, genetic counseling, and obstetric and neonatal management.
- It may be a part of a root cause analysis or quality review process that can improve care for future patients.
- It provides correct diagnoses for statistical reporting and analysis of perinatal care outcomes.

Requesting an autopsy after the death of a newborn must be handled with sensitivity and gentleness. Selecting the right time to introduce the idea is critical. It can be helpful when it is apparent that a newborn is dying, particularly when the underlying cause is uncertain, to introduce the idea of a postmortem examination to the parents. Its value as a means of gaining information that will be helpful in answering their future questions often is perceived as a compelling reason for consent. Involvement of the primary care physician and the mother's obstetrician in the request for autopsy consent also may facilitate the family's acceptance of the idea.

If there is reluctance to consent for a complete examination of the body, consideration can be given to a limited examination, to obtaining specimens of body fluids for microbial culture, genetic analysis, or other analyses as indicated, and to obtaining postmortem imaging studies if such information could further elucidate the cause of death. In all neonatal deaths, every effort should be made to obtain histopathologic examination of the placenta, membranes, and umbilical cord. When an underlying genetic disorder is suspected and premortem testing is incomplete, advance planning for appropriate specimen retrieval with or without a full autopsy should occur. In every instance, the family should receive the final written results of the autopsy and other examinations in a timely fashion in person, if possible, in conjunction with a verbal explanation of the findings.

Each unit should have a formal process for periodic review of all neonatal deaths. In addition, when there has been an unexpected clinical deterioration leading to a death, a contemporaneous review of the specific clinical events and decisions with all the involved staff participating can be helpful to resolve interpersonal conflicts, relieve feelings of guilt or failure, and improve both understanding and team interaction. The attending neonatologist is the best person to lead the debriefing session, although, on occasion, employment of an uninvolved facilitator can be useful. Consultation with legal counsel is advised to determine if the minutes of the debriefing session are immune from future inquiries in a medical–legal process.

Bereavement Follow-up

The responsibility for ongoing bereavement counseling depends on the specific circumstances of the death and on the family's relationship with the physician. Usually, a multidisciplinary approach is best. In general, such counseling should include the following:

- An initial session 4–6 weeks after the death
- Assessment of the grieving process

- Additional genetic services, if indicated
- Review of preliminary autopsy data, if available
- Answers for parents' specific questions
- Education and reassurance regarding the normal grieving process
- Follow-up visits as indicated by the individual family needs
- Referral of family members to bereavement support groups or bereavement counselors

Hospital Discharge of High-Risk Infants

Discharge Planning

The designation "high-risk" encompasses the broad spectrum of medical, neurologic, developmental, and psychosocial outcomes experienced by vulnerable neonatal subgroups described in the following section. Discharge planning for high-risk infants should begin early in hospitalization and includes six critical elements:

1. Parental education and readiness for discharge
2. Completion of appropriate elements of primary care in the hospital
3. Development of a management plan for unresolved medical problems
4. Development of the comprehensive home-care plan
5. Identification and involvement of support services
6. Determination and designation of follow-up care

Discharge planning for infants who have been transported back to community hospitals for convalescent care should follow the same principles, and the care plan should be coordinated between the two units before the transfer of the infant occurs.

Readiness for Hospital Discharge

The decision of when to discharge an infant from the hospital after a stay in the NICU is complex and includes assessment of the infant's physiologic stability, the family's readiness to care for their infant, and the mobilization of appropriate community resources to ensure continuing care and follow-up, including identification of a primary care physician experienced in the care of such infants. The following recommendations are offered as a framework for guiding decisions about the timing of discharge. It is prudent for each institution to establish guidelines that ensure a consistent approach yet allow some flexibility on the basis of physician and family judgment. It is of foremost importance that the infant, family, and community be prepared for the infant to be safely cared for outside the hospital.

Infant Readiness

The infant is considered ready for discharge if, in the judgment of the responsible physician, the following have been accomplished:

- A sustained pattern of weight gain of sufficient duration has been demonstrated.
- The infant has demonstrated adequate maintenance of normal body temperature when fully clothed in an open bed with normal ambient temperature (20–25°C [68–77°F]) for more than 24 hours.
- The infant has established competent feeding by breast or bottle without cardiorespiratory compromise.
- Physiologically mature and stable cardiorespiratory function has been documented for a sufficient duration. The infant should be off caffeine without clinically significant apneic events for a sustained period before discharge, commonly 5–7 days.
- Appropriate immunizations have been administered or arrangements have been made to administer them on an outpatient basis.
- Appropriate metabolic screening has been performed.
- Hematologic status has been assessed and appropriate therapy has been instituted, if indicated.
- Nutritional risks have been assessed and therapy and dietary modification have been instituted, if indicated.
- Hearing evaluation has been completed.
- Funduscopic examinations for red reflex and retinopathy of prematurity have been completed, as indicated or follow-up ensured if such examination is incomplete.
- Neurodevelopmental and neurobehavioral status has been assessed and demonstrated to the parents.
- Cardiorespiratory monitoring while in a car seat has been completed (see also "Safe Transportation of Late-Preterm and Low-Birth-Weight Infants" in Chapter 10).

- Review of the hospital course has been completed, unresolved medical problems have been identified, and plans for follow-up monitoring and treatment have been instituted.
- An individualized home-care plan has been developed with input from all appropriate disciplines.

Family and Home Environmental Readiness

Assessment of the family's caregiving capabilities, resource availability, and home physical facilities has been completed as follows:

- Identification of at least two family caregivers and assessment of their ability, availability, and commitment
- Psychosocial assessment for parenting strengths and risks
- Home environmental assessment that may include an on-site evaluation
- Review of available financial resources and identification of adequate financial support

In preparation for home care of the technology-dependent infant, it is essential to complete an assessment documenting availability of 24-hour telephone access, electricity, safe in-house water supply, and adequate heating. Specific modification of home facilities must have been completed, if needed, to accommodate home-care systems. Plans should be in place for responding to loss of electrical power, heat, or water, and for emergency relocation mandated by natural disaster. Detailed financial assessment and planning are also essential. Caregivers should have demonstrated the necessary capabilities to provide all components of care, including the following:

- Feeding, whether breast, bottle, or alternative technique, including formula preparation or fortification of human milk, if required
- Basic infant care, which includes bathing, skin and genital care, temperature measurement, dressing, and comforting
- Infant cardiopulmonary resuscitation and emergency intervention
- Assessment of clinical status, including understanding and detection of the general early signs and symptoms of illness, as well as the signs and symptoms specific to the infant's condition

- Infant safety precautions, including proper positioning during sleep and proper use of car seats (see also "Parent Education and Psychosocial Factors" in Chapter 10). Encourage limited car seat travel in the first 6 months of life and have an adult ride in the rear seat to observe the infant during extended car travel, if possible.
- Specific safety precautions for the artificial airway, if any; feeding tube; intestinal stoma; infusion pump; and other mechanical and prosthetic devices, as indicated
- Administration of medications, specifically proper storage, dosage, timing, and administration, and recognition of signs of potential toxicity
- Equipment operation, maintenance, and problem solving for each mechanical support device required
- Appropriate technique for each special care procedure required, including special dressings for infusion entry sites, intestinal stomas, or healing wounds; maintenance of an artificial airway; oropharyngeal and tracheal suctioning; and physical therapy, as indicated

Community and Health Care System Readiness

An emergency intervention and transportation plan should be developed, and emergency medical service providers identified and notified, if indicated. Follow-up care needs should be determined, appropriate physicians identified, and appropriate information exchanged, including the following:

- A primary care physician has been identified, and has accepted responsibility for care of the infant.
- Surgical specialty and pediatric medical subspecialty follow-up care requirements have been identified and appropriate arrangements have been made.
- Neurodevelopmental follow-up requirements have been identified and appropriate referrals have been made.
- Home nursing visits for assessment and parent support have been arranged as indicated, and the home care plan has been transmitted to the home health agency.
- For breastfeeding mothers, information on breastfeeding support and availability of lactation specialists has been provided.

Special Considerations

The final decision for discharge, which is the responsibility of the attending physician, must be tailored to the unique constellation of issues posed by each infant's situation. Within this framework, there are four broad categories of high-risk infants that require individual consideration: 1) preterm infants, 2) infants with special health care needs or dependence on technology, 3) infants at risk because of family issues, and 4) infants with anticipated early death.

Preterm Infants

Criteria for hospital discharge of preterm infants should include physiologic stability rather than attainment of a specific weight. The three physiologic competencies generally recognized as essential before discharge are 1) oral feeding sufficient to sustain appropriate growth, 2) the ability to maintain normal body temperature in a home environment, and 3) sufficiently mature respiratory control. These competencies usually are achieved by 36–37 weeks of postmenstrual age; however, infants born earlier in gestation and with more complicated medical courses tend to take longer to achieve these physiologic competencies. Home monitors are rarely indicated (see also "Apnea" earlier in this chapter). Preterm infants should be placed in the supine position for sleeping, and hospitals should model this behavior for parents by positioning infants in the supine position after approximately 32 weeks of postmenstrual age if not contraindicated by medical care needs. Late preterm infants (34–37 weeks of gestation) are at increased risk of feeding problems and hyperbilirubinemia after discharge. These infants require close follow-up after discharge to monitor bilirubin concentrations and weight gain (see also "Discharge of Late Preterm Infants" in Chapter 10).

Infants With Special Health Care Needs or Dependence on Technology

Increasing numbers of infants are being discharged from the hospital with continuing medical problems requiring specialized technologic support. For infants discharged from the NICU, this support is primarily nutritional and respiratory, although additional special services may be necessary.

When infants are unable to achieve adequate oral feedings to sustain growth, alternatives include gavage or gastrostomy feedings, parenteral nutrition, or both. Gavage feeding has a limited role and should be considered only when feeding is the last issue requiring continued hospitalization and the parents or caregivers have demonstrated competence and comfort with this procedure. When little to no progress is being made with oral feedings, gastrostomy tube placement can make hospital discharge feasible and allow the infant to develop competent oral feeding skills if possible. Home parenteral nutrition requires thorough education of caregivers and the availability of a home-care company that is well versed in infant nutritional support and monitoring.

Respiratory support can include supplemental oxygen, tracheostomy, or home ventilation. Home oxygen therapy for infants with BPD has become a fairly common practice, allowing earlier hospital discharge for an otherwise stable infant. Oxygen saturation levels should be assessed intermittently after discharge by the primary care provider or pediatric pulmonologist to ensure sufficient oxygen is being delivered during a range of activities and sleep. Some infants who are discharged on supplemental oxygen also are discharged on a cardiorespiratory monitor or pulse oximeter. Reducing or stopping supplemental oxygen should be supervised by the physician or other health care professional and attempted only when the infant demonstrates acceptable oxygen saturations (greater than 90%) with good growth velocity and sufficient stamina for usual activity. Home care of the infant with a tracheostomy requires extensive parental teaching and coordinated multidisciplinary follow-up care. Infants with tracheostomy should be discharged on a cardiorespiratory monitor in case the airway should become obstructed. If the infant also requires continuing assisted ventilation, home nursing support will be needed for at least part of each day, and the ventilator must have a disconnect alarm.

Infants at Risk Because of Family Issues

Preterm birth, prolonged hospitalization, birth defects, and disabling conditions are known family stressors and risk factors for subsequent family dysfunction and child abuse. An organized approach to planning for discharge may help identify infants who require extra support or whose home environments present unacceptable risks. Adverse social conditions, including lower maternal education, lack of social support or stability, limited prenatal visits, parental discord or history of physical or mental abuse, or concern for parental substance use disorder should prompt awareness of the need for increased support after discharge. Most interventions have focused on multidisciplinary teams that provide follow-up monitoring, including home visits, although the efficacy of these interventions has been difficult to demonstrate. Simultaneous discharge of multiples may put additional stress on an already fragile home situation. Consideration should be given to stagger these discharges, allowing families time to accommodate the additional needs of each baby in the home environment.

Infants With Anticipated Early Death

For many infants with terminal conditions, the best place to spend the last days or weeks is at home. If the family wishes, assisted ventilation can even be withdrawn at home, rather than in the hospital. Preparation to discharge an infant for home hospice care should include arrangements for medical follow-up and home nursing, necessary equipment and supplies, management of pain, and bereavement support for the family. The parents should be given a letter to confirm to health care personnel that the infant should not be resuscitated (see also "Noninitiation or Withdrawal of Intensive Care for High-Risk Infants" in Chapter 10). Involvement of a multidisciplinary hospice or palliative care team before and after discharge can be very helpful to both the health care team and the family.

Hospice care may be chosen by families whose infants have an irreversible, fatal disease. The site for such care may vary with local community resources and family wishes. Enhancing the quality of the remaining life for the neonate and family is more important than the site of care delivery. Although less well studied than for older children, the components of neonatal hospice care are not unlike those established for pediatric hospice care. These components include the following elements:

- Involvement of skilled professionals
- Control of distressing conditions and provision of physical comfort
- Coordinated, multidisciplinary service delivery
- Social support of the family
- Follow-up and bereavement care and counseling

Follow-up Care of High-Risk Newborn Infants

The organization of follow-up care for high-risk infants will vary with the neonatal subgroup being monitored, potential adverse outcomes frequently associated with individual subgroups, and the purpose for ongoing evaluation.

Specific requirements for follow-up care of high-risk neonatal subgroups include the following components:

- Primary care—monitoring of growth and development, preventive care, and guidance
- Supervision of nutrition with special emphasis on achieving appropriate growth parameters and the use of specialized formulas and supplements
- Management of unresolved medical problems
- Early detection of abnormality or delayed developmental progress
- Early intervention and habilitation
- Infant safety
- Parent education
- Evaluation of treatment benefit and complications
- Documentation of outcomes
- Neurosensory follow-up
- Environmental and psychosocial concerns
- Referral to other community resources

Role of the Primary Care Provider

The infant's primary care physician should provide a medical home and share in the responsibility for providing continuity of care with the neonatal level II, level III, or level IV care center. Frequently, the more detailed developmental and psychologic evaluations and the initial management of complex unresolved medical problems are primarily the responsibility of the neonatal level III or level IV care center. As recovery progresses, medical care is increasingly assumed by the primary care physician. The primary care physician likely will assume the responsibility for referral to subspecialty consultation and care. Within any format of shared patient care delivery, it is imperative that all professionals communicate information in a timely manner and share in the planning and execution of the long-term care for infants with multidisciplinary service needs. If the infant is participating in a perinatal follow-up program, the roles of the health care providers in each area should be established.

Surveillance and Assessment

The timing of follow-up visits for high-risk infants will vary with the needs of the individual infant and family. It may be necessary to examine some of these infants weekly or semimonthly at first. Neurologic, developmental, behavioral, and sensory status should be assessed more than once during the first year in high-risk infants to ensure early identification of problems and referral for appropriate interventions. A multidisciplinary perinatal follow-up program is especially valuable in providing these assessments.

Many infants who are born preterm have increased difficulty with emotional and attentional regulation, resulting in irritability, dependency, and other attentional problems. These factors as well as prolonged hospitalization disrupt family relationships, particularly the parent–child relationship. Infants with such a history may be at higher risk of child abuse, and these families benefit from close follow-up and support (for more information on child abuse risk factors, see "Follow-up Care" in Chapter 10).

Growth should be assessed at each follow-up visit—including weight gain, linear growth, and head growth—and plotted on standardized, birth-weight-appropriate growth curves with the appropriate-age correction for gestational age at birth. Review of nutritional intake and calculation of caloric intake are helpful in case management. Inadequate growth or weight gain may require consultation with a dietitian or nutritionist well acquainted with postdischarge needs of the preterm infant, and possible alternative feeding regimens such as placement of a feeding tube.

Physical examination should assess neuromotor, cardiac, pulmonary, gastrointestinal, and nutritional status, as well as the presence of any hernias, anomalies, or orthopedic deformities. Residual scars from invasive procedures during the neonatal course should be monitored for satisfactory healing. On occasion, referral for reconstructive procedures may be necessary.

Medication dosage should be reevaluated, doses increased with weight gain and age, and blood concentrations monitored as indicated. Immunization status should be reviewed, and age-appropriate administration should be maintained. Follow-up audiology and visual assessments should be obtained when indicated. Occasionally, patients who are transferred from their community to regional NICUs may have missed standard state newborn screening examinations or the results may not be readily available. The primary health care provider should ensure these have been completed and are within the accepted range.

Neurologic assessment should include an appraisal of muscle tone, development, protective and deep-tendon reflexes, and visual and auditory responses. In addition, developmental progress should be monitored both by parental report of milestone acquisition and by assessment using a standard developmental screening tool. When neurologic findings are suspect or developmental delays are suspected, children should be referred to either a neonatal follow-up program or an appropriate community program for more in-depth assessment. Infants at greatest risk of adverse neurodevelopmental outcome (eg, those with a birthweight of 1,500 g or less; hypoxic–ischemic encephalopathy or neonatal seizures; hypoxic cardiorespiratory failure; or complex, multiple congenital anomalies) should have formal neurodevelopmental testing with a battery of standardized tests at least at 1 year and 2 years corrected age to monitor development in all domains (gross motor; fine motor and adaptive; visual perceptive and problem solving; hearing, language, and speech; and socialization). Primary care physicians should educate families regarding the importance of formal neurodevelopmental testing and encourage them to complete the assessment, irrespective of the results of developmental screening.

Early Intervention

Intervention programs for high-risk infants have been established under federal legislation to provide early detection of developmental delay and other disabilities. Intervention services may be provided up to 3 years of age for individual infants with confirmed neurodevelopmental delay or other disability. Programs also offer therapeutic guidelines for families, parent support groups, and respite care programs. Although no definitive data confirm the beneficial effects of infant-stimulation programs, early intervention may improve social adaptation, limit residual functional disability, and provide valuable family support.

Bibliography

Adamkin DH. Postnatal glucose homeostasis in late-preterm and term infants. American Academy of Pediatrics Committee on Fetus and Newborn. Pediatrics 2011;127:575–9.

Aher SM, Ohlsson A. Late erythropoietin for preventing red blood cell transfusion in preterm and/or low birth weight infants. Cochrane Database of Systematic Reviews 2014, Issue 4. Art. No. CD004868. DOI: 10.1002/14651858.CD004868.pub4.

Akula VP, Joe P, Thusu K, Davis AS, Tamaresis JS, Kim S, et al. A randomized clinical trial of therapeutic hypothermia mode during transport for neonatal encephalopathy. J Pediatr 2015;166:856-61.e1–2.

Alcohol abuse and other substance use disorders: ethical issues in obstetric and gynecologic practice. Committee Opinion No. 633. American College of Obstetricians and Gynecologists. Obstet Gynecol 2015;125:1529–37.

American Academy of Pediatrics. Pediatric nutrition handbook. 7th ed. Elk Grove Village (IL): AAP; 2013.

American Academy of Pediatrics. Red book: report of the Committee on Infectious Diseases. 30th ed. Elk Grove Village (IL): AAP; 2015.

American Academy of Pediatrics, American Heart Association. Textbook of neonatal resuscitation. 7th ed. Elk Grove Village (IL): AAP; Dallas (TX): AHA; 2016.

American Association of Blood Banks. Standards for blood banks and transfusion services. 30th ed. Bethesda (MD): AABB; 2016.

Antenatal corticosteroid therapy for fetal maturation. Committee Opinion No.677. American College of Obstetricians and Gynecologists. Obstet Gynecol 2016;128:e187–94.

Asti L, Magers JS, Keels E, Wispe J, McClead RE Jr. A quality improvement project to reduce length of stay for neonatal abstinence syndrome. Pediatrics 2015;135:e1494–500.

Ballard RA, Truog WE, Cnaan A, Martin RJ, Ballard PL, Merrill JD, et al. Inhaled nitric oxide in preterm infants undergoing mechanical ventilation. NO CLD Study Group. N Engl J Med 2006;355:343–53.

Barrington KJ, Finer N. Inhaled nitric oxide for respiratory failure in preterm infants. Cochrane Database of Systematic Reviews 2010, Issue 12. Art. No. CD000509. DOI: 10.1002/14651858.CD000509.pub4; 10.1002/14651858.CD000509.pub4.

Baud O, Maury L, Lebail F, Ramful D, El Moussawi F, Nicaise C, et al. Effect of early low-dose hydrocortisone on survival without bronchopulmonary dysplasia in extremely preterm infants (PREMILOC): a double-blind, placebo-controlled, multicentre, randomised trial. PREMILOC trial study group. Lancet 2016;387:1827–36.

Bellieni CV, Tei M, Coccina F, Buonocore G. Sensorial saturation for infants' pain. J Matern Fetal Neonatal Med 2012;25(suppl):79–81.

Bellù R, de Waal KA, Zanini R. Opioids for neonates receiving mechanical ventilation. Cochrane Database of Systematic Reviews 2008, Issue 1. Art. No. CD004212. DOI: 10.1002/14651858.CD004212.pub3; 10.1002/14651858.CD004212.pub3.

Bhutani VK. Phototherapy to prevent severe neonatal hyperbilirubinemia in the newborn infant 35 or more weeks of gestation. Committee on Fetus and Newborn, American Academy of Pediatrics. Pediatrics 2011;128:e1046–52.

Brody AS, Frush DP, Huda W, Brent RL. Radiation risk to children from computed tomography. American Academy of Pediatrics Section on Radiology. Pediatrics 2007;120:677–82.

Cong X, McGrath JM, Cusson RM, Zhang D. Pain assessment and measurement in neonates: an updated review. Adv Neonatal Care 2013;13:379–95.

Cools F, Offringa M, Askie LM. Elective high frequency oscillatory ventilation versus conventional ventilation for acute pulmonary dysfunction in preterm infants. Cochrane Database of Systematic Reviews 2015, Issue 3. Art. No. CD000104. DOI: 10.1002/14651858.CD000104.pub4.

Cummings JJ, Polin RA. Oxygen targeting in extremely low birth weight infants. Committee on Fetus and Newborn [published erratum appears in Pediatrics 2016;138(6)]. Pediatrics 2016;138(2).

De Paoli AG, Clark RH, Bhuta T, Henderson-Smart DJ. High frequency oscillatory ventilation versus conventional ventilation for infants with severe pulmonary dysfunction born at or near term. Cochrane Database of Systematic Reviews 2009, Issue 3. Art. No. CD002974. DOI: 10.1002/14651858.CD002974.pub2.

Delayed umbilical cord clamping after birth. Committee Opinion No. 684. American College of Obstetricians and Gynecologists. Obstet Gynecol 2017;129:e5–10.

Desai RJ, Huybrechts KF, Hernandez-Diaz S, Mogun H, Patorno E, Kaltenbach K, et al. Exposure to prescription opioid analgesics in utero and risk of neonatal abstinence syndrome: population based cohort study. BMJ 2015;350:h2102.

Doyle LW, Ehrenkranz RA, Halliday HL. Early (< 8 Days) Postnatal Corticosteroids for Preventing Chronic Lung Disease in Preterm Infants. Cochrane Database of Systematic Reviews 2014, Issue 5. Art. No. CD001146. DOI: 10.1002/14651858.CD001146.pub4.

Eichenwald EC. Apnea of prematurity. Committee on Fetus and Newborn, American Academy of Pediatrics. Pediatrics 2016;137.

El Shahed AI, Dargaville PA, Ohlsson A, Soll R. Surfactant for meconium aspiration syndrome in term and late preterm infants. Cochrane Database of Systematic Reviews 2014, Issue 12. Art. No. CD002054. DOI: 10.1002/14651858.CD002054.pub3.

Fierson WM. Screening examination of premature infants for retinopathy of prematurity. American Academy of Pediatrics Section on Ophthalmology, American Academy of Ophthalmology, American Association for Pediatric Ophthalmology and Strabismus, American Association of Certified Orthoptists. Pediatrics 2013;131: 189–95.

Finer N, Barrington KJ. Nitric oxide for respiratory failure in infants born at or near term. Cochrane Database of Systematic Reviews 2006, Issue 4. Art. No. CD000399. DOI: 10.1002/14651858.CD000399.pub2; 10.1002/14651858.CD000399.pub2.

Hall ES, Wexelblatt SL, Crowley M, Grow JL, Jasin LR, Klebanoff MA, et al. A multicenter cohort study of treatments and hospital outcomes in neonatal abstinence syndrome. OCHNAS Consortium. Pediatrics 2014;134:e527–34.

Higgins RD, Raju T, Edwards AD, Azzopardi DV, Bose CL, Clark RH, et al. Hypothermia and other treatment options for neonatal encephalopathy: an executive summary of the Eunice Kennedy Shriver NICHD Workshop. Eunice Kennedy Shriver National Institute of Child Health and Human Development Hypothermia Workshop Speakers and Moderators. J Pediatr 2011;159:851–58.e1.

Hospital discharge of the high-risk neonate. American Academy of Pediatrics Committee on Fetus and Newborn. Pediatrics 2008;122:1119–26.

Hudak ML, Tan RC. Neonatal drug withdrawal. Committee on Drugs, Committee on Fetus and Newborn American Academy of Pediatrics [published erratum appears in Pediatrics 2014;133:937]. Pediatrics 2012;129:e540–60.

Jacobs SE, Berg M, Hunt R, Tarnow-Mordi WO, Inder TE, Davis PG. Cooling for Newborns with Hypoxic Ischaemic Encephalopathy. Cochrane Database of Systematic Reviews 2013, Issue 1. Art. No. CD003311. DOI: 10.1002/14651858.CD003311.pub3.

Jobe AH, Bancalari E. Bronchopulmonary dysplasia. Am J Respir Crit Care Med 2001;163:1723–9.

Johnston C, Campbell-Yeo M, Fernandes A, Inglis D, Streiner D, Zee R. Skin-to-skin care for procedural pain in neonates. Cochrane Database of Systematic Reviews 2014, Issue 1. Art. No. CD008435. DOI: 10.1002/14651858.CD008435.pub2.

Kumar P, Denson SE, Mancuso TJ. Premedication for nonemergency endotracheal intubation in the neonate. Committee on Fetus and Newborn, Section on Anesthesiology and Pain Medicine. Pediatrics 2010;125:608–15.

Lamola AA, Bhutani VK, Du L, Castillo Cuadrado M, Chen L. Shen Z, et al. Neonatal bilirubin binding capacity discerns risk of neurological dysfunction. Pediatr Res. 2015;77:334–9.

Maisels MJ, Bhutani VK, Bogen D, Newman TB, Stark AR, Watchko JF. Hyperbilirubinemia in the newborn infant > or =35 weeks' gestation: an update with clarifications. Pediatrics 2009;124:1193–8.

Maisels MJ, Watchko JF, Bhutani VK, Stevenson DK. An approach to the management of hyperbilirubinemia in the preterm infant less than 35 weeks of gestation. J Perinatol 2012;32:660–4.

Management of hyperbilirubinemia in the newborn infant 35 or more weeks of gestation. American Academy of Pediatrics Subcommittee on Hyperbilirubinemia [Published Erratum Appears in Pediatrics 2004;114:1138]. Pediatrics 2004;114:297–316.

Manja V, Lakshminrusimha S, Cook DJ. Oxygen saturation target range for extremely preterm infants: a systematic review and meta-analysis [published erratum appears in JAMA Pediatr 2015;169:507]. JAMA Pediatr 2015;169:332–40.

Moon RY. SIDS and other sleep-related infant deaths: updated 2016 recommendations for a safe infant sleeping environment. Task Force on Sudden Infant Death Syndrome. Pediatrics 2016;138:e20162940.

Morley CJ, Davis PG, Doyle LW, Brion LP, Hascoet JM, Carlin JB. Nasal CPAP or intubation at birth for very preterm infants. COIN Trial Investigators [published erratum appears in N Engl J Med 2008;358:1529]. N Engl J Med 2008;358:700–8.

Morris BH, Oh W, Tyson JE, Stevenson DK, Phelps DL, O'Shea TM, et al. Aggressive vs. conservative phototherapy for infants with extremely low birth weight. NICHD Neonatal Research Network. N Engl J Med 2008;359:1885–96.

Ng E, Taddio A, Ohlsson A. Intravenous midazolam infusion for sedation of infants in the neonatal intensive care unit. Cochrane Database of Systematic Reviews 2012, Issue 6. Art. No. CD002052. DOI: 10.1002/14651858.CD002052.pub2.

Ohls RK, Christensen RD, Kamath-Rayne BD, Rosenberg A, Wiedmeier SE, Roohi M, et al. A randomized, masked, placebo-controlled study of darbepoetin alfa in preterm infants. Pediatrics 2013;132:e119–27.

Ohlsson A, Aher SM. Early erythropoietin for preventing red blood cell transfusion in preterm and/or low birth weight infants. Cochrane Database of Systematic Reviews 2014, Issue 4. Art. No. CD004863. DOI: 10.1002/14651858.CD004863.pub4.

Patrick SW, Dudley J, Martin PR, Harrell FE, Warren MD, Hartmann KE, et al. Prescription opioid epidemic and infant outcomes. Pediatrics 2015;135:842–50.

Papile LA, Baley JE, Benitz W, Cummings J, Carlo WA, Eichenwald E, et al. Hypothermia and neonatal encephalopathy. Committee on Fetus and Newborn. Pediatrics 2014;133:1146–50.

Pillai Riddell RR, Racine NM, Gennis HG, Turcotte K, Uman LS, Horton RE, et al. Non-pharmacological management of infant and young child procedural pain. Cochrane Database of Systematic Reviews 2015, Issue 12. Art. No. CD006275. DOI: 10.1002/14651858.CD006275.pub3.

Polin RA, Carlo WA. Surfactant replacement therapy for preterm and term neonates with respiratory distress. Committee on Fetus and Newborn American Academy of Pediatrics. Pediatrics 2014;133:156–63.

Prevention and management of procedural pain in the neonate: an update. Committee on Fetus and Newborn and Section on Anesthesiology and Pain Medicine. Pediatrics 2016;137:e20154271.

Saugstad OD, Aune D. Optimal oxygenation of extremely low birth weight infants: a meta-analysis and systematic review of the oxygen saturation target studies. Neonatology 2014;105:55–63.

Schmidt B, Anderson PJ, Doyle LW, Dewey D, Grunau RE, Asztalos EV, et al. Survival without disability to age 5 years after neonatal caffeine therapy for apnea of prematurity. Caffeine for Apnea of Prematurity (CAP) Trial Investigators. JAMA 2012;307:275–82.

Shah PS, Herbozo C, Aliwalas LL, Shah VS. Breastfeeding or breast milk for procedural pain in neonates. Cochrane Database of Systematic Reviews 2012, Issue 12. Art. No. CD004950. DOI: 10.1002/14651858.CD004950.pub3.

Shankaran S, Laptook AR, Pappas A, McDonald SA, Das A, Tyson JE, et al. Effect of depth and duration of cooling on deaths in the nicu among neonates with hypoxic ischemic encephalopathy: a randomized clinical trial. Eunice Kennedy Shriver National Institute of Child Health and Human Development Neonatal Research Network. JAMA 2014;312:2629–39.

Stevens B, Yamada J, Ohlsson A, Haliburton S, Shorkey A. Sucrose for analgesia in newborn infants undergoing painful procedures. Cochrane Database of Systematic Reviews 2016, Issue 7. Art. No. CD001069. DOI: 10.1002/14651858.CD001069.pub5.

Suttner DM, Short BL. Neonatal respiratory ECLS. In: Annich G, Lynch W, MacLaren G, Wilson J, Bartlett R, editors. ECMO: extracorporeal cardiopulmonary support in critical care. 4th ed. Ann Arbor (MI): Extracorporeal Life Support Organization; 2012. p. 225–49.

Supplemental therapeutic oxygen for prethreshold retinopathy of prematurity (STOP-ROP), a randomized, controlled trial. I: primary outcomes. Pediatrics 2000;105: 295–310.

Tolia VN, Patrick SW, Bennett MM, Murthy K, Sousa J, Smith PB, et al. Increasing incidence of the neonatal abstinence syndrome in U.S. neonatal ICUs. N Engl J Med 2015;372:2118–26.

Walsh MC, Wilson-Costello D, Zadell A, Newman N, Fanaroff A. Safety, reliability, and validity of a physiologic definition of bronchopulmonary dysplasia. J Perinatol 2003;23:451–6.

Watterberg KL. Policy statement--postnatal corticosteroids to prevent or treat bronchopulmonary dysplasia. American Academy of Pediatrics Committee on Fetus and Newborn. Pediatrics 2010;126:800–8.

Whyte RK, Kirpalani H, Asztalos EV, Andersen C, Blajchman M, Heddle N, et al. Neurodevelopmental outcome of extremely low birth weight infants randomly assigned to restrictive or liberal hemoglobin thresholds for blood transfusion. PINTOS Study Group. Pediatrics 2009;123:207–13.

Resources

American Academy of Pediatrics. Jaundice in newborns - Q&A. Elk Grove Village (IL): AAP; 2009. Available at: https://www.healthychildren.org/English/news/Pages/Jaundice-in-Newborns.aspx. Retrieved November 9, 2016.

American College of Obstetricians and Gynecologists. Immunization for women. Washington, DC: American College of Obstetricians and Gynecologists; 2016. Available at: http://immunizationforwomen.org. Retrieved October 26, 2016.

Centers for Disease Control and Prevention. Advisory Committee on Immunization Practices (ACIP). Atlanta (GA): CDC; 2016. Available at: https://www.cdc.gov/vaccines/acip/. Retrieved November 8, 2016.

Chapter 12

Perinatal Infections

Certain infections that occur in the antepartum or intrapartum period may have a significant effect on the fetus and newborn. Appropriate antepartum and intrapartum care of the mother and subsequent care of the newborn soon after birth is required to a) optimize maternal and fetal health, b) reduce the frequency of vertical and horizontal pathogen transmission, and c) provide pathogen-specific neonatal care. Some infections, such as influenza and varicella, may have more severe outcomes in pregnant women than in other adults. Other infections are of little consequence to the mother and yet may cause severe illness in the fetus or newborn. Communication and cooperation among all perinatal care personnel are essential to obtain the best results (see also "First Visit" in Chapter 6). The infections discussed in this chapter have been selected on the basis of the frequency with which they must be addressed in pregnancy, as well as on the basis of new and evolving information that affects management.

Many of the sections in this chapter refer to vaccination risks, benefits, and recommendations for pregnant women. The American College of Obstetricians and Gynecologists (ACOG) recommends routine assessment of each pregnant woman's immunization status and administration of indicated immunizations. The benefits of nonlive vaccines outweigh any unproven potential concerns. Importantly, evolving data demonstrate both maternal and neonatal protection against an increasing number of aggressive newborn pathogens through the use of maternal immunization programs, suggesting pregnancy is an optimal time to immunize for disease prevention in both women and newborns. There is no evidence of adverse fetal effects from vaccinating pregnant women with an inactivated virus or bacterial vaccines or toxoids, and a growing body of robust data demonstrates safety of such use. Maternal vaccination during pregnancy is particularly important for diseases such as pertussis and influenza because newborns cannot receive vaccines for these conditions until later in infancy. Co-administration of indicated inactivated vaccines during pregnancy (ie, tetanus toxoid, reduced diphtheria toxoid, and acellular pertussis [Tdap] and influenza) is also acceptable, safe, and may optimize effectiveness of immunization efforts. Furthermore, no evidence exists that suggests that any vaccine is associated with an increased risk of autism or adverse effects due to exposure to traces of the mercury-containing preservative thimerosal. It should be remembered, however, that live attenuated vaccines (eg, measles–mumps–rubella [MMR], varicella) do pose a theoretical risk (although never documented or proved) to the fetus and generally should be avoided during pregnancy (see also Chapter 10). All vaccines administered during pregnancy as well as health care provider-driven discussions about the indications and benefits of immunization during pregnancy should be fully documented in the patient's prenatal record. In addition, if a patient declines vaccination, this should be documented in the patient's prenatal record, and the health care provider is advised to revisit the issue of vaccination at subsequent visits. Updated information on vaccination with reference to pregnancy, lactation and general women's and newborn health can be found at www.cdc.gov/vaccines/pregnancy/hcp/guidelines.html and on ACOG's immunization website at www.immunizationforwomen.org/. In addition, the drugs and lactation website LactMed (www.toxnet.nlm.nih.gov/newtoxnet/lactmed.htm) contains information on vaccine administration in lactating women.

Viral Infections

Cytomegalovirus

Cytomegalovirus (CMV) is a ubiquitous double-stranded DNA herpes virus that is transmitted by sexual contact; by body fluids such as saliva, urine and breastmilk; and by blood transfusion and organ transplantation. In infants, children, and adults, after an incubation period of 28–60 days (mean, 40 days), CMV infection induces immunoglobulin M (IgM) antibody production followed by an immunoglobulin G (IgG) antibody response. Viremia can be detected for 2–3 weeks after primary infection (infection in a previously seronegative individual). Although adults with primary CMV infection are usually asymptomatic, individuals may experience a mononucleosis-like syndrome, with fever, chills, myalgias, malaise, leukocytosis, lymphocytosis, abnormal liver function, and lymphadenopathy. After the primary infection, CMV remains latent in host cells and recurrent, or secondary, infection can occur. Secondary infection (intermittent viral excretion in the presence of host immunity) can occur after reactivation of the latent endogenous CMV strain or by reinfection with a different exogenous viral strain.

Prevalence of CMV immunity, in primary or secondary infection, varies significantly by geographic region, socioeconomic status, and ethnicity. The incidence of primary CMV infection among previously seronegative pregnant women in the United States ranges from 0.7% to 4%, with estimates of secondary infection ranging up to 13.5%. Vertical transmission of CMV may occur as a result of transplacental infection after primary or secondary infection, exposure to contaminated genital tract secretions at delivery, or breastfeeding. Most infants with congenital CMV are asymptomatic at birth. Clinical findings of symptomatic congenital CMV infection include jaundice, petechiae, thrombocytopenia, hepatosplenomegaly, growth restriction, myocarditis, and nonimmune hydrops.

Transmission

Cytomegalovirus is the most common congenital infection, occurring in 0.2–2.2% of all newborn infants. The annual cost of treating the permanent disabilities and complications caused by CMV infections in the United States is estimated to be more than $1.86 billion. Transplacental CMV transmission represents the most significant risk of developing clinical sequelae. Cytomegalovirus infection resulting from exposure to infected cervical secretions or breast milk is typically asymptomatic and is not associated with severe neonatal sequelae in the term infant. Among infants who acquire infection from maternal cervical secretions or human milk, preterm infants born before 32 weeks of gestation and with a birth weight less than 1,500 g are at greater risk of CMV disease than are full-term infants. With primary maternal CMV infection, the overall risk of transmission to the fetus is approximately 30–40%. Although vertical transmission may occur at any stage of pregnancy, the risk of transmission is greatest in the third trimester. Transmission rates for primary infection are 30% in the first trimester, 34–38% in the second trimester, and 40–72% in the third trimester. However, more serious fetal sequelae occur after maternal CMV infection during the first trimester. Of those fetuses infected in utero after a primary infection, 12–18% will have signs and symptoms of CMV infection at birth and up to 25% will develop sequelae. Approximately 30% of severely infected infants die, and 65–80% of survivors have severe neurologic morbidity. The incidence of severe fetal infection is much lower after recurrent maternal infection than after primary infection. Vertical transmission after a recurrent infection is 0.15–2%. Infants infected after maternal CMV reactivation generally are asymptomatic at birth. Congenital hearing loss is typically the most severe sequela of secondary infection, and congenital infection after recurrent infection is unlikely to produce multiple sequelae.

Screening

Routine serologic screening of pregnant women for CMV is not recommended. The limitations of maternal IgM antibody screening in differentiating primary from recurrent infection makes the results difficult to use in counseling patients about fetal risk. In addition, maternal immunity does not eliminate the possibility of fetal infection given that up to 75% of congenital CMV infections worldwide may be due to reactivation of latent virus or reinfection with a new viral strain. The lack of a proven treatment to prevent congenital transmission further diminishes the potential benefit of universal screening.

Testing should be considered for term infants with hearing loss demonstrated on newborn hearing screens. A recent trial of extended antiviral therapy for infants with congenital CMV demonstrates modestly improved hearing outcomes, although the extension of these findings to infants with isolated hearing loss is unclear. Testing also may be considered among very-low-birth-weight, premature infants with signs of late-onset sepsis or otherwise unexplained acute thrombocytopenia or cholestasis. Antiviral therapy has not been systematically studied for safety or efficacy in preterm infants, but the recognition of CMV infection may prevent unneeded antibiotic therapy and prompt more intensive neurodevelopmental and hearing follow-up care.

Diagnosis

Congenital CMV may be suspected prenatally after a documented maternal primary infection (more commonly because universal screening is not recommended) or after ultrasound findings suggestive of infection. These findings include abdominal and liver calcifications, hepatosplenomegaly, echogenic bowel or kidneys, ascites, cerebral ventriculomegaly, intracranial calcifications, microcephaly, hydrops fetalis, and growth restriction. Nevertheless, such findings are more likely to be associated with other abnormalities, such as aneuploidy, and the positive predictive value of each of these markers for CMV infection is quite weak. The presence of echogenic bowel, for instance, is only predictive of CMV infection approximately 3% of the time.

After detection of maternal infection or suspected fetal infection based on ultrasound findings, congenital CMV can be detected in the amniotic fluid of infected fetuses by either culture or polymerase chain reaction (PCR). Fetal blood sampling, which is less sensitive than amniotic fluid testing and carries additional risks for the fetus, is not warranted. The sensitivity of a CMV amniotic fluid culture ranges from 70% to 80% compared with a sensitivity of 78% to 98% for PCR (specificity of 92% to 98%). The sensitivity of amniotic fluid testing for prenatal diagnosis of congenital CMV infection is markedly lower if performed before approximately 21 weeks of gestation. Although a positive culture or PCR is highly predictive of congenital infection, the detection of CMV in amniotic fluid does not predict the severity of congenital CMV infection.

Treatment

Currently, no therapies are available for the treatment of maternal or fetal CMV infection. Antiviral medications such as ganciclovir, valganciclovir, and foscarnet are approved by the U.S. Food and Drug Administration (FDA) only for treatment of patients with acquired immunodeficiency syndrome (AIDS) or organ transplants. A recent randomized, placebo-controlled trial in newborn infants with symptomatic congenital CMV disease compared 6 months of valganciclovir therapy with 6 weeks of therapy. At 24 months' follow-up, 6 months of treatment compared with 6 weeks appeared to modestly improve hearing and developmental outcomes, with grade 3 or 4 neutropenia occurring in approximately 25% of treated infants. There are no data regarding the safety or efficacy of ganciclovir or valganciclovir therapy in very-low-birth-weight, preterm infants with congenital or acquired CMV infection.

Antiviral therapy for pregnant women with primary CMV infection to prevent vertical transmission is not recommended. A recent randomized, placebo-controlled trial of CMV hyperimmune globulin to prevent vertical transmission of CMV failed to demonstrate a significant decrease in fetal infection and was associated with a significant increase in pregnancy adverse events, including preterm delivery. Routine use of CMV hyperimmune globulin in pregnant women with a primary CMV infection is not currently recommended. In cases of known maternal CMV infection during pregnancy, referral to a maternal–fetal medicine specialist is warranted.

Enteroviruses

The enteroviruses comprise a group of RNA viruses that includes the polioviruses, Coxsackie viruses, echoviruses, parechovirus and other numbered enteroviruses. Through the widespread use of vaccines, wild-type poliovirus infection has been eliminated from the Western Hemisphere as well as the Western Pacific and European regions. Vaccine-associated paralytic poliovirus has been eliminated in the United States with the use of inactivated poliovirus vaccine rather than the use of live attenuated oral poliovirus vaccine. Nonpolio enteroviral infections are common and are spread by fecal–oral and respiratory routes. Enteroviruses are common and pregnant women are frequently exposed to them, especially during summer and fall months. Most enterovirus infections during pregnancy cause mild or no illness in the mother. However, infection in the third trimester can trigger labor.

Enteroviruses rarely cross the placenta and cause disease in the fetus. Vertical transmission of enteroviruses can occur at or shortly after birth after exposure to virus-containing maternal secretions, including blood, cervical and respiratory secretions, or stool. Signs of an enterovirus infection in the newborn infant generally begin 3–7 days after birth. Newborn infants who acquire infection from their mothers perinatally or within days of birth are at risk of severe disease primarily because such infections are acquired in the absence of a serotype-specific maternally derived antibody. Any infection acquired in the absence of a specific antibody can cause severe disease, including sepsis syndrome, meningoencephalitis, myocarditis, hepatitis, coagulopathy, and pneumonitis.

Diagnosis is confirmed by recovery of the virus from swabs of the throat or rectum and samples of stool, cerebrospinal fluid (CSF), or blood. Diagnostics that are PCR based are more sensitive than viral culture and more reliably detect all types of enteroviruses, some of which are difficult to grow in culture.

No specific therapy is clinically available for neonatal enteroviral infection. Immune globulin given intravenously has been used in life-threatening neonatal infections, suspected viral myocarditis, and enterovirus 71 neurologic disease, but efficacy data are lacking. A recent small trial of pleconaril for neonatal enteroviral sepsis showed a trend to lower mortality among infants confirmed to have enteroviral infection. Hospitalized newborns should be managed with contact precautions.

Hepatitis A Virus

The hepatitis A virus (HAV) is a small RNA virus that can produce either asymptomatic infection or acute illness. Serious effects of HAV infection are uncommon, but patients may require hospitalization and supportive care if encephalopathy, coagulopathy, or severe debilitation occur. Hepatitis A virus has little effect on pregnancy and rarely is transmitted perinatally. The risk of transplacental transmission to the fetus is negligible, and there is no evidence that the virus is a teratogen. The most common mode of transmission is by the fecal–oral route. Diagnosis is confirmed by the demonstration of anti-HAV IgM antibodies in the serum of pregnant women or infants. Vaccines for hepatitis A are highly effective and approved for use during pregnancy, if indicated. Pregnant women with the following risk factors are candidates for hepatitis A vaccination: history of or current intravenous drug use, travel to endemic regions, residence in communities with a high prevalence of hepatitis A, working or having close contact with HAV-infected primates, diagnosis of chronic liver disease such as chronic hepatitis B or receipt of a liver transplant, or receiving clotting factor concentrate for treatment of a clotting disorder. Immunoglobulin is effective for both preexposure and postexposure prophylaxis, does not pose a risk to either a pregnant woman or her fetus, and should be administered during pregnancy if indicated.

Nosocomial outbreaks have been reported in neonatal intensive care units, but these are rare. Prevention of virus spread is based on contact precautions. With appropriate hygienic precautions, breastfeeding by a mother with HAV infection is permissible. Although immunoglobulin has been administered to newborns if the mother's symptoms began 2 weeks before delivery through 1 week after delivery, the efficacy of this practice has not been established.

Hepatitis B Virus

Hepatitis B virus (HBV) is a small DNA virus that contains three principal antigens: 1) hepatitis B surface antigen (HBsAg), 2) hepatitis B core antigen, and 3) hepatitis B e antigen (HBeAg). People acutely infected with HBV may be asymptomatic or symptomatic. Among people with symptomatic HBV infection, the spectrum of signs and symptoms is varied and includes subacute illness with nonspecific symptoms (eg, anorexia, nausea, or malaise), clinical hepatitis with jaundice, or fulminant hepatitis. Transmission of HBV occurs through contact with infected blood or bodily fluids (ie, semen, cervical secretions, and saliva).

Perinatal transmission of HBV infection is highly efficient and generally occurs from exposure to maternal blood during labor and delivery. Transplacental passage of HBV accounts for only approximately 2% of perinatal transmission cases. If appropriate and timely treatment is not instituted, perinatal infection occurs in 5–20% of infants born to mothers positive for

HBsAg alone and 70–90% of infants born to mothers who are both HBsAg positive and HBeAg positive. Acute infection in the third trimester of pregnancy is associated with an 80–90% rate of neonatal infection. More than 90% of infants who are infected perinatally will develop chronic HBV infection, which is associated with a 25% lifetime risk of premature death from liver disease.

Antepartum Screening, Immunization, and Treatment

Because historical information about risk factors identifies less than one half of chronic carriers, serologic testing for HBsAg is recommended for all pregnant women as part of routine prenatal care. When ordering an HBsAg screening test for a pregnant or postpartum patient, ACOG recommends using a test designated as "Prenatal" whenever possible (see Table 12-1 for a list of laboratories offering prenatal-specific HBsAg tests). Laboratory results should be communicated to and available at the delivery hospital to ensure appropriate care for the woman and her infant. Women who have not been screened prenatally, those who are at high risk of infection (eg, intravenous drug users, women with sexually transmitted infections [STIs], multiple sexual partners or recent international travel), and those with clinical hepatitis should be tested at admission for delivery. Women who are HBsAg positive should receive additional tests including: HBeAg, HBV DNA concentration, and ALT (alanine aminotransferase) to assess for chronic HBV infection. Pregnant women with chronic HBV should be informed about transmission risks and ways to prevent newborn infection. Pregnant women with diagnosed chronic HBV infection should be referred for evaluation to a physician experienced in the management of chronic liver disease. Recent studies have demonstrated benefit from antiviral treatment in decreasing the risk of vertical transmission of HBV in women with high viral loads late in pregnancy. HBV-infected women with high viral loads have an increased risk of their infants developing HBV infection despite appropriate immunoprophylaxis with hepatitis B immune globulin (HBIG) and hepatitis B vaccine. Studies are on-going to determine if HBV-infected women with high viral loads should routinely receive antiviral therapy directed at HBV in order to reduce perinatal transmission of HBV. Any use of antiviral therapies in HBV-positive pregnant women must be considered in consultation with infectious disease and hepatology specialists.

Women who are HBsAg negative but who have risk factors for HBV infection should be offered vaccination during pregnancy. The recommended

TABLE 12-1. Screening Pregnant Women for Hepatitis B Virus Infection: Ordering Prenatal Hepatitis B Surface Antigen Tests From Major Commercial Laboratories

Laboratory	Test Option	Test Name	Reflex to Confirmation Test*	Test Code/ID	CPT Code	Web Link
ARUP Laboratories	Panel	Prenatal Reflexive Panel	✓	0095044	87340[†]	http://ltd.aruplab.com/Tests/Pub/0095044
	Stand-alone	Hepatitis B Virus Surface Antigen with Reflex to Confirmation, Prenatal	✓	2007573	87340	http://ltd.aruplab.com/Tests/Pub/2007573
LabCorp	Panel	Prenatal Profile I with Hepatitis B Surface Antigen	✓	202945	80055	https://www.labcorp.com/wps/portal/provider/testmenu/ *(Enter test code or CPT code to search for test)*
	Panel	Hepatitis Profile XIII (HBV Prenatal Profile)	✓	265397	87340[†]	https://www.labcorp.com/wps/portal/provider/testmenu/ (Enter test code or CPT code to search for test)
	Stand-alone	N/A	N/A	N/A	N/A	
Mayo Medical Laboratories	Panel	Prenatal Hepatitis	✓	PHSP	87340[†]	http://www.mayomedicallaboratories.com/test catalog/Overview/5566
	Stand-alone	Hepatitis B Surface Antigen Prenatal, Serum	✓	HBAGP	87340	http://www.mayomedicallaboratories.com/test-test-catalog/Overview/86185

(continued)

TABLE 12-1. Screening Pregnant Women for Hepatitis B Virus (HBV) Infection: Ordering Prenatal Hepatitis B Surface Antigen (HBsAg) Tests from Major Commercial Laboratories *(continued)*

Laboratory	Test Option	Test Name	Reflex to Confirmation Test*	Test Code/ID	CPT Code	Web Link
Quest Diagnostics	Panel	Obstetric Panel	✓	20210	80055	http://www.questdiagnostics.com/testcenter/TestDetail.action?ntc=20210
	Stand-alone	N/A	N/A	N/A	N/A	

*When an HBsAg test result is reactive, laboratories may automatically perform a confirmatory test without additional provider order.

†This CPT code corresponds only to the HBsAg screening component of this laboratory panel; additional CPT codes might be associated with other component tests in this laboratory panel.

Notes: CDC recommends health care providers use prenatal HBsAg tests (vs. nonspecific tests) for pregnant women, which allows for reporting of positive results along with pregnancy status to public health jurisdictions. Refer all HBsAg-positive pregnant women to Perinatal Hepatitis B Prevention Program coordinators for case management of mother and infant: https://www.cdc.gov/vaccines/vpd/hepb/hcp/perinatal-contacts.html.

Laboratories reserve the right to add, modify, or stop performing tests at any time – providers should review any test notifications from laboratories for changes. Information presented in this table is updated by the CDC and available at: http://immunizationforwomen.org/uploads/Prenatal%20HBsAg%20Testing%20Guide%20and%20Algorithm_Final.pdf.

Screening pregnant women for hepatitis B virus (HBV) infection. Atlanta (GA): Washington, DC: CDC; ACOG; 2015. Available at: https://www.cdc.gov/hepatitis/hbv/pdfs/prenatalhbsagtesting.pdf. Retrieved March 7, 2017.

adult dose of HBV vaccine is 10–20 micrograms (1 mL) injected into the deltoid muscle. A series of three doses is required; the second and third doses are given 1 month and 6 months after the first dose. A two-dose schedule, administered at time zero and again 4–6 months later, is available for adolescents aged 11–15 years using the adult dose of the 10-microgram hepatitis B recombinant vaccine.

Hepatitis B vaccine also is recommended for household contacts and sexual partners of chronic carriers of HBV (ie, those who are positive for HBsAg) unless immunity has previously been demonstrated. Nonimmunized sexual partners of individuals with acute HBV infection should receive a single dose of HBIG and should begin an HBV vaccine series if their test results are serologically negative. After delivery, hepatitis B vaccine may be administered to breastfeeding mothers if indicated.

Neonatal Immunization

Universal HBV immunization is recommended for all newborn infants before they leave the hospital. Delivery hospitals should develop policies and procedures that ensure administration of the vaccine as part of the routine care of all medically stable infants with birth weights greater than or equal to 2,000 g by 24 hours of age. Delivery hospitals are strongly encouraged to have a written policy to provide vaccine to every newborn prior to discharge unless there is a parental request to defer immunization and the negative serologic status of the mother is documented in the infant's medical record. Three intramuscular doses are required to provide effective protection. A variety of recombinant single-antigen (monovalent) and combination antigen products are currently available for hepatitis B immunization. Although these contain different amounts of antigen, all are effective; however, only the monovalent preparations can be used for birth doses. Detailed information on different commercial preparations and alternate dosage schedules using these preparations is available in the American Academy of Pediatrics (AAP) Committee on Infectious Diseases Red Book chapter on Hepatitis B.

Figure 12-1 provides recommendations for use of vaccine and HBIG for all infants; Figure 12-2 provides guidance on follow-up care for infants by maternal HBsAg status. The recommendations are summarized here.

Hepatitis B Surface Antigen-Negative Mother. For infants born to women who are known to be HBsAg negative, the first 0.5-mL dose of monovalent vaccine should be administered within 24 hours of birth, and before discharge from the hospital. Depending on the preparations used, the

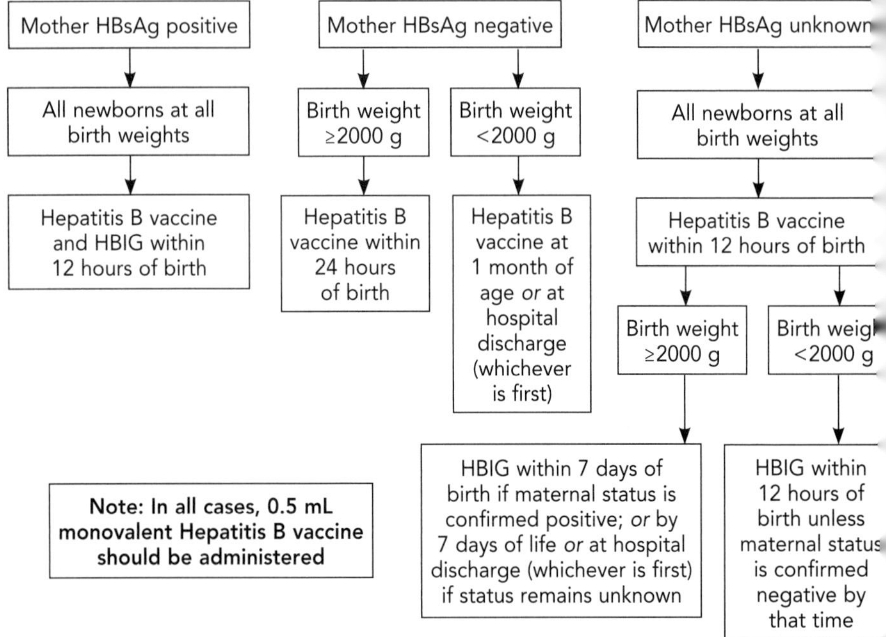

Figure 12-1. Hepatitis B immunoprophylaxis scheme by infant birth weight. Abbreviations: HBsAg, hepatitis B surface antigen; HBIG, hepatitis B immune globulin; anti-HBs, antibody to HBsAg. (Elimination of perinatal hepatitis b: providing the first vaccine dose within 24 hours of birth. American Academy of Pediatrics Committee on Infectious Diseases. Pediatrics 2017:140:e20171870.)

subsequent doses are given 1–2 months later, and the third dose, by 6–18 months of age.

Because of suboptimal immune response in some preterm infants, the current American Academy of Pediatrics recommendation is to delay the start of hepatitis B immunization in low-risk preterm infants (whose mothers are HBsAg negative) who weigh less than 2,000 g at birth until they reach the chronologic age of 30 days, regardless of initial birth weight or gestational age; or by hospital discharge, whichever occurs first. The appropriate dose can be given into the anterolateral thigh muscle of infants.

Hepatitis B Surface Antigen-Positive Mother. Newborns of HBsAg-positive women should receive timely postexposure prophylaxis and follow-up. Both term and preterm infants born to women known to be

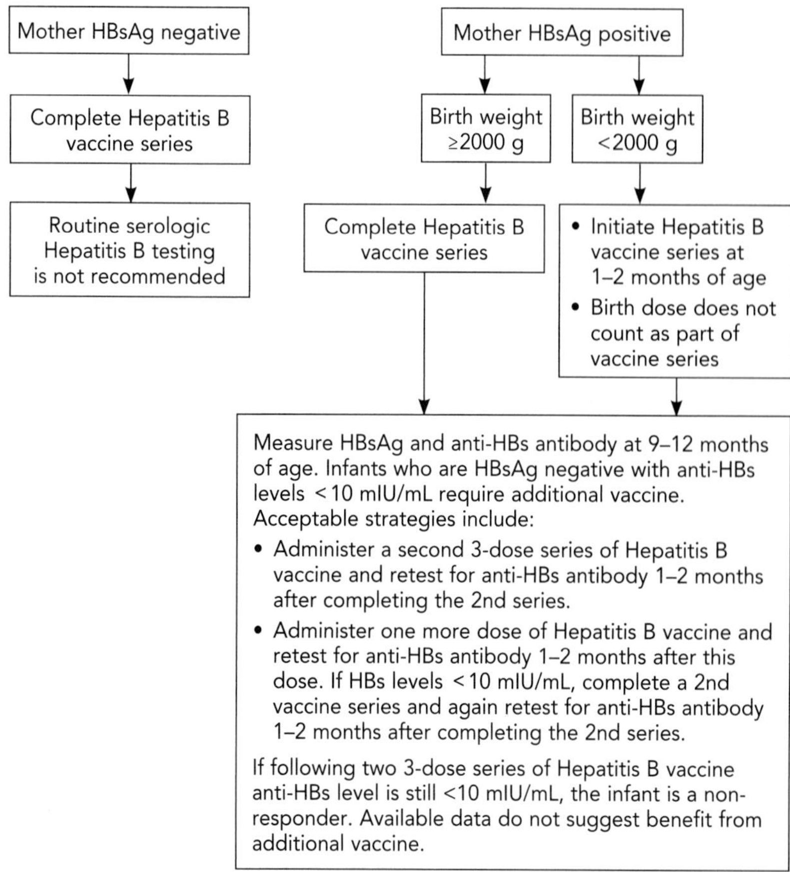

Figure 12-2. Management of infants after administration of hepatitis B vaccine birth dose.

HBsAg positive should receive monovalent hepatitis B vaccine and one 0.5-mL dose of HBIG as soon as possible within 12 hours of birth. Prophylaxis for exposed newborns can prevent perinatal HBV infection in approximately 95% of infants when HBIG is given within 12 hours after birth and the three-dose immunization series is completed. The initial dose of HBV vaccine can be administered concurrently with HBIG but should be given at a different site. No special care of the infant is indicated other than removal of maternal blood to avoid the virus contaminating the skin; in many settings, the infant is fully bathed before administering the intramuscular doses. The second dose of vaccine should be administered at 1–2 months of chronologic age, regardless of the infant's gestational age or birth weight. The third dose should be given at 6 months of age. For preterm infants who weigh less than 2,000 g at birth, the initial vaccine dose is given at birth but is not counted in the required three-dose schedule; therefore, these infants receive four doses: 1) at birth, 2) when their weight reaches 2,000 g or by 1–2 months of age, 3) 1–2 months later, and 4) at 6 months of age.

At 1–3 months after completion of the immunization schedule for newborns of HBsAg-positive women, testing is indicated to ensure immune response or to identify infants who have become chronically infected. If the infant is HBsAg negative and has HBs titers greater than 10 mIU per mL, no further follow-up is needed. If the infant is HBsAg negative and has HBs titers less than 10 mIU per mL, a second three-dose immunization series should be administered and testing again done 1–3 months after completion of the second series. Alternatively, one more dose of vaccine can be administered, and HBs titers checked; if HBs titers remain less than 10 mIU per mL, a full second vaccine series should be completed and HBs titers again tested. There is no evidence that those infants who remain persistent nonresponders after two full vaccine courses would benefit from further doses of the vaccine. Breastfeeding of newborns by HBsAg-positive women poses no additional risk for the transmission of HBV.

Hepatitis B Surface Antigen Status Unknown. Newborns of women whose HBsAg status is unknown should receive HBV vaccine within 12 hours of birth in a dose appropriate for infants born to HBsAg-positive women. The woman's blood should be obtained for testing at hospital admission for delivery. If the woman subsequently is found to be HBsAg positive, the neonate should receive HBIG as soon as possible (within 7 days of birth) and should receive the second and third doses of vaccine as recommended for infants of HBsAg-positive women. For preterm infants born weighing less than 2,000 g, hepatitis B vaccine should be given as soon as possible, and HBIG should be given within 12 hours of birth if the mother has not been documented as HBsAg negative by that time. Both maternal HBsAg test results and the infant's hepatitis vaccine administration should be documented in the infant's medical record.

Hepatitis C Virus

Hepatitis C virus (HCV) is a small RNA virus that has at least six identified, distinct genotypes, with broad geographic variation and widely ranging prognoses for both disease progression and response to therapy. The seroprevalence of HCV among pregnant women in the United States is estimated to be approximately 1–2% but varies in different populations in proportion to risk factors. The primary route of transmission is parenteral exposure to blood and blood products from individuals who are infected with HCV. Sexual transmission among monogamous couples is uncommon, as is transmission among family contacts. In many cases, no source can be identified. The risk of maternal–fetal transmission of HCV ranges from 5% to 6%, is limited to women who are HCV RNA positive, and increases with increasing viral load. The risk is increased for women who are also infected with human immunodeficiency virus (HIV). There are limited data on the safety of invasive procedures (amniocentesis, chorionic villus sampling) among women with HCV infection. Mode of delivery does not affect the risk of perinatal transmission. Newborn infants infected with HCV usually appear healthy. Maternal HCV infection is not a contraindication to breastfeeding unless the mother has cracked and bleeding nipples that could result in infant exposure to maternal blood.

Routine serologic testing during pregnancy for HCV infection is not recommended. Testing should be reserved for women seeking evaluation or care for a sexually transmitted infection (STI), including HIV, or whose histories suggest an increased risk of infection, such as blood transfusions before 1990, intravenous drug use, occupational or recreational percutaneous exposure (eg, tattooing), or mucosal surface blood exposure. Infection with HCV is diagnosed serologically by the presence of HCV antibodies with a third-generation enzyme immunoassay, which has a sensitivity of 97% and specificity of 99%. Positive antibody test results should be confirmed with HCV-specific RNA testing and genotyping. Liver enzyme and function tests should be performed in patients with positive test results for the antibodies because as many as 70% of patients with HCV infection develop chronic liver disease, with cirrhosis ultimately developing in 20–25% of these patients. Multiple antiviral regimens are currently available for the management of chronic HCV infection, and referral to specialty care should be made for further management. The relative merits of treating pregnant women to reduce viral load and decrease risk of vertical transmission should be addressed for women with high HCV RNA levels.

Children born to HCV-positive women should be tested for HCV infection. However, antibody testing should be deferred until at least 18 months of age, when passively transferred maternal HCV antibodies have decreased below detectable levels. If earlier diagnosis of HCV infection is desired, testing for HCV RNA result could be performed at age 1–2 months. This is particularly relevant because many women infected with HCV are at risk for being lost to follow-up. If the HCV RNA result is negative, the HCV antibody test should be performed at 18 months of age. If the HCV RNA result is positive, the infant should be referred to an HCV expert (infectious diseases or gastroenterologist). Currently, no preventive measures are available to lower the risk of vertical HCV infection in infants after birth, and antiviral agents are not currently recommended for postexposure prophylaxis of infants born to women with HCV.

Herpes Simplex Virus

Herpes simplex virus (HSV) is a DNA virus with two distinct species: HSV type 1 (HSV-1) and HSV type 2 (HSV-2). Most genital infections with HSV are caused by HSV-2; however, 20–50% of genital herpes infections are now caused by HSV-1. Genital herpes infection is classified as primary when it occurs in a woman with no evidence of prior HSV infection (ie, seronegative for both HSV-1 and HSV-2), as a nonprimary first episode when it occurs in a woman with a history of heterologous infection (eg, first HSV-2 infection in a woman with prior HSV-1 infection or vice versa), and as recurrent when it occurs in a woman with clinical or serologic evidence of prior genital herpes (of the same serotype). In most adults with unequivocal serologic evidence of HSV-2 infection, the infection has not been diagnosed clinically, indicating that most primary infections are asymptomatic.

Antepartum Management

Women who have primary genital HSV infection in late pregnancy (whether symptomatic or asymptomatic) and who give birth vaginally have a high risk (25–60%) of transmitting the virus to their infants. Similarly, nonprimary first-episode HSV infection occurring late in pregnancy also has a high risk of vertical transmission. The risk of transmission during a vaginal delivery is much lower with recurrent infection (less than 2%). Currently, most newborns infected with HSV are delivered to women who have asymptomatic or unrecognized infections.

Diagnosis. Routine antepartum genital cultures for HSV screening among asymptomatic pregnant patients are not recommended for women with or without a history of HSV. In contrast, all suspected herpes virus infections should be evaluated and confirmed through viral detection techniques (viral culture or nucleic acid-based PCR detection) or by type-specific serologic antibody testing. For patients who do not present with active lesions or whose lesions have negative culture or PCR test results, type-specific serologic assays that accurately distinguish between HSV-1 and HSV-2 antibodies can be useful in confirming a clinical diagnosis of genital herpes (see Table 12-2 for a quick reference guide for blood tests that accurately detect type-specific HSV antibodies). Multiple HSV glycoproteins elicit antibody production, but type-specific assays should be based upon HSV-specific glycoprotein G. Since 2011, the FDA has approved several diagnostic tests for HSV nucleic acid-based detection from oral and genital lesions and one PCR-based test for HSV detection from CSF. The U.S. Food and Drug Administration-approved diagnostics for HSV nucleic acid-based detection and HSV serology can be found at www.accessdata.fda.gov/scripts/cdrh/devicesatfda/index.cfm.

Antiviral Therapy. At the time of the outbreak of a primary herpes infection, antiviral treatment may be administered orally to pregnant women to reduce the duration and the severity of the symptoms as well as reduce the duration of viral shedding. The efficacy of suppressive therapy during pregnancy to prevent recurrences near term has been evaluated in numerous studies. In pregnant women near term, acyclovir or valacyclovir use has been found to reduce the risk of clinical HSV recurrence at delivery and decrease both HSV shedding at delivery and the rate of cesarean delivery for a recurrence of genital herpes. Valacyclovir is metabolized to acyclovir and is twice as bioavailable as acyclovir, allowing for a less frequent dosage; however, the higher cost of valacyclovir may affect adherence. Women with a history of a recurrence of genital herpes should be offered suppressive viral therapy at or beyond 36 weeks of gestation. Acyclovir or valacyclovir can be administered orally to pregnant women with first-episode genital herpes or a severe recurrence of herpes, and intravenous administration is indicated for pregnant women with severe genital HSV infection or with disseminated herpetic infections.

Patient Counseling on Prevention. All pregnant women and their partners should be asked about a history of genital HSV infection. Couples should be educated about the natural history of genital HSV infection and should be advised that, if either partner is infected, they should abstain from sexual contact while lesions or prodromes are present. To minimize the risk of sexual transmission, use of condoms is recommended for HSV-infected

TABLE 12-2. Quick Reference Guide for Blood Tests to Accurately Detect Type-Specific HSV Antibodies

	Biokit HSV-2 Rapid Test (also sold as SureVue HSV-2 Rapid Test by Fischer Health Care)	BioPlex HSV	Captia ELISA	Euroimmun Anti-HSV-1 and Anti-HSV 2 ELISA	Herpe-Select HSV-1 ELISA and Herpe Select HSV-2 ELISA	Herpe-Select 1 and 2 Differentiation Immunoblot	Liaison HSV-2	AtheNA MultiLyte
Supplier	Biokit USA	Bio-Rad Laboratories	Trinity Biotech USA	Euroimmun US LLC	Focus Diagnostics	Focus Diagnostics	DiaSorin	Inverness medical
FDA Approved	1999	2009	2004	2007	2000/2002	2000	2008	2008
Antibodies detected	HSV-2 only	HSV-1 or HSV-2 or both	HSV-1 or HSV-2 or both	HSV-1 or HSV-2	HSV-1 or HSV-2 or both	HSV-1 and/or HSV-2	HSV-1 or HSV-2	HSV-1 and/or HSV-2
Best use of test	POC text to screen or test individuals >3 mo post-exposure	Screening or testing (high volume)	Screening or testing pregnant women or STD clinic patients (moderate volume)	Moderate volume	Screening or testing STD patients or pregnant women (moderate volume)	Low volume	High volume	Screening or testing (moderate to high volume)

Collection method	Finger stick, whole blood, serum in clinic	Blood draw (sent to laboratory)	Blood draw (sent to laboratory)	Blood draw (sent to laboratory)	Blood draw (sent to laboratory)	Blood draw (sent to laboratory)	Blood draw (sent to laboratory)	Blood draw (sent to laboratory)
Test time	10 min	45 min	~2 h	~2 h	~2 h	~2 h	35 min	~2 h
FDA approved for use during pregnancy		Yes	Yes		Yes	Yes		
Test availability	Limited	Limited	Widely available		Widely available			
Website	www.biokitusa.com	www.bio-rad.com	www.trinitybiotech.com	www.euroimmunus.com	www.herpeselect.com	www.herpeselect.com	www.diasorin.com	www.invernessmedicalpd.com
For more information	800-926-3353	800-224-6723	800-325-3424	800-913-2022			800-328-5669	877-546-8633

Abbreviations: FDA, U.S. Food and Drug Administration; POC, point of care; STD, sexually transmitted disease. Adapted from http://www.ashasexualhealth.org. Accessed January 17, 2017.

Reprinted from Kimberlin DW, Baley J, Committee on infectious diseases, Committee on fetus and newborn. Guidance on management of asymptomatic neonates born to women with active genital herpes lesions. Pediatrics;131:e635–46.

individuals when asymptomatic. However, protection provided by condoms is incomplete (estimated to be approximately 50% effective). Susceptible pregnant women should avoid sexual contact during the last 6–8 weeks of gestation if their partners have active genital HSV infections. In addition, oral–genital sexual contact should be avoided in the latter weeks of pregnancy to avoid acquisition of HSV-1 in susceptible individuals.

Intrapartum Management

Women with a history of genital HSV infection should be questioned about recent symptoms and should undergo careful examination of the perineum before delivery. If no lesions are observed, infants can be delivered vaginally. A detailed examination of the cervix is not required because recurrent infections rarely cause isolated cervical lesions.

Cesarean delivery is indicated for all women with active genital HSV lesions or with a typical herpetic prodrome at the time of delivery. In patients with active HSV infection and ruptured membranes at or near term, a cesarean delivery should be performed as soon as the necessary personnel and equipment can be readied. In active HSV infection and premature rupture of membranes remote from term, there is no consensus on the gestational age at which the risks of prematurity outweigh the risks of HSV. When expectant management is elected, treatment with an antiviral drug may be considered. Local neonatal infection can result from the use of fetal scalp electrode monitoring in patients with a history of herpes, even when maternal lesions are not present. However, if there are indications for fetal scalp monitoring, it may be appropriate in a woman who has a history of HSV recurrence and no active lesions.

Contact precautions, use of gown or gloves, and covering of all lesions (in addition to standard precautions), should be used for women with clinically evident or serologically confirmed primary genital HSV infection or non-genital HSV infection in the labor, delivery, recovery, and postpartum care areas. For a recurrence of mucocutaneous lesions, standard precautions are sufficient. Infected family members and others in contact with the infant also should use contact precautions. Health care personnel and the woman herself should use gloves for direct contact with the infected area or with contaminated dressings, and meticulous handwashing is essential. Labor, delivery, and recovery rooms require only routine, careful cleaning and disinfection before using the rooms for other patients.

Neonatal Diagnosis

Neonatal infections are caused by both HSV-1 and HSV-2. Most infants who develop HSV infection acquire the infection during passage through the infected maternal lower genital tract or by ascending infection to the fetus, sometimes even when membranes apparently are intact. Less common sources of neonatal infection include postnatal transmission from the parents, hospital personnel, or other close contact, most often from a nongenital HSV-1 infection (eg, mouth, hands, or around the breasts). Uncommonly, intrauterine transmission occurs, and signs of congenital infection may include in utero growth restriction, microcephaly, hydranencephaly and chorioretinitis.

Several factors influence the risk of vertical transmission of HSV. These include type of maternal infection (primary or recurrent during the pregnancy), maternal type-specific HSV antibody, duration of rupture of membranes, mode of delivery, and neonatal mucosal disruptions such as the use of fetal scalp monitors. Symptomatic neonatal disease may be limited to surface lesions of the skin, eyes, or mouth (SEM disease); may involve the central nervous system as meningoencephalitis (CNS disease); or may involve multiple visceral organs (disseminated disease) and present with symptoms of sepsis. Among women whose newborns acquire HSV infection, 60–80% have no symptoms at the time of delivery and no known personal or partner history of HSV infection. Therefore, clinicians must consider HSV infection among symptomatic newborns even in the absence of maternal lesions or history of infection.

Infants Born to Women With Active Lesions at Delivery. In 2013, the AAP Committee on Infectious Diseases and Committee on the Fetus and Newborn issued a new clinical report containing specific recommendations for the management of newborn infants born to mothers with active HSV genital lesions at the time of delivery. A summary of these recommendations is presented here; consult the full report for detailed management guidelines (http://pediatrics.aappublications.org/content/131/2/e635). The recommendations are the same regardless of mode of delivery because cesarean delivery before rupture of membranes reduces but does not eliminate risk of neonatal HSV disease. In all cases, the infant should be monitored closely for signs of infection and placed on contact precautions. Strict isolation is not required. An infant may stay with the mother in a private room after the mother has been instructed on proper preventive care to reduce postpartum transmission. All maternal genital lesions suggestive of HSV should be tested for HSV by culture and PCR, with typing performed for positive results. This information will be critical to newborn management. Neonatal testing detailed as follows should be performed after 24 hours of age to distinguish neonatal contamination with infected maternal secretions from active replication of the virus, indicating neonatal infection. Two exceptions should be noted. If the delivery was complicated by rupture of membranes longer than 4–6 hours; or if the infant is born prematurely at 37 weeks of gestation or less; neonatal testing and empiric treatment should be initiated immediately after delivery. If any infant becomes symptomatic before 24 hours of age, evaluation and treatment should proceed immediately. Further recommendations are stratified by maternal history of HSV infection.

No Maternal History of Previous Herpes Simplex Virus Infection. Maternal serologies should be obtained to distinguish primary, nonprimary first episode and recurrent disease. After 24 hours of age, HSV surface cultures or PCR should be obtained from the newborn's conjunctivae; mouth; nasopharynx; rectum; and scalp electrode site (if applicable); HSV PCR from blood; CSF cell count, chemistries and HSV PCR; serum ALT. Acyclovir should be administered intravenously (60 mg per kg per day in three divided doses).

- If maternal testing demonstrates recurrent infection and the infant's cultures and PCR result are negative at 48–72 hours, and the infant is clinically well, then acyclovir should be discontinued and the family educated about signs of neonatal HSV infection.
- If maternal testing demonstrates first-episode primary or nonprimary infection, the infant's cultures and PCR result are negative at 48–72 hours, and the infant is clinically well, then acyclovir should be continued for a total of 10 days as preemptive therapy.
- If maternal testing demonstrates recurrent, first-episode primary or nonprimary infection, and the infant is not well or cultures or PCR result confirm HSV infection, acyclovir should be continued for 14 days for localized SEM disease, or for 21 days for disseminated disease, or disease with CNS infection. With CNS disease, CSF should be obtained and retested by HSV PCR near the end of the 21-day course to determine if extended acyclovir therapy is needed. After intravenous therapy is concluded, infants should receive oral acyclovir suppressive therapy for 6 months.

History of Maternal Herpes Simplex Virus Infection. After 24 hours of age, HSV surface cultures or PCR should be obtained from conjunctivae; mouth; nasopharynx; rectum; and scalp electrode site (if applicable) as well as HSV PCR from blood. No empiric therapy should be administered.

- If newborn cultures and PCR result are negative, family should be counseled about signs of infection and infant monitored clinically and discharged at 48–96 hours of life depending on individual hospital virology facilities and reliability of family and local pediatric care.
- If newborn cultures or PCR result are positive or infant becomes symptomatic, CSF studies should be obtained and acyclovir administered intravenously at 60 mg per kg per day in three divided doses. The duration of therapy is guided as described previously, pending the results of CSF studies. After intravenous therapy is concluded, infants should receive oral acyclovir suppressive therapy for 6 months.

Infants Born to Asymptomatic Women With History of Genital Herpes. The risk of HSV infection is extremely low in infants born vaginally to asymptomatic women with a history of genital HSV disease. Such infants should be observed for signs of infection, including both vesicular lesions and nonspecific signs of sepsis. If symptoms develop, neonatal HSV testing and empiric acyclovir therapy should be provided as outlined previously. Neither routine HSV testing, empiric acyclovir therapy, nor contact precautions are recommended for asymptomatic infants. The length of in-hospital observation is empirical and is based on risk factors, local resources, and access to adequate follow-up. Family education should be provided about the signs and symptoms of neonatal HSV infection during the first 6 weeks of life.

Neonatal Treatment

In addition to testing and acyclovir therapy as described here, infants with proven HSV disease should be managed in a facility that provides neonatal intensive care and consultation with an infectious diseases specialist. The infant should be physically segregated and managed with contact precautions for the duration of care, utilizing an isolation room if available. Although HSV infection is more likely to occur at a site of skin trauma, there are no data to guide the timing of elective circumcision of male infants who may have been exposed to HSV at birth.

Contact of Infants With Infected Mothers

A woman with active HSV infection should be educated about her infection and about hygienic measures to prevent postpartum transmission of herpes to her infant. Before touching her newborn, the woman should wash her hands carefully and use a clean barrier to ensure that the infant does not come into contact with lesions or potentially infectious material. If the woman has genital HSV infection, her infant can room with her after she has been instructed in protective measures. Breastfeeding is permissible if the woman has no vesicular herpetic lesions in the breast area and other active cutaneous lesions are covered.

A woman with herpes labialis (cold sore) or stomatitis should not kiss or nuzzle her infant until the lesions have cleared. Careful hand hygiene is important. She should wear a disposable surgical mask when she touches her infant until the lesions have crusted and dried. Herpetic lesions on other skin sites should be covered. Direct contact of an infant with other family members or friends who have active HSV infection should be avoided.

Human Immunodeficiency Virus

Acquired immunodeficiency syndrome (AIDS) is caused by HIV type 1 (HIV-1) and, less commonly, HIV type 2 (HIV-2), a related virus. Human immunodeficiency virus type 2 is extremely uncommon in the United States but is more common in West Africa and South America.

Transmission

Human immunodeficiency virus has been isolated from blood (including lymphocytes, macrophages, and plasma), CSF, pleural fluid, human milk, semen, cervical secretions, saliva, urine, and tears. However, only blood, semen, cervical secretions, and human milk have been implicated epidemiologically in the transmission of infection. Well-documented modes of HIV transmission in the United States are sexual contact (both heterosexual and homosexual), skin penetration by contaminated needles or other sharp instruments, transfusion of contaminated blood products, and mother-to-infant transmission during pregnancy, around the time of labor and delivery, and postnatally through breastfeeding. Before effective perinatal HIV interventions, the risk of infection for an infant born to an HIV- seropositive mother was approximately 25% (range, 12–40%). All pregnant women who are infected with HIV should be offered antiretroviral drug regimens, which can decrease HIV viral loads to undetectable levels. The exact timing of transmission from an infected mother to her infant is uncertain. Most perinatal transmission occurs intrapartum, with lesser contributions from in utero transmission and postpartum transmission from breastfeeding.

Antepartum Management

Medical benefits are derived from pregnant women knowing their HIV serostatus. Demonstrated benefits include early diagnosis and treatment to delay active disease in women and significant reduction in perinatal transmission through early treatment.

Prenatal Screening. All pregnant women should be told that HIV screening is recommended during pregnancy and that an HIV test is part of the routine panel of prenatal tests unless it is declined (opt-out screening). If a woman declines HIV testing, this should be documented in the medical record. Repeat testing in the third trimester (preferably before 36 weeks of gestation) is recommended for women in areas with a high HIV prevalence, women known to be at high risk of acquiring HIV infection, and women who declined testing earlier in pregnancy. Individual state laws vary with respect to HIV testing of pregnant women and newborns and HIV status disclosure. Maternal and neonatal providers should be aware of and comply with their states' legal requirements for perinatal HIV screening. The Centers for Disease Control and Prevention (CDC) updated recommendations for HIV testing in 2014. Pregnant women should be screened using an FDA-approved antibody-antigen test during each pregnancy. Positive results are repeated if recommended by the manufacturer's instructions. Positive test results should be subsequently followed up with a test to distinguish HIV-1 and HIV-2 antibodies and with a nucleic acid-based HIV test.

If the screening and confirmatory test results are both positive, the patient should be given her results in person. The implications of HIV infection and vertical transmission should be discussed with the patient. Additional laboratory evaluation, including CD4 count, HIV viral load, HIV antiretroviral resistance testing, hepatitis C virus antibody, hepatitis B antigen and viral load, complete blood count with platelet count, and baseline chemistries with liver function tests, are useful before prescribing antiretroviral prophylaxis. Coordination of care for the woman and fetus should be done in consultation with a specialist in maternal–fetal medicine and in infectious diseases. Laboratory results should be communicated to and available at the delivery hospital to ensure appropriate care for the woman and her infant.

Maternal Antiretroviral Therapy. Combination antiretroviral (ARV) drug regimens that maximally suppress viral replication are recommended for HIV-1-infected adults. Pregnancy does not preclude the use of these standard antiretroviral regimens. Offering antiretroviral therapy to infected women during pregnancy, either to treat HIV-1 infection or to reduce perinatal transmission or both, should be accompanied by discussion of the known and unknown short-term and long-term benefits and risks of such therapy for affected women and their infants. It is recommended that zidovudine chemoprophylaxis be included in the antiretroviral combination regimen, except in cases of known intolerance. No significant short-term adverse effects have been observed from zidovudine use other than mild, self-limited anemia in the infants. In addition, infants have been monitored for several years and no untoward effects of zidovudine have been observed.

Current recommendations for adults are that plasma viral load determinations be done at baseline and every 3 months or after changes in therapy. Additionally, CD4+ T-lymphocyte counts should be monitored during pregnancy. Because of the rapid advances in this area, refer to the CDC (www.cdc.gov/) and the U.S. Department of Health and Human Services AIDSinfo websites (www.aidsinfo.nih.gov/) for treatment recommendations.

Intrapartum Management

As noted, a substantial proportion of neonatal HIV cases occur as a result of exposure to the virus during labor and delivery. Intrapartum strategies to prevent mother-to-child transmission include expedited HIV antibody testing for women with unknown HIV status during labor and delivery; administration of antepartum, intrapartum, and neonatal antiretroviral prophylaxis; and cesarean delivery performed before the onset of labor and before rupture of membranes in women with viral loads of more than 1,000 copies per milliliter and in HIV-infected women with unknown viral loads.

Rapid HIV Testing. All facilities with maternity or neonatal intensive care services should have rapid (expedited) HIV testing available on a 24-hour basis, with results available within 60 minutes. Ideally rapid testing should use an FDA-approved fourth generation immunoassay that detects HIV-1 and HIV-2 antibodies as well as HIV-1 p24 antigen; such assays can detect acute HIV infection and shorten the period that an acutely infected woman would test negative by antibody screening alone. Information on state laws concerning testing of pregnant women and newborns also should be available at these facilities. Any woman whose HIV status is unknown during labor and delivery should be given a rapid HIV test, unless she declines (opt-out screening), in order to provide an opportunity to begin prophylaxis before delivery if necessary. A negative rapid HIV test result is definitive. A positive HIV test result is not definitive and must be confirmed with supplemental tests, as recommended previously, after delivery. All antiretroviral prophylaxis should be discontinued if the result of supplemental testing concordant with cited guidelines is negative.

If the expedited HIV test result at labor and delivery is positive, the obstetric provider should take the following steps:

1. Tell the woman she may have HIV infection and that her infant also may be exposed.
2. Explain that the rapid test result is preliminary and that false-positive test results are possible.
3. Assure the woman that additional testing will be done to confirm the positive rapid test result.
4. Recommend immediate initiation of antiretroviral prophylaxis for woman and infant, without waiting for the supplemental test results.
5. Tell the woman that she should postpone breastfeeding until the confirmatory result is available because she should not breastfeed if she is infected with HIV.
6. Inform pediatric care providers of positive maternal test results so that they may institute the appropriate neonatal prophylaxis.

Route of Delivery. For HIV-infected women, the combination of ARV therapy and viral load guide decisions for mode of delivery. Recommendations for delivery are available at www.aidsinfo.nih.gov/. Women who are receiving an antepartum combined ARV therapy regimen should continue that regimen on schedule as much as possible during the intrapartum period to provide maximal effect and to minimize the chance of development of drug resistance. The patient's autonomy in making the decision regarding route of delivery should be respected, but as of 2014 recommendations include the following:

- If the woman is known to be adherent to ARV therapy and viral load is known to be less than 1,000 copies per mL in late pregnancy or near delivery, the delivery should be managed without regard to HIV status.

Oral medications can be continued; zidovudine may be administered orally or intravenously.

- If the woman has viral load greater than 1,000 copies per mL, or if the woman is known to have HIV and does not have a known viral load, cesarean delivery at 38 weeks before the onset of labor and rupture of membranes should be recommended. ARV therapy should be continued, with zidovudine administered intravenously.
- If a woman's prenatal ARV therapy regimen does not include zidovudine because of viral resistance, intravenous zidovudine should still be administered intrapartum because of demonstrated efficacy in reducing perinatal transmission even in the presence of documented resistance.

It is clear that the rate of maternal morbidity is higher with cesarean delivery than with vaginal delivery. However, the benefit to the infant outweighs the increased maternal morbidity associated with cesarean delivery (see also "Cesarean Delivery" in Chapter 7).

Because HIV may be present in blood, vaginal secretions, amniotic fluid, and other fluids, standard precautions should be strictly followed during all vaginal and cesarean deliveries. Gloves should be used when handling the infant until blood and amniotic fluid have been removed from the infant's skin.

Postpartum Management

After delivery, HIV-infected women can receive care in the postpartum care unit with the use of standard precautions. Human immunodeficiency virus RNA has been detected in both the cellular and cell-free fractions of human breast milk, and breastfeeding has been implicated in the transmission of HIV infection. Women in developed countries who are infected with HIV should be counseled not to breastfeed and not to donate to milk banks. If HIV has been diagnosed intrapartum, obstetric providers should refer women who are infected with HIV to an infectious disease specialist for further health evaluation including initiation of ARV therapy.

To minimize risk to health care personnel, routine standard precautions should be used when caring for the infant. Prompt and careful removal of blood from the infant's skin is important. There is no need for other special precautions or for isolation of the infant from an HIV-infected mother; rooming-in is acceptable. Gloves should be worn for contact with blood or blood-containing fluids, for procedures that entail exposure to blood, and for diaper changes.

Evaluation and Management of Exposed Newborns

Screening and Antiretroviral Prophylaxis. Umbilical cord blood should not be used for newborn HIV testing because of possible contamination with maternal blood. HIV diagnosis among newborns requires HIV DNA PCR testing. Antibody tests will reflect maternally derived antibody in the newborn period, up to approximately 18 months of age. HIV RNA tests (as used for viral load determination) can return false-negative results among infants receiving ARV prophylaxis. Earliest possible diagnosis should be achieved, because ARV therapy (rather than ARV prophylaxis) is indicated for all HIV-infected infants regardless of clinical symptoms, immune status, or viral load. Current care recommendations for newborns are provided here; both the AAP Red Book and www.aidsinfo.nih.gov/ should be consulted for updates.

- *Infant born to a mother with known HIV infection who received prenatal ARV therapy*: Mother should receive her regular ARV medications (except for stavudine), as well as intravenous zidovudine. After birth, the infant should be bathed to remove maternal blood and secretions. Oral (or intravenous, if warranted by newborn prematurity or illness) ARV prophylaxis should begin as soon as possible, preferably within 12 hours of birth. Currently in the United States, neonatal zidovudine prophylaxis is given for 6 weeks.
- *Infant born to HIV-infected mother who did not receive prenatal ARV treatment*: Infectious disease consultation should be obtained if mother was not treated with ARV before the onset of labor because neonatal postexposure prophylaxis with a 2- or 3-drug ARV regimen is recommended for such infants. HIV DNA PCR should be done by 48 hours to detect in utero transmission. Early determination of infection should be followed by immediate referral to a pediatric infectious disease specialist for initiation of ARV treatment rather than prophylaxis
- *Infant born to a mother with unknown maternal HIV status at birth*: Both the newborn and the mother should have expedited HIV testing performed as soon as possible after birth. The newborn should receive postpartum ARV prophylaxis within 12 hours of birth to reduce the risk of perinatal HIV-1 transmission. If the results of rapid testing are positive, postpartum ARV prophylaxis should be administered until

confirmatory test results are available. Breastfeeding should be withheld pending confirmatory tests. If the maternal confirmatory test results are negative, ARV medications can be stopped and breastfeeding can begin if desired. If the infant or maternal confirmatory test results are positive, infant ARV prophylaxis should continue and the infant should not be breastfed. In such cases, HIV DNA PCR should be performed immediately to determine if in utero transmission has occurred. As stated previously, if this testing confirms in utero transmission, the infant requires referral to a pediatric infectious disease specialist to determine appropriate ARV therapy rather than prophylaxis.

Additional Care. Maternal health information should be reviewed to determine if the infant may have been exposed to maternal coinfections (such as tuberculosis, syphilis, toxoplasmosis, hepatitis B or hepatitis C, cytomegalovirus, or HSV). Diagnostic testing for and treatment of coinfections in the infant should be based on maternal findings and evaluation of the infant. Immunizations should be given to HIV-exposed infants per recommended schedules. If infection is confirmed, guidelines for HIV-infected children should be followed. Both mother and infant should be given prescriptions for HIV medications when they leave the delivery hospital. Because zidovudine is administered every 6 hours to newborns, and pediatric liquid medications can be difficult to obtain in outpatient pharmacies, the infant should not leave the hospital until the mother or guardian has zidovudine pediatric liquid medication in his or her possession. The infant should have an appointment for a postnatal visit by 2 weeks of age to monitor medication adherence and to screen the infant for anemia from zidovudine therapy. Pediatricians should provide counseling to parents and caregivers of HIV-1 exposed infants about HIV-1 infection, including anticipatory guidance on the course of illness, infection control measures, care of the infant, diagnostic tests, and potential drug toxicities.

Diagnostic Testing. Some experts recommend HIV DNA PCR testing for all exposed infants before 48 hours of postnatal age to identify in utero infection; approximately 30–40% of HIV-infected infants will have a positive HIV DNA PCR assay result in samples obtained before 48 hours of age. At minimum, HIV DNA PCR testing should be done within the first 2 weeks of life to facilitate transition from ARV prophylaxis to ARV treatment. Approximately 93% of infected infants have detectable HIV DNA by 2 weeks of age, and approximately 95% of HIV-infected infants have a positive HIV DNA PCR assay result by 1 month of age. In nonbreastfed children younger than 18 months of age, *presumptive* exclusion of HIV infection is based on the following:

- two negative HIV DNA PCR test results, from separate specimens, both of which were obtained at 2 weeks of age or older and one of which was obtained at 4 weeks of age or older; or
- one negative HIV DNA PCR test result from a specimen obtained at 8 weeks of age or older; or
- one negative HIV antibody test result obtained at 6 months of age or older; and
- no other laboratory or clinical evidence of HIV infection (ie, no subsequent positive HIV DNA PCR tests and no AIDS-defining condition for which there is no other underlying condition of immunosuppression).

HIV can be *definitively excluded* in nonbreastfed infants at less than 18 months based on the following:

- at least two negative HIV DNA test results, from separate specimens, both of which were obtained at 1 month of age or older and one of which was obtained at 4 months of age or older;
- at least two negative HIV antibody test results from separate specimens obtained at 6 months of age or older; and
- no other laboratory or clinical evidence of HIV infection (ie, no subsequent virologic positive results and no AIDS-defining condition for which there is no other underlying condition of immunosuppression).

Among infants with two negative HIV DNA PCR test results, many clinicians choose to confirm the absence of antibody (ie, loss of passively acquired natural antibody) to HIV on testing at 12 through 18 months of age.

Pneumocystis jiroveci Pneumonia Prophylaxis. *Pneumocystis jiroveci* (formerly known as *Pneumocystis carinii*) is the most common opportunistic infection in HIV-1-infected infants and children. All HIV-1-exposed infants should be considered for prophylaxis beginning at 4–6 weeks of age. Infants who meet criteria for presumptive or definitive HIV-uninfected status do not require *Pneumocystis pneumonia* (PCP) prophylaxis. Infants with indeterminate status should be given PCP prophylaxis until testing is consistent with presumptive or definitively HIV-uninfected status. Infants in whom HIV-1 is diagnosed should be given PCP prophylaxis until 1 year of age, at which time reassessment is made on the basis of age-specific CD4+ T-lymphocyte count and percentage thresholds.

Human Papillomavirus

Infections caused by the human papillomavirus (HPV) (a DNA virus) are common. More than 100 types of HPV exist, more than 40 of which can infect the genital area. Infection with certain HPV types can cause genital warts and recurrent respiratory papillomatosis (eg, HPV-6 and HPV-11) as well as cervical and anogenital carcinomas (eg, HPV-16 and HPV-18). Most genital HPV infections are sexually transmitted, and most cervical HPV infections are transient and asymptomatic. Persistent infection is more likely with oncogenic serotypes. Clinically asymptomatic HPV infection can lead to dysplastic lesions of the cervix, which can be detected during Pap testing of the cervix. Similar lesions can occur in other genital, anal, and oropharyngeal mucosal sites, and over time, persistent HPV infection can lead to the development of invasive cancer at these sites. Pap testing should begin at 21 years of age in otherwise healthy females. Screening at earlier ages is recommended in the setting of HIV infection, organ transplant, or chronic corticosteroid treatment.

Genital HPV infections may be exacerbated during pregnancy. Papillary lesions (condylomata acuminata) may proliferate on the vulva and in the vagina, and lesions can become increasingly friable during pregnancy. Although genital wart removal can be considered during pregnancy, resolution can be incomplete or poor until after delivery. Multiple approaches can be taken for removal of genital warts but only cryotherapy, laser therapy, and trichloroacetic acid can be used safely during pregnancy. Imiquimod, sinecatechins, podophyllin, and podofilox should not be used during pregnancy. Respiratory papillomatosis can rarely result from vertical transmission of HPV. These lesions are thought to result from aspiration of infectious secretions during passage through the birth canal. There is no proven approach to prevent HPV vertical transmission. Cesarean delivery is not recommended for women with genital HPV unless lesions obstruct the pelvic outlet or risk serious bleeding. Infants born to women with HPV infection should receive routine newborn care and do not require special precautions.

There are three FDA-approved vaccines shown to be effective in preventing HPV infection in adolescents and young adults: 1) bivalent (including types 16 and 18); 2) quadrivalent (including types 1, 6, 16, and 18); and

3) 9-valent (including types 6, 11, 16, 18, 31, 33, 42, 55, 58). None of the preparations contain live virus and all can be given to immunocompromised persons, including those with HIV. As of December 2016, only the 9-valent vaccine is being distributed in the United States. The Advisory Committee on Immunization Practices (ACIP) of the Centers for Disease Control and Prevention recommends HPV vaccination for females and males ages 9–26 years of age. Vaccination is recommended to start at age 11–12 years but may start as young as 9 years of age. Two doses (on schedule 0, 6–12 months) are recommended if vaccination begins at 9–14 years of age; if these two doses are given at an interval of less than 5 months, a third dose is recommended. Three doses (on schedule 0, 1–2 and 6 months) are recommended for vaccination that begins at 15 years or older. Although HPV vaccination in pregnancy is not recommended, neither is routine pregnancy testing before vaccination. Available safety data regarding the inadvertent administration of the vaccine during pregnancy are reassuring. Patients and obstetrician–gynecologists or other health care providers are encouraged to register women exposed to the 9-valent HPV vaccine around the time of fertilization or during pregnancy by contacting the manufacturer. Pregnancy registries for the quadrivalent HPV vaccine and bivalent HPV vaccine have been closed. If the HPV vaccine series was interrupted for pregnancy, the series should be resumed postpartum with the next dose. HPV vaccines can and should be given to breastfeeding women aged 26 years and younger who have not previously been vaccinated. Human papillomavirus vaccines are not currently licensed in the United States for women older than 26 years. Off-label use may be indicated on a case-by-case basis.

Influenza Virus

Influenza A and influenza B viruses are the main types of human influenza virus that are responsible for seasonal influenza epidemics each year. During the course of influenza season, different types and subtypes of influenza viruses can circulate and cause illness. Influenza viruses are spread from person to person primarily through hand-to-hand contact and large-particle respiratory droplet transmission. Contact with respiratory-droplet contaminated surfaces is another possible source of transmission. Uncomplicated influenza illness is characterized by the abrupt onset of constitutional and respiratory signs and symptoms (eg, fever, myalgia, headache, malaise, nonproductive cough, sore throat, and rhinitis) that typically resolve after 3–7 days; however, malaise can persist for up to 14 days.

Pregnant women and young children are at greater risk of serious influenza complications, which can include influenza or secondary bacterial pneumonia, ear infections, sinus infections, dehydration, and worsening of chronic medical conditions, such as congestive heart failure, asthma, or diabetes. Pregnant women also have higher hospitalization and mortality rates than nonpregnant women. Preventing influenza during pregnancy is an essential element of prenatal care, and the most effective strategy for preventing influenza is annual immunization at any gestational age. Obstetrician–gynecologists are an important source of information and advice on immunization for pregnant women and play a crucial role in recommending influenza vaccine to every pregnant woman.

The seasonal trivalent and quadrivalent inactivated influenza vaccines are safe for pregnant women and their fetuses and can be given during any trimester. Live attenuated virus should not be used in pregnant women. The CDC Advisory Committee on Immunization Practices recommends that all women who are pregnant during influenza season (October through May in the United States) receive the trivalent or quadrivalent inactivated influenza vaccine at any point in gestation. The Advisory Committee on Immunization Practices does not preferentially recommend a specific formulation—trivalent or quadrivalent—of the influenza vaccine. Vaccination early in the season is optimal, regardless of gestational age. No study to date has shown an adverse consequence of the inactivated influenza vaccine in pregnant women or their offspring. Thimerosal is a mercury-containing preservative used in multidose vials of the influenza vaccine. Although thimerosal-free formulations of the influenza vaccine are available, there is no scientific evidence that thimerosal-containing vaccines cause adverse effects in children born to women who received vaccines with thimerosal. Hence, ACIP does not indicate a preference for thimerosal-containing or thimerosal-free vaccines for any group, including pregnant women.

In addition to the benefits of immunization for pregnant women, prospective, controlled, randomized trials have demonstrated fewer cases of laboratory-confirmed influenza as well as fewer cases of respiratory illness with fever in infants whose mothers had been immunized compared with women in the control group. Maternal immunity is the only effective prevention strategy in newborns because the vaccine is not approved for use in infants younger than 6 months.

Pregnant and laboring women with suspected or confirmed influenza should be managed with standard and droplet precautions while in the hospital. Newborns that become infected with influenza are at an increased risk for severe complications. To reduce the risk of influenza in the newborn, the CDC recommends that delivery facilities consider temporarily separating the mother who is ill with suspected or confirmed influenza from her baby following delivery during the hospital stay. During separation, mothers who intend to breastfeed may express milk for infant feeding, and all feedings should be provided by a healthy caregiver. The optimal duration for separation has not been established; guidelines used during the 2009 H1N1 pandemic recommended that separation should continue until all of the following were met: a) mother receives antiviral treatment for more than 48 hours; b) mother is afebrile without antipyretics for more than 24 hours, and c) mother is able to control her cough and respiratory secretions. If separation is not possible because of local hospital constraints, the following should be considered: a) physical barriers (eg, a curtain between the mother and newborn); b) keeping the newborn 6 feet or more away from the ill mother; and c) ensuring a healthy adult is present to care for the newborn. If the mother with suspected or confirmed influenza is the only available caregiver, she should wear a face mask and practice hand hygiene before each feeding or other close contact with her newborn. The face mask should remain in place during contact with the newborn. These practices, which are consistent with Droplet Precautions, should continue for at least 7 days after onset of maternal illness. Newborns with influenza requiring neonatal intensive care should be placed in an isolation room and Droplet Precautions instituted.

All health care professionals who care for pregnant women and high-risk newborns should receive seasonal influenza vaccine annually as soon as the vaccine becomes available. All household contacts of newborns (including siblings and other children older than 6 months) and caregivers should receive influenza vaccination. Immunization of pregnant women and immunization of those living with and caring for infants less than 6 months of age is the optimal approach to preventing influenza in young infants. Antiviral chemoprophylaxis can be used in family members or health care providers who for specific reasons cannot be immunized, and who are likely to have ongoing close exposure to infants who are younger than 12 months. Postexposure antiviral chemoprophylaxis can be considered for pregnant women and women who are up to 2 weeks postpartum (including following pregnancy loss) who have had close contact with someone likely to have been infectious with influenza. Because vaccine formulations and antiviral resistance patterns can change over time, all influenza-associated recommendations are updated regularly. Physicians are advised to monitor annual recommendations from CDC (www.cdc.gov/flu/index.htm) and ACOG (www.immunizationforwomen.org).

Human Parvovirus

Parvovirus B19 is a single-stranded DNA virus that causes the childhood exanthema erythema infectiosum, also known as fifth disease. Children typically demonstrate a facial rash, sometimes similar in appearance to a slapped cheek, in addition to possible fever, body rash, and joint pain. In immunocompetent adults, the most common symptoms of parvovirus B19 infection are a reticular rash on the trunk and peripheral arthropathy, although approximately 20% of infected individuals are asymptomatic. Another manifestation of parvovirus B19 infection is transient aplastic crisis, which is more common in those with an underlying hemoglobinopathy. Most infections are mild and most individuals recover completely from parvovirus B19 infection and require only supportive care during the acute phase.

Perinatal Transmission

Transmission of parvovirus B19 most commonly occurs through respiratory secretions and hand-to-mouth contact. The infected person generally is infectious for 5–10 days after exposure before the onset of the rash or other symptoms and is no longer infectious by the time of onset of the rash. In response to infection, IgM and IgG antibodies are produced. The IgM response, which persists for 1 month to several months, is indicative of a recent infection. The IgG antibodies persist indefinitely and, in the absence of IgM, indicate prior infection and lifelong immunity. Prevalence of seropositivity to parvovirus B19 increases with age, and 50–65% of reproductive-aged women are seropositive. The risk of maternal parvovirus B19 infection varies with level of exposure to the infected individual. Exposure to a household member infected with parvovirus B19 is associated with a 50% risk of seroconversion. The risk of transmission in a child-care setting or classroom is lower, approximately 20–50%.

After acute parvovirus B19 infection during pregnancy, rates of maternal-to-fetal transmission range from 17% to 33%. Although most cases of fetal infection resolve spontaneously with no adverse outcomes, fetal parvovirus B19 has been associated with spontaneous abortion, hydrops fetalis, and stillbirth. The rate of fetal loss among women with serologically proven parvovirus B19 infection ranges from 8% to 17% before 20 weeks of gestation to 2–6% after 20 weeks of gestation. In utero, parvovirus B19 infection can lead to nonimmune hydrops fetalis. An estimated 8–10% (potentially up to 18–27%) of cases of nonimmune hydrops fetalis are associated with parvovirus B19 infection. Because the virus is cytotoxic to erythroid precursors, hydrops fetalis most often results from aplastic anemia, although hydrops also can be related to myocarditis or chronic fetal hepatitis. Severe effects are seen most frequently among fetuses when maternal parvovirus B19 infection occurs before 20 weeks of gestation.

The fetus is particularly vulnerable to disease transmission and severe complications in the second trimester because of the mechanisms of viral placental transport and rapid changes in fetal hematopoiesis that occur during this period. Stillbirth that results from maternal infection has occurred from 1 week up to 11 weeks after maternal infection. However, hydrops is unlikely to develop if it has not occurred by 8 weeks after maternal infection.

Long-term neurodevelopmental outcomes are uncertain in fetuses with congenital parvovirus B19 infection who do not succumb to the disease. Earlier studies suggested no long-term adverse effects in fetuses with hydrops that have been transfused after maternal infection; however, a more recent study suggested an increase in neurodevelopmental impairment among fetuses with hydrops who underwent transfusion.

Screening

Routine serologic screening of pregnant women for parvovirus B19 is not recommended. Given the low incidence of seroconversion during pregnancy combined with the variable risk of fetal transmission and subsequent sequelae, targeted screening during pregnancy is not recommended either. Testing should be performed for patients with symptoms consistent with parvovirus B19 infection or for those with exposure to suspected or confirmed acute infections.

Diagnosis and Management

Pregnant women exposed to parvovirus B19 should have serologic screening performed as soon as possible after exposure to determine if they should be monitored for seroconversion.

Women who are IgM negative and IgG positive have evidence of previous exposure and immunity and, thus, are not at risk of transplacental transmission. Women who are IgM positive, regardless of IgG status, should be monitored for potential fetal infection. Women who are IgM and IgG negative are susceptible to parvovirus B19 infection, and serologic testing should be repeated in 4 weeks. If the result of repeat testing demonstrates positive IgM or IgG, these women should be monitored for potential fetal infection.

Fetal infection can be diagnosed using PCR to detect parvovirus B19 DNA in amniotic fluid. Although tests that measure quantitative serum and tissue DNA viral load exist, they are not widely available, and qualitative PCR is used to diagnose fetal infection during pregnancy, with a sensitivity that has been reported to be as high as 100%. Testing for fetal parvovirus B19 infection should be considered when ultrasonography reveals hydrops fetalis.

Pregnant women with acute parvovirus B19 infection should be monitored for the development of fetal anemia using serial ultrasonography. Standard monitoring should include assessment for ascites, placentomegaly, cardiomegaly, hydrops fetalis, and impaired fetal growth. In addition, Doppler assessment of the peak systolic velocity of the fetal middle cerebral artery should be performed because this measure has been identified as an accurate predictor of fetal anemia. However, fetal death can occur without evidence of hydrops fetalis. Serial ultrasonography should be performed every 1–2 weeks for 8–12 weeks after exposure. In the absence of ultrasound evidence of fetal sequelae by 8–12 weeks after exposure, adverse outcomes related to parvovirus B19 infection are highly unlikely.

If hydrops fetalis is present or severe fetal anemia is suspected in the setting of parvovirus B19, fetal blood sampling should be performed to determine the fetal hematocrit in preparation for fetal transfusion. Although there is procedure-related risk, intrauterine transfusion should be considered if severe fetal anemia is present.

Prevention

When outbreaks of parvovirus B19 infection occur in situations in which prolonged, close-contact exposure occurs, such as in schools, homes, or child care centers, options for prevention of transmission are limited. Exposure cannot be eliminated by identifying and excluding individuals with acute parvovirus B19 infection because individuals are infectious before they develop symptoms. Exclusion of pregnant women from the workplace during endemic periods is not recommended. If a pregnant woman is exposed to individuals who are suspected or known to be infected with parvovirus B19, she should report this exposure to her obstetric care providers.

Respiratory Syncytial Virus

Respiratory syncytial virus (RSV), an RNA virus of the family Paramyxoviridae, is a common cause of respiratory infection in infancy and the most common cause of hospitalization for lower respiratory illness in infants (commonly termed "bronchiolitis"). Characteristics that increase the risk of severe RSV lower respiratory tract illness are preterm birth; cyanotic or complicated congenital heart disease, especially conditions causing pulmonary hypertension; chronic lung disease; and immunodeficiency disease or therapy causing immunosuppression at any age.

Transmission

Respiratory syncytial virus usually occurs in annual epidemics during winter and early spring in temperate climates. In North America, RSV season is typically November to April. Regional differences in RSV activity have been documented in certain parts of Alaska and Florida. The virus is spread easily among household and child care contacts, including adults. Transmission usually is by direct or close contact with contaminated secretions, which may occur from exposure to large-particle droplets at short distances (less than 3 feet) or fomites. Enforcement of infection control policies is important to decrease the risk of health care-related transmission of RSV.

Diagnosis and Treatment

Rapid diagnostic assays, including immunofluorescent and enzyme immunoassay techniques for detection of viral antigen in nasopharyngeal specimens, and reverse transcriptase (RT)-PCR for direct viral detection, are available commercially and generally are reliable in infants and young children. Young children with bronchiolitis may be co-infected with other respiratory viruses in as many as 20% of cases. Primary treatment is supportive and includes hydration, careful clinical assessment of respiratory status, including measurement of oxygen saturation, use of supplemental oxygen if needed, suction of the upper airway, and if necessary, intubation and mechanical ventilation. Corticosteroids are not routinely recommended for RSV bronchiolitis. The aerosolized antiviral ribavirin has not been shown to improve outcomes in most pediatric patients, and is reserved for use in life-threatening RSV infections in immunocompromised individuals. Palivizumab (as follows) is not recommended or approved for use in treatment of RSV infection.

Prophylaxis

Prophylaxis to prevent RSV in infants at increased risk of severe disease, particularly those with chronic lung disease receiving medical management on a long-term basis, is available using a humanized mouse monoclonal antibody—palivizumab. Prophylaxis with palivizumab decreases the risk of severe RSV disease and hospitalization by 39–82% among high-risk infants. No study has demonstrated an effect of palivizumab treatment on RSV-attributable mortality or recurrent wheezing. Palivizumab is administered as a maximum of five monthly intramuscular injections (15 mg per kg per dose) during RSV season, with the first dose typically administered in November in most areas of North America; local data in Alaska and Florida may mandate different timing. The AAP issued revised indications for palivizumab use in 2014. According to current AAP recommendations for RSV prophylaxis infants must be less than 12 months old at the beginning of RSV season, and meet one of the following categories:

- Birth at or below 28 6/7 weeks of gestation
- Birth at 29 0/7–31 6/7 weeks of gestation with chronic lung disease of prematurity, defined as requiring supplemental oxygen for at least the first 28 days after birth. Infants who still require mechanical ventilation at 28 days of life will also meet the definition of chronic lung disease. Infants who still require noninvasive respiratory support, but who do not require supplemental oxygen while receiving such support, should be formally evaluated for oxygen dependence at 28 days of age for the purpose of determining the presence of chronic lung disease.
- Infants with hemodynamically significant acyanotic congenital heart disease, such as those receiving medication for congestive heart failure before surgical correction and those infants with moderate-to-severe pulmonary hypertension
- Infants with cyanotic congenital heart disease, after discussion with their cardiologist
- Infants who have undergone cardiac or other solid-organ transplantation
- Infants with severe immunocompromise due to specific medical conditions, after consultation with their immunologist or oncologist
- Infants with pulmonary structural disease or neuromuscular disease that results in chronic lung disease or inability to clear secretions

- Infants with cystic fibrosis who meet the definition of chronic lung disease or who have severe nutritional compromise (not all infants with cystic fibrosis)
- Special consideration may be prudent for Navajo and White Mountain Apache infants in the first year of life
- Infants with chronic lung disease in their second RSV season should receive palivizumab only if they continue to require medical support (chronic corticosteroid therapy, bronchodilator therapy, or supplemental oxygen)

Infants who experience RSV disease should not continue to receive palivizumab, either as treatment or subsequent prophylaxis. Palivizumab is not recommended for infants with trisomy 21 or cystic fibrosis who do not otherwise qualify for palivizumab.

Respiratory syncytial virus can be transmitted in the hospital setting and may cause serious disease in high-risk newborns. The major means to prevent RSV disease in the hospital is strict observance of infection control practices, including identifying and cohorting RSV-infected patients. Palivizumab is not indicated as a control measure for hospital outbreaks of RSV infection.

A critical aspect of RSV prevention is parent education about the importance of avoiding exposure to and transmission of the virus. Preventive measures include limiting, when feasible, exposure to contagious settings, such as child care centers. The importance of hand hygiene should be emphasized in all settings, including the home.

Rubella

The rubella virus is an RNA virus that can manifest clinically as postnatal rubella or congenital rubella syndrome. Before widespread use of the rubella vaccine, rubella was an epidemic disease. More recently, infection has occurred in foreign-born or underimmunized individuals, because endemic rubella has been eliminated from the United States since 2004. Rubella infection can be subclinical. Clinical disease usually is mild, characterized by a generalized erythematous maculopapular rash, lymphadenopathy, and slight fever. Maternal rubella during pregnancy can result in miscarriage, fetal death, or congenital rubella syndrome. The most common manifestations associated with congenital rubella syndrome are ophthalmologic (cataracts, pigmentary retinopathy, microphthalmos, and congenital glaucoma), cardiac (patent ductus arteriosus, peripheral pulmonary artery stenosis), auditory (sensorineural hearing impairment), and neurologic (behavioral disorders, meningoencephalitis, and intellectual disability). Mild forms of congenital rubella syndrome can be associated with few or no obvious clinical manifestations at birth.

Antepartum Management

Surveillance for susceptibility to rubella infection is essential in prenatal care. Each patient should have serologic screening for rubella immunity at the first prenatal visit unless she is known to be immune by 1) documentation of vaccination with one dose of live rubella virus-containing vaccine, 2) laboratory evidence of immunity, or 3) laboratory confirmation of the disease. Seropositive women do not need further testing, regardless of their subsequent history of exposure. If a seronegative pregnant woman is exposed to rubella or develops symptoms that suggest infection, she should be retested for rubella-specific antibody. Specimens should be obtained as soon as possible after exposure, again 2 weeks later, and, if necessary, 4 weeks after exposure. Acute and chronic serum specimens should be tested on the same day in the same laboratory. Detection of rubella-specific IgM antibodies usually indicates recent infection, but false-positive test results can occur. Isolation of the virus from throat swabs establishes the diagnosis of acute rubella.

If rubella is diagnosed in a pregnant woman, she should be advised of the risks of fetal infection, and the choice of pregnancy termination should be discussed. Congenital defects occur in approximately 85% of cases of maternal infection during the first 12 weeks of gestation, and in approximately 50% at 13–16 weeks of gestation. Fetal infection may occur throughout pregnancy, but congenital defects are rare when infection occurs after the 20th week of gestation.

The rubella vaccine is a live attenuated virus and is highly effective with few adverse effects. However, rubella vaccination is not recommended during pregnancy. Women found to be susceptible during pregnancy should be offered vaccination postpartum before discharge from the birthing facility. Breastfeeding is not a contradiction to receiving the rubella vaccine. After immunization, women should be advised to avoid pregnancy for 1 month. However, a woman who becomes pregnant within 1 month of rubella vaccination or who is inadvertently vaccinated in early pregnancy should be counseled that the teratogenic risk to the fetus is very low. Surveillance by the CDC among women who received the rubella vaccine near the time of pregnancy reveals a less than 2% risk of fetal infection and no occurrence of congenital defects. Therefore, receipt of the rubella vaccine during pregnancy is not an indication for termination of pregnancy. All suspected cases of congenital rubella syndrome, whether caused by wild-type virus or vaccine virus infection, should be reported to local and state health departments. A pregnant household member is not a contraindication to vaccination of a child.

Neonatal Management

Infants who show signs of congenital rubella infection or who were born to women with a history of rubella during pregnancy should be managed with contact isolation. Care of the infant should be restricted to personnel who are immune to rubella. Efforts should be made to obtain viral cultures from the infant to document the infection. Infected infants should be considered contagious until 1 year of age unless nasopharyngeal and urine cultures (after 3 months of age) are repeatedly negative for the rubella virus.

Varicella Zoster Virus

Varicella zoster virus (VZV) is a highly contagious DNA herpesvirus that is transmitted by respiratory droplets or close contact. The infection rate among susceptible contacts is 60–90% after exposure. The incubation period after exposure ranges from 10 to 21 days. The period of infectivity begins 48 hours before the rash appears and lasts until the vesicles crust over. The primary infection causes chickenpox, which is characterized by fever, malaise, and a maculopapular pruritic rash that becomes vesicular. After the primary infection, VZV remains dormant in sensory ganglia and can be reactivated to cause a vesicular erythematous skin rash known as herpes zoster, or shingles. The antibody to VZV develops within a few days after the onset of infection, and prior infection with VZV confers lifelong immunity to primary infection.

In pregnancy, varicella may be transmitted across the placenta, which results in congenital or neonatal chickenpox. The risk of congenital varicella syndrome is low (0.4–2%); limited to exposure during early pregnancy (first trimester 0.4%, second trimester 2%, third trimester 0%); and is characterized by skin scarring, limb hypoplasia, chorioretinitis, and microcephaly. Neonatal VZV infection is associated with high mortality when maternal disease develops from 5 days before delivery to 48 hours postpartum, because of the relative immaturity of the neonatal immune system and the lack of protective maternal antibodies. Susceptible pregnant women theoretically can acquire varicella infection from exposure to individuals with herpes zoster infection (shingles). However, transmission is extremely rare because contact with an open cutaneous lesion is required and viral shedding is lower with recurrent varicella infection compared with primary chickenpox.

Antepartum Management

Pregnant women should have their varicella immune status documented at the first prenatal visit by history of natural infection or vaccination. In the absence of either history, VZV IgG antibody can be measured, although commercial assays detect antibody acquired by natural infection more reliably that vaccine-induced antibody. Diagnosis of maternal VZV infection usually is based initially on clinical findings; VZV PCR detection of viral DNA from skin lesions is currently the diagnostic test of choice. Direct fluorescence antibody for detection of viral antigens and viral culture are less sensitive than PCR assays; VZV PCR also can be used to detect virus from saliva in the acute phase of illness, and can distinguish wild-type and vaccine-strain VZV.

Pregnant women who are seronegative for VZV can receive varicella zoster immune globulin (VZIG) within 96 hours of exposure to a person with primary active VZV, although it can be given up until 10 days postexposure. However, there is no evidence that administration of VZIG to a susceptible, pregnant woman will prevent viremia, fetal infection, or congenital varicella syndrome. Because most immunosuppressed persons who receive VZIG after a significant exposure develop modified clinical disease or subclinical infection, it is theoretically possible that VZIG may prevent or suppress clinical disease in the normal woman without preventing fetal infection and disease. In the absence of evidence that VZIG can prevent congenital varicella syndrome or neonatal varicella, the primary indication for VZIG in pregnant women is to prevent complications of varicella in a susceptible adult patient rather than to prevent intrauterine infection.

Varicella during pregnancy can be treated with oral acyclovir to minimize maternal symptoms. Maternal treatment with acyclovir has not been shown to ameliorate or prevent the fetal effects of congenital varicella syndrome. Pregnant women with VZV infection should be advised of pulmonary complications and urged to seek medical care immediately if any pulmonary symptoms develop. Although women with VZV infection during pregnancy are no more likely to develop varicella pneumonia than are other adults, varicella pneumonia is more severe during pregnancy. Maternal varicella complicated by pneumonia should be treated with intravenous acyclovir because intravenous acyclovir may reduce maternal morbidity and mortality associated with varicella pneumonia.

Neonatal Management

Neonatal VZV infection is associated with a high neonatal death rate when maternal disease develops from 5 days before delivery up to 48 hours postpartum because of the relative immaturity of the neonatal immune system and the lack of protective maternal antibody. Varicella zoster immune globulin should be given to infants born to women who develop varicella during this interval, although this does not universally prevent neonatal varicella. Infants who develop varicella within the first 2 weeks of life should be treated with intravenous acyclovir.

Infants born at less than 28 weeks of gestation or less than 1,000 g who are exposed to VZV postnatally are at an increased risk of severe varicella, regardless of maternal history. These infants should receive VZIG regardless of the maternal history of varicella or varicella zoster serostatus. Hospitalized, preterm infants born at 28 weeks of gestation or later who are exposed postnatally to chickenpox and whose mothers have no history of chickenpox also should receive VZIG. If VZIG is unavailable, intravenous immunoglobulin may be given at a dosage of 400 mg per kg once.

Infection Control

Hospitalized women with VZV infection must be kept under airborne and contact precautions. Similar precautions are recommended for infants born to mothers with varicella and should continue during the incubation period (28 days after VZIG administration) if still hospitalized. Infants with VZV infection should be isolated in a private room for the duration of the illness. Infants with congenital VZV infection acquired earlier in gestation do not require special precautions or isolation unless vesicular lesions are present. Hospitalized infants who are exposed postnatally should be isolated from 8 days to 21 days after onset of the rash in the index case.

Immunization

Pregnant women should not be vaccinated, and vaccinated women should be advised to avoid pregnancy for 1 month after each dose because of concern about possible fetal effects. Surveillance data to date on fetal outcomes after inadvertent vaccine exposures, however, have not found any cases of fetal varicella syndrome. Women who do not have varicella immunity should receive the first dose of VZV vaccine in the postpartum period before discharge from the birthing facility. A pregnant household member is not a contraindication to vaccination of a child. A study of nursing mothers and their infants showed no evidence of excretion of vaccine strain in human milk or of transmission to infants who are breastfeeding. Varicella vaccine should be administered to nursing mothers who lack evidence of immunity. (For the most current immunization schedules and recommendations, please visit the CDC's "Vaccines & Immunizations" web page at www.cdc.gov/vaccines/index.html)

West Nile Virus

West Nile virus (WNV) is associated with fever, rash, arthritis, myalgias, weakness, lymphadenopathy, and meningoencephalitis. This virus is carried by mosquitoes and birds and can be transmitted through blood transfusion or organ transplant. Congenital infection can rarely occur. Pregnant women are not at higher risk for West Nile virus infection than nonpregnant women. Most women known to have been infected with West Nile virus during pregnancy have given birth to infants without evidence of infection or clinical abnormalities. In the single known instance of confirmed congenital West Nile virus infection, the mother developed West Nile virus encephalitis during week 27 of gestation, and the infant was born with cystic destruction of cerebral tissue and chorioretinitis. If West Nile virus disease is diagnosed during pregnancy, a detailed examination of the fetus and the newborn infant should be performed. To date, outcomes of 72 pregnancies have been published, with only one fetus having a proven intrauterine infection and subsequent bilateral chorioretinitis. It is unclear whether pregnant women are more susceptible to West Nile virus and whether the disease is more severe. The virus can be transmitted through breast milk, but to date infants infected by this route have been asymptomatic or had mild symptoms. Women with symptoms should not be discouraged from breastfeeding. Pregnant women and breastfeeding mothers should be encouraged to wear protective clothing, minimize their outdoor exposure at dawn and dusk when mosquitoes are most active, and use insect repellant containing N,N-diethyl-3-methylbenzamide (known as DEET) as a preventive measure.

Considerations for Mosquito-Borne Illness

In addition to West Nile virus, several additional mosquito-borne illnesses may affect pregnant women. These include dengue virus, chikungunya virus, and Zika virus. There currently are no vaccines to prevent infections caused by these viruses.

Currently, of the three mosquito-borne viruses discussed here, Zika virus is the only mosquito-borne illness that has been associated with birth defects, specifically microcephaly, brain abnormalities, intracranial calcification, and congenital contractures. Information about Zika virus is rapidly evolving and the most updated information may be found at www.acog.org/zika and www.cdc.gov/zika/pregnancy/index.html. Pregnant women are advised not to travel to areas with Zika risk. If such travel cannot be avoided, advise pregnant women to take all precautions to avoid mosquito bites, including using EPA-approved insect repellant with DEET, covering exposed skin, staying in air-conditioned or screened-in areas, and treating clothing with permethrin. Health care providers should specifically communicate to pregnant women that EPA-registered insect repellents, including those with DEET and permethrin, can be used safely during pregnancy when used as directed on the product label. Pregnant women with partners who have traveled to Zika risk areas are advised to use condoms during sex or to abstain from sex during pregnancy.

Recommendations are rapidly evolving for assessment and testing of pregnant women, their partners, and women and men of reproductive age as well as travel precautions for Zika. For current recommendations, see ACOG's website at www.acog.org/zika. It is important that maternal Zika virus exposure and testing information be available and communicated to the pediatric provider at birth so that appropriate infant testing and management can be implemented in accordance with existing guidance. It is particularly important that this information be conveyed while infants are hospitalized after birth to allow for collection of infant specimens within 2 days of birth.

Mosquito-borne illnesses are an area of evolving guidance based on new information. Obstetric care providers and pregnant women should see the CDC's website for updates on Zika virus, www.cdc.gov/zika; Dengue virus, www.cdc.gov/dengue; and Chikungunya virus, www.cdc.gov/Chikungunya.

Bacterial Infections

Intraamniotic Infection

The American College of Obstetricians and Gynecologists recommends administration of intrapartum antibiotics whenever an intraamniotic infection (also referred to as chorioamnionitis) is suspected or confirmed; such treatment benefits both the mother and the fetus. Suspected intraamniotic infection is diagnosed when maternal intrapartum temperature is greater than or equal to 39.0°C, or maternal intrapartum temperature is 38.0–38.9°C and one additional clinical risk factor, including maternal leukocytosis, purulent cervical drainage, or fetal tachycardia is present. Isolated maternal temperature of 38.0–38.9°C without apparent cause is not considered to be intraamniotic infection. However, given the potential benefits for both mother and fetus, if no obvious source for maternal temperature elevation is apparent, antibiotics are also recommended in the setting of isolated maternal fever. Recommended antibiotics for the treatment of intraamniotic infection are ampicillin and gentamicin, with the addition of metronidazole or clindamycin if cesarean delivery is performed. Clindamycin or vancomycin and gentamicin together are recommended for severe penicillin-allergic women; cefazolin and gentamicin are recommended for women with mild penicillin allergy. Regardless of institutional protocol, when an obstetric provider diagnoses an intraamniotic infection or when other risk factors for early-onset neonatal sepsis are present in labor (eg, maternal fever, rupture of the membranes at more than 18 hours, or preterm birth), communication with the neonatal care team is essential to optimize neonatal evaluation and management.

The most recent CDC published guidelines for the prevention of perinatal GBS disease can be accessed at www.cdc.gov/groupbstrep/guidelines/guidelines.html. Recommendations for GBS screening, indications for intrapartum antibiotic prophylaxis (IAP) (see also Table 12-3), and antibiotic choices for IAP are summarized here.

Indications for GBS screening:

- All pregnant women should be screened for rectovaginal GBS colonization at 35–37 weeks of gestation.
- Women who present in preterm labor, with preterm rupture of membranes, or both, should be screened for GBS colonization. If the woman does not give birth within 5 weeks of screening, GBS screening cultures should be repeated when in true labor, or at 35–37 weeks of gestation.
- Women with GBS bacteriuria or GBS urinary tract infection in the current pregnancy and women with a prior infant affected by GBS disease should be considered GBS-colonized and do not require further GBS testing.

TABLE 12–3. Indications and Nonindications for Intrapartum Antibiotic Prophylaxis to Prevent Early-Onset Group B Streptococcal Disease

Intrapartum GBS Prophylaxis Indicated	Intrapartum GBS Prophylaxis Not Indicated
Previous infant with invasive GBS disease	Colonization with GBS during a previous pregnancy (unless an indication for GBS prophylaxis is present for current pregnancy)
GBS bacteriuria during any trimester of the current pregnancy	GBS bacteriuria during previous pregnancy (unless another indication for GBS prophlaxis is present for current pregnancy)
Positive GBS screening culture result during current pregnancy (unless a cesarean delivery is performed before onset of labor on a woman with intact amniotic membranes)	Cesarean delivery performed before onset of labor on a woman with intact amniotic membranes, regardless of GBS colonization status or gestational age
Unknown GBS status at the onset of labor (culture not done, incomplete, or results unknown) and any of the following: • Delivery at 37 weeks of gestation* • Amniotic membrane rupture at 18 hours or more • Intrapartum temperature greater than or equal to 100.4°F (greater than or equal to 38.0°C)[†] • Intrapartum NAAT[‡] positive for GBS	Negative vaginal and rectal GBS screening culture result obtained at 35–37 weeks of gestation during the current pregnancy, regardless of intrapartum risk factors Negative screening results obtained earlier than 35 weeks of gestation should be repeated if obtained 5 weeks or more before anticipated delivery

Abbreviations: GBS, group B streptococci; NAAT, nucleic acid amplification test.

*Recommendations for the use of intrapartum antibiotics for prevention of early-onset GBS disease in the setting of preterm delivery are included in the complete guidelines, which are available at http://www.cdc.gov/groupbstrep/guidelines/guidelines.html.

[†]If intraamniotic infection is suspected, broad-spectrum antibiotic therapy that includes an agent known to be active against GBS should replace GBS prophylaxis.

[‡]NAAT testing for GBS is optional and may not be available in all settings. If intrapartum NAAT result is negative for GBS but any other intrapartum risk factor (delivery at less than 37 weeks of gestation, amniotic membrane rupture at 18 hours or more, or temperature greater than or equal to 100.4°F [greater than or equal to 38.0°C]) is present, then intrapartum antibiotic prophylaxis is indicated.

Data from Verani JR, McGee L, Schrag SJ. Prevention of perinatal group B streptococcal disease--revised guidelines from CDC, 2010. Division of Bacterial Diseases, National Center for Immunization and Respiratory Diseases, Centers for Disease Control and Prevention. MMWR Recomm Rep 2010;59(RR-10):1–36.

Indications for intrapartum antibiotic prophylaxis administration:

- Women in labor with documented GBS colonization
- Women with preterm labor (less than 37 0/7 weeks of gestation), or preterm premature rupture of membranes, or both, pending determination of true labor and GBS screening results
- Women in labor at term (37 0/7 or more weeks of gestation) with unknown GBS status if specific risk factors arise, including rupture of membranes at 18 hours or more; maternal intrapartum temperature of 38.0°C (100.4°F) or more (if the patient has intraamniotic infection, treat appropriately for both intraamniotic infection and GBS); or if determined to be GBS positive by intrapartum nucleic acid amplification testing

Antibiotics for intrapartum antibiotic prophylaxis:

- Penicillin or ampicillin are the preferred antibiotics for intrapartum antibiotic prophylaxis
- Penicillin-allergic women who DO NOT have a history of anaphylaxis, angioedema, respiratory distress or urticaria following administration of a penicillin or a cephalosporin should receive cefazolin for intrapartum antibiotic prophylaxis
- Penicillin-allergic women who DO have a history of anaphylaxis, angioedema, respiratory distress or urticaria following administration of a penicillin or a cephalosporin should receive clindamycin if GBS sensitivities have been performed and the isolate is sensitive to both clindamycin and erythromycin for intrapartum antibiotic prophylaxis
- Penicillin-allergic women who DO have a history of anaphylaxis, angioedema, respiratory distress or urticaria following administration of a penicillin or a cephalosporin should receive vancomycin for intrapartum antibiotic prophylaxis if sensitivity testing has not been performed or if the isolate is resistant to either clindamycin or erythromycin (unless inducible resistance to clindamycin testing is performed and is negative)
- Only the administration of penicillin, ampicillin, or cefazolin 4 hours or more before delivery can be considered adequate intrapartum antibiotic prophylaxis with respect to newborn risk assessment

Intrapartum antibiotic prophylaxis for GBS disease is not recommended for GBS-colonized women undergoing a planned cesarean delivery in the absence of labor and rupture of membranes, regardless of the gestational age. However, all patients undergoing cesarean delivery should have prophylactic antibiotics administered before the incision to reduce the risk of maternal postoperative infections (see also "Cesarean Delivery" in Chapter 7).

In discussing the role of GBS intrapartum antibiotic prophylaxis with pregnant women, it is important to differentiate the effect of intrapartum antibiotic prophylaxis on decreasing the incidence of GBS-specific neonatal early-onset sepsis versus the lack of effect on recurrent and late-onset GBS disease. Mothers and other caregivers should be educated on three important points. First, GBS intrapartum antibiotic prophylaxis does not decrease the risk of late-onset invasive GBS disease (occurring at 7–90 days of age). Second, there is no known method for the prevention of late-onset neonatal GBS infection. Third, infants who have GBS-specific early-onset neonatal sepsis and receive recommended intravenous antibiotic treatment are at risk of recurrent invasive GBS disease. Approximately 5–6% of infants with GBS-specific early-onset neonatal sepsis will have recurrent disease, usually with the same strain of GBS, because antibiotic treatment cannot decolonize the infant and newborns do not usually mount protective antibody responses to GBS.

Early-Onset Neonatal Sepsis

Early-onset neonatal sepsis (EOS) is defined by the CDC as blood or CSF culture-confirmed infection occurring in the newborn at less than 7 days of age. For the continuously hospitalized very-low-birth-weight infant, EOS is defined as culture-confirmed infection occurring at less than 72 hours of age. Currently, EOS occurs in approximately 0.8 cases per 1,000 live births in the United States. The incidence and case-fatality rate are both strongly influenced by gestational age at birth. Among infants born at 37 weeks of gestation or greater, EOS occurs in approximately 0.5 cases per 1,000 live births. The incidence of EOS among preterm infants is inversely proportional to gestational age, as follows: approximately 30 per 1,000 among infants born at 22–24 weeks of gestation, approximately 10 per 1,000 among those born at 27–28 weeks of gestation, and approximately 1 per 1,000 among infants born at 34–36 weeks of gestation. Case-fatality rates are 2–3% among infants born at 37 weeks of gestation or greater, but 22% among infants born at less than 37 weeks of gestation, with most deaths occurring among the lowest gestational ages. A 10-fold difference in mortality is observed when assessed by birth weight (3.5% for birth weight 1,500 g or greater versus 35% for birth weight less than 1,500 g). Group B streptococcus remains the single most common bacterial cause of EOS, accounting for approximately 35% of all EOS cases. In contrast, gram-negative bacteria are the most common organisms that cause EOS in very-low-birth-weight preterm infants; *Escherichia coli* alone accounts for approximately 40% of EOS cases among these infants.

Prevention of Early-Onset Neonatal Sepsis

Prevention of early-onset neonatal sepsis is based on the recognition of clinical risk factors during labor and delivery; appropriate provision of intrapartum antibiotics; and, where indicated, empiric antibiotic treatment of newborns after birth. Risk factors for early-onset neonatal sepsis include gestational age less than 37 0/7 weeks; maternal intrapartum fever and other signs of intraamniotic infection; prolonged or preterm rupture of membranes; and maternal GBS rectovaginal colonization. Intrapartum antibiotics may be administered reactively, as when there is concern for intraamniotic infection, or prophylactically, as is done for maternal GBS colonization.

Risk Assessment and Empiric Antibiotic Treatment of Early-Onset Neonatal Sepsis

The goal of clinical risk assessment in early-onset neonatal sepsis is to identify high-risk newborns and subsequently prevent the onset or progression of the disease. In assessing risk of early-onset neonatal sepsis, consideration should be given to perinatal risk factors for early-onset neonatal sepsis as outlined here; clinical status of the newborn; and results of laboratory results (if performed). Risk can be assessed by the dichotomous presence/absence of specific factors and conditions, or by using multivariate analysis such as provided in the Neonatal Sepsis Risk Calculator, found at https://neonatalsepsiscalculator.kaiserpermanente.org. Risk is increased by the presence of specific clinical risk factors such as prematurity and by symptoms of illness in the newborn (eg, respiratory distress, metabolic acidosis, hypotension, perinatal depression). Risk can be assessed with adjunctive laboratory diagnostics such as complete blood count (with components of the white blood cell differential) and C-reactive protein. Among infants born ατ 34 weeks or more of gestation, interpretation of the white blood count and differential is best done with consideration of infant age (in hours) at time of testing with use of likelihood ratios for each test. Positive and negative predictive values are dependent on disease incidence and of less value than likelihood ratios among term infants given current incidence of early-onset neonatal sepsis. Among preterm infants, symptoms of illness such as respiratory distress may be due to early-onset neonatal sepsis or more commonly, due to prematurity itself. Laboratory studies can also be difficult to interpret among preterm infants. Leukopenia and neutropenia, for example, are associated with increased risk of early-onset neonatal sepsis but also may be due to the effects of intrauterine stress. The difficulties encountered in attributing clinical status and laboratory values to prematurity or to infection lead to high rates of empiric antibiotic administration among preterm infants. Clinical judgment must be used to determine the risk of early-onset neonatal sepsis (with consideration given to the circumstances of delivery), and the best course of initial therapy among preterm infants. Neonatal empiric antibiotic administration should include ampicillin (providing specific coverage for GBS, as well as for organisms that are not sensitive to cephalosporins, such as enterococci and *Listeria* and an aminoglycoside (commonly gentamicin) to provide coverage for gram-negative organisms. Local data informing antibiotic susceptibility of early-onset neonatal sepsis organisms may affect additional local antibiotic choices. Among infants at the highest risk of early-onset neonatal sepsis (including those who are critically ill), health care providers should consider the individual risks and benefits of obtaining CSF for cell count and culture prior to the institution of empiric antibiotics.

Discharge Education

Neonatal bacterial infection remains a concern after discharge from the delivery hospital. Late-onset bacterial infection is defined as invasive bacterial infection occurring at 7–90 days of age. Pathogens include those associated with early-onset neonatal sepsis, as well as others more common among pediatric outpatients, such as *Staphylococcus aureus* and *Streptococcus pneumoniae*. Mothers and other caregivers should be educated on the signs of infant illness after discharge from the delivery hospital, including fever of 38.0°C (100.4°F) or more, poor feeding, lethargy, breathing difficulties, skin rash or focal erythema, and inconsolability, and should be counseled to seek immediate pediatric care if these occur.

Chlamydial Infection

Chlamydia trachomatis is the most common reportable STI in the United States, with high rates among sexually active adolescents and young adults. Genital chlamydial infection is associated with age younger than 25 years, race and ethnicity, income, marital status, number of sexual partners, and level of education. Most infected women are asymptomatic, but *C trachomatis* may cause urethritis and mucopurulent (nongonococcal) cervicitis. Chlamydial infection also is associated with postpartum endometritis and infertility. Infection may be transmitted from the genital tract of infected women to their infants during birth.

Antepartum Management

All pregnant women younger than 25 years of age or with other risk factors for chlamydia should be screened for chlamydial infection during the first prenatal care visit (see also "Routine Laboratory Testing in Pregnancy" in Chapter 6). A repeat test should be obtained in the third trimester for these women. The diagnosis of *C trachomatis* infection is based on a cell culture, direct fluorescent antibody staining, enzyme immunoassay, DNA probe, or nucleic acid amplification tests (eg, polymerase chain reaction). Nucleic acid amplification tests are the most sensitive diagnostic test and are widely used for genital specimens, but are not FDA-approved for use with conjunctival or respiratory specimens. Use of nucleic acid amplification tests for non-genital specimens may be done with local verification of Clinical Laboratory Improvement Amendments.

Treatment should be administered to women who have known *C trachomatis* infection or whose newborn infants are infected. Women whose sexual partners have nongonococcal urethritis or epididymitis are presumed to be infected and also should be treated. Simultaneous treatment of partners is an important component of the therapeutic regimen. Doxycycline is contraindicated in pregnancy. Ofloxacin and levofloxacin likely present a low risk to the fetus during pregnancy, but animal studies have raised concerns about cartilage damage in newborn offspring. The only recommended regimen for treating *C trachomatis* infection in pregnant women is 1 g azithromycin orally in a single dose. Alternative regimens are amoxicillin (500 mg orally, three times daily for 7 days), erythromycin base (500 mg orally, four times a day for 7 days or 250 mg orally, four times daily for 14 days) or erythromycin ethylsuccinate (800 mg orally, four times daily for 7 days or 400 mg orally, four times daily for 14 days). Erythromycin estolate is contraindicated during pregnancy because of drug-related hepatotoxicity. During pregnancy, a test of cure is recommended 3–4 weeks after completion of treatment regimens to confirm successful treatment.

Neonatal Management

Approximately 50% of infants born to women who have untreated chlamydial infection become colonized with *C trachomatis*. Of these, 25–50% will manifest a purulent conjunctivitis a few days to several weeks after delivery, and 5–20% will develop pneumonia 2–19 weeks after delivery. Infections generally are mild and responsive to antimicrobial therapy. Infants with chlamydial conjunctivitis or pneumonia should be treated with erythromycin base or ethylsuccinate (50 mg per kg per day in 4 divided doses) for 14 days. Limited data suggest azithromycin 20 mg per kg once daily for 3 days may be effective. Topical treatment of conjunctivitis is ineffective. If hospitalized, infants should be managed with standard precautions. An association between orally administered erythromycin and infantile hypertrophic pyloric stenosis has been reported in infants younger than 6 weeks of age. This association requires further study, and currently the AAP continues to recommend erythromycin treatment for neonatal chlamydial infection.

Gonorrhea

Gonorrhea, caused by the gram-negative bacterium *Neisseria gonorrhoeae*, is one of the most commonly reported bacterial STIs. Women younger than 25 years are at highest risk of gonorrhea infection, as are those of African American, Hispanic, Native American, or Alaska Native race or ethnicity. Other risk factors for gonorrhea include a previous gonococcal infection, other STIs, new or multiple sexual partners, inconsistent condom use, commercial sex work, and illicit drug use. Gonococcal infection of the genital tract in females may be asymptomatic; common clinical syndromes are vaginitis, urethritis, endocervicitis, and salpingitis. Asymptomatic infection in females can progress to pelvic inflammatory disease, with tubal scarring that can result in ectopic pregnancy or infertility. Perinatal transmission also can occur, which results in neonatal gonococcal infection.

Antepartum Management

All pregnant women younger than 25 years of age or with other risk factors for gonorrhea should be screened for *N gonorrhoeae* at the first prenatal care visit (see also "Routine Laboratory Testing in Pregnancy" in Chapter 6). A repeat test should be performed in the third trimester for these women. Nucleic acid amplification tests (eg, polymerase chain reaction) are highly sensitive and specific for detecting *N gonorrhoeae* when used on endocervical or vaginal swab and urine specimens. Cultures are the most widely used tests for identifying *N gonorrhoeae* from nongenital sites.

Because of the prevalence of penicillin-resistant, tetracycline-resistant and fluoroquinolone-resistant *N gonorrhoeae,* the recommended treatment for pregnant women infected with *N gonorrhoeae* is dual therapy consisting of ceftriaxone 250 mg in a single intramuscular dose and azithromycin 1 g orally as a single dose. When cephalosporin allergy or other considerations preclude treatment with this regimen and spectinomycin is not available, consultation with an infectious-disease specialist is recommended. A test-of-cure is not recommended routinely in individuals with uncomplicated gonorrhea who are treated with this first-line therapy, except for pharyngeal gonorrhea. Because concurrent infection with *C trachomatis* is common, patients with gonococcal infections should be treated for chlamydial infection (unless it has been excluded) and should be evaluated for co-infection with syphilis, HIV, and other STIs. All cases of gonorrhea must be reported to public health officials.

Neonatal Management

Gonococcal infection in the newborn usually involves the eyes. Antimicrobial prophylaxis soon after delivery is mandated by law or regulation in many states for all newborns, including those born by cesarean delivery (see also "Conjunctival [Eye] Care" in Chapter 10). Infants born to women with active gonorrhea should receive a single dose of ceftriaxone (25–50 mg per kg given intravenously or intramuscularly, not to exceed 125 mg). Single-dose systemic antibiotic therapy is effective treatment for gonococcal ophthalmia and prophylaxis for disseminated disease. In addition to ophthalmia, neonatal disease may include scalp abscess, vaginitis, and systemic disease with bacteremia, arthritis, meningitis, or endocarditis. Infants with clinical gonococcal disease should be hospitalized, and cultures of blood, CSF, eye discharge, or other sites of infection should be obtained. For infants with positive cultures (ie, disseminated infection), the recommended antimicrobial therapy is cefotaxime (50 mg per kg per day, divided into two doses given every 12 hours, or ceftriaxone 25–50 mg per kg intravenously once per day). The duration of recommended antibiotic treatment depends on the site of infection, 7 days for disseminated infection, 10–14 days for meningitis, and 14 days for arthritis. Infected infants should be managed with standard universal precautions. Tests for concomitant infection with *C trachomatis*, congenital syphilis, and HIV infection should be performed.

Listeriosis

The major cause of epidemic and sporadic listeriosis is food-borne transmission of the bacterium *Listeria monocytogenes*. Foods associated with listeria contamination include unpasteurized milk, cheese, and other dairy products; undercooked poultry; prepared meats, such as hot dogs, deli meats, and pâté; and some contaminated fresh fruits and vegetables. Asymptomatic fecal and vaginal carriage can result in sporadic neonatal disease from transplacental or ascending intrauterine infection or from exposure during delivery. Maternal infection has been associated with preterm delivery, in utero fetal demise, and other obstetric complications. Pregnant women may present with a prodromal flu-like illness and clinical concern for decreased fetal movement. Late-onset neonatal infection results from acquisition of the organism during passage through the birth canal or possibly from environmental sources. To prevent pregnancy-related listeria infections, pregnant women are advised not to eat uncooked or undercooked hot dogs and deli meats, refrigerated smoked seafood, unpasteurized dairy products, undercooked foods, or unwashed fresh fruits and vegetables.

Listeria monocytogenes can be recovered on blood agar media from cultures of usually sterile body sites (eg, blood or CSF). Special techniques may be needed to recover *L monocytogenes* from sites with mixed flora (eg, vagina, rectum). Because of morphologic similarity to diphtheroids and streptococci, a culture isolate of *L monocytogenes* can be mistaken for a contaminant or saprophyte. Clinicians should notify their laboratories when listeriosis is suspected to ensure positive cultures are not mistaken for a skin contaminant.

Prompt diagnosis and antibiotic treatment of maternal listeriosis may prevent fetal or perinatal infection. *Listeria monocytogenes* is uniformly sensitive to ampicillin, and there may be a synergistic benefit from adding gentamicin. Signs of listeriosis in the newborn vary widely and often are nonspecific. The clinical picture is similar to that of GBS infection with early-onset and late-onset syndromes. Therapy with intravenous ampicillin and an aminoglycoside is recommended for neonatal infections.

Pertussis

Pertussis, commonly known as whooping cough, is a respiratory infection that initially is manifested as coryza, followed by the onset of paroxysms of cough that last for weeks. Complications in adults include pneumonia, sleep disturbance, rib fracture, and incontinence. In the first 6 months of life, illness is more severe and may present with apnea and bradycardia. Infant complications can include pneumonia, seizures, encephalopathy, and death. Newborns are noted to be protected from infection if high concentrations of passively transferred pertussis-specific antibodies are present.

Immunization During Pregnancy

Universal immunization during pregnancy is recommended to prevent acquisition of pertussis in both mothers and newborns. Immunization with Tdap during pregnancy has been associated with an increase in protective diphtheria and pertussis antibody levels in newborns of vaccinated mothers. Ideally, all women should be up to date with the tetanus toxoid, reduced diphtheria toxoid, and Tdap before pregnancy. With national increases in pertussis disease, currently the Advisory Committee on Immunization Practices and ACOG recommend that all pregnant women should receive Tdap vaccine during each pregnancy regardless of prior immunization history. To maximize the maternal antibody response and passive antibody transfer and levels in the newborn, optimal timing for Tdap administration is between 27 weeks and 36 weeks of gestation, although Tdap may be given at any time during pregnancy. To protect pregnant women who live in geographic regions with epidemics of pertussis, they should be immunized as soon as feasible for their own protection in accordance with local recommendations for nonpregnant adults. Newborn protection will still be garnered from vaccination earlier in the same pregnancy.

A pregnant woman in the third trimester should not be re-vaccinated if she received the vaccine in the first or second trimester. If Tdap is not administered during pregnancy, and if the patient has not previously received an adult booster, Tdap should be administered immediately postpartum to ensure her immunity and to reduce the risk of transmission to the newborn. It is safe to administer Tdap to breastfeeding women

Additional guidelines for the administration of Tdap during pregnancy include the following:

Tetanus Booster—If a tetanus and diphtheria (Td) booster vaccination is indicated during pregnancy (ie, more than 10 years since the previous Td vaccination) for a woman who has previously not received Tdap, then health care providers should administer the Tdap vaccine during pregnancy, preferably at 27–36 weeks of gestation.

Unknown or Incomplete Tetanus Vaccination—To ensure protection against maternal and neonatal tetanus, pregnant women who never have been vaccinated against tetanus should receive three vaccinations containing tetanus and reduced diphtheria toxoids during pregnancy. The recommended schedule is 0, 4 weeks, and 6–12 months. One dose of the Td booster vaccine should be replaced by Tdap, preferably at 27–36 weeks of gestation.

Wound Management—As part of standard wound management care to prevent tetanus, a tetanus toxoid-containing vaccine might be recommended for a pregnant woman if 5 years or more have elapsed since the previous Td booster vaccination. If a Td booster is indicated for a pregnant woman who previously has not received Tdap, health care providers should administer Tdap.

Vaccination of Adolescents and Adults in Contact With Infants

The CDC Advisory Committee on Immunization Practices recommends that adolescents and adults who have or anticipate having contact with an infant younger than 12 months and who have not received Tdap previously should receive a single dose of Tdap to protect against pertussis and reduce the likelihood of transmission. Ideally, this dose should be received at least 2 weeks before contact with the infant.

Neonatal and Infant Management

Infected infants younger than 6 months frequently require hospitalization for supportive care and to manage complications; however, those younger than 3 months account for most of the pertussis-related mortality. Diagnosis is made by culture or PCR, although both may be negative in a previously immunized individual and both require special sampling and handling. Antimicrobial agents given during the early catarrhal stage may lessen the severity of the disease. Antimicrobial treatment does not improve the clinical course once cough occurs, but treatment still is recommended to decrease disease transmission. Azithromycin, clarithromycin, and erythromycin are effective, but azithromycin and clarithromycin are not recommended for infants younger than 6 months and erythromycin may carry risk of infantile hypertrophic pyloric stenosis. For all these reasons, consultation with infectious disease specialists is recommended to diagnose and manage pertussis disease, particularly for infants younger than 6 months.

Tuberculosis

Tuberculosis disease is caused by infection with organisms of the *Mycobacterium tuberculosis* complex (including *Mycobacterium tuberculosis, Mycobacterium bovis* and *Mycobacterium africanum*). Clinical manifestations include feelings of sickness or weakness, weight loss, fever, and night sweats. The symptoms of pulmonary tuberculosis also include cough, chest pain, and hemoptysis. Tuberculosis disease also may affect nonpulmonary organs. The risk of developing active tuberculosis is highest during the 6 months after infection and remains high for 2 years; however, many years can elapse between initial mycobacterial infection and the onset of active tuberculosis. Pregnancy does not change a woman's baseline risk of acquiring infection or progressing from latent infection to tuberculosis disease and does not change the response to treatment. However, pregnancy can complicate the evaluation of constitutional symptoms of tuberculosis disease such as fatigue and weight loss. Once considered rare in the United States, the incidence of tuberculosis has increased considerably in women of childbearing age because risk has increased in the general population. Risk is highest among immigrants to the United States and in urban, low-income areas. In the United States, 80% of disease occurs in Hispanic and nonwhite individuals.

Diagnosis

Screening. Tuberculosis exposure is assessed by the Mantoux tuberculin skin test with purified protein derivative (PPD) or interferon-gamma release assay (IGRA). The PPD consists of intradermal injection of purified mycobacterial protein derivative, with subsequent assessment of immune reaction to these antigens. The PPD response may become positive 2–10 weeks (median 3–4 weeks) after exposure. Previous vaccination with bacille Calmette–Guérin, common in many countries with high prevalence of tuberculosis disease, may cause a false-positive reaction to the PPD. Interferon-gamma release assay tests measure immune response to antigens that are fairly specific to *M tuberculosis* complex. Neither PPD nor interferon-gamma release assays can distinguish latent tuberculosis infection from tuberculosis disease, and a negative result from these tests cannot exclude the possibility of disease. The sensitivity of interferon-gamma release assay is similar to PPD for untreated, confirmed tuberculosis disease, but the specificity is higher because the bacille Calmette–Guérin antigens used are not usually found in the BCG vaccine or nonpathogenic mycobacteria. Interferon-gamma release assay can be used in place of (but not in addition to) PPD in all situations in which a PPD is recommended, including pregnancy. Latent tuberculosis infection is diagnosed in an individual with positive PPD or IGRA test, but with no physical findings of disease and either a normal chest X-ray or only granuloma or calcification in the lung parenchyma, or regional lymph nodes, or both. The purpose of treating latent tuberculosis infection is to prevent progression to tuberculosis disease.

Definitive diagnosis. Tuberculosis disease is diagnosed in an individual with infection who also has signs, symptoms, positive cultures, or radiographic manifestations of *M tuberculosis*. Isolation of *M tuberculosis* by culture from early morning gastric aspirate, sputum, pleural fluid, or other body fluids establishes the diagnosis of active disease. *Mycobacterium tuberculosis* is slow growing, usually requiring 2–10 weeks for isolation from cultured materials. Smears to demonstrate acid-fast bacilli should be performed on sputum and body fluids. Nucleic-acid amplification tests are available to aid in diagnosis, but are only FDA-approved for respiratory specimens.

Antepartum Management

All pregnant women who are at high risk of tuberculosis should be screened with a PPD or IGRA when they begin receiving prenatal care (see also "Routine Laboratory Testing in Pregnancy" in Chapter 6). Women at high risk include those with exposure history that would suggest recent infection; high to moderate risk of reactivation of latent tuberculosis infection incurred by immunocompromising conditions (particularly those involving HIV infection); pregestational diabetes mellitus, dialysis-dependent renal failure; treatment with immunosuppressive agents such as chronic steroids or tumor necrosis factor (TNF)-alpha inhibitors; and foreign-born patients who have emigrated from endemic countries within the past 5 years. Women should be tested during pregnancy even if the intent is not to initiate treatment for latent tuberculosis infection or active disease until after pregnancy. This will avoid missing women who do not return for care after delivery. When the result of a tuberculin skin test or IGRA is positive, the time of conversion is unknown. Evaluation for active disease should include assessment of symptoms and chest radiograph.

Treatment of Latent Tuberculosis Infection. The risk of tuberculosis disease to the pregnant woman and fetus is considered to be higher than the risk of treatment; therefore, if a woman is at high enough risk to be tested, the CDC currently recommends initiating treatment of latent tuberculosis infection during pregnancy. Most experts recommend delaying treatment until the second trimester, but this decision must be made on an individual basis. Of note, women receiving treatment for latent tuberculosis infection before pregnancy should not suspend treatment because of intervening pregnancy. If treatment for latent tuberculosis infection is not initiated during pregnancy, it should begin immediately postpartum. Treatment of latent tuberculosis infection among pregnant women consists of isoniazid either daily or once or twice weekly (using directly observed therapy) for 9 months, with supplemental pyridoxine (vitamin B_6). Isoniazid treatment is compatible with breastfeeding, and breastfed infants not receiving isoniazid themselves do not require supplemental pyridoxine because of maternal treatment.

Treatment of Tuberculosis Disease. If tuberculosis is diagnosed in a pregnant woman, referral to an infectious disease specialist for prompt initiation of multidrug therapy is recommended to protect both the woman and the fetus. Standard therapy includes ethambutol, isoniazid, and rifampin, all of which are compatible with pregnancy. Pyrazinamide is contraindicated for pregnant women in most cases; streptomycin, kanamycin, amikacin, capreomycin, and fluoroquinolones are either relatively contraindicated or contraindicated in pregnancy

Neonatal Management

Congenital tuberculosis is rare in the United States. In utero infection can occur as a result of hematogenous dissemination, which seeds the placenta, or as a result of aspiration of infected amniotic fluid in utero. Neonatal infection may also occur at the time of delivery as a result of aspiration of tubercle bacilli in women with tuberculosis endometritis. The presence of miliary disease or abdominal or pelvic disease in the pregnant women should raise concern for congenital disease in the newborn. If a newborn infant is suspected of having congenital tuberculosis, consultation with an infectious disease expert is mandatory. A PPD (although usually negative), chest radiograph, lumbar puncture, and appropriate cultures should be performed promptly. Treatment of the infant should be initiated promptly with isoniazid, rifampin, pyrazinamide, and an aminoglycoside (eg, amikacin), pending the results of evaluation. The placenta should be examined histologically for granulomata and acid-fast bacilli, and a specimen should be cultured for *M tuberculosis* complex. If meningitis is confirmed, corticosteroids should be added. Drug susceptibility testing of the organism recovered from the mother or household contact, infant, or both should be performed.

Management of a newborn whose mother (or other household contact) is suspected of having tuberculosis is based on individual considerations. Whenever possible, separation of the mother and the infant should be minimized. Recommendations for different circumstances are listed as follows:

- The mother has a positive PPD or IGRA but a negative X-ray result. If the mother is asymptomatic, the infant needs no special evaluation or therapy and no separation of the mother and the infant is required. The newborn may breastfeed regardless of maternal isoniazid therapy. Because the positive PPD or IGRA could be a marker of an unrecognized case of contagious tuberculosis within the household, other household members should be tested and evaluated.
- The mother has an abnormal chest X-ray but no evidence of tuberculosis disease. If the mother's chest X-ray is abnormal but the history, physical examination, sputum smear, and X-ray indicate no evidence of current tuberculosis, the infant can be assumed to be at low risk of *M tuberculosis* infection. The mother should initiate isoniazid therapy for latent tuberculosis infection if it is not already being given at the time of delivery. Separation of mother and infant is not required. Other household members should be tested and appropriately evaluated.
- The mother has clinical or radiographic evidence of contagious tuberculosis disease. The mother should be reported immediately to the public health department so that investigation of all household members can be performed within 7 days. All contacts should have PPD or IGRA, chest X-ray, and physical examination and clinical history. The infant should be evaluated for congenital tuberculosis and the mother should be tested for HIV infection. The mother and the infant should be separated until the mother has been evaluated, mother and infant are receiving appropriate treatment, the mother wears a mask, and the mother understands and is willing to adhere to infection control measures. Once mother and infant are receiving isoniazid, separation is not necessary. If however, the mother has possible multi-drug resistant (MDR) tuberculosis disease or has poor adherence to treatment and

precautions, mother and infant should be separated indefinitely and consideration given to BCG immunization for the infant after HIV has been excluded. Consultation with infectious diseases experts is mandatory to determine when it is safe to resume mother–infant contact in these cases. Women with non-MDR tuberculosis disease who have been treated appropriately for 2 or more weeks and who are not considered contagious can breastfeed. If congenital tuberculosis is excluded, isoniazid is given until the infant is 3–4 months of age, at which time a PPD should be performed. If the PPD is positive, the infant should be reassessed for tuberculosis disease. If disease is not present, isoniazid should be continued for a total of 9 months depending on HIV status. If the PPD is negative and the mother and other family members with tuberculosis have good adherence and response to treatment, and are no longer infectious, isoniazid may be discontinued.

- *Bacille Calmette–Guérin Vaccine.* Bacille Calmette–Guérin vaccine is a live vaccine prepared from attenuated strains of *Mycobacterium bovis.* Although widely used in many countries with high rates of tuberculosis disease, BCG is rarely used in the United States. Immunization in the United States should be considered only for children and health care workers with a negative tuberculin skin test result who are not infected with HIV and who are 1) at high risk of intimate and prolonged exposure to patients with persistently infectious pulmonary tuberculosis or MDR tuberculosis, 2) cannot be removed from the source of exposure, and 3) cannot be placed on long-term preventive therapy.

Spirochetal Infections

Syphilis

Syphilis is a systemic disease caused by infection with the spirochete *Treponema pallidum*. Rates of infection are highest in urban areas and the rural South. In adults, syphilis is more common in individuals with HIV infection. Syphilis disease is divided into primary, secondary, latent (early latent if less than 1 year; late latent if more than 1 year), and tertiary stages. Primary disease is characterized by the presence of painless mucosal ulcers, secondary disease by rash and lymphadenopathy, and latent disease by seroreactivity without signs of disease. Tertiary disease occurs 15–30 years after the initial infection and involves gumma formation and organ damage, often involving the liver and cardiovascular system. Infection of the central nervous system (neurosyphilis) can occur at any stage. Acquired syphilis almost always is contracted through direct sexual contact with ulcerative lesions of the skin or mucous membranes of infected people. Congenital syphilis most often is acquired through hematogenous transplacental infection of the fetus, although direct contact of the infant with infectious lesions during or after delivery also can result in infection. Among women with untreated early syphilis, as many as 40% of pregnancies result in spontaneous abortion, stillbirth, or perinatal death. Transplacental infection can occur throughout pregnancy and at any stage of maternal infection.

Antepartum Management

All pregnant women should be serologically screened for syphilis as early as possible in pregnancy. False-negative serologic test results may occur in early primary infection, and infection may be acquired later in pregnancy. Therefore, in communities and populations with a high prevalence, serologic testing should also be performed at 28–32 weeks of gestation and at again at delivery. Some states require all women to be screened at delivery. *Treponema pallidum* is a fastidious spirochete that cannot be cultured on artificial media. Microscopic dark-field and histologic examinations for spirochetes are most reliable when lesions are present. Syphilis is commonly diagnosed with a combination of nontreponemal and treponemal serology. The specificity of serologic testing is high if both a nontreponemal screening test (Venereal Disease Research Laboratories [VDRL] or rapid plasma reagin [RPR] test result) and a subsequent treponemal serologic test result are reactive. Nontreponemal tests measure antibodies to the lipoidal antigen from *T pallidum*, antibody interaction with host tissues, or both. Treponemal tests include fluorescent treponemal antibody absorbed (FTA-ABS) tests, the *T pallidum* passive particle agglutination (TP-PA) assay, various enzyme immunoassays (EIAs), chemiluminescence immunoassays, immunoblots, or rapid treponemal assays. There are no commercially available nucleic acid-based tests. False-positive nontreponemal test results can occur with pregnancy as well as with infections such as HIV, autoimmune conditions, immunizations, injection drug use, and older age. Primary use of treponemal tests also can be complicated by false-positive test results, as well as detection of prior, treated infection and incompletely treated infection. Therefore, both nontreponemal and treponemal positive screening test results must be confirmed with a complementary confirmatory test.

Pregnant women with syphilis should be treated with a penicillin regimen appropriate to the stage of infection. Primary, secondary, and early latent syphilis are treated with benzathine penicillin G, 2.4 million units intramuscularly. Late latent and tertiary syphilis are treated with 3 doses of benzathine penicillin G, 2.4 million units intramuscularly at weekly intervals. Neurosyphilis is treated with intravenous penicillin for 10–14 days. Although alternate treatment regimens are available for nonpregnant women with penicillin allergy, penicillin G is the only reliable treatment in pregnancy. Alternate regimens are either contraindicated in pregnancy (tetracycline, doxycycline) or ineffective. Erythromycin and azithromycin neither reliably cure maternal infection nor treat an infected fetus. Women who are allergic to penicillin should be desensitized and then treated with penicillin. During treatment, women should be observed for signs of a Jarisch–Herxheimer reaction (an immune response to toxins released when spirochetes die), which may cause fever, nonreassuring fetal status, and preterm labor. For women treated for syphilis during pregnancy, follow-up nontreponemal serologic testing is necessary to assess the effectiveness of therapy. Treated pregnant women with syphilis should have quantitative nontreponemal serologic tests repeated at 28–32 weeks of gestation, at delivery, and according to recommendations for the stage of disease. Serologic titers may be repeated monthly in women at high risk of reinfection or in geographic areas where the prevalence of syphilis is high.

Women with syphilis should be asked about illicit substance use, especially cocaine. Results of the maternal serologic tests and treatment, if given, should be recorded in the newborn infant's medical record and be made available to the infant's pediatrician.

Neonatal Management

No newborn infant should be discharged from the hospital without determination of the mother's serologic status for syphilis. All infants born to seropositive mothers require a careful examination, and a nontreponemal test performed on the infant. An infant should be evaluated for congenital syphilis if he or she is born to a mother with a positive treponemal test result who has one or more of the following conditions:

- Syphilis and HIV infection
- Untreated or inadequately treated syphilis
- Syphilis during pregnancy treated with a nonpenicillin regimen and inadequate regimen, such as erythromycin

- Syphilis during pregnancy treated with an appropriate penicillin regimen that failed to produce the expected fourfold decrease in non-treponemal antibody titer after therapy
- Syphilis treated less than 1 month before delivery (because treatment failures occur, and the efficacy of treatment cannot be assumed without sufficient time for an expected decrease in nontreponemal antibody titer)
- Syphilis treatment not documented
- Syphilis treated before pregnancy but with insufficient serologic follow-up during pregnancy to assess the response to treatment and current infection status

The diagnostic and therapeutic approach to infants delivered to mothers with syphilis is outlined in Figure 12-3. Infant evaluation should include the following:

- Serum VDRL or RPR (same test as mother to facilitate comparison of titers)
- Complete blood cell count and platelet count
- Liver function tests
- Cerebrospinal fluid examination for cell count, protein, and quantitative VDRL

In addition, depending on the results of these tests, evaluation may include the following:

- Chest radiograph and long bone radiographs
- Eye examination
- Neuroimaging
- Auditory brainstem responses

Management decisions are based on the three possible maternal situations: 1) maternal treatment before pregnancy, 2) adequate maternal treatment and response during pregnancy, or 3) inadequate maternal treatment, inadequate maternal response to treatment, or reinfection during pregnancy.

For proven or probable congenital syphilis (based on the infant's physical examination and radiographic and laboratory testing), the preferred treatment is aqueous crystalline penicillin G, administered intravenously. The

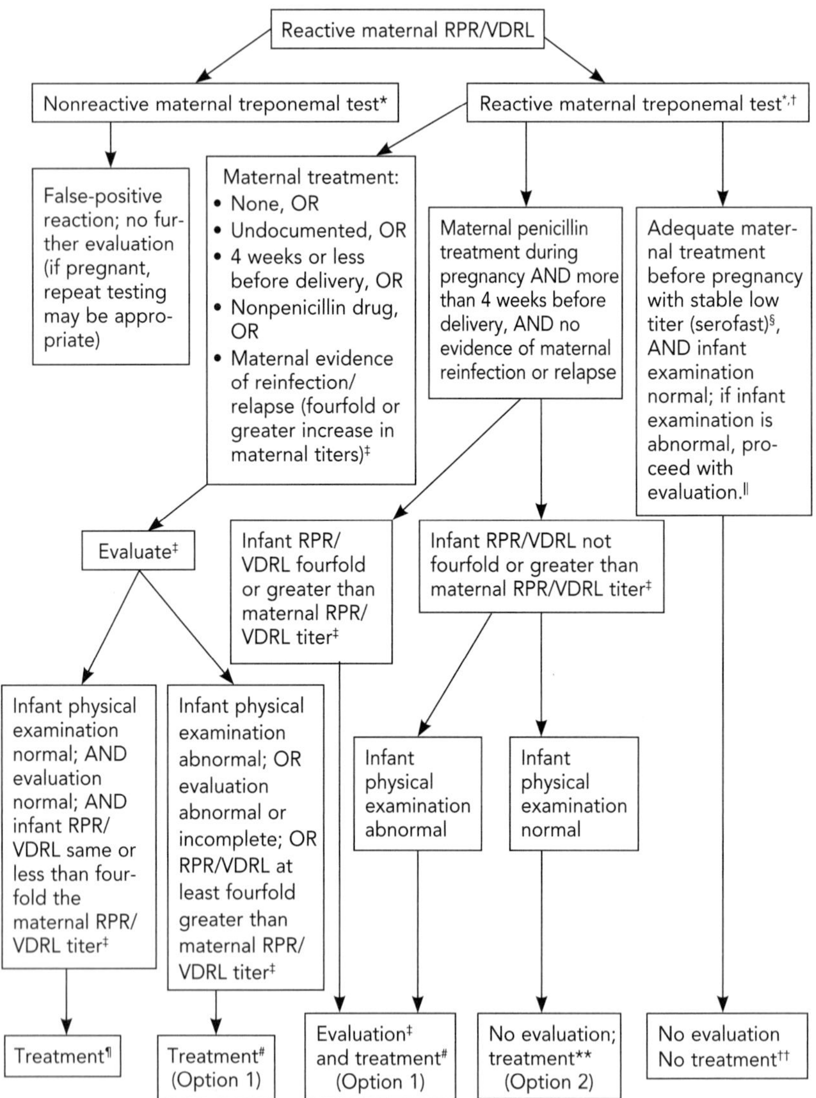

Figure 12-3. Algorithm for evaluation and treatment of infants born to mothers with reactive serologic tests for syphilis. Abbreviations: FTA-ABS, fluorescent treponemal antibody absorption; MHA-TP, microhemagglutination test for antibodies to Treponema pallidum; RPR, rapid plasma reagin; TP-EIA, T pallidum enzyme immunoassay; TP-PA, T pallidum particle agglutination; VDRL, Venereal Disease Research Laboratory.

*FTA-ABS, MHA-TP, TP-EIA, or TP-PA.

†Test for human immunodeficiency virus (HIV) antibody. Infants of HIV-infected mothers do not require different evaluation or treatment.

‡A fourfold change in titer is the same as a change of 2 dilutions. For example, a titer of 1:64 is fourfold greater than a titer of 1:16, and a titer of 1:4 is fourfold lower than a titer of 1:16.

§Women who maintain a VDRL titer 1:2 or less or an RPR 1:4 or less beyond 1 year after successful treatment are considered serofast.

||Complete blood cell and platelet count; cerebrospinal fluid examination for cell count, protein, and qualitative VDRL; other tests as clinically indicated (eg, chest radiographs, long bone radiographs, eye examination, liver function tests, neuroimaging, and auditory brainstem response).

¶Treatment (option 1 or option 2, below), with many experts recommending treatment option 1. If a single dose of benzathine penicillin G is used, then the infant must be fully evaluated, full evaluation must be normal, and follow-up must be certain. If any part of the infant's evaluation is abnormal or not performed, or if the cerebrospinal fluid analysis is rendered uninterpretable, then a 10-day course of penicillin is required.

#Treatment option 1: Aqueous penicillin G, 50,000 units/kg, intravenously, every 12 hours (1 week of age or younger) or every 8 hours (older than 1 week); or procaine penicillin G, 50,000 units/kg, intramuscularly, as a single daily dose for 10 days. If 24 or more hours of therapy are missed, the entire course must be restarted.

**Treatment option 2: Benzathine penicillin G, 50,000 units/kg, intramuscularly, single dose.

††Some experts would consider a single intramuscular injection of benzathine penicillin (treatment option 2), particularly if follow-up is not certain.

American Academy of Pediatrics. Red book: report of the Committee on Infectious Diseases, 29th. Elk Grove Village (IL): American Academy of Pediatrics; 2012.

dosage should be based on chronologic age rather than gestational age and is 50,000 units per kg, intravenously, every 12 hours (for infants 1 week of age or younger) or every 8 hours (for infants older than 1 week). Alternatively, procaine penicillin G, 50,000 units per kg can be administered intramuscularly as a single daily dose for 10 days. No treatment failures have occurred with this formulation despite its low CSF concentrations. When the infant is at risk of congenital syphilis because of inadequate maternal treatment or response to treatment or reinfection during pregnancy but the infant's physical examination, radiographic imaging, and laboratory analyses are normal (including an infant RPR/VDRL either the same as or less than fourfold higher than the maternal RPR/VDRL; see Figure 12-3 for examples), some experts would treat the infant with a single dose of penicillin G benzathine (50,000 units per kg intramuscularly), but most still would prefer 10 days of treatment. If more than 1 day of therapy is missed, the entire course should be restarted. Data supporting use of other antimicrobial agents (eg, ampicillin) for treatment of congenital syphilis are not available. When possible, a full 10-day course of penicillin is preferred, even if ampicillin initially was provided for possible sepsis. Use of agents other than penicillin requires close serologic follow-up to assess adequacy of therapy.

Infants who have a normal physical examination and a serum quantitative nontreponemal serologic titer less than fourfold the maternal titer are at minimal risk of syphilis if they are born to mothers who completed appropriate penicillin treatment for syphilis during pregnancy more than 4 weeks before delivery, and if the mother has no evidence of reinfection or relapse. Although a full evaluation may be unnecessary, these infants should be treated with a single intramuscular injection of penicillin G benzathine because fetal treatment failure can occur despite adequate maternal treatment during pregnancy. Alternatively, these infants may be examined carefully, preferably monthly, until their nontreponemal serologic test results are negative.

Infants who have a normal physical examination and a serum quantitative nontreponemal serologic titer less than fourfold the maternal titer, whose mother's treatment was adequate before pregnancy, and whose mother's nontreponemal serologic titer remained low and stable before and during pregnancy and at delivery (VDRL less than 1:2; RPR less than 1:4) require no evaluation. Some experts, however, would treat with penicillin G benzathine as a single intramuscular injection if follow-up is uncertain. All infants who have reactive serologic tests for syphilis or were born to mothers who were seroreactive at delivery should receive careful follow-up evaluations during regularly scheduled well-child care visits at 2, 4, 6, and 12 months of age. Serologic nontreponemal tests should be performed every 2–3 months until the nontreponemal test becomes nonreactive.

Lyme Disease

Lyme disease is caused by a spirochete (*Borrelia burgdorferi*) transmitted by the bite of a deer tick. The early localized stage of the disease is characterized by a distinctive "bull's-eye" skin lesion (erythema migrans) that occurs in 60–80% of patients and nonspecific, flu-like symptoms. Early disseminated disease can result in multiple erythema migrans several weeks after a tick bite, cranial nerve palsies (especially cranial nerve VII) or carditis within 4–6 weeks after the onset of early signs and symptoms. A late manifestation of Lyme disease is relapsing arthritis, usually pauciarticular and affecting large joints. Patients in the later stages of Lyme disease usually will be seropositive, but false-positive and false-negative test results are common.

Suspicion of early maternal infection is based on a history of exposure to tick bites, the presence of the distinctive erythema migrans rash, and nonspecific, flu-like symptoms. Adequately treated patients may never develop antibodies to spirochetes. Because congenital infection occurs with other spirochetal infections, there has been concern that an infected pregnant woman could transmit *B burgdorferi* to her fetus. However, Lyme disease is not thought to produce a congenital infection syndrome. No causal relationship between maternal Lyme disease and abnormalities of pregnancy and congenital disease caused by *B burgdorferi* has been documented. No evidence shows that Lyme disease can be transmitted through breast milk. The infant's health care provider should be informed when maternal disease is suspected.

Recommended treatment of suspected early disease in pregnant women is amoxicillin, 500 mg three times per day, for 2–3 weeks. For women who are allergic to penicillin, erythromycin is recommended for 2–3 weeks. For patients who are unable to tolerate erythromycin, cefuroxime axetil is an alternative for patients with immediate and anaphylactic hypersensitivity to penicillin who have undergone penicillin desensitization. Multiple other regimens are recommended for later stages of Lyme disease.

The best preventive measure is to avoid heavily wooded areas. If entrance into such areas is necessary, long-sleeved shirts and long pants tucked in at the ankle are helpful. Prophylactic antibiotic therapy for deer tick bites is not recommended routinely.

Parasitic Infections

Malaria

Although malaria mainly is confined to tropical areas of Africa, Asia, and Latin America, international travel and migration have made malaria a disease to consider in developed countries. Transmission is possible in certain parts of the United States, but the vast majority of U.S. cases are found in individuals who have returned from international travel. The classic symptoms are high fever with chills, rigors, sweats, and headache.

Severe malaria can manifest as potentially fatal neurologic, renal, respiratory or cardiovascular failure, as well as anemia and hypoglycemia. Malaria infection may be more severe in pregnant women and also may increase the risk of adverse outcomes of pregnancy, including spontaneous abortion, stillbirth, preterm birth, and low birth weight. Because of the risk to both the woman and the fetus, and because no chemoprophylactic regimen is completely effective, pregnant women (or women likely to become pregnant) should avoid travel to malaria-endemic areas. If travel to a malaria-endemic area is necessary, appropriate consultation should be sought for chemoprophylaxis recommendations based on the malaria species and drug-resistance patterns prevalent in that area. Health care professionals should check the CDC website, www.cdc.gov/travel when providing pretravel malaria advice or evaluating a febrile returned traveler.

Congenital malaria is rare. Signs and symptoms resemble those of neonatal sepsis. Definitive diagnosis (of the mother and the infant) relies on identification of the parasite on stained blood films. Both thick and thin films should be examined. Treatment of infection is based on the infecting species, possible drug resistance, severity of disease, and parasitic burden. If malaria is a diagnostic consideration in a pregnant woman or newborn, consultation with appropriate specialists is recommended for optimal patient management.

Toxoplasmosis

Toxoplasmosis is caused by the intracellular parasite *Toxoplasma gondii. Toxoplasma gondii* exists in several forms: a trophozoite, which is the invasive form, and a cyst or an oocyst, which are latent forms. Human infection is acquired by consumption of cysts in undercooked meat from infected animals, consumption of insect-contaminated food, contact with oocysts from the feces of infected cats (the only definitive hosts), or contact with infected materials or insects in soil. Infection with *T gondii* usually is asymptomatic, although after an incubation period of 5–18 days, some nonspecific symptoms may occur. In the immunocompetent adult, the clinical course is benign and self-limited. Most often, toxoplasmosis presents as asymptomatic cervical lymphadenopathy, with symptoms occurring in only 10–20% of infected adults. Other symptoms include fever, malaise, night sweats, myalgias, and hepatosplenomegaly. Parasitemia can occur after infection, which in pregnant women can seed the placenta and cause subsequent fetal infection. Congenital transmission of *T gondii* from an infected woman results in an overall risk of congenital toxoplasmosis ranging from 20% to 50% without treatment. The later in pregnancy that the infection occurs, the more likely transmission is to occur. The rate of vertical transmission increases from 10% to 15% in the first trimester to 25% in the second trimester and to more than 60% in the third trimester. The severity of fetal infection depends on gestational age at the time of transmission. The earlier the fetus is infected, the more severe the disease. Most infected infants do not have clinical signs of infection at birth, but as many as 90% will develop sequelae, including chorioretinitis and subsequent severe visual impairment, hearing loss, or severe neurodevelopmental delay. Other clinical manifestations of congenital toxoplasmosis include rash, hepatosplenomegaly, ascites, fever, periventricular calcifications, ventriculomegaly, and seizures.

Immunoglobulin M antibodies appear soon after acute infection and reach maximum levels in 1 month. Immunoglobulin G antibodies appear after IgM antibodies, are detectable within a few weeks after infection, and confer immunity. High titers of IgG and IgM may persist for years.

Antepartum Management

Routine serologic screening of pregnant women for toxoplasmosis is not recommended. There are many challenges involved in routine screening, including a relatively low seroprevalence (approximately 38% of pregnant women have evidence of prior toxoplasmosis infection), which means that most women are susceptible to infection; relatively low incidence of acute infection; lack of standardized serologic assays outside of reference laboratories; and cost. In the United States, prenatal screening for toxoplasmosis should be limited to women who are immunosuppressed or human immunodeficiency virus (HIV)-positive.

The diagnosis of maternal infection is based on serologic test results for the detection of *Toxoplasma*-specific antibodies. Both IgG and IgM testing should be used for the initial evaluation of patients suspected to have toxoplasmosis. A negative IgM test result and a positive IgG test result are indicative of remote infection and pose no concern for fetal transmission in an immunocompetent woman. A negative IgM test result essentially excludes recent infection, but a positive IgM test result is difficult to interpret because *Toxoplasma*-specific IgM antibodies may persist for many months or years after acute infection. In addition, false-positive test results are common with commercially available kits. Immunoglobulin G avidity testing may be helpful in determining the timing of infection among pregnant women. Before making treatment recommendations, confirmation of diagnosis should be made based on results obtained in a reference laboratory. Additional information on laboratory diagnosis of toxoplasmosis is available from the CDC website at www.cdc.gov/dpdx and www.pamf.org/serology/clinicianguide.html.

Treatment of the pregnant woman with acute toxoplasmosis reduces but does not eliminate the risk of congenital infection but may reduce congenital disease severity. In the presence of acute maternal infection, consultation with an expert in maternal–fetal medicine or infectious diseases should be obtained. Pregnant women who are acutely infected with toxoplasmosis should be treated with spiramycin to reduce transplacental parasitic transfer. Spiramycin is a macrolide antibiotic that concentrates in, but does not readily cross, the placenta. Use of spiramycin after confirmatory testing in a reference laboratory generally requires assistance from the FDA because the drug is not commercially available in the United States. Fetal infection with toxoplasmosis should be treated with a combination of pyrimethamine, sulfadiazine, and folinic acid because this regimen more effectively eradicates parasites in the placenta and fetus than spiramycin alone and can lessen the severity of disease in the affected fetus.

Neonatal Management

A definitive diagnosis of congenital toxoplasmosis can be made prenatally by detecting parasite DNA in amniotic fluid by PCR. Serial prenatal ultrasound examinations can detect evolving evidence of fetal infection such as visceral calcifications and ventriculomegaly. Congenital toxoplasmosis can be diagnosed serologically by the detection of antitoxoplasma-specific IgM or immunoglobulin A antibodies soon after birth or by the persistence of antitoxoplasma IgG beyond 12 months of age. If the diagnosis is suspected but unconfirmed at the time of birth, ophthalmologic, auditory, and neurologic examinations should be performed.

For healthy appearing infants and for those with clinical signs of congenital toxoplasmosis, treatment with pyrimethamine and sulfadiazine (supplemented with folinic acid) is recommended for 1 year. Additional medications and different treatment timing may be recommended depending on the extent of symptomatic disease. Alternate regimens may be used if sulfonamide compounds are not tolerated. Eye and brain disease may require additional treatment with corticosteroids. Infants with congenital toxoplasmosis should be managed in consultation with infectious disease specialists. Additional professional and patient information is available on the CDC website at www.cdc.gov/parasites/toxoplasmosis/ and detailed treatment information is available in the AAP Red Book.

Infections with High-Risk Infection Control Issues, Emerging Infections, and Bioterrorism

A number of infectious diseases are of intermittent concern to U.S. citizens, primarily because of the spread of emerging infections from international travel or from bioterrorist threats. Infectious agents in this category include *Bacillus anthracis* (cause of anthrax), viral hemorrhagic fever agents (eg, Ebola, Lassa, Marburg viruses), coronaviruses (eg, the viruses causing Middle East respiratory syndrome [MERS] and severe acute respiratory syndrome [SARS]) and smallpox. When there is a specific concern for one of these potentially fatal infections, perinatal providers must partner with local public health officials as well as hospital infection control and emergency preparedness personnel to arrange appropriate care. Specific medical information on individual agents will not be provided here because recommended therapies, vaccines, and infection control practices evolve quickly. The CDC website (www.cdc.gov/), particularly the Division of High-Consequence Pathogens and Pathology (DHCPP) section (www.cdc.gov/ncezid/dhcpp/index.html), should be consulted for the most current information. Perinatal providers should partner with hospital officials to ensure that institutional preparedness plans for high-risk infections and toxic exposure include consideration of the specific needs of pregnant women and newborns.

Bibliography

Abzug MJ, Michaels MG, Wald E, Jacobs RF, Romero JR, Sanchez PJ, et al. A randomized, double-blind, placebo-controlled trial of pleconaril for the treatment of neonates with enterovirus sepsis. National Institute of Allergy and Infectious Diseases Collaborative Antiviral Study Group. J Pediatric Infect Dis Soc 2016;5:53–62.

American Academy of Pediatrics. Red book: report of the Committee on Infectious Diseases. 30th ed. Elk Grove Village (IL): AAP; 2015.

Class II special controls guidance document: herpes simplex virus types 1 and 2 serological assays. Guidance for Industry and Food and Drug Administration Staff. Silver Spring (MD): Food and Drug Administration; 2011. Available at: http://www.fda.gov/downloads/MedicalDevices/DeviceRegulationandGuidance/GuidanceDocuments/UCM227597.pdf. Retrieved November 16, 2016.

Cytomegalovirus, Parvovirus B19, Varicella Zoster, and Toxoplasmosis in pregnancy. Practice Bulletin No. 151. American College of Obstetricians and Gynecologists [published erratum appears in Obstet Gynecol 2016;127:405]. Obstet Gynecol 2015;125:1510–25.

Elimination of perinatal hepatitis b: providing the first vaccine dose within 24 hours of birth. American Academy of Pediatrics Committee on Infectious Diseases. Pediatrics 2017:140:e20171870.

Havens PL, Mofenson LM. Evaluation and management of the infant exposed to HIV-1 in the United States. American Academy of Pediatrics Committee on Pediatric AIDS [published erratum appears in Pediatrics 2012;130:1183–4]. Pediatrics 2009;123:175–87.

Hendricks KA, Wright ME, Shadomy SV, Bradley JS, Morrow MG, Pavia AT, et al. Centers for Disease Control and Prevention Expert Panel meetings on prevention and treatment of anthrax in adults. Workgroup on Anthrax Clinical Guidelines. Emerg Infect Dis 2014;20.

Higgins RD, Saade G, Polin RA, Grobman WA, Buhimschi IA, Watterberg K, et al. Evaluation and management of women and newborns with a maternal diagnosis of chorioamnionitis: summary of a workshop. Chorioamnionitis Workshop Participants. Obstet Gynecol 2016;127:426–36.

Human papillomavirus vaccination. Committee Opinion No. 704. American College of Obstetricians and Gynecologists. Obstet Gynecol 2017;129:e173–8.

Infant feeding and transmission of human immunodeficiency virus in the United States. Committee on Pediatric AIDS. Pediatrics 2013;131:391–6.

Influenza vaccination during pregnancy. Committee Opinion No. 608. American College of Obstetricians and Gynecologists. Obstet Gynecol 2014;124:648–51.

Kimberlin DW, Baley J. Guidance on management of asymptomatic neonates born to women with active genital herpes lesions. Committee on Infectious Diseases and Committee on Fetus and Newborn. Pediatrics 2013;131:e635–46.

Kimberlin DW, Jester PM, Sanchez PJ, Ahmed A, Arav-Boger R, Michaels MG, et al. Valganciclovir for symptomatic congenital cytomegalovirus disease. National Institute of Allergy and Infectious Diseases Collaborative Antiviral Study Group. N Engl J Med 2015;372:933–43.

Madhi SA, Cutland CL, Kuwanda L, Weinberg A, Hugo A, Jones S, et al. Influenza vaccination of pregnant women and protection of their infants. Maternal Flu Trial (Matflu) Team. N Engl J Med 2014;371:918–31.

Management of herpes in pregnancy. ACOG Practice Bulletin No. 82. American College of Obstetricians and Gynecologists. Obstet Gynecol 2007;109:1489–98.

Management of pregnant women with presumptive exposure to Listeria monocytogenes. Committee Opinion No. 614. American College of Obstetricians and Gynecologists. Obstet Gynecol 2014;124:1241–4.

Markowitz LE, Dunne EF, Saraiya M, Lawson HW, Chesson H, Unger ER. Quadrivalent human papillomavirus vaccine: recommendations of the Advisory Committee on Immunization Practices (ACIP). Centers for Disease Control and Prevention (CDC), Advisory Committee on Immunization Practices (ACIP). MMWR Recomm Rep 2007;56:1–24.

Meaney-Delman D, Zotti ME, Creanga AA, Misegades LK, Wako E, Treadwell TA, et al. Special considerations for prophylaxis for and treatment of anthrax in pregnant and postpartum women. Workgroup on Anthrax in Pregnant and Postpartum Women. Emerg Infect Dis 2014;20.

O'Leary DR, Kuhn S, Kniss KL, Hinckley AF, Rasmussen SA, Pape WJ, et al. Birth outcomes following west nile virus infection of pregnant women in the United States: 2003-2004. Pediatrics 2006;117:e537–45.

Prenatal and perinatal human immunodeficiency virus testing: expanded recommendations. Committee Opinion No. 635. American College of Obstetricians and Gynecologists. Obstet Gynecol 2015;125:1544–7.

Prevention of early-onset group B streptococcal disease in newborns. Committee Opinion No. 485. American College of Obstetricians and Gynecologists. Obstet Gynecol 2011;117:1019–27.

Puopolo KM, Draper D, Wi S, Newman TB, Zupancic J, Lieberman E, et al. Estimating the probability of neonatal early-onset infection on the basis of maternal risk factors. Pediatrics 2011;128:e1155–63.

Recommendations for use of antiretroviral drugs in pregnant HIV-1-infected women for maternal health and interventions to reduce perinatal HIV transmission in the United States. Panel on Treatment of HIV-Infected Pregnant Women and Prevention of Perinatal Transmission. Rockville (MD): National Institutes of Health; 2016. Available at: http://aidsinfo.nih.gov/contentfiles/lvguidelines/PerinatalGL.pdf. Retrieved November 16, 2016.

Revello MG, Lazzarotto T, Guerra B, Spinillo A, Ferrazzi E, Kustermann A, et al. A randomized trial of hyperimmune globulin to prevent congenital cytomegalovirus. CHIP Study Group. N Engl J Med 2014;370:1316–26.

Schrag SJ, Farley MM, Petit S, Reingold A, Weston EJ, Pondo T, et al. Epidemiology of invasive early-onset neonatal sepsis, 2005 to 2014. Pediatrics 2016;138:e20162013.

Stoll BJ, Hansen NI, Sanchez PJ, Faix RG, Poindexter BB, Van Meurs KP, et al. Early onset neonatal sepsis: the burden of group B streptococcal and E. coli disease continues. Eunice Kennedy Shriver National Institute of Child Health and Human Development Neonatal Research Network [Published Erratum Appears in Pediatrics 2011;128:390]. Pediatrics 2011;127:817–26.

U.S. Preventive Services Task Force. Syphilis infection in pregnancy: summary. Rockville (MD): USPSTF; 2009. Available at: http://www.uspreventiveservicestaskforce.org/Page/Document/ClinicalSummaryFinal/syphilis-infection-in-pregnancy-screening. Retrieved March 7, 2017.

Update on immunization and pregnancy: tetanus, diphtheria, and pertussis vaccination. ACOG Committee Opinion No. 566. American College of Obstetricians and Gynecologists. Obstet Gynecol 2013;121:1411–4.

Updated guidance for palivizumab prophylaxis among infants and young children at increased risk of hospitalization for respiratory syncytial virus infection. American Academy of Pediatrics Committee on Infectious Diseases, American Academy of Pediatrics Bronchiolitis Guidelines Committee [published erratum appears in Pediatrics 2014;134:1221]. Pediatrics 2014;134:415–20.

Verani JR, McGee L, Schrag SJ. Prevention of perinatal group B streptococcal disease--revised guidelines from CDC, 2010. Division of Bacterial Diseases, National Center for Immunization and Respiratory Diseases, Centers for Disease Control and Prevention. MMWR Recomm Rep 2010;59(RR-10):1–36.

Viral hepatitis in pregnancy. ACOG Practice Bulletin No. 86. American College of Obstetricians and Gynecologists. Obstet Gynecol 2007;110:941–56.

Winter K, Cherry JD, Harriman K. Effectiveness of prenatal tetanus, diphtheria, and acellular pertussis vaccination on pertussis severity in infants. Clin Infect Dis 2017;64:9–14.

Winter K, Nickell S, Powell M, Harriman K. Effectiveness of prenatal versus postpartum tetanus, diphtheria, and acellular pertussis vaccination in preventing infant pertussis. Clin Infect Dis 2017;64:3–8.

Workowski KA, Bolan GA. Sexually transmitted diseases treatment guidelines, 2015. Centers for Disease Control and Prevention [published erratum appears in MMWR Recomm Rep 2015;64:924]. MMWR Recomm Rep 2015;64:1–137.

Zaman K, Roy E, Arifeen SE, Rahman M, Raqib R, Wilson E, et al. Effectiveness of maternal influenza immunization in mothers and infants [published erratum appears in N Engl J Med 2009;360:648]. N Engl J Med 2008;359:1555–64.

Resources

AIDSinfo: offering information on HIV/AIDS treatment, prevention, and research. Rockville (MD): National Institutes of Health; 2016. Available at: http://www.aidsinfo.nih.gov. Retrieved November 16, 2016.

American Academy of Pediatrics. Red book: report of the Committee on Infectious Diseases. 30th ed. Elk Grove Village (IL): AAP; 2015.

American College of Obstetricians and Gynecologists. Immunization for women. Washington, DC: American College of Obstetricians and Gynecologists; 2016. Available at: http://immunizationforwomen.org. Retrieved October 26, 2016.

Division of High-Consequence Pathogens and Pathology (DHCPP). Atlanta (GA): CDC; 2017. Available at: https://www.cdc.gov/ncezid/dhcpp/index.html. Retrieved March 7, 2017.

Guidelines for vaccinating pregnant women. Atlanta (GA): CDC; 2016. Available at: https://www.cdc.gov/vaccines/pregnancy/hcp/guidelines.html. Retrieved December 20, 2016; March 7, 2017.

Centers for Disease Control and Prevention. Cytomegalovirus (CMV) and congenital CMV infection. Atlanta (GA): CDC; 2016. Available at: http://www.cdc.gov/cmv/congenital-infection.html. Retrieved November 16, 2016.

Centers for Disease Control and Prevention. Listeria (Listeriosis). Atlanta, GA: CDC; 2016. Available at: https://www.cdc.gov/listeria. Retrieved October 28, 2016.

Centers for Disease Control and Prevention. Parasites - Toxoplasmosis (Toxoplasma Infection): Toxoplasmosis & pregnancy FAQs. Atlanta (GA): CDC; 2015. Available at: http://www.cdc.gov/parasites/toxoplasmosis/gen_info/pregnant.html. Retrieved November 16, 2016.

Centers for Disease Control and Prevention. Vaccines and immunizations. Atlanta (GA): CDC; 2016. Available at: http://www.cdc.gov/vaccines. Retrieved October 26, 2016.

Morof DF, Carroll ID. Advising travelers with specific needs: pregnant travelers. In: Centers for Disease Control and Prevention. CDC health information for international travel 2016. New York (NY): Oxford University Press; 2016. Available at: http://wwwnc.cdc.gov/travel/yellowbook/2016/advising-travelers-with-specific-needs/pregnant-travelers. Retrieved November 16, 2016.

United States Department of Agriculture Food Safety and Inspection Service. Protect your baby and yourself from Listeriosis. Washington, DC: USDA; 2013. Available at: http://www.fsis.usda.gov/wps/portal/fsis/topics/food-safety-education/get-answers/food-safety-fact-sheets/foodborne-illness-and-disease/protect-your-baby-and-yourself-from-listeriosis/ct_index. Retrieved November 16, 2016.

Updated guidance for palivizumab prophylaxis among infants and young children at increased risk of hospitalization for respiratory syncytial virus infection. American Academy of Pediatrics Committee on Infectious Diseases, American Academy of Pediatrics Bronchiolitis Guidelines Committee [Published erratum appears in Pediatrics 2014;134:1221]. Pediatrics 2014;134:415–20.

Verani JR, McGee L, Schrag SJ. Prevention of perinatal group B streptococcal disease--revised guidelines from CDC, 2010. Division of Bacterial Diseases, National Center for Immunization and Respiratory Diseases, Centers for Disease Control and Prevention. MMWR Recomm Rep 2010;59(RR-10):1–36.

Chapter 13

Infection Control

Serious hospital-acquired infection of the mother–newborn dyad is rare. However, when colonization with certain organisms occurs, the outcome may be devastating for the newborn, the mother, or both. Many of the nosocomial infections that occur in intensive care units are caused by pathogens acquired from the hospital environment (ie, health care-associated infections). Health care-associated infections result in increased morbidity and mortality, prolonged lengths of hospital stay, and increased medical costs.

Definition of Health Care-Associated Infection

Health care-associated infection is defined as an infection that is acquired in the hospital while receiving treatment for other conditions. This definition should be applied consistently to allow uniform reporting and analysis of health care-associated infections. The infection control committee of each hospital should work with perinatal care personnel to ensure that appropriate surveillance of health care-associated infection is being performed. For obstetric patients, a health care-associated infection can be defined broadly as one that is not present or incubating when the patient is admitted to the hospital and occurs more than 48 hours after hospitalization. Many cases of urinary tract infection that occur postpartum are health care-associated. Risk factors associated with health care-associated infection in the infant include preterm birth, the presence of invasive devices (intravascular catheters, endotracheal tubes, orogastric tubes, urinary catheters, drains), exposure to broad-spectrum antibiotic agents, parenteral nutrition, overcrowding and poor staffing ratios, administration of steroids and histamine-2 receptor blockers, and acuity of underlying illness.

Prevention and Control of Infections

Prevention of infections requires a multifaceted approach. This includes cleaning and decontamination of the environment, using meticulous patient care techniques, practicing hand hygiene, promoting breastfeeding (unless contraindicated because of maternal infection; see also "Contraindications to Breastfeeding" in Chapter 10), limiting the number of invasive procedures (eg, central lines), limiting the number of visitors, grouping together (cohorting) infants colonized with the same pathogen, and judicious use of antimicrobial therapy.

Labor and Delivery Admission Policy

The pediatric health care provider should be notified of all mothers admitted to the antepartum obstetrics unit who are colonized with or are chronic carriers of a potentially infectious organism that may be transmitted vertically to the newborn (eg, human immunodeficiency virus [HIV], hepatitis B [HBV] or hepatitis C virus [HCV], HSV, influenza, methicillin-resistant staphylococcus [MRSA], vancomycin-resistant enterococcus) or may be associated with a congenital infection. Group A streptococci and group B streptococci (GBS) are pathogens that may be indigenous to the female genital tract. Both may cause serious, life-threatening infections in the mother and newborn. There are national guidelines for the management of GBS colonization in the mother (see "Bacterial Infections" in Chapter 12).

Nursery Admission Policies

Infants transferred from another hospital and those who require rehospitalization within a few days of being discharged home ideally should be admitted to the newborn unit. Infants with suspected infectious diseases should be admitted to specialized areas whenever possible where additional transmission precautions (airborne, contact, droplet) can be provided to minimize the risks of spreading the infection to others.

Routine culturing of infants' respiratory or gastrointestinal tracts, or skin for surveillance purposes is not recommended, but cultures from lesions or sites of infection should be taken to identify the etiology. When clusters of infections caused by a single strain of bacteria are noted, appropriate personnel, such as hospital infection control professionals, should be notified. During an outbreak of infection, routine surveillance cultures of infants and nursery staff can be useful. It is important to document organisms colonizing all infants residing in the area where the outbreak occurred so that appropriate isolation and cohorting procedures can be undertaken. Routine screening for specific pathogens, such as MRSA, may be done as part of an institution's infection control program, but more research is needed to determine the circumstances in which this surveillance is most beneficial.

Standard Precautions

The Centers for Disease Control and Prevention (CDC) recommend that standard precautions be used for all patients. Standard precautions are intended to prevent transmission of bloodborne pathogens, recognizing the importance of all body fluids, secretions, excretions, and contaminated items in the transmission of health care-associated pathogens. These precautions apply to the following: blood, semen, vaginal secretions, cerebrospinal fluid, synovial fluid, pleural fluid, pericardial fluid, peritoneal fluid, amniotic fluid, saliva in dental procedures, any body fluid that is visibly contaminated with blood, and all body fluids in situations in which it is difficult or impossible to differentiate between body fluids. When exposure to blood or body fluids is possible, standard precautions include practicing hand hygiene before and after examining patients; wearing gloves (in addition to practicing hand hygiene); using masks, eye protection, and face shields; and wearing nonsterile gowns.

Disposal of equipment or materials contaminated with blood or other potentially infectious material always should be accomplished using standard precautions and careful hand hygiene practices. Instruments should not be shared, and each patient's bedside should be considered a separate, clean environment.

The federal Occupational Safety and Health Administration (OSHA) has issued regulations designed to minimize the transmission of HIV, HBV, and other potentially infectious organisms in the workplace. The OSHA guidelines are available at: www.osha.gov/SLTC/bloodbornepathogens/index.html. The regulations apply to all employees in physicians' offices, hospitals, medical laboratories, and other health care facilities where workers reasonably could be anticipated to come into contact with blood and other potentially infectious material. The OSHA regulations require employers to implement an exposure-control plan to minimize employees' exposure to bloodborne and infectious pathogens. The plan must contain the following components:

- Personal protective equipment for employees exposed to blood and other body fluids

- Housekeeping requirements
- Provision of HBV vaccination to employees
- Postexposure evaluation and follow-up procedures
- Employee training
- Use of warning labels
- Record-keeping requirements
- Adoption of certain work practice controls (eg, hand hygiene facilities, safer medical devices, such as needleless systems and sharps with engineered sharps protection)

These requirements are enforced by OSHA or, in the case of states with OSHA-approved comparable job safety and health plans, by state agencies. Violations are punishable by fines.

Health Standards for Personnel

Obstetric, nursery, and neonatal intensive care unit (NICU) personnel, as well as others who have significant contact with newborns, should be as free of transmissible infectious diseases as possible. Each hospital should establish written policies and procedures for assessing the health of personnel assigned to perinatal care services, restricting their contact with patients when necessary, maintaining their health records, and requiring staff to report any potentially infectious illness they may have. These policies and procedures should address screening for immunity to measles, rubella, mumps, varicella zoster, HBV, pertussis, tetanus, diphtheria, and exposure to tuberculosis. The frequency of and need for screening employees should be determined by local epidemiologic data. Personnel with active tuberculosis should be restricted from patient contact until adequate treatment has occurred and noninfective status has been verified. Vaccinations protect both staff and patients and may reduce health care costs. Immunization against measles, mumps, rubella, varicella, tetanus, diphtheria, pertussis, and HBV should be recommended to all susceptible, nonpregnant hospital personnel. In addition, tetanus, diphtheria, pertussis, HBV, and inactivated influenza vaccines should be recommended to all susceptible pregnant hospital personnel. Offering annual influenza immunization to all health care providers is strongly encouraged. Given the communicability of influenza, obstetric and pediatric care practices should consider alternative prevention strategies (eg, wearing a mask) during peak influenza season for staff who are unable or unwilling to receive influenza vaccination.

Bloodborne pathogens, such as HBV, hepatitis C virus, and HIV may be transmitted from infected patients to health care workers as well as from infected health care workers to patients. To reduce the risk of transmission, all practicing obstetric and neonatal care providers should receive the HBV vaccine. Health care providers infected with HBV, HCV, or HIV are advised to follow the updated recommendations from the Society for Healthcare Epidemiology of America regarding infection control measures, supervision, and periodic testing (available at: www.jstor.org/stable/pdf/10.1086/650298.pdf). The recommendations provide a framework within which to consider such cases; however, each case should be independently considered by an expert review panel. Such an expert panel may include the following: the health care provider's personal physician, an infectious disease specialist, a health care professional with expertise in the procedures performed by the health care provider, state or local public health official(s), and a hospital epidemiologist or other member of the infection control committee of the hospital.

Individuals with a respiratory, cutaneous, mucocutaneous, or gastrointestinal infection should not have direct contact with newborns. Personnel with exudative skin lesions or weeping dermatitis should refrain from all direct patient care and should not handle patient care equipment until the condition resolves. Personnel in contact with newborns should report personal infections, inability to perform adequate hand hygiene (eg, because of casts or braces), and other conditions to their immediate supervisors and should be medically examined by employee health to determine suitability for patient contact. Decisions regarding the exclusion of staff members from obstetric and nursery areas should be made on an individual basis. Employee health policies should be worded and applied in a way to ensure that personnel feel free to report infectious problems without fear of repercussions.

Transmission of HSV from infected personnel to infants in newborn nurseries is rare. Personnel with cold sores who have direct contact with newborns should cover their lesions and carefully observe hand hygiene policies. Transmission of HSV infection from personnel with genital lesions is not likely. Personnel with herpetic hand infections (herpetic whitlow) should not participate in patient care until the lesions have healed.

Nursery personnel can be exposed to infants excreting cytomegalovirus. Acquisition of cytomegalovirus infection from infants is minimized by adherence to standard precautions. Women of childbearing age who work in neonatal units should be counseled about the relatively low risk of exposure should they become pregnant. A routine program of serologic testing of obstetric and nursery hospital employees for immunity to cytomegalovirus is not recommended.

Employee education regarding standard precautions and other proper infection control techniques should occur regularly. All personnel should be required to follow strictly established infection control procedures.

Personnel who care for women during pregnancy and the postpartum period and their infants should collaborate with hospital infection control personnel in conducting and reviewing the results of surveillance programs for health care-associated infections. This type of monitoring provides information about any unusual problems or clusters of infection, the risks associated with certain procedures or techniques, and the success of specific preventive measures. It also can reveal temporal trends, allow comparison with other obstetric and neonatal units by using standard definitions, and provide feedback to responsible personnel working in these units.

Hand Hygiene

Proper hand hygiene before and after each patient contact is the single most effective method for reducing health care-associated infections. In 2009, the World Health Organization (WHO) published new consensus recommendations for hand hygiene. The WHO guidelines provide a comprehensive overview of hand hygiene in health care and evidence-based and consensus-based recommendations for successful implementation and are available at http://apps.who.int/iris/bitstream/10665/44102/1/9789241597906_eng.pdf. The American Academy of Pediatrics has also published guidance on infection control and hand hygiene based on the WHO recommendations (available at: http://pediatrics.aappublications.org/content/120/3/650.long).

Dress Codes

Each hospital should establish dress codes for personnel who enter the labor, delivery, and nursery areas. Protective, long-sleeved gowns should be worn by all personnel who have direct contact with the sterile field during vaginal deliveries, obstetric surgical procedures, and surgical procedures in the nursery or NICU (eg, central line insertion). Hospital policies regarding sterile areas should be established and maintained. It has become commonplace for medical care providers to wear surgical scrubs to and from work. This has engendered controversy regarding the efficacy and safety of laundering surgical scrubs at home versus the hospital. According to the CDC, "the risk of actual disease transmission from soiled linen is negligible." It is further stated by the CDC that, "in the home, normal washing and drying cycles including 'hot' and 'cold' cycles are adequate to ensure patient safety." To date, there are no data indicating that there is any significant difference between home and hospital laundering of scrubs.

Some hospitals have approved more flexible dress codes for personnel who work in birthing rooms. However, based on the CDC's standard precautions for the prevention of infection with bloodborne pathogens, it is recommended that all health care workers who perform or assist in deliveries wear sterile gloves, gowns, surgical masks, and eye protection during the procedure. Wearing aprons or gowns made of impervious material during cesarean delivery may provide additional protection. Gloves should be worn when handling the placenta or the newborn until blood and amniotic fluid have been removed from the newborn's skin. Hands should be washed immediately before putting gloves on and after gloves are removed or when skin surfaces are contaminated with blood. Studies have demonstrated that the routine use of cover gowns is not necessary in the nursery or NICU.

Gowns and gloves should be worn when an infant is colonized with a resistant or invasive pathogen, consistent with appropriate isolation requirements. Additional personal protective equipment may be required on the basis of isolation requirements of the specific pathogen or clinical condition and the activity or procedure to be performed.

Caps, beard bags, and masks should be worn during certain surgical procedures, including umbilical vessel catheterization and insertion of central lines. Long hair should be restrained so that it does not touch the newborn or equipment during patient examinations or treatments. Masks should be worn so that they cover both the nose and the mouth, and they should be discarded as soon as they are removed from the nose and mouth. High-efficiency, disposable masks should be used, but even these masks remain effective only for a few hours.

Sterile gloves should be used during deliveries and all invasive procedures performed in either the obstetric or the nursery area. Disposable, nonsterile gloves may be useful in the care of patients in isolation or in the performance of procedures that may result in contamination of the hands.

Obstetric Considerations

The areas where cesarean deliveries and tubal ligations are performed are operating rooms and are subject to all policies pertaining to such facilities. Therefore, all individuals present should wear appropriate operating room attire. For those in the sterile surgical field, this attire includes clean scrub clothing, sterile operating room gowns, caps, masks, eye protection, gloves, and shoe covers. For those not involved with the surgical field, a sterile operating room gown is not required, but caps and masks should be worn. The surgical field should be prepared and draped according to standard recommendations. Preoperative clipping of hair very close to the skin is preferred to shaving.

Intrauterine pressure catheters (for monitoring contractions or for amnioinfusion) or internal fetal electrodes (for fetal heart rate monitoring) should be inserted and maintained in accordance with standard sterile techniques. Fluids used with pressure catheters should be sterile. To minimize the chance of contamination, the packages containing the devices should be opened only at the time of their use, and proper sterile techniques should be followed during their handling and insertion. Disposable items should be used whenever possible.

Neonatal Considerations

Prevention of Catheter-Related Bloodstream Infections

Catheter-related bloodstream infections are the most common hospital-acquired infections in the NICU. Maximum sterile barrier precautions (ie, cap, mask, sterile gown, sterile gloves, and sterile drapes) during the insertion of central venous catheters, including all umbilical catheters, substantially reduce the incidence of catheter-related bloodstream infections compared with sterile gloves and small drapes.

Extraluminal contamination of the intracutaneous tract is believed to be responsible for catheter-related infections that occur in the week after placement. Catheters are more mobile during the first week after insertion and can slide in and out of the insertion site, drawing organisms down into the catheter tract. Techniques to reduce the likelihood of extraluminal contamination include proper hand hygiene, aseptic catheter insertion (including use of a maximal sterile barrier for catheter insertion and care), use of a topical antiseptic, and use of sterile dressing. Both chlorhexidine (2%) and povidone iodine are recommended for skin antisepsis in infants 2 months or older.

However, the U.S. Food and Drug Administration states that chlorhexidine should be used with care in premature infants or infants younger than 2 months of age because of the concern of irritation and chemical burns. Although transparent dressings permit easier inspection of the catheter site, they have no proven benefit in reducing infection. Catheter sites must be monitored visually or by palpation on a daily basis and should be redressed and cleaned on a regular basis, or if soiled, or showing evidence of loosening of the dressing. In infants, there are no data indicating that tunneled catheters have a lower risk of infection than nontunneled catheters.

After the first week of placement, intraluminal colonization after hub manipulation and contamination is responsible for most catheter-related bloodstream infections. Tubing used to administer blood products or lipid emulsions should be changed daily. Tubing used to infuse dextrose and amino acids should be replaced every 4–7 days. It is important to remove all central venous catheters when they are no longer essential. Many NICUs remove central catheters when the volume of enteral feedings reaches 80–100 mL per kg per day.

An intravascular catheter should be removed promptly if signs of device-associated infection occur. Each unit should have a written policy on the procedures governing the use and proper removal of these catheters. Arterial cannulas and catheters present a risk of acquired infection, especially when used for obtaining blood samples. Samples should be obtained aseptically, with precautions to avoid contamination of the system and with the realization that the risk of infection is increased when using the cannula or catheter.

Meticulous attention should be given to aseptic techniques of fluid administration. Total parenteral nutrition generally is safe, but it has been associated with infection, including bacteremia and fungemia. A multidisciplinary team approach involving pharmacists, nurses, and physicians is strongly recommended to reduce the incidence of infections and other complications. The hospital pharmacy should establish a system to ensure a satisfactory and safe means of providing sterile, unpreserved fluids to the nursery areas. All solutions intended for parenteral infusion should be compounded in the hospital pharmacy, including those containing heparin. The CDC has no recommendations for the duration of infusion (hang time) of intravenous fluids, including lipid-free parenteral nutrition fluids. However, the CDC does recommend infusion of lipid-containing parenteral nutrition fluids should be completed within 24 hours of hanging the fluid. Infusion of lipid emulsions alone should be completed within 12 hours of hanging the fluid. Infusions of blood products should be completed within 4 hours of hanging the product. Flush solutions should be kept at room temperature no longer than 8 hours before being used or discarded. They should be labeled clearly with the time of opening or preparation. Single-use prefilled saline or heparin flushes also may be used. Solutions with benzyl alcohol are contraindicated in newborns because their use may lead to severe metabolic acidosis, encephalopathy, and death.

Care bundles have been shown to be an effective strategy for reducing the incidence of catheter-related bloodstream infections in NICU patients. Care bundles are groups of interventions (extrapolated from studies in adults or recommendations from professional organizations) that are likely to be effective. This multifaceted approach has reduced the incidence of health care-associated sepsis in each center or groups of centers where it has been implemented.

Guidelines for the prevention of umbilical catheter-related infections have been published and are summarized as follows:

- Remove and do not replace umbilical artery catheters if any signs of central line-associated bloodstream infection, vascular insufficiency in the lower extremities, or thrombosis are present.
- Remove and do not replace umbilical venous catheters if any signs of central line-associated bloodstream infection or thrombosis are present.
- Cleanse the umbilical insertion site with an antiseptic before catheter insertion. Avoid tincture of iodine because of the potential effect on the neonatal thyroid. Other iodine-containing products (eg, povidone iodine) can be used.
- Do not use topical antibiotic ointment or creams on catheter insertion sites because of the potential to promote fungal infections and antimicrobial resistance.
- Add low doses of heparin (0.25–1.0 unit/mL) to the fluid infused through an umbilical arterial catheter.
- Remove umbilical arterial catheters as soon as possible. Optimally, umbilical artery catheters should not be left in place for more than 5 days.
- Umbilical venous catheters should be removed as soon as possible but can be used up to 14 days if managed aseptically.

- A malfunctioning umbilical catheter may be replaced if there is no other indication for catheter removal and the total duration of catheterization has not exceeded 5 days for an umbilical artery catheter or 14 days for an umbilical vein catheter.

Prevention of Health Care-Associated Pneumonia

The CDC published guidelines for preventing health care-associated pneumonia in all patient populations in 2003. Although these guidelines were not specifically designed to address the unique issues facing mechanically ventilated newborns and the definition of health care-associated pneumonia in newborns is controversial, many of the recommendations are relevant to all patient populations. General concepts in the CDC document are as follows:

- Staff education and involvement in infection prevention—All health care providers should receive appropriate information relating to the epidemiology of and infection control procedures for preventing health care-associated pneumonia. There should be procedures in place, including performance of appropriate infection control activities, to ensure worker competency. Staff should be involved with implementation of interventions to prevent health care-associated pneumonia using performance-improvement tools and techniques.
- Infection and microbiologic surveillance—Surveillance for health care-associated pneumonia should be performed to determine trends and help identify outbreaks or other problems. Routine surveillance cultures of patients or equipment should not be performed.
- Prevention of transmission of microorganisms—Risks of acquisition of microorganisms that could result in health care-associated pneumonia can be reduced by proper sterilization or disinfection and maintenance of equipment and devices, and prevention of person-to-person transmission of bacteria by use of standard precautions as well as other isolation practices, when appropriate.
- Modifying host risk of infection—Aspiration is a major risk for the development of health care-associated pneumonia. Devices, such as endotracheal tubes, tracheostomy tubes, or enteral tubes, should be removed from patients as soon as clinically appropriate. In the absence of medical contraindications, the head of the bed should be elevated at an angle of 30–45 for mechanically ventilated patients. A comprehensive oral-hygiene program should be followed for the patient.

Suctioning practices may influence tracheal colonization. The use of closed-suctioning systems allows endotracheal suctioning without disconnecting patients from the ventilator. Closed-suctioning methods reduce physiologic disruptions (hypoxia and decrease in heart rate), and NICU nurses judged them to be easier to use than an open system. Closed-suctioning systems provide an opportunity for bacterial contamination when pooled secretions in the lumen are reintroduced into the lower respiratory tract with repeat suctioning. However, closed-suctioning systems could potentially reduce environmental contamination of the endotracheal tube. In studies evaluating mechanically ventilated adults, airway colonization was more common when closed-suctioning systems were used, but ventilator-associated pneumonia rates were equal to or slightly less than the rates in patients cared for with open systems. The CDC recommendations do not endorse one system over the other, and there is no recommendation addressing the frequency at which closed-suctioning systems should be changed.

Using a nonsupine position may reduce the risk of ventilator-associated pneumonia. Tracheal colonization from oropharyngeal contamination is less common in infants on mechanical ventilation when the infants are placed in a lateral position on the bed as compared with the supine position. Keeping the endotracheal tube and the ventilator circuit in a horizontal position might reduce tracking of oropharyngeal secretions down into the lower respiratory tract. The lateral position also is associated with reduced aspiration of gastric secretion into the trachea.

Prophylactic Antibiotic Therapy for Prevention of Health Care-Associated Infection

The efficacy of prophylactic antibiotic therapy for the prevention of infection in newborns has not been documented. Antibiotic prophylaxis in newborns is strongly discouraged except for specific indications (eg, ophthalmic antibiotics for prevention of ophthalmia neonatorum). The relative frequencies of documented infections in newborns, etiologic agents, and patterns of antimicrobial susceptibility should be monitored by the infection control committee in collaboration with the unit's medical director. These data should guide the selection of antibiotics to be used for treating suspected infection while awaiting the results of cultures. The best tolerated, narrowest spectrum, and most effective antibiotic regimen should be selected for this purpose based on the accumulated data on the antibiotic sensitivity patterns of microbial isolates. Antibiotics should be discontinued when culture results are negative. The indiscriminate and injudicious use of either systemic or topical antibiotics promotes the emergence of resistant strains of bacteria, making subsequent therapy for clinical infections more difficult and dangerous. Duration of initial antibiotic therapy longer than 5 days has been associated with an increased risk of necrotizing enterocolitis and mortality.

Maternal Postpartum Infections

The newborn need not be isolated from a mother with a postpartum infection in most circumstances. Women with abscesses or infected or draining wounds should have appropriate cover dressings and should wash their hands frequently before handling the baby. If it is not possible to cover the infected or draining wound completely, the infant should be placed in a separate room. Gloves and, with some infections, gowns should be worn by staff during all contact with infected patients.

Mothers with communicable diseases that are likely to be transmitted to their newborns should be separated from the newborns until the infection is no longer communicable, based on the natural history of the infection and the effectiveness of therapy in eliminating the contagion. A mother with postpartum fever that does not have a specific, communicable cause may feed and care for her newborn. With the exception of certain infections (see also "Contraindications to Breastfeeding" in Chapter 10), breastfeeding rarely is contraindicated because of maternal infection. A mother can care for her newborn if

- she feels well enough to handle the infant.
- she demonstrates effective hand hygiene techniques.
- she avoids contact of the infant with contaminated clothes, linen, dressings, or pads.

A woman with a respiratory tract infection should be made aware that the infection can be transmitted not only by droplets but also by contact with contaminated hands and fomites. Therefore, she should practice strict hand hygiene techniques and appropriately handle or dispose of contaminated tissues and any other items that may have come in contact with infectious secretions. If needed, she can wear a surgical mask to reduce the chance of droplet spread to her newborn.

Postpartum women who are infected with nonobstetric-related communicable diseases should be treated according to the precautions and isolation techniques required by the specific disease. If the required guidelines cannot be followed safely in the obstetric unit, the patient should be transferred to the appropriate unit where such care can be provided.

Cohorting During Epidemics

During hospital epidemics, a comprehensive program of infection control is required. Even if an intensive investigation is not indicated, the results of the control measures should be evaluated to ensure that they have been effective and that the problem has been resolved. Because many infections become apparent only after newborns leave the hospital, each hospital should establish procedures to be used during a suspected or confirmed epidemic for disease surveillance of recently discharged newborns. Hospital infection control personnel and appropriate public health officials should be notified promptly about suspected or confirmed epidemics.

Newborns with overt infection and those who are colonized with that pathogen should be identified rapidly and placed in cohorts—separate areas where newborns with similar exposure or illness receive care. If rapid identification of these newborns is not possible, separate cohorts should be established for newborns with disease, those who have been exposed, those who have not been exposed, and those who are newly admitted. The success of cohort programs depends largely on the willingness and ability of nursery and ancillary personnel to adhere strictly to the cohort system and to follow established infection control practices.

Newborn Infections

The isolation requirements for a newborn who has an infection or is suspected of having an infection depend on the type of infection, the condition of the newborn, the type of care required, the available space and facilities, the ratio of available nurses to patients, and the size and type of the clinical service. Other factors to be considered include the clinical manifestations of the infection, the source and possible modes of its transmission, and the number of colonized or infected newborns.

Isolation. In many instances (notable exceptions are neonatal varicella zoster virus infection or epidemics of bacterial infection), infected newborns do not need to be placed in a separate room, if certain criteria are met:

- Sufficient nursing and medical staff are on duty to provide comprehensive care.

- Adequate sinks for handwashing are available in each nursery room or area and alcohol-based hand hygiene solutions are available at all entry points and at each bed space.
- Continuing instruction is provided about the ways in which infections spread.
- If multiple infants are kept in a single room, a 4–6-foot aisle is open between infant stations.

Physical separation with assignment of separate health care personnel for each area is best. In 2007, the CDC recommended new isolation guidelines for hospitalized patients (available at: www.cdc.gov/infectioncontrol/pdf/guidelines/isolation-guidelines.pdf). These guidelines outline transmission-based precautions for patients who are infected or colonized with pathogens that are spread by airborne, droplet, or contact routes. Isolation categories, with examples, are listed in Table 13-1.

TABLE 13-1. Transmission-Based Precautions for Hospitalized Patients*

Category of Precautions	Single-Patient Room	Respiratory Tract and Mucous Membrane Protection	Gowns	Gloves
Airborne	Yes, with negative air-pressure ventilation, 6–12 air exchanges per hour, ± HEPA filtration	Respirators: N95 or higher level	No†	No†
Droplet	Yes‡	Surgical masks§	No†	No†
Contact	Yes‡	No	Yes	Yes

Abbreviation: HEPA, high-efficiency particulate air

*These recommendations are in addition to those for standard precautions for all patients.

†Gowns and gloves may be required as a component of standard precautions (eg, for blood collection or during procedures likely to cause blood splashes or if there are skin lesions containing transmissible infectious agents).

‡Preferred. Cohorting of children infected with the same pathogen is acceptable if a single-patient room is not available, a distance of more than 3 feet between patients can be maintained, and precautions are observed between all contacts with different patients in the room.

§Masks should be donned on entry into the room.

Reprinted from American Academy of Pediatrics. Red book: report of the Committee on Infectious Diseases. 30th ed. Elk Grove Village (IL): AAP; 2015.

Forced-air incubators filter incoming air, but they do not filter the air that is discharged from the incubator into the nursery. Therefore, they are satisfactory for limited protective isolation of infants, but they should not be relied on to prevent transmission of microorganisms from infected infants to others.

When an isolation room is deemed necessary (eg, for patients with highly contagious infections), blinds, windows, and other structural items must allow for ease of regular room cleaning. An intercom should be provided. Air from this room should be exhausted to the outside and not to the nursery or NICU.

Gastroenteritis, Abscess, Viral Respiratory Infection, or Cutaneous Infection. Contact precautions should be observed when treating patients with viral respiratory infection, gastroenteritis, cutaneous infections, or draining lesions or abscesses that cannot be contained adequately by a dressing. All personnel should use gowns and disposable gloves when providing direct patient care. If the patient has a viral respiratory infection, masks are also needed. Contaminated items should be properly discarded, and gowns and gloves should be discarded before leaving the room. The environment may be heavily contaminated with the infecting microorganism, and these organisms often are transmitted on the hands of personnel to other newborns. If more than one newborn is infected, a cohort approach should be taken (see also "Cohorting During Epidemics" earlier in this chapter).

Congenital Infections. Standard precautions provide adequate isolation for most congenital infections, with two exceptions: 1) congenital rubella, which requires droplet isolation, and 2) suspected herpetic infection, which requires contact isolation.

Viral Infections. Many viruses, such as respiratory syncytial virus, coxsackie viruses, or echoviruses, spread rapidly among infants and personnel in a nursery. Such viral infections can be serious in newborns, sometimes resulting in death. Because infants may shed selected viruses after their clinical illness has been resolved, they can be reservoirs of infection. It is believed that enteroviruses and respiratory syncytial virus are transmitted predominantly by direct or indirect contact by the hands of personnel that become contaminated with virus-containing secretions or with contaminated environmental surfaces or fomites.

Newborns with confirmed or possible infections caused by a viral agent that could be transmitted by the airborne route should be separated from other infants by transfer from the nursery area, rooming-in with the mother, or enclosure of all other infants in the area in incubators.

Multidrug-Resistant Organisms. Although the CDC reports a decrease in health care-associated infection with invasive MRSA, infection with MRSA and other multidrug-resistant organisms continues to be an important public health care problem. Infants infected with multidrug-resistant organisms or MRSA should be isolated, and contact precautions should be observed.

Environmental Control

The responsible physicians and the nurse managers of the obstetric and nursery areas should work with infection control personnel and other appropriate groups (eg, representatives of the respiratory therapy service, central supply, and housekeeping) to establish an environmental control program for the labor, delivery, and nursery areas. This program should include specific procedures in a written policy manual for cleaning and disinfection or sterilization of patient care areas, equipment, and supplies. The CDC guidelines on disinfection and sterilization in health care facilities are available at: www.cdc.gov/infectioncontrol/guidelines/disinfection/index.html. Consultation for specific details and problems should be encouraged. Nursing supervisors should ensure that these procedures are carried out correctly.

General Housekeeping

Cleaning should be conducted in the following time sequence:

1. Patient areas
2. Accessory areas
3. Adjacent halls

It is not known whether floor bacteria are a source of health care-associated infection, but regular cleaning prevents the accumulation of pathogenic bacteria. Disinfectant–detergents have been shown to be more effective than soap and water alone in cleaning floors, although hospital floors are recontaminated rapidly after disinfection. Available disinfectant–detergents may differ in effectiveness.

During the cleaning process, dust should not be dispersed into the air. Removal of dust by a dry vacuum machine followed by wet vacuuming is effective in cleaning and disinfecting hospital floors. Once dust has been removed, scrubbing with a mop and a disinfectant–detergent solution should be sufficient to clean and disinfect floors. Mop heads should be machine laundered and thoroughly dried daily.

Cabinet counters, work surfaces, and similar horizontal areas may be subject to heavy contamination during routine use. These areas should be cleaned once per day and between patient use with a disinfectant–detergent and clean cloths. Application of friction during cleaning is important to ensure physical removal of dirt and contaminating microorganisms. Surfaces that are contaminated by patient specimens or accidental spills should be cleaned carefully and disinfected.

Walls, windows, and storage shelves may be reservoirs of pathogenic microorganisms if visibly soiled or if dust and dirt are allowed to accumulate. These areas and similar noncritical surfaces should be scrubbed periodically with a disinfectant–detergent solution as part of the general housekeeping program.

Faucet aerators may be useful to reduce water splashing in sinks, but they are extremely susceptible to contamination with a variety of hydrophilic bacteria. For this reason, removing aerators permanently may be preferred. Sinks should be sufficiently deep and have backsplashes to prevent splashing of hands with water pooled in the sink drain, a source of bacterial growth. Sinks should be scrubbed clean daily with a disinfectant–detergent; drain traps should not need routine cleaning or disinfection. Foot-operated sinks or sinks without handles operated by motion sensors are preferred. The walls and floor surrounding the sinks should be covered with easily cleanable surfaces.

Written policies should be established for the removal and disposal of solid waste. Sturdy plastic liners should be used in trash receptacles; these liners should be sealed before they are removed from the trash receptacles. In patient care areas, trash receptacles should be cleaned and disinfected regularly. Potentially infectious material requires special handling and disposal.

Dedicated housekeeping personnel should be assigned to clean the nursery. If the nursery is small, they also may be assigned to work in the obstetric areas or other clean areas of the hospital. The nursery should be cleaned daily at an appropriate time. Intensive care units ideally should be cleaned when traffic is minimal.

Cleaning and Disinfecting Patient Care Equipment

Incubators, Open Care Units, and Bassinets

After an infant has been discharged, the care unit used by that infant should be thoroughly cleaned and disinfected. A disinfectant–detergent registered by the U.S. Environmental Protection Agency should be used for this purpose. Manufacturers' directions for use of a disinfectant–detergent should be followed carefully. A bassinet or incubator should never be cleaned when occupied. Infants who remain in the nursery for an extended period should be transferred periodically, as per hospital policy, to a different, disinfected unit.

When a care unit is being cleaned and disinfected, all detachable parts should be removed and scrubbed meticulously. If the incubator has a fan, it should be cleaned and disinfected; the manufacturer's instructions should be followed to avoid equipment damage. The air filter should be maintained as recommended by the manufacturer. Mattresses should be replaced when the surface covering is broken; such a break precludes effective disinfection or sterilization. Mattresses may be sterilized by heat or gas. Incubator portholes and porthole cuffs and sleeves are contaminated easily and often heavily; cuffs should be replaced on a regular schedule or cleaned and disinfected frequently with freshly prepared mild soap or quaternary ammonium disinfectant- detergent solution. Incubators not in use should be dried thoroughly by running the incubator hot without water in the reservoir for 24 hours after disinfection.

Evaporative humidifiers in incubators usually do not produce contaminated aerosols, but contaminated water reservoirs may be responsible for direct, rather than airborne, transmission of infection. Reservoirs should be filled with sterile water only, and they should be drained and refilled with sterile water every 24 hours. In many areas of the United States and in hospitals with a central ventilation system, environmental humidity levels may be sufficiently high to eliminate the need for additional humidification in most cases, and water reservoirs may be left dry.

Nebulizers, Water Traps, and Respiratory Support Equipment

Nebulizers and attached tubing should be replaced by clean, sterile equipment (or equipment that has been subjected to high-level disinfection) in accordance with established hospital policy. Failure to replace tubing may result in contamination of freshly cleaned equipment. Water traps also should be replaced regularly by autoclaved or disinfected equipment. Only sterile water should be used for nebulizers or water traps; residual water should be discarded when these containers are refilled. Water condensed in tubing loops should be removed and discarded and should not be allowed to reflux into the container.

Other Equipment

Cleaning and disinfection or sterilization of equipment should be performed between patients. Equipment that is used for only one patient should be replaced, cleaned, and disinfected or sterilized according to an established schedule. Disposable equipment should be replaced with approximately the same frequency as reusable equipment. Disposable equipment never should be reused. Resuscitators, face masks, laryngoscopes, eye speculums, and other items used in direct contact with newborns should be dismantled, thoroughly cleaned, and sterilized, if possible. Alternately, the equipment may be subjected to high-level disinfection with liquid chemicals or by pasteurization. Equipment, such as tubing for respiratory or oxygen therapy, should be sterilized or discarded after use. In-line, closed suctioning systems are thought to reduce the risk of spreading potential pathogens from the airway of intubated patients. Stethoscopes and similar types of diagnostic instruments should be wiped with iodophor or alcohol before use. Standard precautions should be used when any type of suctioning is performed.

Bibliography

American Academy of Pediatrics. Red book: report of the Committee on Infectious Diseases. 30th ed. Elk Grove Village (IL): AAP; 2015.

Benitz WE, Wynn JL, Polin RA. Reappraisal of guidelines for management of neonates with suspected early-onset sepsis. J Pediatr 2015;166:1070–4.

Centers for Disease Control and Prevention. MRSA tracking. Methicillin-resistant staphylococcus aureus. Atlanta (GA): CDC; 2016. Available at: https://www.cdc.gov/mrsa/tracking/index.html. Retrieved November 17, 2016.

Environmental Protection Agency. Antimicrobial pesticides. Washington, DC: EPA; 2016. Available at: https://www.epa.gov/pesticides/antimicrobial-pesticides. Retrieved November 16, 2016.

Henderson DK, Dembry L, Fishman NO, Grady C, Lundstrom T, Palmore TN, et al. SHEA guideline for management of healthcare workers who are infected with hepatitis B virus, hepatitis C virus, and/or human immunodeficiency virus. Society for Healthcare Epidemiology of America. Infect Control Hosp Epidemiol 2010;31:203–32.

Hepatitis B, hepatitis C, and human immunodeficiency virus infections in obstetrician-gynecologists. Committee Opinion No. 655. American College of Obstetricians and Gynecologists. Obstet Gynecol 2016;127:e70–4.

Infection prevention and control in pediatric ambulatory settings. American Academy of Pediatrics Committee on Infectious Diseases. Pediatrics 2007;120:650–65.

Jurkovich P. Home- versus hospital-laundered scrubs: a pilot study. MCN Am J Matern Child Nurs 2004;29:106–10.

O'Grady NP, Alexander M, Burns LA, Dellinger EP, Garland J, Heard SO, et al. Guidelines for the prevention of intravascular catheter-related infections. Healthcare Infection Control Practices Advisory Committee (HICPAC). Clin Infect Dis 2011;52:e162–93.

Pittet D, Allegranzi B, Boyce J. The World Health Organization guidelines on hand hygiene in health care and their consensus recommendations. World Health Organization World Alliance for Patient Safety First Global Patient Safety Challenge Core Group of Experts. Infect Control Hosp Epidemiol 2009;30:611–22.

Polin RA. Management of neonates with suspected or proven early-onset bacterial sepsis. Committee on Fetus and Newborn. Pediatrics 2012;129:1006–15.

Polin RA, Denson S, Brady MT. Epidemiology and diagnosis of health care-associated infections in the NICU. Committee on Fetus and Newborn, Committee on Infectious Diseases. Pediatrics 2012;129:e1104–9.

Polin RA, Denson S, Brady MT. Strategies for prevention of health care-associated infections in the NICU. Committee on Fetus and Newborn, Committee on Infectious Diseases. Pediatrics 2012;129:e1085–93.

Polizzi J, Byers JF, Kiehl E. Co-bedding versus traditional bedding of multiple-gestation infants in the NICU. J Healthc Qual 2003;25:5-10; quiz 10–1.

Sehulster L, Chinn RY. Guidelines for environmental infection control in health-care facilities. Recommendations of CDC and the Healthcare Infection Control Practices Advisory Committee (HICPAC). CDC HICPAC [published erratum appears in MMWR Morb Mortal Wkly Rep 2003;52:1025–6]. MMWR Recomm Rep 2003;52(RR-10):1–42.

Siegel JD, Rhinehart E, Jackson M, Chiarello L. 2007 Guideline for isolation precautions: preventing transmission of infectious agents in healthcare settings. Healthcare Infection Control Practices Advisory Committee (HICPAC). Atlanta (GA): Centers for Disease Control and Prevention; 2007. Available at: http://www.cdc.gov/infection control/pdf/guidelines/isolation-guidelines.pdf. Retrieved November 17, 2016.

Resources

Influenza vaccination during pregnancy. Committee Opinion No. 608. American College of Obstetricians and Gynecologists. Obstet Gynecol 2014;124:648–51.

United States Environmental Protection Agency (EPA). Washington, DC: EPA; 2016. Available at: https://www3.epa.gov. Retrieved November 17, 2016.

World Health Organization. WHO guidelines on hand hygiene in health care: first global patient safety challenge clean care is safer care. Geneva: WHO; 2009. Available at: http://apps.who.int/iris/bitstream/10665/44102/1/9789241597906_eng.pdf. Retrieved November 17, 2016.

Appendix A

The American College of Obstetricians and Gynecologists' Antepartum Record and Postpartum Form

The American College of Obstetricians and Gynecologists
WOMEN'S HEALTH CARE PHYSICIANS

Patient Addressograph

ANTEPARTUM RECORD

Date: – – ID #:

Hospital of Delivery:

Name:

LAST FIRST MIDDLE

Newborn Care Provider:	Referred By:
Primary Care Provider/Group:	Address:
Final EDD:	
Birth Date: – – Age: Race: Marital Status: S M W D Sep	Address: Zip: Phone: (1) (2)
Occupation: Education: (Last Grade Completed)	E-Mail:
Language: Ethnicity:	Insurance Carrier/Medicaid #:
Partner: Phone:	Policy #:
Father Of Baby: Phone:	Emergency Contact: Phone:

Total Preg:	Full Term:	Premature:	Ab, Induced:	Ab, Spontaneous:	Ectopics:	Multiple Births:	Living:

Menstrual History

Lmp ☐ Definite ☐ Approximate (Month Known)
☐ Unknown ☐ Normal Amount/Duration
☐ Final: ______

Duration: Q ______ Days
Prior Menses: ______ Date

Frequency: Q ______ Days
Contraception at conception ☐ Yes ☐ No

Menarche: ______ (Age Onset)
Hcg + ___/___/___

Past Pregnancies (Last Five)

Date Month/ Year	GA Weeks	Length Of Labor	Birth Weight	Sex M/F	Type Of Delivery	Anes	Place Of Delivery	Breastfeeding Duration	Lactation Consult Needed Yes/No	Comments/ Complications

Medical History

	P*	F*	Detail Positive Remarks Include Date & Treatment		P*	F*	Detail Positive Remarks Include Date & Treatment
A. Drug/Latex Allergies/ Reactions				17. Dermatologic Disorders			
B. Allergies (Food, Seasonal, Environmental)				18. Operations/Hospitalizations (Year & Reason)			
1. Neurologic/Epilepsy				19. Gyn Surgery (Year & Reason)			
2. Thyroid Dysfunction				20. Anesthetic Complications			
3. Breast Disease/Breast Surgery				21. History Of Blood Transfusions			
4. Pulmonary (TB, Asthma)				22. Infertility			
5. Heart Disease				23. Art (IVF Or FET)			
6. Hypertension				24. History of Abnormal Pap			
7. Cancer				25. History of STI			
8. Hematologic Disorders				26. Psychiatric Illness			
9. Anemia				27. Depression/Postpartum Depression			
10. Gastrointestinal Disorders				28. Trauma/Violence			Prepreg / Preg / # Years Use
11. Hepatitis/Liver Disease				29. Tobacco (Smoked, Chewed, ENDS, Vaped) (AMT/Day)			
12. Kidney Disease/UTI				30. Alcohol (AMT/Wk)			
13. Deep Vein Thrombosis				31. Drug Use (Including Opioids) (Uses/Wk)			
14. Diabetes (Type 1 Or Type 2)				32. Polycystic Ovary Syndrome			
15. Gestational Diabetes				33. Other			
16. Autoimmune Disorders							

*P= Personal F= Family

COMMENTS: ______

 (AA128) 12345/09876

Patient Name:		Birth Date: – –	ID No.:	Date: – –

Genetic Screening*				
Condition	Patient	Partner	Other	Relationship
Congenital Heart Defect				
Neural Tube Defect				
Hemoglobinopathy Or Carrier				
Cystic Fibrosis				
Chromosome Abnormality				
Tay-Sachs				
Hemophilia				
Intellectual Disability/Autism				
Recurrent Pregnancy Loss/Stillbirth				
Other Structural Birth Defect				
Other Genetic Disease (eg, PKU, Metabolic Disease, Muscular Dystrophy)				

Teratogen Exposures Since LMP/Conception	Yes	No	Details/Date
Prescription Medications			
Over The Counter Medications			
Alcohol			
Illicit Drugs			
Maternal Diabetes			HGB A1C
Other			
Uterine Anomaly/DES			

*If a patient has been screened for a genetic disorder previously, the results should be documented but the test should not be repeated.

COMMENTS/COUNSELING: ______

Infection History	Yes	No		Yes	No
1. Live with Someone with TB or Exposed to TB			6. HIV Infection		
2. Patient or Partner has History of Genital Herpes			7. History Of Hepatitis		
3. Rash or Viral Illness Since Last Menstrual Period			8. Recent Travel History Outside Of Country		
4. Prior GBS-Infected Child			9. Other (See Comments)		
5. History of STIS: (Check All That Apply) ☐ Gonorrhea ☐ Chlamydia ☐ HPV ☐ Syphilis ☐ PID					

COMMENTS: ______

______ INTERVIEWER'S SIGNATURE: ______

Immunizations	Yes (Month/Year) ___/___	No	If No, Vaccine Indicated?*	Immunizations	Yes (Month/Year) ___/___	No	If No, Vaccine Indicated?*
TDAP (Each pregnancy, between 27–36 weeks)				Hepatitis A (When Indicated)			
Influenza† (Each pregnancy as soon as vaccine is available)				Hepatitis B (When Indicated)			
Varicella†				Meningococcal (When Indicated)			
MMR (Rubella-containing vaccine)†				Pneumococcal (When Indicated)			
HPV							

*Yes/No & date to be administered

†All live vaccines are contraindicated in pregnancy, including the live intranasal influenza, MMR, and varicella vaccines. All women who will be pregnant during influenza season (October through May) should receive inactivated influenza vaccine at any point in gestation. Administer the HPV, MMR, and varicella vaccines postpartum if needed. The Tdap vaccine can be given postpartum if the woman has never received it as an adult and did not get it during pregnancy.

Initial Physical Examination

Date: ___/___/___ BP/Prepregnancy Weight: ______ Height: ______ BMI: ______

1. Heent		Normal	Abnormal	11. Vulva		Normal		Condyloma		Lesions
2. Teeth		Normal	Abnormal	12. Vagina		Normal		Inflammation		Discharge
3. Thyroid		Normal	Abnormal	13. Cervix		Normal		Inflammation		Lesions
4. Breasts		Normal	Abnormal	14. Uterus Size	___	Weeks				Fibroids
5. Lungs		Normal	Abnormal	15. Adnexa		Normal		Mass		
6. Heart		Normal	Abnormal	16. Rectum		Normal		Abnormal		
7. Abdomen		Normal	Abnormal	17. Clinical Pelvimetry		Concerns		No Concerns		
8. Extremities		Normal	Abnormal							
9. Skin		Normal	Abnormal							
10. Lymph Nodes		Normal	Abnormal							

COMMENTS (Number and explain abnormals): ______

______ EXAM BY: ______

 (AA128) 12345/09876

Patient Addressograph

Patient Name:	Birth Date: – –	ID No.:	Date: – –

Drug Allergy:________	Latex Allergy ☐ Yes ☐ No	Postpartum Contraception Method:________ Counseled About LARC? ☐ Yes ☐ No
Is Blood Transfusion Acceptable? ☐ Yes ☐ No		Antepartum Anesthesia Consult Planned ☐ Yes ☐ No

Problems	**Plans**	**Resolved?**
1.		
2.		
3.		
4.		
5.		

Medication List (Including Opioids)	**Start Date**	**Stop Date**
1.	– –	– –
2.	– –	– –
3.	– –	– –
4.	– –	– –
5.	– –	– –

EDD Confirmation					**Pregnancy Weight Gain**	
Lmp:	– –	=	= EDD	– –	Prepregnancy Weight	
Initial Exam:	– –	=	Wks = EDD	– –	Height	
Ultrasonography:	– –	=	Wks = EDD	– –	BMI	
Final Edd:	– –		IVF Transfer:	– –	Estimated Weight Gain	
Initialed By:					Recommended Weight Gain	

Prepregnancy Weight ________

BMI ________

Date	Weeks Gest. (Best Est.)	Weight	Blood Pressure	Urine (Albumin/Glucose)	Pain Scale* (0–10)	Fetal Movement	Preterm Labor Signs/Symptoms: +=Present O=Absent	FHR	Fundal Height (CM)/EFW	Presentation	Edema	Cervix Examination (DIL/EFF STA.) Length On Ultrasonography	Next Appointment	Provider (Initials)	Comments:
- -															
- -															
- -															
- -															
- -															
- -															
- -															
- -															
- -															
- -															
- -															
- -															
- -															

*Describe the intensity of discomfort ranging from 0 (no pain) to 10 (worst possible pain).

 (AA128) 12345/09876

ANTEPARTUM RECORD (FORM C, page 3 of 12)

Patient Addressograph

Patient Name:		Birth Date: - -	ID No.:	Date: - -

Laboratory and Screening Tests | **Comments/Additional Labs**

Initial Labs	**Date**	**Result**	**Reviewed**
Blood Type	- -	A B AB O	
D (Rh) Type	- -		
Antibody Screen	- -		
Complete Blood Count	- -	HCT/HGB: ______ % ______ g/dL MCV:______________ PLT:______________	
VDRL/RPR (Syphilis)	- -		
Urine Culture/Screen	- -		
HBsAg	- -		
HIV Testing	- -	Pos. Neg. Declined	
Chlamydia (When Indicated)	- -		
Gonorrhea (When Indicated)	- -		
Rubella Immunity	- -		
Other:			
Supplemental Labs	**Date**	**Result**	
Hemoglobin Electrophoresis	- -	AA AS SS AC	
PPD/Quanta (When Indicated)	- -		
Pap Test (When Indicated)	- -		
HPV (When Indicated)	- -		
Early Diabetes Screen (When Indicated)	- -	Pos. Neg. Declined	
Varicella Immunity (When Indicated)	- -		
Cystic Fibrosis	- -	Pos. Neg. Declined	
Spinal Muscular Atrophy	- -	Pos. Neg. Declined	
Fragile X	- -	Pos. Neg. Declined	
Tay-Sachs	- -	Pos. Neg. Declined	
Canavan Disease	- -	Pos. Neg. Declined	
Familial Dysautonomia	- -	Pos. Neg. Declined	
Genetic Screening Tests (See Form B)	- -	Pos. Neg. Declined	
Other:			

8–20-Week Aneuploidy Screening	**Date Test Performed**	**Result**
Aneuploidy Screening Offered	- -	Accepted Declined GA Too Advanced
1st Trimester Aneuploidy Screening	- -	Pos Neg
2nd Trimester Serum Screening	- -	Pos Neg
Integrated Screening	- -	Pos Neg
Cell-Free DNA	- -	Pos Neg
CVS	- -	Karyotype: 46,XX Or 46,XY/Other______ Array
Amniocentesis	- -	Karyotype: 46,XX Or 46,XY/Other______ Array
Amniotic Fluid (AFP)	- -	Normal Abnormal
Other:		

(continued)

PROVIDER SIGNATURE (AS REQUIRED): ________________________________

 (AA128) 12345/09876

ANTEPARTUM RECORD (FORM D, page 4 of 12)

Patient Addressograph

Patient Name:		Birth Date: – –	ID No.:	Date: – –

Laboratory and Screening Tests *(continued)*				Comments/Additional Labs
Late Pregnancy Labs and Screening	**Date**	**Result**	**Reviewed**	
Tdap Vaccination (Every Pregnancy; 27–36 Weeks)	– –			
Complete Blood Count	– –	HCT/HGB:_______ % ______ g/dL MCV:________________ PLT:________________		
Diabetes Screen (24–28 Weeks)	– –			
GTT (If Screen Abnormal)	– –	_____Fbs _____1 Hour _____2 Hours _____3 Hours		
D (Rh) Antibody Screen (When Indicated)	– –			
Anti-D Immune Globulin (Rhlg) Given (28 Wks Or Greater) (When Indicated)	– –	________________ Signature		
Complete Blood Count	– –	Hct/Hgb:_______ % ______ g/dL MCV:________________ PLT:________________		
Ultrasonography (18–24 Weeks) (When Indicated)	– –			
HIV (When Indicated)*	– –			
VDRL/RPR (Syphilis) (When Indicated)	– –			
Gonorrhea (When Indicated)	– –			
Chlamydia (When Indicated)	– –			
Group B Strep (35–37 Weeks)	– –			
Resistance Testing If Penicillin Allergic	– –			
Other:				

*Check state requirements before recording results.

Comments

____

____

____

____

____

____

____

____

____

PROVIDER SIGNATURE (AS REQUIRED): ________________________________

 (AA128) 12345/09876

ANTEPARTUM RECORD (FORM D, page 5 of 12)

Patient Addressograph

Patient Name:		Birth Date: – –	ID No.:	Date: – –

Plans/Education
By Trimester. Initial And Date When Discussed.

	NA	Date	Follow-Up Needed	Referral	Comments
First Trimester					
Psychosocial Screening					
Desire For Pregnancy		– –			
Depression / Anxiety (Should Be Performed At Least Once During Perinatal Period)		– –			
Alcohol		– –			
Tobacco (Smoked, Chewed, ENDS, Vaped) Cessation Counseling (Ask, Advise, Assess, Assist, And Arrange)		– –			
Illicit/Recreational Drugs/Substance Use (Parents, Partner, Past, Present)*		– –			
Intimate Partner Violence		– –			
Barriers To Care		– –			
Unstable Housing		– –			
Communication Barriers		– –			
Nutrition		– –			
Wic Referral		– –			
Environmental/Work Hazards		– –			
Anticipatory Guidance					
Anticipated Course Of Prenatal Care		– –			
Nutrition Counseling; Special Diet; Dietary Precautions (Mercury, Listeriosis)		– –			
Weight Gain Counseling		– –			
Toxoplasmosis Precautions (Cats/Raw Meat)		– –			
Use Of Any Medications (Including Supplements, Vitamins, Herbs, Or Otc Drugs)		– –			
Sexual Activity		– –			
Exercise		– –			
Dental Care/Refer to Dentist		– –			
Avoidance Of Saunas Or Hot Tubs		– –			
Seat Belt Use		– –			
Childbirth Classes/Hospital Facilities		– –			
Breastfeeding		– –			
Fetal Testing					
Indications For Ultrasonography		– –			
Screening For Aneuploidy		– –			
Second Trimester					
Anticipatory Guidance					
Signs And Symptoms Of Preterm Labor		– –			
Selecting A Newborn Care Provider		– –			
Reproductive Life Planning & Contraception		– –			
Postpartum Care Planning		– –			
Psychosocial Screening					
Tobacco (Smoked, Chewed, ENDS, Vaped) Cessation Counseling (Ask, Advise, Assess, Assist, And Arrange)		– –			
Depression / Anxiety (Should Be Performed At Least Once During Perinatal Period)		– –			
Intimate Partner Violence		– –			

(continued)

*Data from Ewing H. A practical guide to intervention in health and social services with pregnant and postpartum addicts and alcoholics: theoretical framework, brief screening tool, key interview questions, and strategies for referral to recovery resources. Martinez (CA): The Born Free Project, Contra Costa County Department of Health Services; 1990.

 (AA128) 12345/09876

Patient Addressograph

Patient Name:		Birth Date: – –	ID No.:	Date: – –

Plans/Education *(continued)*

By Trimester. Initial And Date When Discussed.

	NA	Date	Follow-Up Needed	Referral	Comments
Third Trimester					
Birth Preferences					
Pain Management Plans		– –			
Trial Of Labor After Cesarean Counseling		– –			☐ TOLAC ☐ Elective RCS
Labor Support Person(S)		– –			
Immediate Postpartum Larc		– –			☐ Implant ☐ LNG-IUS ☐ Copper IUD
Circumcision Preference		– –			☐ Yes ☐ No
Infant Feeding Intention		– –			☐ Exclusive ☐ Mixed ☐ Formula
Anticipatory Guidance					
Fetal Movement Monitoring		– –			
Signs And Symptoms Of Preeclampsia		– –			
Labor Signs		– –			
Cervical Ripening/Labor Induction Counseling		– –			
Postterm Counseling		– –			
Infant Feeding		– –			
Newborn Education (Newborn Screening, Immunizations, Jaundice, SIDS/Safe Sleeping Position, Car Seat)		– –			
Family Medical Leave Or Disability Forms		– –			
Postpartum Depression		– –			
Psychosocial Screening					
Tobacco (Smoked, Chewed, ENDS, Vaped) Cessation Counseling (Ask, Advise, Assess, Assist, And Arrange)		– –			
Depression / Anxiety (Should Be Performed At Least Once During Perinatal Period)		– –			
Intimate Partner Violence		– –			
Postpartum					
Screening					
Depression / Anxiety (Should Be Performed At Least Once During Perinatal Period)		– –			
Infant Feeding Problems		– –			
Birth Experience		– –			
Glucose Screen (If Gdm)		– –			
Anticipatory Guidance					
Infant Feeding		– –			
Pelvic Muscle Exercise/Kegel		– –			
Return To Work / Milk Expression		– –			
Weight Retention		– –			
Optimal Birth Spacing		– –			
Postpartum Sexuality		– –			
Exercise		– –			
Nutrition		– –			
Cardiometabolic Risk (If Gdm / Ghtn)		– –			
Transition Of Care					
Referral Made To Primary Care Provider		– –			
Pregnancy Complications Documented In Medical Record		– –			
Written Recommendations For Follow-Up Communicated To Patient And To Pcp		– –			

ANTEPARTUM RECORD (FORM E, page 7 of 12)

(AA128) 12345/09876

Patient Addressograph

Patient Name:		Birth Date: - -	ID No.:	Date: - -

Plans/Education *(continued)*
By Trimester. Initial And Date When Discussed.

Requests

	Date	Initials	
Tubal Sterilization Consent Signed (If Desired).	- -		
History And Physical Have Been Sent To Hospital, If Applicable.	- -		
Update With Group B Streptococcus Results Sent.	- -		

Comments

 (AA128) 12345/09876

Patient Addressograph

Patient Name:		Birth Date: – –	ID No.:	Date: – –

Plans/Education Notes

(AA128) 12345/09876

Patient Addressograph

Name:		
LAST	FIRST	MIDDLE
ID#:	EDD:	

Prenatal Visits

Prepregnancy Weight ________

BMI ________

Date	Weeks Gest. (Best Est.)	Weight	Blood Pressure	Urine (Albumin/Glucose)	Pain Scale* (0–10)	Fetal Movement	Preterm Labor Signs/Symptoms: +=Present O=Absent	FHR	Fundal Height (CM)/EFW	Presentation	Edema	Cervix Examination (DIL./EFF. STA.) Length On Ultrasonography	Next Appointment	Provider (Initials)	Comments:
- -															
- -															
- -															
- -															
- -															
- -															
- -															
- -															
- -															
- -															
- -															
- -															
- -															

*Describe the intensity of discomfort ranging from 0 (no pain) to 10 (worst possible pain).

Progress Notes

PROVIDER SIGNATURE (AS REQUIRED): ________________________________

 (AA128) 12345/09876

ANTEPARTUM RECORD (FORM F, page 10 of 12)

Patient Addressograph

Name:		
LAST	FIRST	MIDDLE
ID#:	EDD:	

Prenatal Visits

Prepregnancy Weight ______

BMI ______

Date	Weeks Gest. (Best Est.)	Weight	Blood Pressure	Urine (Albumin/Glucose)	Pain Scale* (0–10)	Fetal Movement	Preterm Labor Signs/Symptoms: +=Present O=Absent	FHR	Fundal Height (CM)/EFW	Presentation	Edema	Cervix Examination (DIL/EFF STA.) Length On Ultrasonography	Next Appointment	Provider (Initials)	Comments:
- -															
- -															
- -															
- -															
- -															
- -															
- -															
- -															
- -															
- -															
- -															
- -															
- -															

*Describe the intensity of discomfort ranging from 0 (no pain) to 10 (worst possible pain).

Progress Notes

PROVIDER SIGNATURE (AS REQUIRED): ______

 (AA128) 12345/09876

ANTEPARTUM RECORD (FORM F, page 11 of 12)

Patient Addressograph

Patient Name:	Birth Date: – –	ID No.:	Date: – –

Progress Notes

PROVIDER SIGNATURE (AS REQUIRED): ______________________

 (AA128) 12345/09876

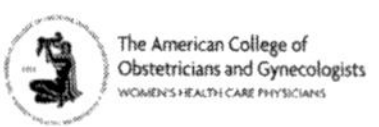

Patient Addressograph

POSTPARTUM CARE PLAN

To be developed prenatally by the patient and her maternity provider and revised as needed after delivery.

Name:

LAST FIRST MIDDLE

Care Team	
Primary Maternal Provider/Group:	Care Coordinator:
	Home Visitor:
PCP:	MFM:
Infant Medical Provider:	Consultant:
Lactation Support:	Consultant:

Postpartum Visits

Early Visit (Indication) _____ /_____ /_____ At: ____________________

☐ Hypertension ☐ Depression/Anxiety ☐ Wound Check ☐ Lactation Difficulties ☐ Medication Titration ☐ Other: ____________

Comprehensive Visit _____ /_____ /_____ At: ____________________

Reproductive Life Plan	
Number Of Children Desired:	Timing Of Next Pregnancy:

Contraceptive Plan

☐ BTL ☐ Implant ☐ LNG-IUS ☐ Copper IUD ☐ Depot Medroxyprogesterone Acetate (DMPA) ☐ Combined Ocp ☐ Progesterone Only Pill

☐ Vasectomy ☐ Condoms ☐ Diaphragm ☐ Lactational Amenorrhea ☐ Natural Family Planning ☐ Other

Immediate Postpartum LARC?

☐ Desires ☐ Declines ☐ Unsure

Infant Feeding Plan

☐ Exclusive Breastfeeding For _____ Months ☐ Mixed Feeding ☐ Formula

Community Resources

☐ WIC Peer Counselor ☐ Mothers' Groups ☐ Lactation Warmline ☐ Return To Work Resources

Pregnancy Complications

Complication __________	Follow-Up Scheduled	Result
☐ GDM	Glucose Screen: _____ /_____ /_____	_____ MG/DL (Fasting) _____ MG/DL (Post 75 G Load)
☐ Preeclampsia ☐ GHTN	BP Check _____ /_____ /_____	_____ /_____ MM HG
☐ Other:		

Mental Health

Risk For Postpartum Depression/Anxiety	Screening (Should Be Performed At Least Once During Perinatal Period)
☐ High ☐ Medium ☐ Low	Date: _____ /_____ /_____ Result:

Postpartum Problems

☐ Perineal/C-Section Wound Pain ☐ Urinary Incontinence ☐ Fecal Incontinence ☐ Dyspareunia/Reduced Sexual Desire ☐ Fatigue/Sleep Issues

Referrals/Interventions:

Chronic Health Conditions

Problem	Plan
1.	
2.	
3.	
4.	

(AA197) 12345/54321

Patient Addressograph

POSTPARTUM FORM

Name: LAST FIRST MIDDLE

ID#: EDD:

Discharge Date: – –

Delivery Information

Delivery At______weeks		Labor	Anesthesia	Postpartum Contraception		
☐ Vaginal	☐ Cesarean	☐ None	☐ None	BTL	☐ Yes	☐ No
☐ Svd	☐ Primary (For:________)	☐ Spontaneous	☐ Local/Pudendal	Implant	☐ Yes	☐ No
☐ Vacuum	☐ Repeat (For:________)	☐ Induced	☐ Epidural	LNG-IUS	☐ Yes	☐ No
☐ Forceps		☐ Augmented	☐ Spinal	Copper IUD	☐ Yes	☐ No
☐ Episiotomy	☐ Uterine Incision		☐ General	Depot Medroxyprogesterone Acetate (DMPA)	☐ Yes	☐ No
☐ Lacerations	☐ Low Transverse		☐ Other:	Combined OCP	☐ Yes	☐ No
☐ Tolac	☐ Low Vertical			Progesterone-Only Pill	☐ Yes	☐ No
	☐ Classical			Vasectomy	☐ Yes	☐ No
				Condoms	☐ Yes	☐ No
				Diaphragm	☐ Yes	☐ No
				Lactational Amenorrhea	☐ Yes	☐ No
				Natural Family Planning	☐ Yes	☐ No
				Other: ________		
				Delivered By: ________		

Postpartum Information

Complications

☐ None ☐ Hemorrhage ☐ Infection ☐ Hypertension ☐ Diabetes ☐ Other: ________

Discharge Information

Neonatal Information

Name Of Baby: ________

Sex
☐ Female ☐ Male
Circumcision ☐ Yes ☐ No

Birth Weight: ________ g

Disposition
☐ Home With Mother ☐ In Hospital
☐ Transfer ☐ Neonatal Death
☐ Stillbirth ☐ Other:________

Complications/Anomalies:

Newborn Care Provider: ________

Seen By Newborn Care Provider Before Discharge
☐ Yes ☐ No

Received Hepatitis B Birth Dose Prior to Hospital Discharge ☐ Yes ☐ No

Maternal Information

Maternal Age:________ Gravity And Parity:________

Regarding Smoking, Chewing, Using A Nicotine Delivery System (ENDS), and Vaping
☐ Does Not Use ☐ Quit During Pregnancy
☐ Current User

HGB/HCT Level: ________

Medications: ________

HIV Status* Known ☐ Yes ☐ No
☐ POS
☐ NEG

Feeding Method ☐ Breast ☐ Bottle

Diagnostic Studies Pending:

Secondary Diagnosis/Preexisting Conditions
☐ Asthma ☐ Hypertension
☐ Diabetes ☐ Other: ________

Immunizations Given
☐ Anti-D Immune Globulin
☐ Tdap Or TD ☐ HPV (When Indicated)
☐ No, Received During Pregnancy
☐ No, Received Before Pregnancy
☐ Patient Declined

☐ Influenza ☐ Varicella
☐ No, Received During Pregnancy ☐ Other:________
☐ Patient Declined
☐ MMR (When Indicated)

Infant Status: ________

☐ If Neonatal Death, Bereavement Counseling

Follow-Up Appt: ________

Date: ____ /____ /____

Location: ________

Other: ________

*Check state requirements before recording results.

Interim Contacts Or Hospitalizations

Date	Comment

PROVIDER SIGNATURE (AS REQUIRED): ________

 (AA197) 12345/54321

Patient Addressograph

Postpartum Visit

Date: – –

Feeding Method:

Contraception Method

- Tubal Sterilization ☐ Yes ☐ No
- Intrauterine Device (IUD) ☐ Yes ☐ No
- Depot Medroxyprogesterone Acetate (DMPA) ☐ Yes ☐ No
- Implant ☐ Yes ☐ No
- Oral Contraceptives ☐ Yes ☐ No
- Other: ____

Postpartum Depression Screening:

Intimate Partner Violence Screening:

Discuss Tobacco (Smoked, Chewed, ENDS, Vaped) Relapse Prevention Techniques:

Infant Health:

Interim History:

Follow-Up Lab Studies Ordered

☐ Yes ☐ No Postpartum HCB/HCT: ____

☐ Yes ☐ No Postpartum Glucose Screening If Patient Had Gestational Diabetes: ____

☐ Yes ☐ No Other Studies Requested: ____

Physical Examination

BP:____ WT:____ BMI:____

Breasts	☐ Normal	☐ Abnormal:	____
Abdomen	☐ Normal	☐ Abnormal:	____
External Genitalia	☐ Normal	☐ Abnormal:	____
Vagina	☐ Normal	☐ Abnormal:	____
Cervix	☐ Normal	☐ Abnormal:	____
Uterus	☐ Normal	☐ Abnormal:	____
Adnexa	☐ Normal	☐ Abnormal:	____
Rectal-Vaginal	☐ Normal	☐ Abnormal:	____

Pap Test ☐ Yes ☐ No If No, Due: ____

Allergies:

Immunization Update:

Medications/Contraception:

☐ Dispensed

Interval Care Recommendations

For General Health Promotion:

Plans For Future Pregnancies:

For Reproductive Health Promotion:

Repeat Glucose Screening Needed? ☐ Yes ☐ No

If Yes, Has Patient Been Counseled? ☐ Yes ☐ No

Date Of Repeat Testing:

Return Visit:

Referrals:

Examined By:

Comments

PROVIDER SIGNATURE (AS REQUIRED): ____

 (AA197) 12345/54321

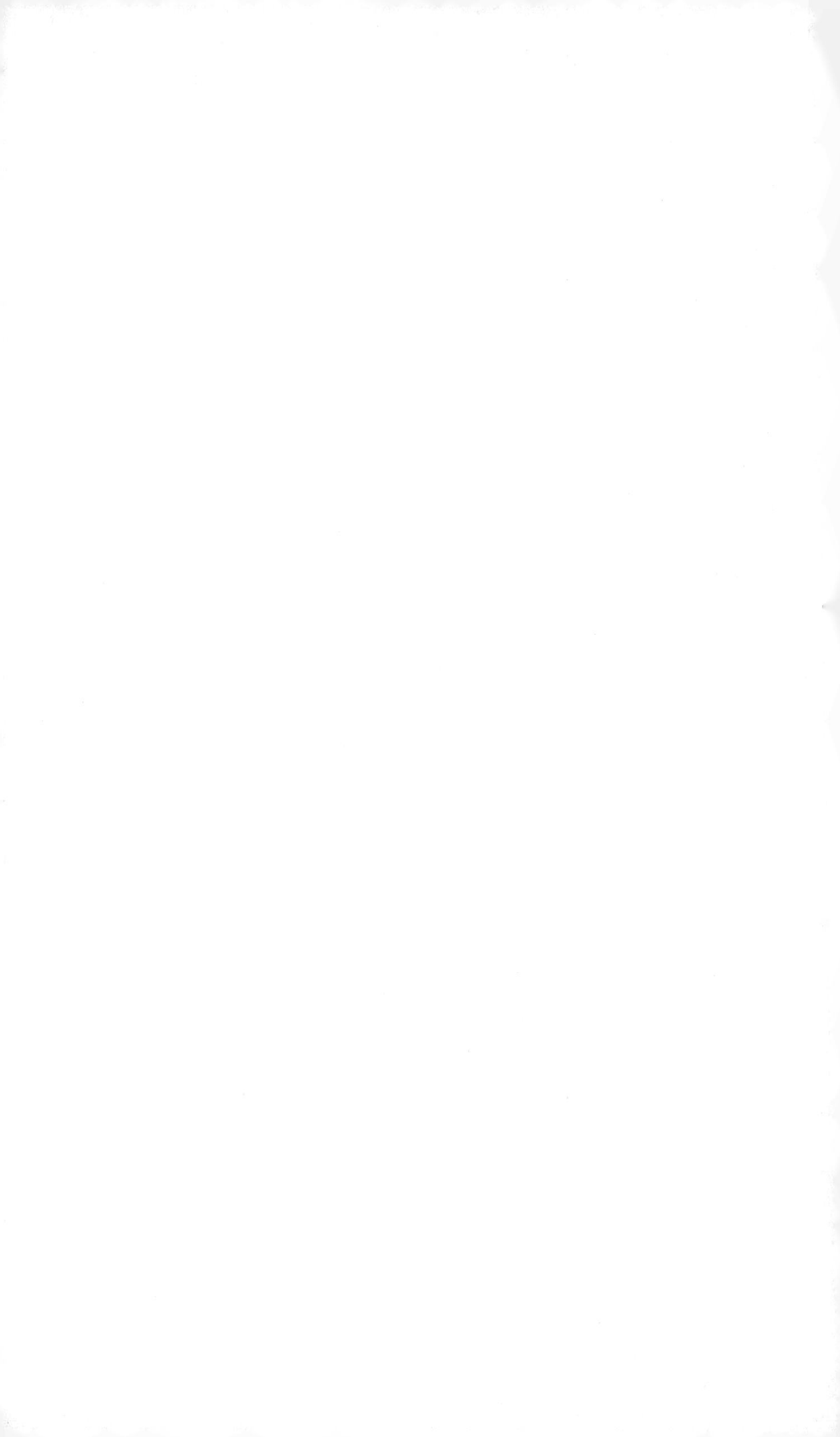

Appendix B

Early Pregnancy Risk Identification for Consultation

Risk Factor	Recommended Consultation*
Medical history and conditions	
Asthma	
Symptomatic on medication	Obstetrician–gynecologist
Severe (multiple hospitalizations)	MFM subspecialist
Cardiac disease	
Cyanotic, prior MI, aortic stenosis, pulmonary hypertension, Marfan syndrome, prosthetic valve, AHA Class II or greater	MFM subspecialist
Other	Obstetrician–gynecologist
Pregestational diabetes	MFM subspecialist
Drug and alcohol use	Obstetrician–gynecologist
Epilepsy (on medication)	Obstetrician–gynecologist
Family history of genetic problems (Down syndrome, Tay–Sachs disease, PKU)	MFM subspecialist
Hemoglobinopathy (SS, SC, S-thal)	MFM subspecialist
Hypertension	
Chronic, with renal or heart disease	MFM subspecialist
Chronic, without renal or heart disease	Obstetrician–gynecologist
Prior pulmonary embolus or deep vein thrombosis	MFM subspecialist
Psychiatric illness	Obstetrician–gynecologist
Pulmonary disease	
Severe obstructive or restrictive	MFM subspecialist
Moderate	Obstetrician–gynecologist

(continued)

Early Pregnancy Risk Identification for Consultation *(continued)*

Risk Factor	Recommended Consultation*
Renal disease	
Chronic, creatinine 3 or greater with or without hypertension	MFM subspecialist
Chronic, other	MFM subspecialist
Requirement for prolonged anticoagulation	MFM subspecialist
Severe systemic disease	MFM subspecialist
Obstetric history and conditions	
Age 35 years or older at delivery	Obstetrician–gynecologist
Cesarean delivery, prior classical or vertical incision	Obstetrician–gynecologist
Cervical insufficiency	Obstetrician–gynecologist
Prior fetal structural or chromosomal abnormality	MFM subspecialist
Prior neonatal death	Obstetrician–gynecologist
Prior fetal death	Obstetrician–gynecologist
Prior preterm delivery or preterm PROM	Obstetrician–gynecologist
Prior low birth weight (less than 2,500 g)	Obstetrician–gynecologist
Second-trimester pregnancy loss	Obstetrician–gynecologist
Uterine leiomyomata or malformation	Obstetrician–gynecologist
Initial laboratory tests	
HIV	
Symptomatic or low CD4 count	MFM subspecialist
CDE (Rh) or other blood group isoimmunization (excluding ABO, Lewis)	MFM subspecialist
Initial examination—condylomata (extensive, covering vulva or vaginal opening)	Obstetrician–gynecologist

Abbreviations: AHA, American Heart Association; HIV, human immunodeficiency virus; MFM, maternal–fetal medicine; MI, myocardial infarction; PKU, phenylketonuria; PROM, premature rupture of membranes.

*At the time of consultation, continued patient care should be determined to be by collaboration with the referring care provider or by transfer of care.

Modified with permission from March of Dimes Birth Defects Foundation, Committee on Perinatal Health. Toward improving the outcome of pregnancy: the 90s and beyond. White Plains, New York: March of Dimes Birth Defects Foundation, 1993.

Appendix C

Ongoing Pregnancy Risk Identification for Consultation

Risk Factor	Recommended Consultation*
Medical history and conditions	
Drug or alcohol use	Obstetrician–gynecologist
Proteinuria (2+ by catheter sample, unexplained by urinary tract infection)	Obstetrician–gynecologist
Pyelonephritis	Obstetrician–gynecologist
Severe systemic disease that adversely affects pregnancy	MFM subspecialist
Obstetric history and conditions	
Blood pressure elevation (diastolic 90 mm or greater Hg), no proteinuria	Obstetrician–gynecologist
Fetal growth restriction suspected	Obstetrician–gynecologist
Fetal abnormality suspected by ultrasonography	MFM subspecialist
Fetal demise	Obstetrician–gynecologist
Gestational age 41 weeks (to be seen by 42 weeks)	Obstetrician–gynecologist
Gestational diabetes mellitus	Obstetrician–gynecologist
Herpes, active lesions 36 weeks	Obstetrician–gynecologist
Hydramnios by ultrasonography	Obstetrician–gynecologist; if severe MFM subspecialist
Hyperemesis, persisting beyond first trimester	Obstetrician–gynecologist
Multiple gestation	Obstetrician–gynecologist
Oligohydramnios by ultrasonography	Obstetrician–gynecologist
Preterm labor, threatened, less than 37 weeks	Obstetrician–gynecologist
Premature rupture of membranes	Obstetrician–gynecologist
Vaginal bleeding 14 weeks or greater	Obstetrician–gynecologist

(continued)

Ongoing Pregnancy Risk Identification for Consultation *(continued)*

Risk Factor	Recommended Consultation*
Examination and laboratory findings	
Abnormal MSAFP (low or high)	Obstetrician–gynecologist
Abnormal Pap test result	Obstetrician–gynecologist
Anemia (Hct less than 28%, unresponsive to iron therapy)	Obstetrician–gynecologist
Condylomata (extensive, covering labia and vaginal opening)	Obstetrician–gynecologist
HIV	
Symptomatic or low CD4 count	MFM subspecialist
Other	
CDE (Rh) or other blood group isoimmunization (excluding ABO, Lewis)	MFM subspecialist

Abbreviations: Hct, hematocrit; HIV, human immunodeficiency virus; MFM, maternal–fetal medicine; MSAFP, maternal serum alpha-fetoprotein.

*At the time of consultation, continued patient care should be determined to be by collaboration with the referring care provider or by transfer of care.

Modified with permission from March of Dimes Birth Defects Foundation, Committee on Perinatal Health. Toward improving the outcome of pregnancy: the 90s and beyond. White Plains, New York: March of Dimes Birth Defects Foundation, 1993.

Appendix D

Granting Obstetric Privileges

Granting Privileges

The following list has been developed to aid in granting privileges to those health care providers within the facility to perform obstetric and gynecologic procedures. The granting of privileges at any level in obstetrics and gynecology is based on satisfaction of criteria for the specified procedures. Criteria for granting privileges must be applied consistently regardless of the applicant's specialty. As stated, the granting of clinical privileges must be based on training, experience, and demonstrated current clinical competence. The educational requirements assume that applicants have achieved a doctor of medicine or doctor of osteopathy degree. Except as otherwise noted, prerequisites for each category of privileges are listed as follows:

Training

- Successful completion of an Accreditation Council for Graduate Medical Education (ACGME)-accredited residency program in obstetrics–gynecology

Certification

- Board certification (or active candidate) by the American Board of Obstetrics and Gynecology or the American Osteopathic Board of Obstetrics and Gynecology
- Maintenance of Certification, if applicable

Reappraisal (recredentialing/reprivileging) (2-year cycle) should require:

- Review of quality improvement file:
  - — trending
  - — sentinel events
  - — other problems with specific procedures

- Review of level of activity:
  — total number of cases
  — total number of complications
  — outcomes
- If the credentials committee determines that the number of cases performed within the cycle is insufficient for adequately assessing competency, it may recommend that the individual be proctored and evaluated for a designated period until competency is demonstrated. However, if the physician has privileges at another institution for the particular procedure, then the individual must provide credentialing data from that hospital for review by the credentials committee and may not require proctoring.

I. Obstetric Privileges

A. Basic Level Obstetric Privileges

1. Privileges may include:
   a. Management of labor
   b. Pudendal and local anesthesia
   c. Fetal assessment, antepartum and intrapartum, including limited obstetric ultrasound examination
   d. Induction of labor
   e. Internal fetal monitoring
   f. Normal cephalic delivery, including use of vacuum extraction and outlet forceps
   g. Episiotomy and repair, including third-degree lacerations
   h. Management of common intrapartum problems
   i. Exploration of vagina, cervix, and uterus
   j. Emergency breech delivery
   k. Management of common postpartum problems
   l. First-assist at cesarean delivery
   m. Circumcision

B. Specialty Level Obstetric Privileges

1. Privileges may include:
   a. All basic level obstetric privileges
   b. Management of normal and abnormal labor and delivery (including premature labor, breech presentation, cesarean delivery, vaginal delivery after previous cesarean delivery,

cephalopelvic disproportion, nonreassuring fetal status, use of amniotomy and oxytocin, and midforceps delivery)

   c. Management of medical or surgical complications of pregnancy
   d. Diagnostic amniocentesis
   e. Cesarean hysterectomy
   f. Hypogastric artery ligation
   g. Vaginal cerclage or treatment of incompetent cervix
   h. External version of breech presentation
   i. Obstetric ultrasonography—complete
   j. Midforceps rotation
   k. Regional anesthesia as determined by training and local practice
2. Board certification (or active candidate) by the American Board of Obstetrics and Gynecology in maternal–fetal medicine may be considered

C. Subspecialty Level Obstetric Privileges

1. Privileges may include:
   a. All basic and specialty obstetric privileges
   b. Intrauterine fetal transfusion
   c. Intrauterine fetal surgery
   d. Chorionic villus sampling
   e. Percutaneous umbilical sampling
2. Training should include documentation of specialized post-residency training
3. Subspecialty certification (or active candidate) by the American Board of Obstetrics and Gynecology in maternal–fetal medicine may be considered

II. Credentialing for Family Physicians

A. Obstetric Privileges for Family Physicians

1. Privileges may include:
   a. Management of labor
   b. Pudendal and local block anesthesia
   c. Fetal assessment, antepartum and intrapartum, including limited obstetric ultrasound examination
   d. Internal fetal monitoring
   e. Normal cephalic delivery

f. Management of common intrapartum problems
g. Exploration of vagina, cervix, and uterus
h. Emergency breech delivery
i. Management of common postpartum problems
j. First-assist at cesarean delivery

2. Family physicians requesting these privileges must demonstrate:
   a. Successful completion of obstetric training as delineated in the special requirements for residency training in Family Medicine by the Accreditation Council for Graduate Medical Education
   b. If transferring from another institution, documentation of current competence as supported by ongoing clinical practice and quality review data
   c. Maintenance of board certification (or active candidate) by the American Board of Family Physicians

B. Advanced Obstetric Privileges for Family Physicians
1. Privileges may include:
   a. Operative vaginal delivery, including low forceps or vacuum extraction
   b. Induction of labor
   c. Management of high-risk pregnancy
2. Family physicians requesting these privileges must demonstrate:
   a. Additional intensive experience taught by or in collaboration with obstetrician–gynecologists (1). In programs where obstetrician–gynecologists are not available, these skills should be taught by appropriately skilled and credentialed family physicians.
   b. The assignment of hospital privileges is a local responsibility, and privileges should be granted on the basis of training, experience, and demonstrated current clinical competence. All physicians should be held to the same standards for granting privileges, regardless of specialty, in order to ensure the provision of high-quality patient care. Prearranged, collaborative relationships should be established to ensure ongoing consultations, as well as consultations needed for emergencies.

      The standard of training should allow any physician who receives training in a cognitive or surgical skill to meet the criteria for privileges in that area of practice. Provisional privileges in primary care, obstetric care, and cesarean delivery should be granted regardless of specialty as long as training criteria and experience are documented. All physicians should be subject to a proctorship period to allow demonstration of ability and current competence. These principles should apply to all health care systems.

c. Privileges recommended by the department of family practice shall be the responsibility of the department of family practice. Similarly, privileges recommended by the department of obstetrics and gynecology shall be the responsibility of the department of obstetrics and gynecology. When privileges are recommended jointly by the departments of family practice and obstetrics and gynecology, they shall be the joint responsibility of the two departments.

Requests for New Privileges

New Equipment and Technology

New equipment or technology usually improves health care, provided that practitioners and other hospital staff understand the proper indications for usage. Problems can arise when staff perform duties or use equipment for which they are not trained. It is imperative that all staff be properly trained in the use of the advanced technology or new equipment.

Privileges for new skills should be granted only when the appropriate training has been completed and documented and the competency level has been achieved with adequate supervision. That is, each physician requesting additional privileges for new equipment or technology should be evaluated by answering the following questions:

1. Does the hospital have a mechanism in place to ensure that necessary support for the new equipment or technology is available?
2. Has the physician been adequately trained, including hands-on experience, to use the new equipment or to perform the new technology?
3. Has the physician adequately demonstrated an ability to use the new equipment or perform the new technology? This may require that the physician undergo a period of proctoring or supervision, or both. If no one on staff can serve as a proctor, the hospital may either require reciprocal proctoring at another hospital or grant temporary privileges to someone from another hospital to supervise the applicant.

Specifically, if the new privileges were not included in residency training, the applicant must:

1. Complete a preceptorship with a physician already credentialed to perform the procedures of that skill level; the preceptorship should require the applicant to perform the designated surgery with the preceptor acting as first assistant.
2. Provide a list of cases satisfactorily completed under supervision at each skill level, as defined by the local institution.
3. Submit a letter from the preceptor documenting that the procedures were completed in a satisfactory manner and that the applicant is competent to perform the procedures independently at the designated skill level.

If there is no experienced surgeon on the hospital staff who is able to serve as a preceptor for advanced or new surgical procedures, a supervised preceptorship must be arranged. This may be done by scheduling a number of cases from physicians requiring credentialing and inviting a credentialed surgeon from another institution to serve as a surgical consultant.

After a Period of Inactivity

The American Medical Association (AMA) defines physician reentry as "a return to clinical practice in the discipline in which one has been trained and certified following an extended period of inactivity" (2). This section will not address inactivity that results from discipline or impairment.

There are several reasons why a physician might take a leave of absence from clinical practice, such as family leave (maternity and paternity leave and child care); personal health reasons; career dissatisfaction; alternate careers such as administration; military service; or humanitarian leave. Traditionally, women were more likely to experience career interruptions; however, recent research shows that younger cohorts of male physicians also take on multiple roles and express intentions to adjust their careers accordingly (2).

When physicians request reentry after a period of inactivity, a general guideline for evaluation would be to consider the physician as any other new applicant for privileges. This would include evaluation of the following:

1. Demonstration that a minimum number of hours of continuing medical education has been earned during the period of inactivity. It is also important to meet any board certification requirements during the absence.

2. In accordance with the medical staff bylaws, supervision by a proctor appointed by the department chair for a minimum number and defined breadth of cases during the provisional period, evaluating and documenting proficiency.
3. A time-sensitive, focused review of cases as required by the departmental quality improvement committee may be completed as appropriate.

The area of skills assessment may prove challenging if the previous guidelines, number 2 and number 3, are not felt to be adequate. But, there are several options to consider:

1. Residency Training Programs

   Benefits: More locations are available, providing structured didactic programs, and implementing competency assessment. Participating in these programs can provide a source of manpower to help compensate for restricted residency work hours.

   Drawbacks: Many hospitals with residency programs have only a limited number of cases available for training. Reentry programs must not negatively affect the residency training program (ie, if someone is being brought into a reentry program in an institution that has a residency program, the Residency Review Committee must be notified with an explanation as to how it will not negatively affect the residents).

2. Simulation Centers

   Benefits: These centers can help supplement hands-on clinical experience and may be more geographically accessible. The use of simulation centers for reentry into practice is a new concept. This training may precede and supplement proctored clinical experience.

   Drawbacks: Currently there is a limited number of functioning simulation centers, although this number should continue to expand. Cost is another drawback.

3. Physician Reentry Program (PREP)

   Benefits: Well-designed PREP systems should be consistent with the current continuum of medical education and meet the needs of the reentering physician.

   Drawbacks: Only a few PREP systems are offered nationally; thus, cost and location are considerable obstacles in using these programs.

An underlying assumption is that physicians do not necessarily lose competence in all areas of practice with time. Competencies such as patient communication and professionalism may not decline. Therefore, a reentry program should target those areas where physicians are more likely to have lost relevant skills or knowledge, or where skills and knowledge need to be updated (3).

Finally, it is extremely important for physicians considering a leave of absence or major change in practice activities to think in advance about options should they wish to return. At a minimum, licensure and continuing medical education activities should be maintained. Working part-time during an absence helps to maintain a minimal amount of competency.

References

1. American Academy of Family Physicians, American College of Obstetricians and Gynecologists. AAFP–ACOG joint statement on cooperative practice and hospital privileges. Leawood (KS): AAFP; Washington, DC: ACOG; 1998.
2. Mark S, Gupta J. Reentry into clinical practice: challenges and strategies. JAMA 2002;288:1091–6.
3. American Medical Association. Report 6 of the Council on Medical Education (A-08): physician reentry. Chicago (IL): AMA; 2008. Available at: http://www.ama-assn.org/sites/default/files/media-browser/public/council-on-med-ed/cmerpt-6a-08.pdf. Retrieved June 24, 2009.

Quality and Safety in Women's Health Care. 2nd ed. Washington, DC: American College of Obstetricians and Gynecologists; 2010.

Appendix E

Glossary of Midwifery Organizations and Terms

There is wide variability in the legal status and level of practice authority of midwives across the United States. The different titles for midwives can be confusing, as can the different credentialing standards for midwives and different professional associations and grassroots organizations.

Seven organizations are responsible for midwifery education, certification, accreditation, and professional association in the United States:

- Professional associations: American College of Nurse-Midwives, National Association of Certified Professional Midwives, and Midwives Alliance of North America
- Certification bodies: American Midwifery Certification Board and North American Registry of Midwives
- Educational accreditors: Accreditation Commission for Midwifery Education and Midwifery Education Accreditation Council

There are three separate midwifery credentials in the United States: certified nurse-midwives (CNM), certified midwives, and certified professional midwives. Each credential accepts different levels of education, training, and experience and the qualifications of midwives who use the certified professional midwife designation can vary markedly. This glossary is provided for information and reference purposes to clarify these various requirements, qualifications, and standards. It is inclusive of the range of midwifery terms, including nurse-midwifery, and is representative of current activity across the country. Listings are alphabetical and include a website address where applicable. The year an organization was formed and when a term first came into use is also noted.

American Association of Birth Centers: A nonprofit, multidisciplinary membership organization founded by Childbirth Connection (formerly Maternity Center Association) more than 25 years ago. It was formerly known as the National Association of Childbearing Centers. The American Association of Birth Centers establishes national standards and accreditation for birth centers and advocates federally and in the states for birth center reimbursement and other concerns. www.birthcenters.org

American College of Nurse–Midwives (ACNM): Professional organization for CNMs and certified midwives established in 1955. The American College of Nurse–Midwives sets competencies and standards for academic preparation and clinical practice. These meet and exceed the global competencies and standards for the practice of midwifery as defined by the International Confederation of Midwives. www.midwife.org

Accreditation Commission for Midwifery Education: Educational accreditor for CNMs and certified midwives. The Accreditation Commission for Midwifery Education is one of only two accrediting agencies for midwifery education recognized by the U.S. Department of Education. Programs accredited by the Accreditation Commission for Midwifery Education meet and exceed standards set by the International Confederation of Midwives.

American Midwifery Certification Board, Inc.: Certification board for CNMs and certified midwives. This board was formerly called the ACNM Certification Council, Inc. In 1997, American Midwifery Certification Board opened its national certification exam to nonnurse graduates of midwifery education programs and issued the first certified midwife credential. Certified nurse–midwives and certified midwives must demonstrate that they meet the *Core Competencies for Basic Midwifery Practice* and practice in accordance with ACNM *Standards for the Practice of Midwifery*. As of 2010, a graduate degree is required for entry into clinical practice for both CNMs and certified midwives. Certified nurse–midwives and certified midwives must recertify every 5 years through the American Midwifery Certification Board and meet specific continuing education requirements. www.amcb-midwife.org

Certified Midwife: A midwife who undergoes the same certification process as a CNM, but whose training does not include education in nursing. The professional association for certified midwives is the ACNM. In 1996, the ACNM adopted standards for the certification of direct-entry midwives to be known as certified midwives. Certified midwives pass the same certification exam as CNMs, and earn a master's degree. To maintain their credential, certified midwives recertify every 5 years through the American Midwifery Certification Board. Competencies and standards are consistent with or exceed the global competencies and standards defined by the International Confederation of Midwives. Certified midwives are relatively few in number and practice legally in only a handful of states including New Jersey, New York, and Rhode Island. New York had the first certified midwife training program and was the first state to recognize the certified midwife credential. It is the only state that has one unified framework for licensing all midwives, both CNMs and certified midwives.

Certified Nurse–Midwife (CNM): A midwife who is educated in the two disciplines of nursing and midwifery. Certified nurse–midwives are the only category of midwives who are trained and licensed as advance practice nurses. The professional association for CNMs is the ACNM. Certified nurse–midwives earn a master's degree, complete a midwifery education program accredited by the Accreditation Commission for Midwifery Education, and pass a national certification examination administered by the American Midwifery Certification Board. To maintain their credential, CNMs recertify every 5 years through the American Midwifery Certification Board. Competencies and standards are consistent with or exceed the global competencies and standards defined by the International Confederation of Midwives. Certified nurse–midwives comprise the majority of midwives in the United States and are licensed in all 50 states and the District of Columbia. Certified nurse–wives practice encompasses primary health care for women; gynecologic and family planning services; prepregnancy care; pregnancy, childbirth, and postpartum care; and normal newborn care. Certified nurse–midwives admit, manage, and discharge patients; order and interpret laboratory and diagnostic tests; have prescriptive authority for most drugs and third-party reimbursement including Medicaid; and practice independently or in collaborative practice with physicians in diverse settings such as hospitals, birth centers, ambulatory care clinics, private offices, community and public health systems, and homes.

Certified Professional Midwife (also licensed midwives, licensed direct-entry midwives, and registered midwives): There is no single standard for education of certified professional midwives. Both apprentice-trained midwives and midwives with some formal academic training use the CPM credential without distinction. Most certified professional midwives are trained in one-on-one apprenticeships and self-study with no university or hospital-based education or training. A high school diploma was not required until 2012. The certified professional midwife credential was developed in the mid-1990s jointly by the Midwives Alliance of North America, the North American Registry of Midwives and the Midwifery Education Accreditation Council. There are two professional associations for certified professional midwives: the National Association of Certified Professional Midwives and the Midwives Alliance of North America. Certified professional midwives practice legally in more than half of the states by mandatory licensure, registration, or permit. In a few states, licensure is voluntary. Most states use the certified professional midwife credential or the North American Registry of Midwives examination as the basis for licensure. Certified professional midwives practice outside the hospital primarily in homes.

Childbirth Connection: Established in 1918, Childbirth Connection (formerly Maternity Center Association) is a national nonprofit organization whose mission is to improve the quality of maternity care through research, education, advocacy, and policy. www.childbirthconnection.org

Citizens for Midwifery, Inc.: A nonprofit, volunteer, grassroots organization founded by several mothers in 1996 to promote certified professional midwives and the Midwives Model of Care™ (see also Midwives Models of Care™). The organization is active federally and in the states. www.cfmidwifery.org

Collaborative Practice: A comprehensive, dynamic system of patient-centered health care delivered by a multidisciplinary team. [*NOTE: This definition is from the glossary section of the 1995 document, American College of Obstetricians and Gynecologists' Guidelines for Implementing Collaborative Practice. The following definition, approved by the American College of Obstetricians and Gynecologists' Executive Board, appears on page one of that document:* Collaborative practice in the health care of women is a comprehensive, dynamic system of patient-centered health care delivered by a multidisciplinary team. The team consists of obstetrician–gynecologists and other health care professionals who function within their educational preparation and scope of practice. These team members work together, utilizing mutually agreed upon guidelines and policies that define the individual and shared responsibilities of each member. Although the responsibilities of obstetrician–gynecologists place them in the role of ultimate authority because of their education and training, the contributions of each team member are valued and important to the quality of patient outcomes. The concept of a team guided by one of its own members and the acceptance of shared responsibility for outcomes promote shared accountability.]

Direct-Entry Midwives (licensed direct-entry midwives, licensed midwives, registered midwives): A midwife who enters the profession of midwifery directly without earning a nursing degree. Both certified professional midwives and certified midwives are considered direct-entry midwives, although their level of education and training varies markedly. (See also "Certified Midwife," "Certified Professional Midwife," and "Lay Midwife".)

International Confederation of Midwives: The global leadership organization for midwives that sets standards for midwifery education, regulation and professional association. The International Confederation of Midwives, in collaboration with the International Federation of Gynecology and Obstetrics (FIGO), first published a definition of midwife in 1972; it was later endorsed by the World Health Organization (WHO). In 2011, the International Confederation of Midwives updated its essential competencies for basic midwifery practice—including its definition of a midwife—and developed and adopted new global standards for midwifery education and regulation. This framework helps countries, including the United States, evaluate, upgrade, and strengthen their midwifery workforce. The International Confederation of Midwives recommends that all midwives worldwide use a common title, meet a common, minimum education and training standard, and be licensed and regulated. The International Confederation of Midwives' baseline education standards include a curriculum that is 40% theory and 50% practice; 3-years of direct-entry training and 18 months of postnursing or other training; and time limited certification. Here in the United States, the Accreditation Commission for Midwifery Education- and the Midwifery Education Accreditation Council-accredited education programs meet or exceed the International Confederation of Midwives' standards; nonaccredited midwifery education pathways, including the Portfolio Evaluation Process apprenticeship program for certified professional midwives, do not meet the International Confederation of Midwives' standards. The International Conferedation of Midwives, WHO, and FIGO stress the importance of a formal education and accreditation process as a means to ensure skilled practitioners. www.internationalmidwives.org

Lay Midwife: Often used incorrectly, this term refers to an unlicensed midwife. In some states still today, any "lay" person may attend or assist a woman giving birth, but in a gratuitous, nonprofessional, nonbusiness capacity. These "lay" midwives typically act outside of state recognition and oversight and, in fact, are not licensed by the state.

Midwives Alliance of North America: One of two professional associations for certified professional midwives. Midwives Alliance of North America is a grassroots alliance founded in 1982 representing midwives of diverse educational backgrounds. In the 1980s, Midwives Alliance of North America developed the first national certifying exam for direct-entry midwives and in 1986 launched a national registry of midwives. Its members include certified professional midwives, certified nurse–midwives, licensed midwives, and "lay" midwives. Midwives Alliance of North America Core Competencies delineate the content areas for certified professional midwife practice. www.mana.org

Midwifery Education Accreditation Council: Educational accreditor for academically trained certified professional midwives. The Midwifery Education Accreditation Council is one of only two accrediting agencies for midwifery education recognized by the U.S. Department of Education. Standards for accreditation were developed in the 1990s. The Midwifery Education Accreditation Council requires that midwifery schools incorporate the *Core Competencies* adopted by the Midwives Alliance of North America and the clinical experience requirements and essential knowledge and skills identified by the North American Registry of Midwives. www.meacschools.org

Midwives Model of Care™: The standard of care for certified professional midwives established by the Midwives Alliance of North America, the North American Registry of Midwives, and the Midwifery Education Accreditation Council.

National Association of Certified Professional Midwives: One of two professional associations for certified professional midwives established in 2001. www.nacpm.org

North American Registry of Midwives: The certification body for both apprentice-trained and academically-trained certified professional midwives established in 1987 by the Midwives Alliance of North America. The North American Registry of Midwives is accredited by the National Commission for Certifying Agencies, the accrediting body of the National Organization for Competency Assurance. The National Commission for Certifying Agencies accredits many health care credentials including the CNM. The North American Registry of Midwives administers certification for certified professional midwives who are qualified to provide the Midwives Model of Care™; recertification is required every 3 years. Many states use the North American Registry of Midwives' certification exam as the basis for licensure. www.narm.org

Portfolio Evaluation Process: A 3–5 year apprenticeship program for certified professional midwives. The Portfolio Evaluation Process does not grant a degree and is not eligible for U.S. Department of Education accreditation. Certified professional midwives trained through the Portfolio Evaluation Process must complete the North American Registry of Midwives' written and skills exam for certification.

Skilled Birth Attendant: WHO, International Confederation of Midwives, and the FIGO define the skilled birth attendant as "an accredited health professional who has been educated and trained to proficiency in the skills needed to manage normal (uncomplicated) pregnancies, childbirth and the immediate postnatal period, and in the identification, management and referral of complications in women and newborns." (See their 2004 joint statement, The Critical Role of the Skilled Attendant.) www.internationalmidwives.org

Traditional Birth Attendant: These practitioners historically have served women and families in distinct cultural or religious groups. They may practice without a license and lack formal education and credentials. The World Health Organization, the International Confederation of Midwives, and FIGO define the traditional birth attendant as the "traditional, independent (of the health care system), nonformally trained, and community-based provider of care during pregnancy, childbirth and the postnatal period." www.internationalmidwives.org

United States Midwifery Education, Regulation, and Association: A collaboration of the seven major U.S. midwifery organizations to strengthen and align U.S. midwifery with the worldwide standards set by the International Confederation of Midwives in 2011. The seven midwifery organizations in the United States with responsibility for midwifery education, certification, accreditation, and professional association are Accreditation Commission for Midwifery Education, American College of Nurse–Midwives, American Midwifery Certification Board, Midwifery Education Accreditation Council,

Midwives Alliance of North America, National Association of Certified Professional Midwives, and the North American Registry of Midwives. Each organization agreed to conduct a gap analysis comparing the International Confederation of Midwives' global standards with comparable U.S. standards, competencies, regulations, and association capacity.

United States Midwifery Education, Regulation, and Association Bridge Certificate: A bridge certificate program to elevate the education and training of certified professional midwives who lack accredited education and do not meet the global standards set by the International Confederation of Midwives. Developed by the seven major U.S. midwifery groups and administered by the North American Registry of Midwives, the bridge certificate became operational in fall 2015. Applicants must complete 50 hours of accredited coursework within 5 years of application in specified categories, including birth emergency skills training and advanced life support in obstetrics courses and emergency skills in pregnancy, birth, immediate postpartum, and newborn care. At the present time, the bridge certificate is voluntary. It is not required for recertification by the North American Registry of Midwives and certified professional midwives already licensed in a state are not required to undergo bridge training. Effective January 2020, Maine is the first state to require the bridge certificate for certified professional midwives licensure. www.narm.org/midwifery-bridge-certificate.

Appendix F

Standard Terminology for Reporting of Reproductive Health Statistics in the United States*

The adoption of standard definitions and reporting requirements for reproductive health statistics will provide an improved basis for standardization and uniformity in the design, implementation, and evaluation of intervention strategies. The reduction of maternal and infant mortality and the improvement of the health of our nation's women and infants are the ultimate goals. The collection and analysis of reliable statistical data are an essential part of in-depth investigations and incorporate case finding, individual review, and analysis of risk factors. These studies could then yield valuable clinical information for practitioners, aiding them in improved case management for patients at high risk, which would result in decreased morbidity and mortality.

Both the collection and the use of statistics have been hampered by lack of understanding of differences in definitions, statistical tabulations, and reporting requirements among state, national, and international bodies. Misapplication and misinterpretation of data may lead to erroneous comparisons and conclusions. For example, specific requirements for reporting of fetal deaths often have been misinterpreted as implying a weight or gestational age for viability. Distinctions can and should be made among the definition of an event, the reporting requirements for the event, and the statistical tabulation and interpretation of the data. The definition indicates the meaning of a term (eg, live birth, fetal death, or maternal death). A reporting

*Different states use different birth weight and gestational age criteria to define fetal death. The Committee on Obstetric Practice of the American College of Obstetricians and Gynecologists recommends that perinatal mortality statistics be based on a gestational weight of 500 g.

requirement is that part of the defined event for which reporting is mandatory or desired. Statistical tabulations connote the presentation of data for the purpose of analysis and interpretation of existing and future conditions. The data should be collected in a manner that will allow them to be presented in different ways for different users. Adjustments should be made for variations in reporting before comparisons among data are attempted.

If information is collected and presented in a standardized manner, comparisons between the new data and the data obtained by previous reporting requirements can be delineated clearly and can improve public understanding of reproductive health statistics. For ease in assimilating this information, this appendix is divided into three sections: 1) definitions, 2) statistical tabulations, and 3) reporting requirements and recommendations. Some of the definitions and recommendations are a departure from those currently or historically accepted; however, these recommendations were agreed on by an inter-organizational group that was brought together in the mid-1980s to review terminology related to reproductive health issues.

Definitions*

Birth Weight: The weight of a fetus or neonate determined immediately after delivery or as soon thereafter as feasible. It should be expressed to the nearest gram.

> High birth weight—Any neonate, regardless of gestational age whose birth weight is greater than 4,000 g.
>
> Low birth weight—Any neonate, regardless of gestational age, whose weight at birth is less than 2,500 g. Low birth weight is further subdivided as moderately low birth weight (1,500–2,499 g), very low birth weight (less than 1,500 g), and extremely low birth weight (less than 1,000 g).

Fetal Death: Death before the complete expulsion or extraction from the mother of a product of conception, irrespective of the duration of pregnancy that is not an induced termination of pregnancy. The death is indicated by the fact that, after such expulsion or extraction, the fetus does not breathe

---

*These definitions are for statistical purposes and are not intended to affect clinical management. Appropriate assessment of fetal maturity for purposes of clinical management is delineated in Chapter 6.

or show any other evidence of life, such as beating of the heart, pulsation of the umbilical cord, or definite movement of voluntary muscles. Heartbeats are to be distinguished from transient cardiac contractions; respirations are to be distinguished from fleeting respiratory efforts or gasps.

For statistical purposes, fetal deaths are further subdivided as early fetal death (20–27 weeks of gestation) or late fetal death (28 weeks of gestation). The term stillbirth also is used to describe fetal deaths at 20 weeks of gestation or more. Fetuses that die in utero before 20 weeks of gestation are categorized specifically as miscarriages.

Gestational Age: The period of time between fertilization and birth, written with both weeks and days. It is calculated by one of two ways:

Last menstrual period (LMP)—The number of weeks and days that have elapsed between the first day of the last normal menstrual period (not the presumed time of fertilization) and the date of delivery, irrespective of whether the gestation results in a live birth or a fetal death

Best obstetrical estimate—The number of weeks and days calculated by using the best obstetrical estimated due date (EDD) based on the following formula:

Gestational Age = (280 – [EDD – Reference Date])/ 7

EDD: Estimated due date

Reference Date: Date on which you are trying to determine gestational age

Beginning with U.S. 2014 data, the National Center for Health Statistics transitioned to using the obstetric estimate of gestation at delivery, replacing the measure based on the date of the last menstrual period. This transition was made because of increasing evidence of the greater validity of the obstetric estimate of gestation of delivery compared with the last menstrual period-based measure.

Gestational Age Categories:

Term—37 weeks and 0 days using best EDD. It is further divided into the following categories:

Early term—37 weeks and 0 days through 38 weeks and 6 days

Full term—39 weeks and 0 days through 40 weeks and 6 days

Late term—41 weeks and 0 days through 41 weeks and 6 days

Postterm—Greater than or equal to 42 weeks and 0 days

Preterm—Less than 37 weeks and 0 days

Late preterm—34 weeks and 0 days through 36 weeks and 6 days

Moderately preterm—32 weeks and 0 days through 36 weeks and 6 days

Very preterm—28 weeks and 0 days through 31 weeks and 6 days

Extremely preterm—Less than 28 weeks and 0 days

Infant Death: A live birth that results in death within the first year (less than 365 days) is defined as an infant death. Infant deaths are further subdivided as early neonatal (less than 7 days), late neonatal (7–27 days), neonatal (less than 28 days), or postneonatal (28–364 days).

Live Birth: The complete expulsion or extraction from the mother of a product of conception, irrespective of the duration of pregnancy, which, after such expulsion or extraction, breathes or shows any other evidence of life, such as beating of the heart, pulsation of the umbilical cord, or definite movement of voluntary muscles, regardless of whether the umbilical cord has been cut or the placenta is attached. Heartbeats are to be distinguished from transient cardiac contractions; respirations are to be distinguished from fleeting respiratory efforts or gasps.

*Maternal Death**: The death of a woman from any cause related to or aggravated by pregnancy or its management (regardless of the duration or site of pregnancy), but not from accidental or incidental causes.

Direct obstetric death—The death of a woman resulting from obstetric complications of pregnancy, labor, or the puerperium; from interventions, omissions, or treatment; or from a chain of events resulting from any of these.

Indirect obstetric death—The death of a woman resulting from a previously existing disease or a disease that developed during pregnancy, labor, or the puerperium that did not have direct obstetric causes, although the physiologic effects of pregnancy were partially responsible for the death.

---

*Death occurring to a woman during pregnancy or after its termination from causes not related to the pregnancy or to its complications or management is not considered a maternal death. Nonmaternal deaths may result from accidental causes (eg, auto accident or gunshot wound) or incidental causes (eg, concurrent malignancy).

In 1987, the Centers for Disease Control and Prevention (CDC) collaborated with the Maternal Mortality Special Interest Group of the American College of Obstetricians and Gynecologists (the College), the Association of Vital Records and Health Statistics, and state and local health departments to initiate the National Pregnancy Mortality Surveillance System. The CDC–College Maternal Mortality Study Group introduced two terms, which are being used by the CDC and increasingly by some states and researchers. The study group differentiates between pregnancy-associated and pregnancy-related deaths.

Pregnancy-Associated Death: The death of any woman, from any cause, while pregnant or within 1 calendar year of termination of pregnancy, regardless of the duration and the site of pregnancy.

Pregnancy-Related Death: A pregnancy-associated death resulting from complications of the pregnancy itself, the chain of events initiated by the pregnancy that led to death, or aggravation of an unrelated condition by the physiologic or pharmacologic effects of the pregnancy that subsequently caused death.

Induced Termination of Pregnancy: The purposeful interruption of an intrauterine pregnancy with the intention other than to produce a liveborn infant, and which does not result in a live birth. This definition excludes management of prolonged retention of products of conception after fetal death.

Statistical Tabulations

Statistical tabulations for vital events related to pregnancy provide the medical and statistical community with valuable information on reproductive health and generate data on trends apparent in this country and worldwide. This information often is disaggregated and used to examine specific events over time or within selected geographic locations. In informing the public about health issues, media sources often report various statistical measures. Heightened public interest in health-related issues makes it essential that the medical community understand and have the capacity to interpret these statistics.

The following explanations of statistical tabulations are intended to provide the reader with a better understanding of the measures used for events related to reproduction:

Rate: A measure of the frequency of some event in relation to a unit of population during a specified time period, such as a year; events in the numerator of the rate occur to individuals in the denominator. Rates express the risk of the event in the specified population during a particular time. Rates generally are expressed as units of population in the denominator (eg, per 1,000, per 100,000). For example, the 2015 teenage birth rate was 22.3 live births per 1,000 women aged 15–19 years.

Ratios: A term that expresses a relationship of one element to a different element (where the numerator is not necessarily a subset of the denominator). A ratio generally is expressed per 1,000 or per 100,000 of the denominator element. For example, the pregnancy-related mortality ratio for 2011 was 17.8 pregnancy-related deaths per 100,000 live births.

In the formulae that follow, the term *period* refers to a calendar year.

Live Birth Measures

These measures are designed to show the rate at which childbearing is occurring in the population. The crude birth rate, which relates the total number of births to the total population, indicates the effect of fertility on population growth. The general fertility rate is a more specific measure of fertility because it relates the number of births to the population at risk, namely, women of childbearing age (assumed to be aged 15–44 years). An even more specific set of rates, the age-specific birth rate, relates the number of births to women of specific ages directly to the total number of women in that age group. Formulae for these measures are as follows:

$$\text{Crude birth rate} = \frac{\text{Number of live births to women of all ages during a calendar year} \times 1{,}000}{\text{Total estimated mid-year population}}$$

$$\text{General fertility rate} = \frac{\text{Number of live births to women of all ages during a calendar year} \times 1{,}000}{\text{Estimated mid-year population of women aged 15–44 years}}$$

$$\text{General pregnancy rate} = \frac{\text{Number of live births + number of fetal deaths + number of induced terminations of pregnancy during a calendar year} \times 1{,}000}{\text{Estimated mid-year population of women aged 15–44 years}}$$

$$\text{Age-specific birth rate} = \frac{\text{Number of live births to women in a specific age group during a calendar year} \times 1{,}000}{\text{Estimated mid-year population of women in same age group}}$$

$$\text{Total fertility rate} = \text{The sum of age-specific birth rates of women at each age group 10–14 through 45–49.}$$

Five-year age groups are used; therefore, the sum is multiplied by 5. This rate also can be computed by using single years of age.

Because the birth weight of the infant is included on the birth certificate, it is possible to tabulate and focus an analysis on selected groups of live births, for example, those weighing 500 g or more. Births can be tabulated by where they occur. Therefore, they can be shown by place of occurrence, by place of residence, and by kind of setting of delivery, such as at a hospital or home. Most tabulations of vital statistics are routinely calculated by place of residence of the mother, but they could be tabulated on another basis as well. What is essential, however, is that the classification be the same for all events under consideration for a specific measure.

Fetal Mortality Measures

The population at risk of fetal mortality is the number of live births plus the number of fetal deaths in a year. Fetal death indices, defined by a minimum weight and gestational age, indicate the magnitude of late pregnancy losses.

It is recognized that most states report fetal deaths that occur later in gestation or at 20 weeks of gestation or greater.

$$\text{Fetal death rate} = \frac{\text{Number of fetal deaths (x weight or more) during a period} \times 1{,}000}{\text{Number of fetal deaths (x weight or more) + number of live births during the same period}}$$

$$\text{Fetal death ratio} = \frac{\text{Number of fetal deaths (x weight or more) during a period} \times 1{,}000}{\text{Number of live births during the same period}}$$

Perinatal Mortality Measures

Perinatal death is not a reportable vital event, per se, but is used for statistical purposes. Indices of perinatal mortality combine fetal deaths and live births with only brief survival (up to a few days or weeks) on the assumption that similar factors are associated with these losses. The population at risk is the total number of live births plus fetal deaths, or alternatively, the number of live births. Perinatal mortality indices can vary as to age of the fetus and the infant who is included in the particular tabulation. However, the concept itself cuts across all the calculations.

$$\text{Perinatal mortality rate} = \frac{\begin{array}{c}\text{Number of infant deaths of less than} \\ \text{x days + number of fetal deaths} \\ \text{(with stated or presumed weight of y} \\ \text{or more) during the same period} \times 1{,}000\end{array}}{\begin{array}{c}\text{Number of live births} \\ \text{during the same period}\end{array}}$$

When perinatal death rates based on gestational age are calculated, the number of weeks of a stated or presumed gestational age can be substituted for weight in the formulae. When comparisons based on gestational age are desired, the generally accepted breakdown is as follows:

- Perinatal period I includes infant deaths occurring at less than 7 days and fetal deaths with a stated or presumed period of gestation of 28 weeks or more.
- Perinatal period II includes infant deaths occurring at less than 28 days and fetal deaths with a stated or presumed period of gestation of 20 weeks or more.
- Perinatal period III includes infant deaths occurring at less than 7 days and fetal deaths with a stated or presumed gestation of 20 weeks or more.

Perinatal measures can be specific for race and other characteristics. Perinatal events can be tabulated by where they occur. Therefore, they can be shown by place of occurrence, by place of residence, and by place of delivery, such as at a hospital or home. Most tabulations of vital statistics are routinely calculated by place of residence of the woman, but they could be tabulated by place of occurrence. What is essential, however, is that the classification be the same for all events under consideration for a specific measure.

Indices of infant mortality are designed to show the likelihood that live births with certain characteristics will survive the first year of life or, conversely, will die during the first year of life. For infant mortality, the population at risk is approximated by live births that occur in a calendar year. The infant mortality rate of different population groups can be compared, such as that between white and black infants. Interest sometimes focuses on two different periods in the first year of an infant's life, such as the very early period when the infant is younger than 28 days (up through 27 days, 23 hours, and 59 minutes from the moment of birth), called the neonatal period; and the later period starting at the end of the 28th day up to, but not including, age 1 year (364 days, 23 hours, and 59 minutes), called the postneonatal period. Accordingly, two indices reflect these differences, namely, the neonatal mortality rate and the postneonatal mortality rate.

$$\text{Infant mortality rate} = \frac{\text{Number of infant deaths (neonatal and postneonatal) during a period} \times 1{,}000}{\text{Number of live births during the same period}}$$

$$\text{Neonatal mortality rate} = \frac{\text{Number of neonatal deaths during a period} \times 1{,}000}{\text{Number of live births during the same period}}$$

$$\text{Postneonatal mortality rate} = \frac{\text{Number of postneonatal deaths during a period} \times 1{,}000}{\text{Number of live births during the same period}}$$

Maternal Mortality Measures

Measures of maternal mortality are designed to indicate the likelihood that a pregnant woman will die from complications of pregnancy, childbirth, or the puerperium. Accordingly, the population at risk is an approximation of the population of pregnant women in a year; the approximation usually is taken to be the number of live births. Maternal mortality can be examined in terms of characteristics of the woman, such as age, race, and cause of death. The maternal mortality rate measures the risk of death from deliveries and complications of pregnancy, childbirth, and the puerperium.

The group exposed to risk consists of all women who have been pregnant at some time during the period. Therefore, the population at risk should theoretically include all fetal deaths (reported and unreported), all induced terminations of pregnancy, and all live births. Because most states do not require the reporting of all fetal deaths and a large number of states still do not require reporting of induced terminations of pregnancy, the entire population at risk cannot be included in the denominator. Therefore, the total number of live births has become the generally accepted denominator. It is recommended that when complete ascertainment of the denominator (ie, the number of pregnant women) is achieved, a modified maternal mortality rate should be defined, in addition to the traditional rate. The rate is most frequently expressed per 100,000 live births:

$$\text{Maternal mortality rate} = \frac{\text{Number of deaths attributed to maternal conditions during a period} \times 100{,}000}{\text{Number of live births during the same period}}$$

Death rates for specified maternal causes are computed by restricting the numerator to the specified cause. The maternal mortality rates specific for race and age groups are computed by appropriately restricting both the numerator and the denominator to the specified group. Caution should be used in interpreting rates in small geographic areas; it may not be possible to generate race-specific and age-specific rates.

For statistical comparisons with the World Health Organization (WHO), it is recommended that two tabulations of statistics be prepared: 1) maternal deaths within 42 days of the end of pregnancy (WHO); and 2) maternal deaths with no time limitation for comparison within the United States.

The CDC uses the following statistical measures of pregnancy-related mortality:

$$\text{Pregnancy mortality rate} = \frac{\text{Number of pregnancy-related deaths during a period} \times 100{,}000}{\text{Number of pregnancies (live births, fetal deaths, induced and spontaneous abortions, ectopic pregnancies, and molar pregnancies)}}$$

$$\text{Pregnancy mortality ratio} = \frac{\text{Number of pregnancy-related deaths during a period} \times 100{,}000}{\text{Number of live births during the same period}}$$

Measures of Induced Termination of Pregnancy

Measures of induced pregnancy termination parallel those of fetal deaths but refer to induced events. The population at risk of induced termination of pregnancy is taken to be live births in a year, which is used as a surrogate measure of pregnancies. Because this is not actually the total population at risk, this measure generally is considered to be a ratio.

$$\text{Induced termination of pregnancy ratio I} = \frac{\text{Number of induced terminations occurring during a period} \times 1{,}000}{\text{Number of live births occurring during the same period}}$$

Another measure is one that, by also including an estimate of pregnancies that do not result in live births, more closely approximates the population at risk:

$$\text{Induced termination of pregnancy ratio II} = \frac{\text{Number of induced terminations occurring during a period} \times 1{,}000}{\text{Number of induced terminations of pregnancies + live births + reported fetal deaths during the same period}}$$

Still a third measure is a rate that provides information on the probability that a woman of a certain age or race will have an induced termination of pregnancy:

$$\text{Induced termination of pregnancy rate} = \frac{\text{Number of induced terminations occurring during a period} \times 1{,}000}{\text{Female population aged 15–44 years}}$$

Reporting Requirements and Recommendations

Reporting requirements for vital events related to reproductive health enable the collection of data that are essential to the calculation of statistical tabulations to examine trends and changes at the local, state, and national levels. The data used in statistical tabulations may be only a portion of those collected, because of the need for consistency in a tabulation and because of the variations in reporting requirements from state to state. For instance, although a few states require that all fetal deaths, regardless of length of gestation, be reported, statistical tabulations of fetal death rates by the National Center for Health Statistics use only those fetal deaths occurring at 20 weeks or more of gestation.

Live Birth

It generally is recognized that all states report all live births, as defined in the definitions section of this document. It is recommended that all live births be reported, regardless of birth weight, length of gestation, or survival time.

Fetal Death

Reporting requirements for fetal deaths vary somewhat from state to state. At present, most states require reporting of fetal deaths by gestational age. It generally is recognized that birth weight can be measured more accurately than can gestational age. The 1992 revision of the Model State Vital Statistics Act and Regulations* recommends reporting of all spontaneous losses occurring at 350 g or more or, if weight is unknown, 20 completed weeks of gestation or more. It must be emphasized that a specific birth weight criterion for reporting of fetal deaths does not imply a point of viability and should be chosen instead for its feasibility in collecting useful data. Furthermore, 25 states have adopted the requirement of reporting deaths of 20 weeks or more of gestation. Currently, all state fetal death report forms include birth weight and gestational age.

Perinatal Mortality

Perinatal mortality indices generally combine fetal deaths and live births that survive only briefly (up to a few days or weeks). Because reporting requirements of fetal deaths vary from state to state, perinatal mortality reporting also will vary (see definitions of perinatal periods in "Perinatal Mortality Measures" earlier in this appendix).

As with fetal deaths, it is recommended that perinatal mortality be weight specific. However, for purposes of comparability, knowledge of gestational age (based on last menstrual period) should be collected.

---

*In 2011, the Model Law Revision workgroup completed its work on evaluating and revising the 1992 Model State Vital Statistics Act and Regulations. The proposed revision of the Model Law was still under review by the U.S. Department of Health and Human Services at the time of printing of *Guidelines for Perinatal Care*, Eighth Edition.

Infant Mortality

All states require that all infant deaths (neonatal plus postneonatal), as defined in the section "Definitions" in this appendix, be reported. Infant deaths by birth weight and gestational age are routinely available for the United States. Because birth weight and gestational age are reported on the birth certificate, it is possible to obtain this information on infant deaths by linking together the birth certificate and the death certificate for the same infant. At present, all states link birth and death certificates. National linked birth certificate and infant death certificate files are now available from the National Center for Health Statistics.

Maternal Mortality

Every state is required to report all maternal deaths. Case finding, together with individual review and analysis of risk factors contributing to maternal deaths, is of the highest importance for understanding causes and risk factors for maternal deaths. Collection of data regarding these rare events is critical, when combined, as it should be, with educational review by those closest to the case, usually the obstetrician–gynecologists in the hospital and the surrounding region. Such analysis can yield clinical information about risk factors associated with, for example, detection and treatment of ectopic pregnancies or with anesthesia. This clinical information can then be gathered and exchanged to help practitioners identify risk factors that contribute to maternal death and associated conditions.

Induced Termination of Pregnancy

The United States has no national system for reporting induced termination of pregnancy. State health departments vary greatly in their approaches to the compilation of these data, from compiling no data to periodically requesting hospitals, clinics, and physicians performing the procedures to voluntarily report total number of procedures performed; requiring (by legislative or regulatory authority) hospitals, clinics, and physicians to periodically report aggregate level data on number or number and characteristics of procedures; or requiring (by legal or regulatory authority) hospitals, clinics, and physicians to periodically report individual data on each procedure performed.

Since 1969, the CDC Division of Reproductive Health has published an annual Abortion Surveillance Report based on data provided from state health departments, when available, and from data voluntarily provided to the CDC from hospitals and clinics in states with no data available from health departments. In addition to information on the number and characteristics of induced terminations of pregnancy, the Abortion Surveillance Report contains information from the CDC abortion mortality surveillance, which was begun with the cooperation of state health departments in 1972. Investigation and review of each related death by epidemiologists in the Division of Reproductive Health result in improved detailed nosological identification of abortion mortality by type of risk.*

Since 1977, the National Center for Health Statistics has analyzed the induced terminations of pregnancy occurring in states in which individual reports of induced termination are submitted to state vital registration offices. In addition, the Alan Guttmacher Institute, a private organization, publishes information on induced termination that it obtains from a nationwide survey of health care providers of induced termination.

Collecting information on the number of induced terminations of pregnancy, the characteristics of women having such procedures, and the number and characteristics of all deaths related to induced termination of pregnancy would be extremely valuable in identifying and evaluating risk factors for specific population groups and for the public in general. By gathering these data, studies could be instituted that would examine clinical issues and then results could be shared with practitioners. Knowing the outcomes could further the body of knowledge and ultimately reduce the risks.

Rates of Vaginal Births After Cesarean Delivery

Two methods for defining vaginal birth after cesarean delivery (VBAC) rates are proposed:

$$\text{VBAC rate} = \frac{\text{Total number of VBACs}}{\begin{array}{c}\text{Total number of women with prior cesarean}\\ \text{deliveries, including women who were}\\ \text{candidates for a trial of labor but declined}\\ \text{and women who were not candidates}\end{array}} \times 100$$

*The CDC Abortion Surveillance Report includes information on events categorized by the CDC as abortions (legal, illegal, and spontaneous). Although this terminology predates the recommendations in this document and is at variance with the definition herein, it has been commonly used and understood to include induced termination of pregnancy.

$$\text{Trial of labor success rate} = \frac{\text{VBAC}}{\text{Number of women who had a trial of labor after cesarean delivery}} \times 100$$

Clearly, these rates are interrelated. However, calculations based on the rates as defined allow a more accurate comparison of practice between health care providers and institutions.

Current Reporting Requirements

The general live birth, infant death, fetal death, and induced termination of pregnancy reporting requirements, as of 2014 (Table F-1 and Figure F-1), should be brought into conformity with the recommendations in this report.

Table F-1. Reporting Requirements for Fetal Death According to State or Reporting Area, 2015

Criteria	State and Reporting Area
Gestational age criteria only	
All periods	Colorado, Georgia, Hawaii, New York,[a] Rhode Island, Virginia, Virgin Islands
16 weeks or greater	Pennsylvania
20 weeks or greater	Alabama, Alaska, California, Connecticut, Florida, Illinois, Indiana, Iowa, Kansas, Maine, Maryland,[b] Minnesota, Nebraska, Nevada, New Jersey, New Mexico[c], North Carolina, North Dakota, Ohio, Oklahoma, Oregon, Texas, Utah, Vermont,[d] Washington, West Virginia, Wyoming
5 months or greater	Puerto Rico
Both gestational age and birth weight criteria	
20 weeks or greater or 350 g or more	Arizona, Idaho, Kentucky, Louisiana, Massachusetts, Mississippi, Missouri, New Hampshire, South Carolina, Tennessee, Wisconsin, Guam
20 weeks or greater or 400 g or more	Michigan
20 weeks or greater or 500 g or more	District of Columbia

(continued)

Table F-1. Reporting Requirements for Fetal Death According to State or Reporting Area, 2015 *(continued)*

Criteria	State and Reporting Area
Birth weight criteria only	
350 g or more	Arkansas,[e] Delaware,[e] Montana[e,d]
500 g or more	South Dakota

[a]Includes New York City, which has separate reporting.

[b]If gestational age is unknown, weight of 500 g or more.

[c]If gestational age is unknown, weight of 350 g or more.

[d]If gestational age is unknown, weight of 400 g or more, 15 oz or more.

[e]If weight is unknown, ≥20 weeks' completed gestation.

Data source: National Center for Health Statistics, National Vital Statistics Reports.

Reproduced from Barfield WD. Standard terminology for fetal, infant, and perinatal deaths. Committee on Fetus and Newborn. Pediatrics 2016;137:e20160551.

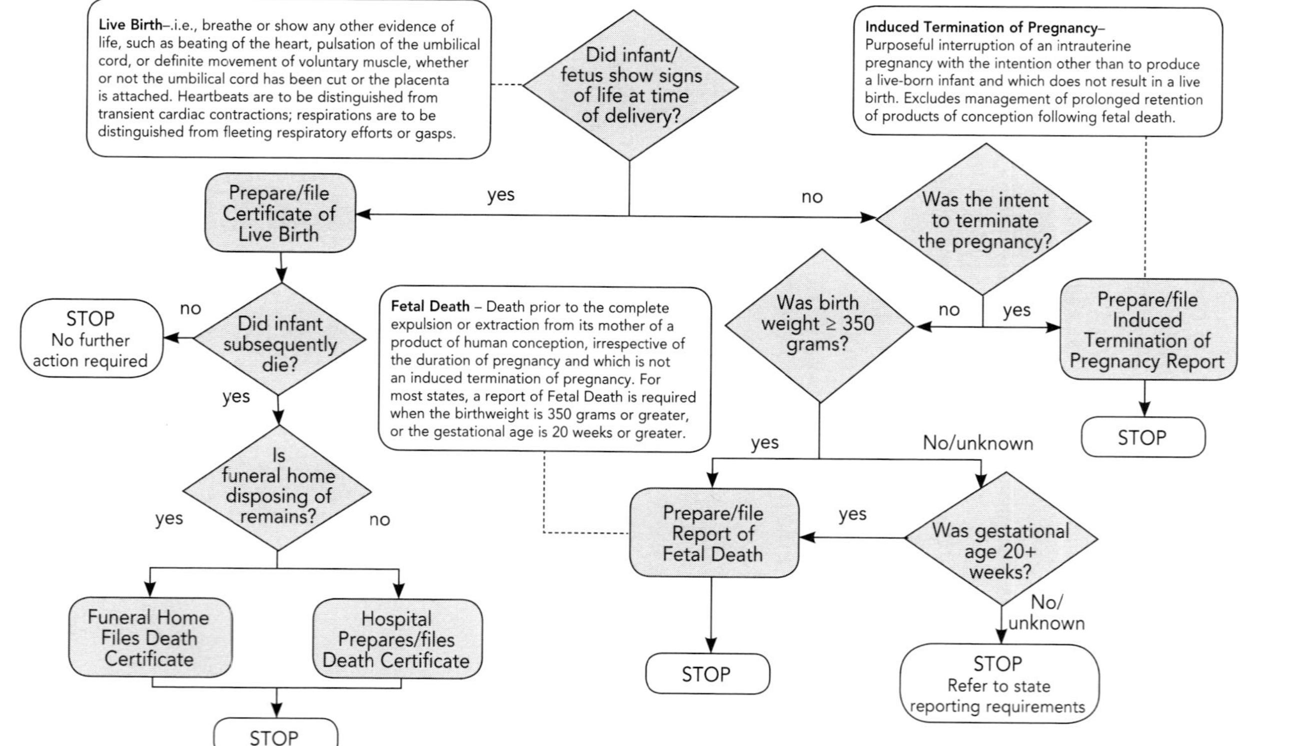

Figure F-1. Hospital Guidelines for Reporting Live Births, Infant Deaths, Fetal Deaths, and Induced Terminations of Pregnancy. (Modified from the National Association for Public Health Statistics and Information Systems [http://www.naphsis.org]. Reprinted from: Barfield WD. Standard terminology for fetal, infant, and perinatal deaths. Committee on Fetus and Newborn. Pediatrics 2016;137:e20160551.)

Bibliography

American College of Obstetricians and Gynecologists. ReVitalize: obstetric data definitions. Washington, DC: American College of Obstetricians and Gynecologists; 2017. Available at: https://www.acog.org/-/media/Departments/Patient-Safety-and-Quality-Improvement/2014reVITALizeObstetricDataDefinitionsV10.pdf. Retrieved December 2, 2016.

Barfield WD. Standard terminology for fetal, infant, and perinatal deaths. Committee on Fetus and Newborn. Pediatrics 2016;137:e20160551.

Hamilton BE, Martin JA, Osterman MJ. Births: preliminary data for 2015. Natl Vital Stat Rep 2016;65(3):1–15.

Kowaleski J. State definitions and reporting requirements for live births, fetal deaths, and induced terminations of pregnancy. 1997 revision. Hyattsville (MD): National Center for Health Statistics; 1997. Available at: http://www.cdc.gov/nchs/data/misc/itop97.pdf. Retrieved December 2, 2016.

Martin JA, Osterman MJ, Kirmeyer SE, Gregory EC. Measuring gestational age in vital statistics data: transitioning to the obstetric estimate. Natl Vital Stat Rep 2015;64(5):1–20.

National Center for Health Statistics. Model state vital statistics act and regulations. Hyattsville (MD): NCHS; 1992. Available at: https://www.cdc.gov/nchs/data/misc/mvsact92b.pdf. Retrieved December 2, 2016.

World Health Organization. International statistical classification of diseases and related health problems. 10th Revision. Geneva: WHO; 2016. Available at: http://www.who.int/classifications/icd/en/. Retrieved December 2, 2016.

World Health Organization. Preterm birth: fact sheet. Geneva: WHO; 2016. Available at: http://www.who.int/mediacentre/factsheets/fs363/en/. Retrieved December 2, 2016.

Appendix G

Emergency Medical Treatment and Active Labor Act

In 1986, Congress enacted the Emergency Medical Treatment and Active Labor Act (EMTALA) to ensure that everyone who seeks medical help from a hospital emergency department receives appropriate screening and treatment, regardless of his or her ability to pay. All hospitals participating in Medicare must meet these requirements.

Patient Screening

All hospitals that participate in the Medicare program and have a dedicated emergency department must comply with EMTALA's requirements for patient screening and transfer. The regulations define a dedicated emergency department as any department or facility of the hospital that meets one of the following criteria:

- It is licensed by the state as an emergency room or emergency department.
- The hospital presents the facility or department to the public as available to provide care for emergency medical conditions without an appointment.
- In the previous year it provided at least one third of its entire outpatient visits for urgent treatment of emergency medical conditions.

Labor and delivery units and psychiatry departments can meet these criteria and, therefore, be covered by EMTALA.

Anyone who requests an examination or treatment for a medical condition at the hospital must be provided a screening examination without regard to his or her ability to pay. Under EMTALA, an emergency medical condition is one with symptoms severe enough that, if the patient does not receive immediate care, there is a reasonable expectation that one of the following consequences could occur:

- The patient's health would be in serious jeopardy.
- The patient would experience serious impairment of a bodily function.
- The patient would experience serious dysfunction of a bodily organ or part.

Special requirements apply for screening pregnant women in the emergency department.

- The health of the fetus must be considered in deciding whether a pregnant patient has an emergency medical condition.
- A pregnant patient having contractions is in "true labor" and, therefore, must be determined to have an emergency medical condition unless a physician, certified nurse–midwife, or other qualified medical professional certifies that she is in false labor.
- A pregnant patient having contractions also has an emergency medical condition if transferring her to another facility would threaten her health or the health of the fetus.
- If the patient has been observed and diagnosed with false labor, she does not have an emergency medical condition.
- If it is determined that a pregnant patient having contractions has an emergency medical condition, EMTALA considers that she is not stabilized until the baby and placenta are delivered.

The hospital can determine whether a physician must perform screening examinations or whether another type of health care provider is qualified.

The requirement to provide a screening examination is not limited to patients who come to the emergency department. In general, anyone who requests an examination or treatment for an emergency medical condition anywhere on the hospital property is entitled to EMTALA protections. Similarly, EMTALA protections may be triggered if a prudent layperson observer would believe that the individual is suffering from an emergency medical condition. In contrast, if an individual is registered as an outpatient of the hospital and she presents on hospital property but not to the emergency department, the hospital does not incur an EMTALA obligation to provide a medical screening examination for that individual if she has started a scheduled course of outpatient care.

If a patient has an emergency medical condition, there are two options depending on the circumstances and the hospital's capabilities:

1. Treat and stabilize the patient.
2. Transfer the patient to another hospital that is better able to provide the necessary care.

Criteria for Transferring Patients

Most of the time, EMTALA prohibits transfer of an unstable patient. However, an unstable patient can be transferred to another hospital under the following conditions:

- She requests the transfer. She must be informed of her rights to stay at the hospital, along with the risks and benefits of transfer, including the fact that she is not medically stable. The request must be documented in writing.
- The hospital does not have the facilities or personnel to provide the care she needs. There must be a signed certification containing a summary of the risks and benefits of transfer.
- If a physician is not physically present in the emergency department at the time of the transfer of a patient, a qualified medical person can sign the certification described previously after consulting with a physician who authorizes the transfer. The physician must countersign the certification as contemporaneously as possible.

If a transfer to another hospital is recommended but the patient refuses, the following steps should be taken:

- Inform the patient of the benefits of the transfer and the risks of remaining at the current hospital.
- Include in the medical record a description of the proposed transfer and the reason(s) for recommending the transfer.
- Make every reasonable attempt to document in writing the patient's informed refusal of the transfer, indicating that the patient has been informed of the risks and benefits of the transfer and the reasons for the patient's refusal.

Interhospital Care and Transport System

All facilities involved in the transferring and receiving of patients must work together to specify how they will accomplish the following:

- Comply with relevant local, state, and federal regulations.
- Obtain informed consent before moving the patient.
- Develop formal agreements outlining each hospital's procedures and responsibilities for patient care.
- Provide patient identification during transport.
- Use patient care orders, guidelines, and verbal communication during transport.
- Educate staff at all facilities about the interhospital care and transport system.

Referring Hospital Responsibilities

If a patient is being transferred to another facility, the referring hospital is responsible for the patient until she arrives at the receiving hospital. Obligations include the following:

- Evaluating and stabilizing the patient, minimizing the risks to the patient's health
- Ensuring that the receiving hospital has agreed to the transfer and has adequate space and qualified staff to treat the patient
- Executing the transfer through the use of qualified personnel and transportation equipment
- Providing all available medical records

Receiving Hospital Responsibilities

The hospital that receives patients from other facilities is responsible for coordinating the transport system and making sure transferred patients are provided appropriate care. Receiving hospitals must have plans in place to prevent bed shortages. A receiving hospital cannot refuse a transfer if it has space and qualified staff available.

General Requirements

The following general requirements should be met:

- Medical records related to transfers must be retained by both the transferring and receiving hospitals for 5 years from the date of the transfer.
- Hospitals are required to report to the Centers for Medicare and Medicaid Services or the state survey agency within 72 hours from the time of the transfer any time they have reason to believe they may have received a patient who was transferred in an unstable medical condition.
- Hospitals are required to post signs in areas such as entrances, admitting areas, waiting rooms, and emergency departments with respect to their obligations under the patient screening and transfer law.
- Hospitals also are required to post signs stating whether the hospital participates in the Medicaid program under a state-approved plan. This requirement applies to all hospitals, not only those that participate in Medicare.
- Hospitals must keep a list of physicians who are on call after the initial examination to provide treatment to stabilize a patient with an emergency medical condition.
- Hospitals must keep a central log of all individuals who come to the emergency department seeking assistance and the result of each individual's visit.
- A hospital may not delay providing appropriate medical screening to inquire about payment method or insurance status.

Enforcement and Penalties

Physicians and hospitals violating these federal requirements for patient screening and transfer are subject to civil monetary penalties of up to $50,000 for each violation and to termination from the Medicare program. Hospitals are prohibited from penalizing physicians who report violations of the law or who refuse to transfer an individual with an unstabilized emergency medical condition.

Appendix H

American Academy of Pediatrics Policy Statements and American College of Obstetricians and Gynecologists' Committee Opinions and Practice Bulletins

American Academy of Pediatrics

Committee on Bioethics

American Academy of Pediatrics Committee on Bioethics: Guidelines on foregoing life-sustaining medical treatment. Pediatrics 1994;93:532–6.

Committee on Drugs

Hudak ML, Tan RC. Neonatal drug withdrawal. Committee on Drugs, Committee on Fetus and Newborn American Academy of Pediatrics [published erratum appears in Pediatrics 2014;133:937]. Pediatrics 2012;129:e540–60.

Sachs HC. The transfer of drugs and therapeutics into human breast milk: an update on selected topics. Committee on Drugs. Pediatrics 2013;132:e796–809.

Committee on Early Childhood, Adoption, and Dependent Care

Borchers D. Families and adoption: the pediatrician's role in supporting communication. American Academy of Pediatrics Committee on Early Childhood, Adoption, and Dependent Care. Pediatrics 2003;112:1437–41.

Committee on Environmental Health

Best D. Technical report—secondhand and prenatal tobacco smoke exposure. American Academy of Pediatrics Committee on Environmental Health, Committee on Native American Child Health, Committee on Adolescence. Pediatrics 2009;124:e1017–44.

Tobacco use: a pediatric disease. Committee on Environmental Health, Committee on Substance Abuse, Committee on Adolescence, and Committee on Native American Child Health [published erratum appears in Pediatrics 2010;125:861]. Pediatrics 2009;124:1474–87.

Committee on Fetus and Newborn

Controversies concerning vitamin K and the newborn. American Academy of Pediatrics Committee on Fetus and Newborn. Pediatrics 2003;112:191–2.

Hospital discharge of the high-risk neonate. American Academy of Pediatrics Committee on Fetus and Newborn. Pediatrics 2008;122:1119–26.

Levels of neonatal care. American Academy of Pediatrics Committee on Fetus and Newborn. Pediatrics 2012;130:587–97.

Prevention and management of procedural pain in the neonate: an update. Committee on Fetus and Newborn and Section on Anesthesiology and Pain Medicine. Pediatrics 2016;137:e20154271.

Adamkin DH. Postnatal glucose homeostasis in late-preterm and term infants. American Academy of Pediatrics Committee on Fetus and Newborn. Pediatrics 2011;127:575–9.

Barfield WD. Standard terminology for fetal, infant, and perinatal deaths. Committee on Fetus and Newborn. Pediatrics 2016;137:e20160551.

Batton DG. Clinical report—Antenatal counseling regarding resuscitation at an extremely low gestational age. Committee on Fetus and Newborn. Pediatrics 2009;124:422–7.

Bell EF. Noninitiation or withdrawal of intensive care for high-risk newborns. American Academy of Pediatrics Committee on Fetus and Newborn. Pediatrics 2007;119:401–3.

Benitz WE. Hospital stay for healthy term newborn infants. Committee on Fetus and Newborn, American Academy of Pediatrics. Pediatrics 2015;135:948–53.

Bhutani VK. Phototherapy to prevent severe neonatal hyperbilirubinemia in the newborn infant 35 or more weeks of gestation. Committee on Fetus and Newborn American Academy of Pediatrics. Pediatrics 2011;128:e1046–52.

Cummings J. Antenatal counseling regarding resuscitation and intensive care before 25 weeks of gestation. Committee on Fetus and Newborn. Pediatrics 2015;136: 588–95.

Cummings JJ, Polin RA. Oxygen targeting in extremely low birth weight infants. Committee on Fetus and Newborn [published erratum appears in Pediatrics 2016;138(6)]. Pediatrics 2016;138(2).

Eichenwald EC. Apnea of prematurity. Committee on Fetus and Newborn, American Academy of Pediatrics. Pediatrics 2016;137.

Engle WA, Tomashek KM, Wallman C. "Late-preterm" infants: a population at risk. Committee on Fetus and Newborn, American Academy of Pediatrics [published erratum appears in Pediatrics 2008;121:451]. Pediatrics 2007;120:1390–401.

Feldman-Winter L, Goldsmith JP. Safe sleep and skin-to-skin care in the neonatal period for healthy term newborns. Committee on Fetus and Newborn and Task Force on Sudden Infant Death Syndrome. Pediatrics 2016;138:10.1542/peds.2016,1889. Epub 2016 Aug 22.

Kumar P, Denson SE, Mancuso TJ. Premedication for nonemergency endotracheal intubation in the neonate. Committee on Fetus and Newborn, Section on Anesthesiology and Pain Medicine. Pediatrics 2010;125:608–15.

Papile LA, Baley JE, Benitz W, Cummings J, Carlo WA, Eichenwald E, et al. Hypothermia and neonatal encephalopathy. Committee on Fetus and Newborn. Pediatrics 2014;133:1146–50.

Polin RA. Management of neonates with suspected or proven early-onset bacterial sepsis. Committee on Fetus and Newborn. Pediatrics 2012;129:1006–15.

Polin RA, Carlo WA. Surfactant replacement therapy for preterm and term neonates with respiratory distress. Committee on Fetus and Newborn American Academy of Pediatrics. Pediatrics 2014;133:156–63.

Polin RA, Denson S, Brady MT. Epidemiology and diagnosis of health care-associated infections in the NICU. Committee on Fetus and Newborn, Committee on Infectious Diseases. Pediatrics 2012;129:e1104–9.

Polin RA, Denson S, Brady MT. Strategies for prevention of health care-associated infections in the NICU. Committee on Fetus and Newborn, Committee on Infectious Diseases. Pediatrics 2012;129:e1085–93.

Wallman C. Advanced practice in neonatal nursing. Committee on Fetus and Newborn. Pediatrics 2009;123:1606–7.

Watterberg KL. Policy statement—postnatal corticosteroids to prevent or treat bronchopulmonary dysplasia. American Academy of Pediatrics, Committee on Fetus and Newborn. Pediatrics 2010;126:800–8.

Committee on Genetics

Folic acid for the prevention of neural tube defects. American Academy of Pediatrics. Committee on Genetics. Pediatrics 1999;104:325–7.

Maternal Phenylketonuria. American Academy of Pediatrics Committee on Genetics. Pediatrics 2008;122:445–9.

Kaye CI, Accurso F, La Franchi S, Lane PA, Hope N, Sonya P, et al. Newborn screening fact sheets. Committee on Genetics. Pediatrics 2006;118:e934–63.

Committee on Hospital Care

Patient- and family-centered care and the pediatrician's role. Committee on Hospital Care and Institute for Patient- and Family-Centered Care. Pediatrics 2012;129:394–404.

Committee on Infectious Diseases

Infection prevention and control in pediatric ambulatory settings. American Academy of Pediatrics Committee on Infectious Diseases. Pediatrics 2007;120:650–65.

Updated guidance for palivizumab prophylaxis among infants and young children at increased risk of hospitalization for respiratory syncytial virus infection. American

Academy of Pediatrics Committee on Infectious Diseases, American Academy of Pediatrics Bronchiolitis Guidelines Committee [Published erratum appears in Pediatrics 2014;134:1221]. Pediatrics 2014;134:415–20.

Kimberlin DW, Baley J. Guidance on management of asymptomatic neonates born to women with active genital herpes lesions. Committee on Infectious Diseases and Committee on Fetus and Newborn. Pediatrics 2013;131:e635–46.

Elimination of perinatal hepatitis b: providing the first vaccine dose within 24 hours of birth. American Academy of Pediatrics. Committee on Infectious Diseases. Pediatrics 2017;140:e20171870.

Committee on Injury, Violence, and Poison Prevention

Bull MJ, Engle WA. Safe transportation of preterm and low birth weight infants at hospital discharge. Committee on Injury, Violence, and Poison Prevention and Committee on Fetus and Newborn, American Academy of Pediatrics. Pediatrics 2009;123:1424–9.

Committee on Nutrition

Baker RD, Greer FR. Diagnosis and prevention of iron deficiency and iron-deficiency anemia in infants and young children (0–3 years of age). Committee on Nutrition American Academy of Pediatrics. Pediatrics 2010;126:1040–50.

Committee on Pediatric AIDS

Infant feeding and transmission of human immunodeficiency virus in the United States. Committee on Pediatric AIDS. Pediatrics 2013;131:391–6.

Havens PL, Mofenson LM. Evaluation and management of the infant exposed to HIV-1 in the United States. American Academy of Pediatrics Committee on Pediatric AIDS [published erratum appears in Pediatrics 2012;130:1183–4]. Pediatrics 2009;123:175–87.

Committee on Pediatric Emergency Medicine Task Force on Terrorism

Markenson D, Reynolds S. The pediatrician and disaster preparedness. American Academy of Pediatrics Committee on Pediatric Emergency Medicine Task Force on Terrorism. Pediatrics 2006;117:e340–62.

Committee on Practice and Ambulatory Medicine

2017 recommendations for preventive pediatric health care. Committee on Practice and Ambulatory Medicine, Bright Futures Periodicity Schedule Workgroup. Pediatrics 2017.

Donahue SP, Baker CN. Procedures for the evaluation of the visual system by pediatricians. Committee on Practice and Ambulatory Medicine, American Academy of Pediatrics, Section on Ophthalmology, American Academy of Pediatrics, American Association of Certified Orthoptists, American Association for Pediatric Ophthalmology and Strabismus, American Academy of Ophthalmology. Pediatrics 2016;137.

Committee on Psychosocial Aspects of Child and Family Health

Cohen GJ. The prenatal visit. Committee on Psychosocial Aspects of Child and Family Health. Pediatrics 2009;124:1227–32.

Committee on Substance Abuse

Williams JF, Smith VC. Fetal alcohol spectrum disorders. Committee on Substance Abuse. Pediatrics 2015;136:e1395–406.

Joint Committee on Infant Hearing

Year 2007 position statement: principles and guidelines for early hearing detection and intervention programs. American Academy of Pediatrics, Joint Committee on Infant Hearing. Pediatrics 2007;120:898–921.

Muse C, Harrison J, Yoshinaga-Itano C, Grimes A, Brookhouser PE, Epstein S, et al. Supplement to the JCIH 2007 position statement: principles and guidelines for early intervention after confirmation that a child is deaf or hard of hearing. Joint Committee on Infant Hearing of the American Academy of Pediatrics. Pediatrics 2013;131:e1324–49.

Medical Home Initiatives for Children with Special Needs Project Advisory Committee

The medical home. Medical Home Initiatives for Children with Special Needs Project Advisory Committee. American Academy of Pediatrics. Pediatrics 2002;110:184–6.

Newborn Screening Authoring Committee

Newborn screening expands: recommendations for pediatricians and medical homes—implications for the system. American Academy of Pediatrics Newborn Screening Authoring Committee. Pediatrics 2008;121:192–217.

Section on Breastfeeding

Breastfeeding and the use of human milk. Section on Breastfeeding. Pediatrics 2012;129:e827–41.

Wagner CL, Greer FR. Prevention of rickets and vitamin d deficiency in infants, children, and adolescents. American Academy of Pediatrics Section on Breastfeeding, American Academy of Pediatrics Committee on Nutrition [published erratum appears in Pediatrics 2009;123:197]. Pediatrics 2008;122:1142–52.

Section on Ophthalmology

Fierson WM. Screening examination of premature infants for retinopathy of prematurity. American Academy of Pediatrics Section on Ophthalmology, American Academy of Ophthalmology, American Association for Pediatric Ophthalmology and Strabismus, American Association of Certified Orthoptists. Pediatrics 2013;131: 189–95.

Section on Radiology

Brody AS, Frush DP, Huda W, Brent RL. Radiation risk to children from computed tomography. American Academy of Pediatrics Section on Radiology. Pediatrics 2007;120:677–82.

Section on Tobacco Control

Farber HJ, Nelson KE, Groner JA, Walley SC. Public policy to protect children from tobacco, nicotine, and tobacco smoke. Section on Tobacco Control. Pediatrics 2015;136:998–1007.

Nelson KE. Clinical practice policy to protect children from tobacco, nicotine, and tobacco smoke. Section on Tobacco Control. Pediatrics 2015;136:1008–17.

Section on Transport Medicine

Insoft RM, Schwartz HP, Romito J, editors. Guidelines for air and ground transport of neonatal and pediatric patients. American Academy of Pediatrics. Section on Transport Medicine. 4th ed. Elk Grove Village (IL): American Academy of Pediatrics; 2015.

Section on Transport Medicine. American Academy of Pediatrics. Elk Grove Village (IL): American Academy of Pediatrics; 2016. Available at: https://www.aap.org/en-us/about-the-aap/committees-councils-sections/section-transport-medicine/pages/default.aspx. Retrieved October 18, 2016.

Subcommittee on Hyperbilirubinemia

Management of hyperbilirubinemia in the newborn infant 35 or more weeks of gestation. American Academy of Pediatrics Subcommittee on hyperbilirubinemia [published erratum appears in Pediatrics 2004;114:1138]. Pediatrics 2004;114:297–316.

Ip S, Chung M, Kulig J, O'Brien R, Sege R, Glicken S, et al. An evidence-based review of important issues concerning neonatal hyperbilirubinemia. American Academy of Pediatrics Subcommittee on Hyperbilirubinemia. Pediatrics 2004;114:e130–53.

Task Force on Circumcision

Circumcision policy statement. American Academy of Pediatrics Task Force on Circumcision. Pediatrics 2012;130:585–6.

Task Force on Sudden Infant Death Syndrome

Moon RY. SIDS and other sleep-related infant deaths: evidence base for 2016 updated recommendations for a safe infant sleeping environment. Task Force on Sudden Infant Death Syndrome. Pediatrics 2016;138:e20162940.

Other Publications

American Academy of Pediatrics. Pediatric nutrition handbook. 7th ed. Elk Grove Village (IL): American Academy of Pediatrics; 2013.

American Academy of Pediatrics. Red book: report of the Committee on Infectious Diseases. 30th ed. Elk Grove Village (IL): American Academy of Pediatrics; 2015.

American Academy of Pediatrics. Recommendations for preventive pediatric health care. Elk Grove Village (IL): AAP; 2016. Available at: https://www.aap.org/en-us/Documents/periodicity_schedule.pdf. Retrieved November 2, 2016.

American Academy of Pediatrics Committee on Fetus and Newborn; American College of Obstetricians and Gynecologists Committee on Obstetric Practice. The Apgar Score. Pediatrics 2015;136:819–22 and Obstet Gynecol 2015;126:e52–5.

American Academy of Pediatrics, American Heart Association. Textbook of neonatal resuscitation. 7th ed. Elk Grove Village (IL): Dallas (TX): AAP; AHA; 2016.

American College of Obstetricians and Gynecologists' Committee Opinions

Committee on Adolescent Health Care

Adolescent pregnancy, contraception, and sexual activity. Committee Opinion No. 699. American College of Obstetricians and Gynecologists. Obstet Gynecol 2017;129:e142–9.

Human papillomavirus vaccination. Committee Opinion No. 704. American College of Obstetricians and Gynecologists. Obstet Gynecol 2017;129:e173–8.

Committee on Ethics

The limits of conscientious refusal in reproductive medicine. ACOG Committee Opinion No. 385. American College of Obstetricians and Gynecologists. Obstet Gynecol 2007;110:1203–8.

Human immunodeficiency virus. ACOG Committee Opinion No. 389. American College of Obstetricians and Gynecologists. Obstet Gynecol 2007;110:1473–8.

Informed consent. ACOG Committee Opinion No. 439. American College of Obstetricians and Gynecologists. Obstet Gynecol 2009;114:401–8.

Multifetal pregnancy reduction. Committee Opinion No. 553. American College of Obstetricians and Gynecologists. Obstet Gynecol 2013;121:405–10.

Committee on Genetics

Family history as a risk assessment tool. Committee Opinion No. 478. American College of Obstetricians and Gynecologists. Obstet Gynecol 2011;117:747–50.

Newborn screening and the role of the obstetrician–gynecologist. Committee Opinion No. 616. American College of Obstetricians and Gynecologists. Obstet Gynecol 2015;125:256–60.

Microarrays and next-generation sequencing technology: the use of advanced genetic diagnostic tools in obstetrics and gynecology. Committee Opinion No. 682. American College of Obstetricians and Gynecologists. Obstet Gynecol 2016;128:e262–8.

Carrier screening in the age of genomic medicine. Committee Opinion No. 690. American College of Obstetricians and Gynecologists. Obstet Gynecol 2017;129: e35–40.

Carrier screening for genetic conditions. Committee Opinion No. 691. American College of Obstetricians and Gynecologists. Obstet Gynecol 2017;129:e41–55.

Counseling about genetic testing and communication of genetic test results. Committee Opinion No. 693. American College of Obstetricians and Gynecologists. Obstet Gynecol 2017;129:e96–101.

Committee on Gynecologic Practice

The importance of preconception care in the continuum of women's health care. ACOG Committee Opinion No. 313. American College of Obstetricians and Gynecologists. Obstet Gynecol 2005;106:665–6.

Routine human immunodeficiency virus screening. Committee Opinion No. 596. American College of Obstetricians and Gynecologists. Obstet Gynecol 2014;123: 1137–9.

Hepatitis B, hepatitis C, and human immunodeficiency virus infections in obstetrician–gynecologists. Committee Opinion No. 655. American College of Obstetricians and Gynecologists. Obstet Gynecol 2016;127:e70–4.

Committee on Health Care for Underserved Women

Methamphetamine abuse in women of reproductive age. Committee Opinion No. 479. American College of Obstetricians and Gynecologists. Obstet Gynecol 2011;117:751–5.

Cultural sensitivity and awareness in the delivery of health care. Committee Opinion No. 493. American College of Obstetricians and Gynecologists. Obstet Gynecol 2011;117:1258–61.

At-risk drinking and alcohol dependence: obstetric and gynecologic implications. Committee Opinion No. 496. American College of Obstetricians and Gynecologists. Obstet Gynecol 2011;118:383–8.

Tobacco use and women's health. Committee Opinion No. 503. American College of Obstetricians and Gynecologists. Obstet Gynecol 2011;118:746–50.

Intimate partner violence. Committee Opinion No. 518. American College of Obstetricians and Gynecologists. Obstet Gynecol 2012;119:412–7.

Opioid abuse, dependence, and addiction in pregnancy. Committee Opinion No. 524. American College of Obstetricians and Gynecologists. Obstet Gynecol 2012;119: 1070–6.

Access to postpartum sterilization. Committee Opinion No. 530. American College of Obstetricians and Gynecologists. Obstet Gynecol 2012;120:212–5.

Nonmedical use of prescription drugs. Committee Opinion No. 538. American College of Obstetricians and Gynecologists. Obstet Gynecol 2012;120:977–82.

Breastfeeding in underserved women: increasing initiation and continuation of breastfeeding. Committee Opinion No. 570. American College of Obstetricians and Gynecologists. Obstet Gynecol 2013;122:423–8.

Exposure to toxic environmental agents. Committee Opinion No. 575. American College of Obstetricians and Gynecologists. Obstet Gynecol 2013;122:931–5.

Effective patient–physician communication. Committee Opinion No. 587. American College of Obstetricians and Gynecologists. Obstet Gynecol 2014;123:389–93.

Access to contraception. Committee Opinion No. 615. American College of Obstetricians and Gynecologists. Obstet Gynecol 2015;125:250–5.

Reproductive life planning to reduce unintended pregnancy. Committee Opinion No. 654. American College of Obstetricians and Gynecologists. Obstet Gynecol 2016;127:e66–9.

Health literacy to promote quality of care. Committee Opinion No. 676. American College of Obstetricians and Gynecologists. Obstet Gynecol 2016;128:e183–6.

Committee on Obstetric Practice

American College of Obstetricians and Gynecologists. Scheduled cesarean delivery and the prevention of vertical transmission of HIV infection. ACOG Committee Opinion 234. Washington, DC: ACOG; 2000.

Amnioninfusion does not prevent meconium aspiration syndrome. ACOG Committee Opinion No. 346. American College of Obstetricians and Gynecologists. Obstet Gynecol 2006;108:1053.

Oral intake during labor. ACOG Committee Opinion No. 441. American College of Obstetricians and Gynecologists. Obstet Gynecol 2009;114:714.

Magnesium sulfate before anticipated preterm birth for neuroprotection. Committee Opinion No. 455. American College of Obstetricians and Gynecologists. Obstet Gynecol 2010;115:669–71.

Placenta accreta. Committee Opinion No. 529. American College of Obstetricians and Gynecologists. Obstet Gynecol 2012;120:207–11.

Maternal–fetal surgery for myelomeningocele. Committee Opinion No. 550. American College of Obstetricians and Gynecologists. Obstet Gynecol 2013;121:218–9.

Hospital disaster preparedness for obstetricians and facilities providing maternity care. Committee Opinion No. 555. American College of Obstetricians and Gynecologists. Obstet Gynecol 2013;121:696–9.

Cesarean delivery on maternal request. Committee Opinion No. 559. American College of Obstetricians and Gynecologists. Obstet Gynecol 2013;121:904–7.

Medically indicated late-preterm and early-term deliveries. Committee Opinion No. 560. American College of Obstetricians and Gynecologists. Obstet Gynecol 2013;121:908–10.

Nonmedically indicated early-term deliveries. Committee Opinion No. 561. American College of Obstetricians and Gynecologists. Obstet Gynecol 2013;121:911–5.

Update on immunization and pregnancy: tetanus, diphtheria, and pertussis vaccination. ACOG Committee Opinion No. 566. American College of Obstetricians and Gynecologists. Obstet Gynecol 2013;121:1411–4.

Effective patient–physician communication. Committee Opinion No. 587. American College of Obstetricians and Gynecologists. Obstet Gynecol 2014;123:389–93.

Preparing for clinical emergencies in obstetrics and gynecology. Committee Opinion No. 590. American College of Obstetricians and Gynecologists. Obstet Gynecol 2014;123:722–5.

Labor induction or augmentation and autism. Committee Opinion No. 597. American College of Obstetricians and Gynecologists. Obstet Gynecol 2014;123:1140–2.

Influenza vaccination during pregnancy. Committee Opinion No. 608. American College of Obstetricians and Gynecologists. Obstet Gynecol 2014;124:648–51.

Management of pregnant women with presumptive exposure to Listeria monocytogenes. Committee Opinion No. 614. American College of Obstetricians and Gynecologists. Obstet Gynecol 2014;124:1241–4.

Screening for perinatal depression. Committee Opinion No. 630. American College of Obstetricians and Gynecologists. Obstet Gynecol 2015;125:1268–71.

Prenatal and perinatal human immunodeficiency virus testing: expanded recommendations. Committee Opinion No. 635. American College of Obstetricians and Gynecologists. Obstet Gynecol 2015;125:1544–7.

First-trimester risk assessment for early-onset preeclampsia. Committee Opinion No. 638. American College of Obstetricians and Gynecologists. Obstet Gynecol 2015;126:e25–7.

The Apgar score. Committee Opinion No. 644. American College of Obstetricians and Gynecologists. Obstet Gynecol 2015;126:e52–5.

Physical activity and exercise during pregnancy and the postpartum period. Committee Opinion No. 650. American College of Obstetricians and Gynecologists. Obstet Gynecol 2015;126:e135–42.

Magnesium sulfate use in obstetrics. Committee Opinion No. 652. American College of Obstetricians and Gynecologists. Obstet Gynecol 2016;127:e52–3.

Guidelines for diagnostic imaging during pregnancy and lactation. Committee Opinion No. 656. American College of Obstetricians and Gynecologists. Obstet Gynecol 2016;127:e75–80.

The obstetric and gynecologic hospitalist. Committee Opinion No. 657. American College of Obstetricians and Gynecologists. Obstet Gynecol 2016;127:e81–5.

Optimizing support for breastfeeding as part of obstetric practice. Committee Opinion No. 658. American College of Obstetricians and Gynecologists. Obstet Gynecol 2016;127:e86–92.

Optimizing postpartum care. Committee Opinion No. 666. American College of Obstetricians and Gynecologists. Obstet Gynecol 2016;127:e187–92.

Hospital-based triage of obstetric patients. Committee Opinion No. 667. American College of Obstetricians and Gynecologists. Obstet Gynecol 2016;128:e16–9.

Immediate postpartum long-acting reversible contraception. Committee Opinion No. 670. American College of Obstetricians and Gynecologists. Obstet Gynecol 2016;128:e32–7.

Perinatal risks associated with assisted reproductive technology. Committee Opinion No. 671. American College of Obstetricians and Gynecologists. Obstet Gynecol 2016;128:e61–8.

Antenatal corticosteroid therapy for fetal maturation. Committee Opinion No.677. American College of Obstetricians and Gynecologists. Obstet Gynecol 2016;128: e187–94.

Immersion in water during labor and delivery. Committee Opinion No. 679. American College of Obstetricians and Gynecologists. Obstet Gynecol 2016;128:e231–6.

Disclosure and discussion of adverse events. Committee Opinion No. 681. American College of Obstetricians and Gynecologists. Obstet Gynecol 2016;128:e257–61.

Delayed umbilical cord clamping after birth. Committee Opinion No. 684. American College of Obstetricians and Gynecologists. Obstet Gynecol 2017;129:e5–10.

Approaches to limit intervention during labor and birth. Committee Opinion No. 687. American College of Obstetricians and Gynecologists. Obstet Gynecol 2017;129: e20–8.

Management of suboptimally dated pregnancies. Committee Opinion No. 688. American College of Obstetricians and Gynecologists. Obstet Gynecol 2017;129: e29–32.

Emergent therapy for acute-onset, severe hypertension during pregnancy and the postpartum period. Committee Opinion No. 692. American College of Obstetricians and Gynecologists. Obstet Gynecol 2017;129:e90–5.

Planned home birth. Committee Opinion No. 697. American College of Obstetricians and Gynecologists. Obstet Gynecol 2017;129:e117–22.

Committee on Patient Safety and Quality Improvement

Patient safety in obstetrics and gynecology. ACOG Committee Opinion No. 447. American College of Obstetricians and Gynecologists. Obstet Gynecol 2009;114: 1424–7.

Patient safety in the surgical environment. Committee Opinion No. 464. American College of Obstetricians and Gynecologists. Obstet Gynecol 2010;116:786–90.

Partnering with patients to improve safety. Committee Opinion No. 490. American College of Obstetricians and Gynecologists. Obstet Gynecol 2011;117:1247–9.

Communication strategies for patient handoffs. Committee Opinion No. 517. American College of Obstetricians and Gynecologists. Obstet Gynecol 2012;119: 408–11.

Fatigue and patient safety. Committee Opinion No. 519. American College of Obstetricians and Gynecologists. Obstet Gynecol 2012;119:683–5.

Effective patient-physician communication. Committee Opinion No. 587. American College of Obstetricians and Gynecologists. Obstet Gynecol 2014;123:389–93.

Preparing for clinical emergencies in obstetrics and gynecology. Committee Opinion No. 590. American College of Obstetricians and Gynecologists. Obstet Gynecol 2014;123:722–5.

Health literacy to promote quality of care. Committee Opinion No. 676. American College of Obstetricians and Gynecologists. Obstet Gynecol 2016;128:e183–6.

American College of Obstetricians and Gynecologists' Practice Bulletins

American College of Obstetricians and Gynecologists. Prevention of Rh D alloimmunization. ACOG Practice Bulletin 4. Washington, DC: ACOG; 1999.

Pregestational diabetes mellitus. ACOG Practice Bulletin No. 60. American College of Obstetricians and Gynecologists. Obstet Gynecol 2005;105:675–85.

Management of alloimmunization during pregnancy. ACOG Practice Bulletin No. 75. American College of Obstetricians and Gynecologists. Obstet Gynecol 2006;108: 457–64.

Postpartum hemorrhage. ACOG Practice Bulletin No. 76. American College of Obstetricians and Gynecologists. Obstet Gynecol 2006;108:1039–47.

Hemoglobinopathies in pregnancy. ACOG Practice Bulletin No. 78. American College of Obstetricians and Gynecologists. Obstet Gynecol 2007;109:229–37.

Management of herpes in pregnancy. ACOG Practice Bulletin No. 82. American College of Obstetricians and Gynecologists. Obstet Gynecol 2007;109:1489–98.

Viral hepatitis in pregnancy. ACOG Practice Bulletin No. 86. American College of Obstetricians and Gynecologists. Obstet Gynecol 2007;110:941–56.

Asthma in pregnancy. ACOG Practice Bulletin No. 90. American College of Obstetricians and Gynecologists. Obstet Gynecol 2008;111:457–64.

Use of psychiatric medications during pregnancy and lactation. ACOG Practice Bulletin No. 92. American College of Obstetricians and Gynecologists. Obstet Gynecol 2008;111:1001–20.

Anemia in pregnancy. ACOG Practice Bulletin No. 95. American College of Obstetricians and Gynecologists. Obstet Gynecol 2008;112:201–7.

Management of stillbirth. ACOG Practice Bulletin No. 102. American College of Obstetricians and Gynecologists. Obstet Gynecol 2009;113:748–61.

Intrapartum fetal heart rate monitoring: nomenclature, interpretation, and general management principles. ACOG Practice Bulletin No. 106. American College of Obstetricians and Gynecologists. Obstet Gynecol 2009;114:192–202.

Induction of labor. ACOG Practice Bulletin No. 107. American College of Obstetricians and Gynecologists; Obstet Gynecol 2009;114:386–97.

Vaginal birth after previous cesarean delivery. Practice Bulletin No. 115. American College of Obstetricians and Gynecologists. Obstet Gynecol 2010;116:450–63.

Management of intrapartum fetal heart rate tracings. Practice Bulletin No. 116. American College of Obstetricians and Gynecologists. Obstet Gynecol 2010;116: 1232–40.

Use of prophylactic antibiotics in labor and delivery. ACOG Practice Bulletin No. 120. American College of Obstetricians and Gynecologists. Obstet Gynecol 2011;117: 1472–83.

Long-acting reversible contraception: implants and intrauterine devices. Practice Bulletin No. 121. American College of Obstetricians and Gynecologists. Obstet Gynecol 2011;118:184–96.

Thromboembolism in pregnancy. Practice Bulletin No. 123. American College of Obstetricians and Gynecologists. Obstet Gynecol 2011;118:718–29.

Prediction and prevention of preterm birth. Practice Bulletin No. 130. American College of Obstetricians and Gynecologists. Obstet Gynecol 2012;120:964–73.

Antiphospholipid syndrome. Practice Bulletin No. 132. American College of Obstetricians and Gynecologists. Obstet Gynecol 2012;120:1514–21.

Fetal growth restriction. Practice Bulletin No. 134. American College of Obstetricians and Gynecologists. Obstet Gynecol 2013; 121:1122–33.

Gestational diabetes mellitus. Practice Bulletin No. 137. American College of Obstetricians and Gynecologists. Obstet Gynecol 2013;122:406–16.

Inherited thrombophilias in pregnancy. Practice Bulletin No. 138. American College of Obstetricians and Gynecologists. Obstet Gynecol 2013;122:706–17.

Thyroid disease in pregnancy. Practice Bulletin No. 148. American College of Obstetricians and Gynecologists. Obstet Gynecol 2015;125:996–1005.

Cytomegalovirus, parvovirus B19, varicella zoster, and toxoplasmosis in pregnancy. Practice Bulletin No. 151. American College of Obstetricians and Gynecologists [published erratum appears in Obstet Gynecol 2016;127:405]. Obstet Gynecol 2015;125:1510–25.

Operative vaginal delivery. Practice Bulletin No. 154. American College of Obstetricians and Gynecologists. Obstet Gynecol 2015;126:e56–65.

Obesity in pregnancy. Practice Bulletin No 156. American College of Obstetricians and Gynecologists. Obstet Gynecol 2015;126:e112–26.

Prenatal diagnostic testing for genetic disorders. Practice Bulletin No. 162. American College of Obstetricians and Gynecologists. Obstet Gynecol 2016;127:e108–22.

Screening for fetal aneuploidy. Practice Bulletin No. 163. American College of Obstetricians and Gynecologists. Obstet Gynecol 2016;127:e123–37.

Prevention and management of obstetric lacerations at vaginal delivery. Practice Bulletin No. 165. American College of Obstetricians and Gynecologists. Obstet Gynecol 2016;128:e1–15.

Multifetal gestations: twin, triplet, and higher-order multifetal pregnancies. Practice Bulletin No. 169. American College of Obstetricians and Gynecologists. Obstet Gynecol 2016;128:e131–46.

Critical care in pregnancy. Practice Bulletin No. 170. American College of Obstetricians and Gynecologists. Obstet Gynecol 2016;128:e147–54.

Management of preterm labor. Practice Bulletin No. 171. American College of Obstetricians and Gynecologists. Obstet Gynecol 2016;128:e155–64.

Premature rupture of membranes. Practice Bulletin No. 172. American College of Obstetricians and Gynecologists. Obstet Gynecol 2016;128:e165–77.

Obstetric analgesia and anesthesia. Practice Bulletin No. 177. American College of Obstetricians and Gynecologists. Obstet Gynecol 2017;129:e73–89.

Shoulder Dystocia. Practice Bulletin No. 178. American College of Obstetricians and Gynecologists. Obstet Gynecol 2017;129:e123–33.

Other Publications

American College of Obstetricians and Gynecologists. Access to reproductive health care for women with disabilities. In: Special issues in women's health. Washington, DC: ACOG; 2005. p. 39–59.

American College of Obstetricians and Gynecologists. Collaboration in practice: implementing team-based care. Washington, DC: American College of Obstetricians and Gynecologists; 2016. Available at: http://www.acog.org/Resources-And-Publications/Task-Force-and-Work-Group-Reports/Collaboration-in-Practice-Implementing-Team-Based-Care. Retrieved September 30, 2016.

American College of Obstetricians and Gynecologists. Guidelines for women's health care: a resource manual. 4th ed. Washington, DC: American College of Obstetricians and Gynecologists; 2014.

American College of Obstetricians and Gynecologists. Hypertension in pregnancy. Washington, DC: American College of Obstetricians and Gynecologists; 2013. Available at: http://www.acog.org/Resources-And-Publications/Task-Force-and-Work-Group-Reports/Hypertension-in-Pregnancy. Retrieved November 2, 2016.

American College of Obstetricians and Gynecologists. Quality and safety in women's health care. 2nd ed. Washington, DC: American College of Obstetricians and Gynecologists; 2010.

Safe prevention of the primary cesarean delivery. Obstetric Care Consensus No. 1. American College of Obstetricians and Gynecologists. Obstet Gynecol 2014;123:693–711.

Levels of maternal care. Obstetric Care Consensus No. 2. American College of Obstetricians and Gynecologists. Obstet Gynecol 2015;125:502–15.

Periviable birth. Obstetric Care Consensus No. 4. American College of Obstetricians and Gynecologists. Obstet Gynecol 2016;127:e157–69.

Severe maternal morbidity: screening and review. Obstetric Care Consensus No. 5. American College of Obstetricians and Gynecologists. Obstet Gynecol 2016;128: e54–60.

Genetics and molecular diagnostic testing. Technology Assessment No. 11. American College of Obstetricians and Gynecologists. Obstet Gynecol 2014; 123:394–413.

Appendix I

Website Resources

Agency for Healthcare Research and Quality
Available at: www.ahrq.gov

American Academy of Pediatrics
Available at: www.aap.org

American College of Medical Genetics and Genomics
Available at: www.acmg.net

American College of Obstetricians and Gynecologists
Available at: www.acog.org

American Dental Association
Available at: www.ada.org

American Medical Association
Available at: www.ama-assn.org

American Psychiatric Association
Available at: www.psych.org

Association for Professionals in Infection Control and Epidemiology.
Available at: www.apic.org

Association of Air Medical Services
Available at: www.aams.org

Association of Women's Health, Obstetrics and Neonatal Nurses
Available at: www.awhonn.org

Centers for Disease Control and Prevention
Available at: www.cdc.gov

College of American Pathologists
Available at: www.cap.org

ECRI Institute
Available at: www.ecri.org

Guttmacher Institute
Available at: www.guttmacher.org

Immunization for Women
Available at: www.immunizationforwomen.org

Institute for Healthcare Improvement
Available at: www.ihi.org

Institute for Patient- and Family- Centered Care
Available at: www.ipfcc.org

March of Dimes
Available at: www.marchofdimes.org

National Association of Neonatal Nurses
Available at: www.nann.org

National Center for Health Statistics
Available at: www.cdc.gov/nchs

National Heart Lung and Blood Institute
Available at: www.nhlbi.nih.gov

National Institutes of Health
Available at: www.nih.gov

The Joint Commission
Available at: www.jointcommission.org

Index

Page numbers followed by italicized letters *b*, *f*, and *t* indicate boxes, figures, and tables, respectively.

A

B

C

F

I

O

S

U

W

X

Y

Z